The art and science of mental health

WITHDRAWN

WITHDRAWN

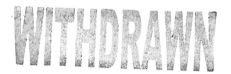

The art and science of mental health nursing

A textbook of principles and practice

Edited by Ian Norman and Iain Ryrie

Open University Press

Open University Press
McGraw-Hill Education
McGraw-Hill House
Shoppenhangers Road
Maidenhead
Berkshire
England
SL6 2QL

email: enquiries@openup.co.uk
world wide web: www.openup.co.uk

and Two Penn Plaza, New York, NY 10121-2289, USA

First published 2004

A catalogue record of this book is available from the British Library

ISBN 0 335 21242 5 (pb) 0 335 21588 2 (hb)

Library of Congress Cataloging-in-Publication Data
CIP data applied for

Typeset by RefineCatch Limited, Bungay, Suffolk
Printed in the UK by Bell & Bain Ltd, Glasgow

To our families: Denise and Sophie, Tom and Doris

Contents

Contributors

Peter Ashton, Senior Lecturer, School of Nursing, Midwifery and Health Studies, University of Wales, Bangor, UK.

Robin Basu, Medical Director, Surrey Oaklands NHS Trust, Epsom, Surrey, UK.

Geoff Brennan, City Nurse Researcher, City University, St Bartholomew School of Nursing and Midwifery, London, UK.

Daniel Bressington, Tutor-practitioner in Medication Management, The South London and Maudsley NHS Trust and the Institute of Psychiatry, King's College London, UK.

Alison Carolan, CAT practitioner, Team Leader, Rehabilitation Service for Eating Disorders, Bromley, Kent, UK.

Jacqueline Curthoys, Publisher and manic depressive, London, UK.

Joe Curran, Principal Cognitive Behavioural Therapist, Sheffield Care Trust, Department of Cognitive and Behavioural Psychotherapies, Michael Carlisle Centre, Sheffield, UK.

Philip Fennell, Professor of Law, Cardiff Law School, UK.

Richard Ford, Director, National Institute for Mental Health in England, South-East Development Centre, Basingstoke, UK.

Catherine Gamble, Consultant Nurse in Psychosocial Interventions, Oxfordshire Mental Health Care Trust, Oxford, UK.

Lina Gega, Senior Lecturer, Mental Health Section, Florence Nightingale School of Nursing and Midwifery, King's College London, UK.

Richard Gray, MRC Fellow in Health Services Research, Institute of Psychiatry, King's College London, UK.

Kevin Gournay, Professor of Psychiatric Nursing, Health Services Research Department, Institute of Psychiatry, King's College London, UK.

Sue Gurney, Lecturer, European Institute of Nursing Studies, University of Surrey, Guildford, UK.

Simon Houghton, Principal Psychotherapist, Specialist Psychotherapy Services, Sheffield Case Trust, Sheffield, UK.

John Keady, Senior Lecturer in Nursing Research, School of Nursing, Midwifery and Health Studies, University of Wales, Bangor, UK.

Cheryl Kipping, Consultant Nurse, Dual Diagnosis, Social Services Department, University Hospital Lewisham, Lewisham, UK.

Steve Morgan, Practice Development Consultant for Mental Health, Blackheath, London, UK.

Ian Noonan, Lecturer-practitioner, Mental Health Section, Florence Nightingale School of Nursing and Midwifery, King's College London, and South London and Maudsley NHS Trust, UK.

Ian Norman, Professor of Nursing and Inter-disciplinary Care and Head of the Mental Health Section, Florence Nightingale School of Nursing and Midwifery, King's College London, UK.

Kingsley Norton, Medical Director, Henderson Hospital, Sutton, Surrey, UK.

Steve Onyett, Professor of Mental Health, University of the West of England, and Development Manager-Mental Health South West, NHSE-South West, Bristol, UK.

Leah Ousley, Lecturer-practitioner, Wathwood Hospital Regional Secure Unit, Nottinghamshire Health Care NHS Trust, UK.

Shaun Parsons, Lecturer in Clinical Psychology, University of Newcastle, Newcastle-upon-Tyne, UK.

Rachel Perkins, Clinical Director of Adult Mental Health Services and Consultant Clinical Psychologist, South West London and St George's Mental Health NHS Trust, London, UK.

Hagen Rampes, Consultant Psychiatrist and Honorary Clinical Senior Lecturer, Barnet, Enfield and Haringey Mental Health NHS Trust, Middlesex, UK.

Julie Repper, Senior Research Fellow, University of Sheffield and Lead Research Nurse, Community Health Sheffield NHS Trust, UK.

Paul Rogers, MRC fellow, Health Services Research Department, Institute of Psychiatry and Division of Psychiatry, Bristol University, UK.

Iain Ryrie, Head of Research, Sainsbury Centre for Mental Health, King's College London, UK.

Susan Sookoo, Lecturer, Mental Health Section, Florence Nightingale School of Nursing and Midwifery, King's College London, UK.

Gill Todd, Clinical Nurse Leader, Eating Disorder Unit, Bethlem Royal Hospital, Beckenham, Kent, UK.

Marc Thurgood, Lecturer-practitioner, Mental Health Section, Florence Nightingale School of Nursing and Midwifery, King's College London and South London and Maudsley NHS Trust, UK.

Janet Treasure, Consultant Psychiatrist and Professor of Psychiatric Medicine, Department of Psychiatry, GKT Medical School, King's College London, UK.

Keith Tudor, Psychotherapist, Supervisor and Trainer in private practice, and mental health consultant, Director, Temenos, Sheffield, UK.

Andrew Wetherell, Co-director, ARW Mental Health Training and Consultancy, Essex, UK.

Phil Woods, Partnerships in Care Senior Lecturer in Forensic Mental Health Nursing, Mental Health Section, Florence Nightingale School of Nursing and Midwifery, King's College London, UK.

Preface

Our aim has been to produce a comprehensive textbook for mental health nurses and students in training, which takes account of the diversity of mental health nursing as a practice discipline and the contemporary context in which nurses practice. In so doing we have sought to avoid the tendency of debates within academic nursing, and some other textbooks, to present a restrictive concept of mental health nursing as a uni-dimensional activity – typically as an 'art' concerned with nurses' therapeutic relationships with 'people' in distress, or as a 'science', concerned with evidence-based interventions that can be applied to good effect by nurses, often working in what might be seen as extended roles, to 'patients' with defined mental illness. In reality, practising nurses must be artists and scientists simultaneously and they need to find ways of integrating these elements while meeting policy directives for mental health services and service users' demands. This book seeks to be a resource to practising nurses to help them to meet this remit.

Thus it seems to us that any contemporary account of the profession needs to establish its case within three broad parameters:

- professional diversity;
- national policy; and
- service users' expectations.

Professional diversity

We avoid aligning the discipline of mental health nursing to any one theoretical perspective but, rather, acknowledge the breadth and complexity of the perspectives upon which mental health nurses draw in their work. The title of this book reflects our aim, therefore, which is to provide an integrative account of the discipline that accommodates its many origins, influences and practices. To assist this process we introduce a schema in Chapter 1 which integrates explanatory models of mental disorder and demonstrates each one's crucial, though partial, contribution to our understanding of the human condition. We contend that all mental health nursing, whatever its origin or theoretical basis, can be mapped onto this schema. Further, no one part of the schema is, in itself, adequate to deal with people's needs in relation to mental health and mental illness.

National policy

The NHS and social care provision have long been subject to government policy. As a consequence professionals who work in these organizations must be expected to adjust their practice to meet contemporary demands.

To assist them in this we have grounded this textbook in the National Service Frameworks (NSFs) for Mental Health and Older People (DH 1999, 2001), and subsequent policy documents, which provide a blueprint for the development of mental health services in the United Kingdom (UK) over the next decade and beyond. The *NSF for Mental Health* is a particularly important policy document which, for the first time in our professional lifetimes, sets out a comprehensive agenda for mental health services that incorporates mental health promotion, primary care and secondary care, and acknowledges that the whole system of mental health care must be made to work if there are to be real benefits to service users. Together with related mental health policy reforms this has major implications for the work of mental health nurses. Chapter 4 deals with mental health policy specifically, and subsequent chapters shape their content with respect to the NSFs for Mental Health and Older People. This necessarily emphasizes a UK perspective, but we have tried to produce a text that is not too parochial and which can cross geographical boundaries.

Service-user perspectives

An important tenet that underpins this textbook is our belief that mental health nursing is concerned with helping people find meaning and purpose in their lives, and assisting them in the process of recovery. Nurses cannot respectfully assist in this process unless we are prepared to hear service users' accounts of their difficulties and to understand their own preferences for a meaningful life. This fact is so central to understanding how mental health nurses can help that we have sought to make it explicit throughout the book, rather than confine it to a single chapter. Thus, each contributor incorporates user perspectives into their chapter. The terminology used to describe recipients of mental health services does however vary between contributors. There are chapters that use the term 'patient' and others that refer to 'service user' or to 'clients'; these terms tell us something about the perspective that the contributor brings to bear on their work. Following the introduction of the schema in Chapter 1, which integrates explanatory models of mental disorder, it follows that all perspectives are valid though each is partial. We have, therefore, chosen not to standardize these terms (into service user, for example), but have allowed contributors to speak for themselves.

Content and organization

The book is divided into five parts. Part 1, Foundations, deals with the historical origins and contemporary basis of mental health nursing. Chapter 1 explores aetiological theories for understanding mental illness, and this is followed in Chapter 2 by a detailed account of mental health promotion. Chapter 3 examines the origins and orientations of mental health nursing, and Chapter 4 presents the policy and service context within which nurses practise. A further chapter deals with rehabilitation and recovery as a fundamental orientation for contemporary care (Chapter 5) and the final chapter in this section (Chapter 6), provides an overview of the legal and ethical frameworks within which nurses must work.

Part 2, Interventions, includes six chapters that represent the main therapeutic approaches available to nurses in their work. Two chapters are devoted to assessment (Chapters 7 and 8), and one chapter examines the concept of therapeutic milieu in the context of contemporary inpatient care settings (Chapter 9). The other chapters in this part of the book deal with psychosocial, pharmacological and complementary therapies (Chapters 10, 11 and 12, respectively).

Part 3, Applications, examines the major challenges confronting those who use mental health services and outlines evidence-based interventions available to the mental health nurse. Each of the nine chapters in this section is oriented to a particular type or group of disorders that a person can experience (Chapters 13–21).

Part 4, Core procedures, covers the fundamental processes of mental health nursing care. The chapters here have a very practical orientation. They are concerned with the 'know-how' of mental health nursing, with the skills needed by nurses working in partnership with clients in any care setting. Chapters 22 and 23 discuss how to engage clients in treatment and work with them to identify and solve their problems. Chapters 24, 25 and 26 are concerned with the practical application of behavioural and cognitive techniques with clients and the management of their medication; these chapters demonstrate application of some of the interventions previously discussed in Part 2. Chapters 27 and 28 are concerned with the therapeutic management of psychiatric emergencies; of aggression and violence and attempted suicide and self-harm.

Part 4, Future directions, is devoted to the organization and development of mental health care. Respective chapters examine whole systems service provision (Chapter 29) and anticipated future developments for mental health nursing (Chapter 30).

Each chapter is preceded by an overview which outlines its scope and content and concludes with a set of bullet points to summarize the main points, questions for reflection and discussion and an annotated bibliography which points the reader towards more detailed reading. Case studies are used within some chapters to illustrate the practical application of the material. Though written primarily for mental health nurses and nursing students the book should provide also a useful reference for other health care professionals, lay carers and for people with mental health problems.

The book's contributors have been chosen to reflect the many diverse professional perspectives within mental health care. All are experts in their field and in writing their chapter each was asked to draw upon their specialist knowledge and practice rather than try to relate their subject to a narrow definition of mental health nursing.

Without the commitment and patience of each author, this book would not have been written. We are grateful to each of them for taking time out of their busy lives to produce their chapters. This book will have been successful if it goes some small way to helping mental health nurses draw upon an up-to-date knowledge base, and to become skilful and sensitive practitioners who work in partnership with service users to help them regain control over their lives.

Ian Norman and Iain Ryrie

References

Department of Health (1999) *The National Service Framework for Mental Health*. London: Department of Health.

Department of Health (2001) *The National Service Framework for Older People*. London: Department of Health.

Foreword

The 2003 annual NHS workforce census shows that there are currently 39,383 qualified whole time equivalent mental health nurses working in the NHS (DH 2004). This is the largest single professional group working in mental health services and their training and subsequent contribution to the care of people who experience mental illness is, therefore, of paramount importance. In view of this I am delighted to be associated with this exciting new textbook for mental health nurses, which is dedicated to the development of a profession that is fit for modern practice.

Drawing on the knowledge and experience of some 36 contributors – all experts within their respective fields – this major work reflects three central themes of the current change agenda facing mental health services; specifically the importance of incorporating users' preferences in the development and delivery of services, redesign of services to deliver specialist functions, and integrating health and social need into holistic packages of care that support service users to live meaningful lives in their local communities.

The editors are careful not to sideline user preferences into a single chapter or section. A few chapters have been written in partnership with service users and all chapters incorporate a user perspective regarding the interventions that are being discussed. Consequently, there is a strong sense throughout this textbook of nurses working in partnership with the people who use mental health services.

The myriad specialist functions that nurses can perform are evident throughout and are brought together in Steve Onyett's chapter that deals with functional teams and whole systems service delivery. It is increasingly clear that the specialist skills nurses bring to one service setting may no longer be easily transferable to other specialist settings. There is evidence in the authorship of chapters and their content that nurses increasingly identify with teams and functions, and the professionals they work alongside in those teams, rather than with their own professional group alone. I believe this is a necessary step to realizing the potential locked into our health and social care professions and this textbook admirably demonstrates nursing's contribution to the continued development of specialist services.

The third theme I have highlighted is the integration of health and social need into holistic packages of care that support service users to live meaningful lives in their local communities. This is perhaps our greatest challenge and requires new ways of thinking that go beyond traditional health and social care practices. We need, for example, to find ways of working with communities to reduce the stigma associated with mental illness, and to develop socially inclusive practices for people that have experienced mental health difficulties. The chapter by Rachel Perkins and Julie Repper is dedicated to this task and deals specifically with the concept of *recovery* as a foundation for nursing practice. Similarly, Ian Norman and Iain Ryrie in their final chapter provide cogent examples of socially inclusive nursing in relation to the National Service Framework (DH 1999) standards. I believe that any contemporary textbook relating to mental health care must demonstrate a working knowledge of socially inclusive practice, and the editors have secured the contribution of two leading writers in this field, whose perspective they have managed to weave throughout the book.

I have also been struck by the editors avoiding a temptation to throw babies out with bath water! Although we are facing new horizons in mental health care we must be careful not to abandon what is known to be effective. The therapeutic milieu, which was overlooked as services moved into the community is reinterpreted for a contemporary workforce. Psychiatric medication, for all its deleterious consequences for some service users, is necessary and helpful for some people in some situations. Similarly, there are examples in the service user literature of electro-convulsive therapy benefiting some people. Treatments such as these can be overlooked in an era of psychosocial interventions, yet they remain part of the treatment repertoire. Norman and Ryrie have not overlooked this fact and are careful to produce a comprehensive text that draws on a historical as well as a contemporary evidence base.

In addition to these observations on specific content I commend this book for the clarity with which it presents the nursing profession as a whole. I admit to having previously been unsure about the limits of nursing and its 'proper function'. However, Norman and Ryrie provide an integrative account of the discipline that accommodates many origins, influences and practices. I feel sure this will be of considerable benefit to undergraduate nursing students and to qualified nurses engaged in professional development activities. I also believe that the book is necessary reading for those who train our nursing workforce. Finally, as my own experience testifies, there is much in this book that is of relevance to non-nursing health and social care staff, lay carers and service users. On this basis I am delighted to have been invited to write this foreword and commend this book to all mental health nurses and to those who deliver or receive care in partnership with them.

Dr Andrew McCulloch
Chief Executive, Mental Health Foundation

References

Department of Health (1999) *The National Service Framework for Mental Health.* London: DH.

Department of Health (2004) *NHS Hospital and Community Health Service Non-Medical Workforce Census: England 30 September 2003: Detailed Results.* Leeds: DH.

PART 1
Foundations

1

The origins and expression of psychological distress

Iain Ryrie and Ian Norman

Chapter overview

The origins and expression of psychological distress arise from the broad spectrum of conscious and unconscious mental activity that we might refer to simply as human experience. Psychological distress, to some degree at least, is necessary for people to function. Without it we may find ourselves in situations that threaten our lives, but which we are unable to do anything about because we fail to register the distress that such situations should engender. There is a point, though, at which the experience of psychological distress can become the experience of disorder (or illness) and it is these shades of the spectrum that we explore in this opening chapter. Of course, where the boundary is drawn or which shades of human experience constitute disorder is open to debate. We do not draw conclusions in this respect but encourage the reader to consider an integrated explanation of human experience, and thus, of mental disorders. Different models or ways of understanding psychological distress and disorder are therefore described both as singular explanations but also as building blocks for a more integrated view of these phenomena. Systems that classify disordered experiences are presented, and the prevalence and symptoms of key disorders are described. The chapter also includes service-user perspectives on the systems currently employed to classify their human experience.

In summary this chapter covers:

- models of mental disorder;
- integrating models of mental disorder;
- the classification of mental disorder;
- incidence of mental disorder and key symptoms;
- user perspectives.

Models of mental disorder

Experiencing 'mental health' or having a 'mental illness' may appear as two distinct, separate states of being. Such dualistic thought may also appear advantageous. The boundary it represents provides a point of exclusion beyond which we can place our fears of the unknown. 'Madness' becomes distinct from 'sanity', and for the majority, 'madness' is not within 'us' but belongs to 'them'. This seems a comforting position to pursue, but is human experience quite so linear?

'Mental health' is in fact inseparable from 'mental illness'. They do not exist independently of one another, in the same way as night can only be understood in relation to day, black to white, up to down, happy to sad, and of course, back to front. These pairs of opposites each describe the same phenomenon of interest but do so from different perspectives, which is the very antithesis of a boundary that distinguishes two separate entities. 'Mental health' and 'mental illness' are terms of relation, not of reality, and the reality they describe is human experience.

We begin this text with such a cautionary note since the history of mental illness is a history of exclusion, separation, distinction and 'otherness' (Tudor 1996). What we present in the following pages are the approaches different schools have taken to explaining the aetiology of mental disorder. We examine also a number of treatment implications for each of the models. However, this should not be viewed as a definitive account of the terrain within which mental health nursing operates. Professional interest should necessarily incorporate mental health or 'well-being', and for this reason we recommend this chapter is read in conjunction with Tudor's chapter on health promotion (Chapter 2).

So, as we describe different models, or ways of understanding mental disorder, it is important to beware of the artificial boundaries such distinctions draw. To identify professionally with only these shades of the spectrum of human experience is to miss something vital about the human condition. If as nurses we focus only on disorder and illness, what chance is there to promote the mental health of those who endeavour to live a fulfilling life in spite of an illness or disorder?

The disease model

Before examining the disease model it is necessary to deal with the general meaning attributed to disease. Kendall (1975) has reviewed disease definitions in psychiatry, which range from the purely subjective (for example, personal suffering) to the purely objective (for example, the presence of an identifiable pathogen). This latter interpretation tends to predominate and is defined by Scadding (1967) as the presence of abnormal phenomena displayed by a group within a species, that sets the group apart from its species in so far as the disease places them at a biological disadvantage. In lay terms, a disease is only present if it harms the individual or reduces his or her capacity to reproduce (Tyrer and Steinberg 1998).

We may all feel comfortable with the idea of physical disease, such as a cancer, a damaged heart valve, or a pathogen that can be transmitted between people. We can probably also agree that these conditions do, more or less, place individuals at some sort of disadvantage. Disease theorists similarly attribute mental disorders, or psychiatric illnesses, to physiological and chemical changes in the individual, particularly in the brain but also in other parts of the body (Tyrer and Steinberg 1998).

Thus we can understand clearly the basis for disorders of perception and cognition among say, people with dementia or those who have suffered brain injuries. Observable physiological changes in brain structure have correlates in human behaviour. The disease model extends beyond these organic conditions to explain disorders such as depression, which can be attributed to changes in serotonin levels or to some other chemical fluctuation. Similarly, schizophrenia can be attributed to chemical abnormalities, and more recently to physiological differences such as the size of the temporal lobe in the human brain (Gournay 1996).

The disease model, following traditional medicine, endeavours to identify through scientific objectivity the presence of a stable phenomenon that we call 'mental illness'. Clinical syndromes become refined into diagnoses, which are essentially codes for heterogeneous, and often unstable collections of symptoms (Craig 2000). Objectivity in psychiatry is at best quite 'fuzzy', but remains the gold standard. Such a gold standard affords incredible power to its possessor. Clinical syndromes and diagnoses are codified languages, available only to those who have willingly immersed themselves in that particular paradigm. They can provide an efficient means to communicate complex phenomena, but only to those in the know.

The treatment armoury of the disease theorist is also elitist, being available only to the qualified practitioner. Medicines are prescribed to balance chemical imbalances, electroconvulsive therapy is administered to shunt neural pathways into shape, positron emission tomography may be requested to check those temporal lobes and, in the most extreme of cases, pieces of the brain may be removed.

A consistent criticism of the disease model is the possibility that people with mental disorders can become passive recipients of treatment and the nurse or doctor an authority on the person's experience. However, this is not a consequence of the disease model per se, but reflects something of the way in which practitioners apply their knowledge. Passive receipt of care can accompany any model if practitioners fail to speak to people as people, but instead believe they are dealing with symptoms, syndromes or a collection of behavioural problems. We see no reason why the disease model cannot take account of the person behind the symptoms or syndrome, and indeed in our experience this has largely been the case, though not always so.

Some commentators have questioned the validity of associations between human physiology, brain chemistry and mental disorder. In fact there are both weak and strong arguments of this type. The 'strong' camp rejects outright any attempt to reduce human experience to physiological and chemical structures, and tends therefore to reject the disease model. In contrast, the 'weak' camp acknowledges the contribution of the physical sciences to our understanding of mental disorder but maintains that they are insufficient to explain adequately the phenomenon of interest. For example, some people with schizophrenia do appear to have ventricular enlargement, but others do not (Van Horne and McManus 1992).

The case for and against a physiological 'disease' explanation for mental disorders has been rehearsed in the academic literature (cf. Gournay 1996; Dawson 1997, 1998; Provencher *et al.* 1997; Barker *et al.* 1998; Keen 1999; Burnard and Hannigan 2000, Wilkin 2001). We refer readers to these to draw their own conclusions.

The psychodynamic model

The psychodynamic model is more accurately described as a style of human interaction and understanding that draws on a broad philosophy, which includes clinical, biological and evolutionary theory as well as religion and the arts (Tyrer and Steinberg 1998). Psychodynamic practice may conjure an image of the psychoanalyst listening to their patient's stream of consciousness as the patient lies on a couch at their side. This may occur but the psychodynamic model has many branches including some forms of family therapy, group therapies and art therapy (Tyrer and Steinberg 1998).

Common to all psychodynamic approaches, which delineates them from other psychotherapeutic perspectives (for example, behaviour therapy), is their primary focus on the ideas and feelings behind the words and actions that constitute human behaviour. Psychiatric disorders are not viewed as illnesses with disease-based aetiologies but as conflicts between different levels of mental functioning. Of critical importance here are the conscious and unconscious levels. Substantial amounts of mental activity that occur beyond our awareness are believed to determine much of our behaviour.

Human development is important in this respect since a person's early experiences can produce a particular *gestalt* or view of the person and their world, which they will take with them into adult life. This *gestalt* will include mental tricks and mechanisms to protect the person's sense of self. Problems may arise if our *gestalt*, that we necessarily cling to, is at odds with the real circumstances we find ourselves in as adults.

Let us take the simple example of a man whose childhood was coloured by restraint, control, uncertainty and occasional pleasure. Then as an adult he works hard to please others, to demonstrate control and restraint in the expectation that doing for others will bring occasional pleasure. If this man was a priest then we may feel his *gestalt* fits his real circumstances. But suppose this man spent his life struggling to forge a career in marketing or merchant banking, or in the stock market to please his father? Though a simplistic example you may agree that conflict is likely to dominate this man's experience. Conflict between his personal aspirations and the expectations of others. Conflict between his working alliances and the impossibility of any harmony in such a work environment. Conflict between his relative failings as a merchant banker and his father's exacting standards. He may not be conscious of these specific conflicts but will nevertheless be affected by them as unconscious mental activity tries to reconcile the irreconcilable. Quite literally, the psychodynamic therapist views psychological distress as the upshoots of unconscious thought (Tyrer and Steinberg 1998). This simple principle is central to most if not all psychodynamic therapies.

Different theories have been put forward within the psychodynamic tradition to explain different human experiences, but the founding father of the psychodynamic school was Sigmund Freud (1856–1939). Freud was a biological thinker interested primarily in an organism's attraction to pleasure and repulsion from pain. Application of the pain/pleasure continuum to the human mind and its development led Freud to divide mental life into the *id*, *ego* and *superego*. The id represents our basic primitive instincts, present at birth, which tend toward the pursuit of pleasure or gratification. As we pursue gratification we become aware also of an external reality separate from ourselves and this realization necessitates the formulation of a self or ego. Others in our world have helped shape the external reality in terms of laws, rules and social expectations. This realization leads to the development of the superego, which is more easily understood as our conscience.

So we have needs (id), wishes (ego) and a conscience (superego) and, perhaps not surprisingly, psychological distress arises from the struggles that take place between them. Many of these struggles take place in the unconscious and Freudian analysts are concerned with healing the radical split between the conscious and unconscious, thereby creating a strong and healthy ego that is an accurate and acceptable self-image.

Freud's contemporaries and his followers have built subsequently upon his work to elaborate the psychodynamic school. Carl Jung (1875–1961) studied under Freud, who designated Jung his successor and crown prince. However, after less than ten years of collaboration they fell out over theoretical disagreements and never spoke to each other again! While Freud had dedicated his work to the ego level of personal functioning, Jung was more inclined to examine transpersonal levels of human awareness. For Jung there were aspects of a person that appeared to transcend or go beyond the person, and this premise was incomprehensible to Freud, whose work had been confined to the realms of the ego or self.

Jung had studied the great mythologies of the world, particularly their totems, ancient symbols, images and mythological motifs. What he discovered was that these images appeared with some regularity in the dreams and fantasies of modern Europeans, the majority of whom had never been exposed to these myths. His basic premise was that these primordial images, or *archetypes* as he called them, are common to all people. They do not belong to single individuals but are in fact transindividual or transcendent of the self.

Jung called this deep layer of the psyche, in which the archetypes reside, the 'collective unconscious'. Notice this is not individual consciousness but is something that resides deep within us all. According to Jung these archetypes live on, whether we are aware of them or not, and continue to move us deeply in creative but also destructive ways. As an example, Jungian therapists are interested in people's key dreams and understanding the symbolism within them with recourse to ancient mythology. Knowing what mythological images have meant over time to the human race as a whole enables people to understand what the images may mean in their experience of the *collective unconscious*. It follows that through such conscious integration people are no longer forcibly moved by unconscious archetypes. Therefore, though related to Freud's ideas, Jung extended them beyond the organism to the cultural context within which the organism lives and used this context (or collective unconscious) to understand the psychic distress encountered by people.

Melanie Klein (1882–1960) is another key psychodynamic theorist whose work focused on the first two to three months of a child's life at a time when she believed the ego struggles to differentiate between itself and external reality. Unable to comprehend that good and bad can be present in the same object the infant assumes the *paranoid position* in which all things are either good or bad but never both. When able to comprehend that these qualities do exist in a single object (for example both the mother's love and her chastisement) the infant experiences this new discovery and moves to the *depressive position*. Therefore in Kleinian terms the experience and acceptance of depression is considered a maturational step necessary for personal growth (Tyrer and Steinberg 1998).

The influence of these early works on more contemporary psychodynamic therapies such as 'humanistic therapy', 'drama therapy', 'art therapy' and some forms of counselling is without doubt (Tyrer and Steinberg 1998). Equally, the psychodynamic tradition has influenced mental health nursing, particularly through the works of Hildegard Peplau and Annie Altschul (cf. Chapter 3; see also annotated bibliography).

The behavioural model

The behavioural model has a scientific basis in Learning Theory. Symptoms are considered to be learned habits arising from the interaction between external events or stressors and an individual's personality. Persistent, distressing symptoms are considered maladaptive responses rather than being markers for some underlying disease or illness. For the behaviour therapist the symptoms and their associated behaviours *are* the disorder (Tyrer and Steinberg 1998).

Learning theory posits that two forms of conditioning are responsible for the formation of symptoms; *classical* and *operant*. Classical conditioning refers to a neutral stimulus that becomes associated with an unrelated but established stimulus response sequence. Seminal experimental work in this area was conducted by the Russian physiologist Pavlov (1927) who conditioned dogs to salivate in response to a bell rather than to the established stimulus of food. Initially food was provided to the animals when a bell sounded. After several such trials the animals would salivate at the sound of the bell even when unaccompanied by food.

Operant conditioning results from behaviour rather than as the consequence of a stimulus. Skinner (1972) conducted seminal work in this field with a box in which one or more levers could be pressed. Rats would be placed in the box and through natural curiosity they would eventually press one or all of the levers. When the appropriate lever was pressed food would be deposited in the box. Gradually the rats would learn to continually press the appropriate lever until their appetites were satisfied. Thus it is not a neutral stimulus or the manipulation of an experimenter that conditioned the rats, but their own behaviour.

But how do these theories relate to the development of human behavioural problems? Take a simple example involving a phobia or fear of spiders in a parent of a family with children. When the parent encounters a spider their response may be at odds with the threat that a spider poses. They may appear to panic, perhaps scream and will certainly try to avoid the spider. It is possible that the children in this family will also develop a similar response since they have been subject to the classical conditioning of the parent. Thus they may learn to fear and avoid spiders, which can become self-perpetuating as their fear confirms the danger spiders pose, and their avoidance obviates any opportunity to realize that spiders pose no threat.

The behaviour therapist is interested in replacing maladaptive responses with adaptive behaviour patterns. This is usually done by gradually removing the fear response through such techniques as graded exposure and systematic desensitization. So the parent in our example may first be encouraged to imagine spiders, then view pictures of them in a book, followed by seeing them in a jar across the room, then holding the jar and finally holding the spider. Each of these stages will invoke a fear response but these will gradually subside if the person is encouraged to remain with the present situation through which they learn that spiders are actually quite harmless.

An important principle of behaviour therapy is a collaborative working partnership between client and therapist. A person's behaviour is part of their own responsibility and not something that can be handed over to a doctor to sort out (Tyrer and Steinberg 1998). The therapist does not view the person as being abnormal or ill, but regards them as an equal partner in an unlearning, or new learning process. Furthermore, behaviour therapists see this partnership as critical if the individual is to maintain and develop their new adaptive behaviours once therapy has finished.

This approach to managing human behaviour has had a major influence on mental health nursing, for example, through the work of Isaac Marks (Marks *et al.* 1978; Marks 1987) who, though not a nurse, has championed nurse behaviour therapists. Their contribution to health care has been evaluated by Gournay *et al.* (2000) and is described by Rogers *et al.* in Chapter 15.

The cognitive model

Put simply, the cognitive model posits that people interpret their thoughts, which in turn are the main determinants of behaviour (Tyrer and Steinberg 1998). This stands in sharp contrast to the behavioural or disease models, which do not accommodate the cognitive mechanisms involved in behaviour and illness. For the cognitive therapist primacy is given to errors or biases in thinking and it is these dysfunctional thought patterns that create mental disorders.

An important framework used by many cognitive therapists is the ABC model first described by Ellis (1962). A stands for 'activating event', B stands for 'beliefs' about the 'activating event', and C stands for the emotional or behavioural 'consequence' that follows B, given A. Thus, a person who comes across a spider (activating event) may think it harmless or dangerous (beliefs) and will either continue their usual activity or be unable to do so (consequence).

While the behavioural model focuses on the fear response, or consequence in the above example, the crux of the problem according to the cognitive model rests in the beliefs that people hold. Repetitive thoughts (ruminations) can lead to persistent actions (rituals), which can prevent normal functioning. Significant change in a person's mental health necessarily involves significant change in their cognitions (Tyrer and Steinberg 1998).

Though the reverse of the behavioural model, the two are rarely in major conflict. Open, collaborative working partnerships are established by respective therapists, and in the case of cognitive therapy, the client is encouraged to explore their thinking patterns and consider more appropriate and adaptive thoughts that fit the evidence. Furthermore, a growing discipline of cognitive behavioural therapy has emerged in recent decades (Trower *et al.* 1988; Hawton *et al.* 1989; Curwen *et al.* 2000). This trend is evident also in the practice of mental health nursing (cf. Chapters 10 and 25).

The cognitive model is the youngest of those described and it remains to be seen how it may develop and to what ends. Of contemporary interest, however, is the use of this model to manage distressing delusions, hallucinations and feelings of paranoia that people may experience in the course of a mental disorder (Kingdon and Turkington 1993; Chadwick *et al.* 1996).

The social model

The social model is concerned with the influence of social forces as the causes or precipitants of mental disorder. While the psychodynamic model is principally concerned with the individual and their personal relations, the social model focuses on the person in the context of their society as a whole (Tyrer and Steinberg 1998).

Evidence that social forces are central to the aetiology of mental disorder can be traced to the work of Emile Durkheim (1897) who demonstrated that social factors, particularly isolation and the loss of social bonds, were predictive of suicide. We may be more familiar with associations between poor living circumstances in deprived geographical areas and the incidence of physical health problems (Whitehead 1992). However, this relationship holds also for mental disorders, perhaps because the associated deprivation is usually accompanied by unemployment, loss of social role and a subsequent sense of alienation from mainstream society (Hirsch 1988; Thornicroft 1991).

At the heart of this model is the premise that we are all prone to mental disturbance when unpleasant events strike us without warning. This fact led Holmes and Rahe (1967) to develop the Social Readjustment Rating Scale, which attributes a severity score to 42 life events according to the degree of change or adaptation they produce in people. Perhaps not surprisingly, bereavement, divorce and starting a new job are high on the list.

There is an intuitive appeal to the social model since we are all likely to have experienced major upheavals in our lives that may have caused us to feel psychological distress. Anxiety and low mood, for example, may be experienced in the run up to a series of exams or in response to the frustrations associated typically with moving house. The social model provides also a rationale for the origin of other types of psychological distress in which delusions, hallucinations and an apparent loss of contact with reality occur. For example, it is known that unexpected life events are associated with the onset of schizophrenia (Brown and Birley 1968). Furthermore, the levels of critical 'expressed emotion' experienced by a person with schizophrenia from family members is predictive of the severity of the person's condition and, in particular, the likelihood of relapse (Falloon 1995).

Proponents of the social model do not have fixed ideas about what constitutes a psychiatric illness. Indeed, the model is concerned that labelling people with a psychiatric illness may create a disorder itself (Tyrer and Steinberg 1998). All symptoms and behaviour have to be understood in the context of the society from which they emanate. There are no independent, objective criteria for mental disorder according to the social model, only a boundary line between normal and abnormal that has been set by society.

Supporters of the social model aim to help people take up an acceptable role in society once more, rather than to correct a chemical imbalance or recondition specific behaviours (Tyrer and Steinberg 1998). This may involve social skills training (Liberman *et al.* 1993), some systemic family therapies (Barker 1981) and more general family interventions involving education on the influence of critical 'expressed emotion' (Brooker and Butterworth 1991; Lam *et al.* 1993; Falloon 1995). Gournay (1995) has reviewed the use of these interventions by mental health nurses.

The social model has experienced something of a renaissance in recent years with its basic premise reflected in Standard One of the NSF for Mental Health (DH 1999), which acknowledges that mental health problems can arise from the adverse effects of social exclusion. Subsequent work has been conducted through the Department of Health (2001) and the Sainsbury

Centre for Mental Health's Citizenship and Community Programme (Bates 2002) to tackle these adverse effects. The former outlines a process that will enable groups and agencies to contribute to the promotion of public mental health. The latter is focused more specifically on strategies to make social inclusion a reality for people with severe mental health problems. The mental health charity MIND has also reprinted their 1999 inquiry into social exclusion and mental health problems (MIND 1999). Additionally, there have been recent discussion papers on the modernization of the social model in mental health (Duggan *et al.* 2002), and critiques of the role of the media in perpetuating a perception of the mentally ill as violent and dangerous (Paterson and Stark 2001).

Gender and ethnicity

We have chosen to introduce gender and ethnicity at this point since their relationship to mental disorder may be best understood from the perspective of the social model of mental disorders. This is not to say that hormonal differences do not exist between the genders, and these may contribute to differential experiences of mental disorder, but more important perhaps is the observation that differential treatment of women in our society has been a consistent feature of its history.

Gender

The literature consistently reports fewer women to be in receipt of specialist mental health services than men (for example, Repper and Perkins 1995; Owen and Milburn 2001). Though this may reflect a lower prevalence of mental disorder among women, evidence suggests that the phenomenon is a marker for the diagnostic practices and expectations of practitioners, which are different for men than for women (Ussher 1991). For example, Perkins and Rowland (1991) identified a tendency for male patients to be encouraged to find employment, while women were more likely to be expected to improve their self-care and domestic skills. Further, it is known that most women are reluctant to share facilities with male patients, whom they often experience as threatening (Repper and Perkins 1995). Whether or not these reasons are sufficient to explain the under-representation of women in specialist mental health services, it remains that women are a minority group whose needs are often overlooked. Owen and colleagues consider these issues in depth and propose strategies to improve mental health services for women (Owen *et al.* 1998, Owen and Milburn 2001).

A key experience that predominantly affects women and which contributes to mental health problems is domestic violence. Not only does this bring anguish to the women involved, but there is now evidence of lifelong effects on children who witness such violence (Hall and Lynch 1998). Furthermore, abused women may not approach relevant services for help, partly through the fear of retribution from their partners but also because to do so would threaten their social roles, for example as mother, housekeeper, wife, etc.

Ramsay *et al.* (2002) have recently completed a systematic review of domestic violence with particular emphasis on the role of health care workers in screening for this form of abuse. From this it is far from clear that screening per se is advantageous and further evidence is needed to elicit the benefits of specific interventions.

Ethnicity

The flow of people across continents, which is an increasingly common feature of modern life, provides a clear example of how social forces can affect a person's mental health. Many of these people will have fled unimaginable psychological and physical pain in an attempt to find respite and asylum. This group is particularly vulnerable to mental health problems. Post-traumatic stress disorder is commonly reported and the risk of suicide is also raised in this group (DH 1999).

Within established UK communities there is evidence also of interactions between ethnicity and mental health. For example, young Asian women have a relatively high rate of suicide which, though poorly understood, has been attributed to conflicts between parental expectations and the aspirations of children who develop in a Western culture (NHS Centre for Reviews and Dissemination 1996). However, of all the ethnic groups that make up modern Britain, the Black African-Caribbean population's experience provides a salutary lesson on the effect of social forces on mental health.

A consistent finding in the literature has been the differential experiences of African-Caribbeans in mental health services compared with others in our communities. Their care pathways are problematic and are more often characterized by compulsory admissions to hospital, police involvement prior to admission, the administration of medications by force, and contentious staff–user interactions (Goater *et al.* 1999, Thornicroft *et al.* 1999). They are also more likely to receive a diagnosis of schizophrenia and less likely than other social groups to receive diagnoses of depression or other affective disorders (Harrison *et al.* 1989; Lloyd and Moodley 1992).

What social forces might account for these differentials? African-Caribbeans are afforded poorer housing, experience higher levels of unemployment and draw a lower average income per household than their white counterparts (Modood *et al.* 1998). Further, approximately one third of young black men between the ages of 20 and 24 are unemployed, and for the African-Caribbean population at large, unemployment is approximately three times greater than it is among white communities (Sainsbury Centre for Mental Health (SCMH) 2002).

The social model posits that the experiences of African-Caribbean communities in the UK are sufficient to engender mental health problems. However, these differentials are not just a feature of everyday life but extend into the arena of mental health care itself. For example, psychiatrists have been found to more frequently view black people as violent (Lewis *et al.* 1990), and racial stereotyping of this kind (not only by psychiatrists but by mental health nurses and other staff, too), significantly influences patient management (Spector 2001). Thus, there are community features associated with deprivation that African-Caribbean people experience, which we know affect their mental health, and there are the attitudes of some health care professionals, which compound the experience of mental ill-health. The Sainsbury Centre for Mental Health (SCMH) has recently completed a major qualitative inquiry into this phenomenon, which they have termed 'circles of fear' (SCMH 2002). A wide-ranging programme is needed to break these circles of fear, the main aims of which should be to:

- ensure that Black service users are treated with respect and that their voices are heard;
- deliver early intervention and early access to services to prevent escalation of crises;
- ensure that services are accessible, welcoming, relevant and well-integrated with the community;
- increase understanding and effective communication on both sides including creating a culture that allows people to discuss race and mental health issues; and
- deliver greater support and funding to services led by the Black community.

Integrating models of mental illness

There are key features that appear to differentiate each of the models we have described. For example, the disease model is concerned with physical, biological and chemical markers of mental illness. These markers can be observed and measured, and are, therefore, representative of an *objective* orientation. In contrast, the cognitive model deals with internal thought processes unique to individuals. This orientation is therefore primarily *subjective*.

There is a further difference to note. The behavioural model is concerned with *a person*'s behaviour. Attention to this alone will suffice for the behaviour therapist. This model is clearly orientated to the *self*. In contrast, the social model is concerned not with *self* but with forces beyond a person's control in the society in which they live. This orientation we have called *community*.

These two dimensions, *subjective–objective* and *self–community*, are used to formulate a four-quadrant schema (Figure 1.1). We have positioned each of the models in their respective quadrants. Thus, the disease model, which is concerned with a person's biophysiological profile is upper right (*objective–self*). Similarly, the behavioural model, which deals with a person's observable behaviours is also upper right. The cognitive model however, is upper left (*subjective–self*) since its primary focus is on the internal thought processes of the individual.

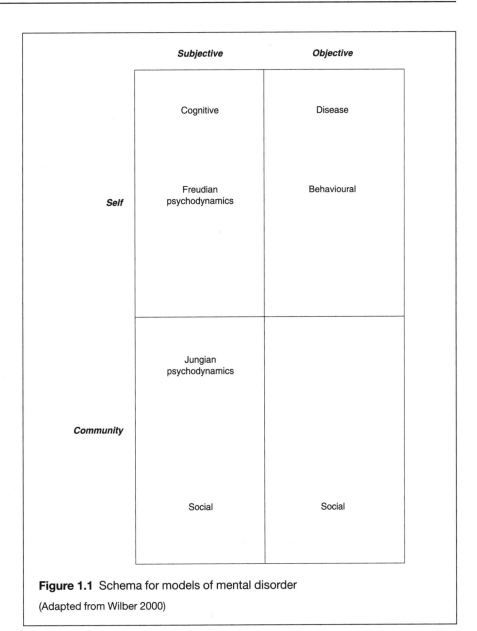

Figure 1.1 Schema for models of mental disorder

(Adapted from Wilber 2000)

Freudian psychodynamics are certainly upper left (*subjective–self*) dealing as they do with our inner world and specifically our sense of self. However, as we have seen, Jungian psychodynamics are premised on a transcendent self, borne of intersubjective culture and mythology (community). For this reason we feel inclined to position Jung in the lower left quadrant (*subjective–community*). Finally, the social model is certainly community oriented but straddles both lower quadrants. Unemployment and poverty are quantifiable attributes, and each is associated with mental disorder. This interpretation of the social model reflects the lower right quadrant (*objective–community*). On the other hand, intersubjective experiences such as kinship and expressed emotion are also associated with mental disorder. This interpretation reflects the lower left quadrant (*subjective–community*).

Figure 1.1 illustrates the general orientation of different schools of thought in explaining the aetiology of mental disorder and points of comparison and contrast. But things are more complex than appear here, and there is certainly blurring across the quadrants. Cognitive behavioural therapy is a good example, since cognitive therapists might argue that although they deal initially with unique internal thought processes, they endeavour to alter these with recourse to external, observable evidence (*objective–self*). Nevertheless, it remains true that they are primarily concerned with, and rooted in, a person's subjective experience. And, anyway, we would wish to encourage integration (blurring) in the minds of our readers. All models have something to contribute to our contemporary understanding of mental disorders precisely because human experience is made up of a subjective and objective sense of self, and a subjective and objective sense of community.

We suggest, therefore, that the models of mental disorder considered here have many more points in common than difference because they each tap into a limited but, nevertheless, vital aspect of human experience. This stands in contrast to the literature that often reflects an egocentric discourse in which opposing camps endeavour to discredit each other. Beware the academic or practitioner who works hard to undermine any one of these models. They will probably have reason to suggest an alternative (complementary) model, but are likely to be in error regarding the model(s) they try to deny. Human experience arises from all four quadrants and mental health nurses need to draw upon all of them in their practice rather than discount some but not others on grounds of preference or prejudice. We return to this basic schema (Figure 1.1) when describing the assessment of mental health and illness in Chapter 7.

The stress vulnerability model

An integrated, second-order model has been developed by Zubin and Spring (1977) to specifically explain the aetiology of schizophrenia. Incorporating all other models, it has as its common denominator the relationship between stress and vulnerability. Stress is the variable that influences the manifestation of symptoms and a person's vulnerability represents their predisposition to such manifestations.

Two types of stress are at play here. The first is known as ambient stress and reflects the general concerns and pressures that we all face in our everyday lives. Although such stressors are necessary for us to function and perform some people experience more ambient stress than others; we have referred to this previously in our discussion of family interventions and levels of critical expressed emotion. The second type of stress arises from life events and again we are familiar with these, following an earlier reference to Holmes and Rahe's (1967) Social Readjustment Rating Scale.

Similarly, there are two types of vulnerability. The first is inborn and will likely include genetic loading and the neurophysiology of the person. The second is acquired and will be specific to an individual's life experiences but may include perinatal complications, maladaptive learned behaviours or thought patterns, and adolescent peer interactions (Zubin and Spring 1977). Notice that these descriptions include features from the single models previously described and can, therefore, be mapped according to the four quadrants in Figure 1.1: for example, vulnerability can be upper left (thought patterns) or upper right (genetic loading) but also lower left (adolescent peer interactions).

Zubin and Spring's (1977) central hypothesis is that the interface between an individual's vulnerability and the stress they experience in the course of their lives is the basis for the development or otherwise of schizophrenic symptomatology. There will, of course, be a range of vulnerabilities in any population, with some people being extremely prone to illness even when experiencing relatively mild levels of stress, to those whose vulnerability is so low that they are able to tolerate high levels of stress for significant periods without any trace of psychiatric symptoms.

Since its publication in 1977 this model has had considerable impact in the field of mental health care. It offers hope to those who experience mental disorders because it suggests that coping mechanisms can be acquired to counter the effects of stress and thus reduce the risk of continued illness or relapse. The model is also of considerable value to mental health staff, since it provides a rationale for the use of psychosocial as well as medicinal interventions, and nursing has significantly developed its psychosocial skills base as a result (Gournay 1995).

A contemporary perspective

Our recommendation that mental health nurses familiarize themselves with these models of mental disorder and employ an integrated perspective in practice is supported by the *NSF for Mental Health* (DH 1999). Each of the single models described above is reflected to varying degrees within this national policy document. We make some of these connections explicit.

Standard 1: mental health promotion

The rationale for this standard is that 'mental health problems can result from the range of adverse effects associated with social exclusion . . .' (p. 4). Here we see evidence of a social explanation for mental health problems and the recommended interventions are directed towards populations and communities as well as individuals.

Standards 2 and 3: primary care and access to services

Recommendations are made regarding the use of medication, electroconvulsive therapy, cognitive therapy, cognitive behavioural therapy and focused psychoanalytic therapy for individuals who present with depression. Cognitive behavioural therapy is recommended also for anxiety disorders. The disease, psychoanalytical, behavioural and cognitive models are evident in these recommendations.

Standards 4 and 5: effective services for people with severe mental illness

Though concerned primarily with care processes, interventions are recommended that variously reflect all the models of mental disorder previously described; these interventions include anti-psychotic medication, cognitive therapy, family interventions and vocational services.

Standard 6: caring about carers

This standard is concerned with assessing the needs of carers and ensuring services are provided to meet those needs. Implicit is the recognition that the stress of caring can affect the carer's own physical and mental health. These associations are supported by the social model of mental disorder.

Standard 7: preventing suicide

Suicide prevention is, in part, achieved by the recommendations made under standards 1–6 and therefore involves interventions that stem from each of the models.

The classification of mental disorder

Systems for classifying mental disorder or 'illness' stem from the medical model, which as Tyrer and Steinberg (1998) point out is not an aetiological model itself but an approach to diagnosing individual disorder. In a general sense all models apply this process, with exception perhaps of the social model, although the systems that are used for classification purposes vary between models. For example, when discussing the cognitive model we described Ellis's (1962) ABC framework for defining specific cognitive problems that arise between an activating event and the behavioural or cognitive consequence. Problem-oriented statements can be constructed from such an analysis, which represent one approach to classification. For example, 'When I make eye contact with strangers in public (Activating event), I believe they immediately think bad of me (Belief), and therefore I avoid social interaction (Consequence).' This statement classifies a cognitive or behavioural problem depending on your perspective.

Medical diagnosis is another classification system, which represents the dominant frame of reference for most mental health workers internationally. These diagnoses are described in two classification systems; the *International Classification of Disease* (ICD-10 World Health Organization (WHO) 1992);

and the *Diagnostic and Statistical Manual for Mental Disorders* (DSM-IV American Psychiatric Association (APA) 1994). In the UK our primary frame of reference is ICD-10, which is described below. DSM-IV is described in more detail in Chapter 2. But first we draw out some differences between the two systems.

Ideally each diagnosis should be mutually exclusive and stand independently of other symptoms associated with other diagnoses. Rarely in practice is this achieved. More often than not a range of symptoms may indicate the relevance of two or more diagnoses. This point is particularly pertinent to the ICD-10 classification system, which uses a single axis upon which to select diagnoses for an individual's disorder. If more than one is selected they may appear to contradict each other (Tyrer and Steinberg 1998). However, psychiatric diagnoses are based on a hierarchical system so that each disorder can manifest symptoms present in disorders lower down the hierarchy, but not above it (Sturt 1981). For example, an individual who experiences persistent low mood may receive a diagnosis of *depression*. However, if the low mood is accompanied by delusional thought patterns, a diagnosis of *schizoaffective disorder* will take precedence over a diagnosis of depression.

In contrast to the single-axis approach of ICD-10 there is an increasing tendency to use multi-axial approaches in which clinical diagnosis is only one part. Thus, in DSM-IV the clinical diagnosis is axis 1, personality status is described in axis 2, and developmental delay, intellectual status, physical health, social functioning and reactions to stress are all separate axes. This approach allows several descriptors to be attributed to an individual's symptoms and their general condition.

Before examining ICD-10 diagnostic categories it is important to stress that any classification system classifies syndromes and conditions, but not individuals. We may all suffer from one or more disorders of either a mental or physical nature at different times in our lives. It is meaningless, therefore, as well as stigmatizing, to use such labels to describe people. A person should never be equated with a disorder, physical or mental (WHO 2001).

ICD-10 diagnostic categories

Table 1.1 presents the main diagnostic groupings in ICD-10 together with their key features. The table presents an overview and we refer readers to subsequent chapters for more detailed accounts of many of these conditions. Equally, we would recommend an examination of the WHO (1992) classification manual, particularly Chapter 5, which provides detailed information on all 100 categories of classification (though a proportion of these remain unused at present).

Psychoses and neuroses

The terms 'psychoses' and 'neuroses' are second-order classifications that group several of the conditions in Table 1.1. The psychoses are disorders in

Table 1.1 ICD-10 classification of mental and behavioural disorders

Diagnostic groupings	Key features
F00–F09 Organic mental disorders including dementias and delirium	Brain dysfunction resulting in disturbances of cognition, mood, perception and/or behaviour
F10–F19 Psychoactive substance use including intoxication, abuse, dependence and withdrawal states	Typically present when substance use interferes with a person's physical, mental or social functioning to the detriment of their well-being
F20–F29 Schizophrenia, schizotypal, delusional and schizoaffective disorders	Mental states characterized by distortions of thinking, perception and mood, but not due to an organic condition
F30–F39 Mood (affective) disorders including depression, manic disorder and bipolar disorders	The key symptom is a disturbance in mood though other features will also be present associated with this mood change for example social isolation accompanying depression
F40–F48 Neurotic, stress-related and somatoform disorders including phobias, obsessive compulsive disorder and stress reactions	A range of symptoms may be present including tension, anxiety, problems with concentration and ritualistic behaviours
F50–F59 Behavioural syndromes including eating disorders, sleep disorders and post-partum mental disorders	Symptoms vary according to the condition, for example weight loss with certain eating disorders. However, physiological and hormonal factors appear to play a part in these conditions
F60–F69 Disorders of adult personality and behaviour including personality disorders, gender identity disorders and impulse disorders	Disorders in which clinically significant behaviour patterns are persistent and reflect the person's lifestyle and way of interacting with others
F70–F79 Mental retardation of varying degrees from mild to profound	Usually manifest by the impairment of skills associated with intelligence
F80–F89 Disorders of psychological development including autism, speech disorders, disorders in scholastic skills and developmental disorders of motor functions	Originating in infancy or childhood these disorders delay the development of functions related to maturation of the central nervous system
F90–F98 Behavioural and emotional disorders of childhood including conduct disorders and hyperkinetic disorders	Only common features are an onset early in life and a fluctuating or unpredictable course

(Adapted from WHO 1992; and Tyrer and Steinberg 1998)

which '. . . people's capacity to recognize reality, their thinking processes, judgements and communications are seriously impaired, together with the presence of delusions and hallucinations' (Craig 2000: 54). In turn, these are divided into 'organic' and 'functional' psychoses. The former are represented by the group F00–F09 in Table 1.1 in which pathological processes affecting the brain result in psychotic symptoms. The functional psychoses are group F20–F29 and include schizophrenia and delusional disorders but also affective psychoses in which a primary disturbance of mood is accompanied by psychotic symptoms. In keeping with the hierarchical nature of diagnosis, any disorder in the F30–F39 group that incorporates psychotic symptoms will be elevated to a diagnosis within the F20–F29 group.

Individuals who experience neuroses are different from the general population only in the degree of the symptoms they experience. Thus, anxiety and low mood are common to our experience of life. Indeed we would hope that anxiety is present to some degree before, say, an important exam, in order to enhance our performance. However, if this anxiety becomes so great that it debilitates us, so that we cannot even attend the exam, then this may indicate a neurotic mental disorder. Therefore, in contrast to the psychoses, in which a person's grasp of reality is uncertain, the neuroses are characterized by the heightening of normal human experiences but to levels that interfere with our ability to function. The neuroses are represented by groups F30–F39 and F40–F48 in Table 1.1.

A group that falls outside of the psychoses/neuroses divide are the personality disorders represented by F60–F69. Personality is a familiar concept and one that we may all use to describe friends and colleagues. We may, for example, say that someone is always cheerful or shy. However, the personality disorders contained in F60–F69 are indicative of people who appear to habitually behave in ways that lead them into conflict with society. These deeply ingrained maladaptive behavioural patterns have been classified into different types of personality disorder including obsessive, avoidant, schizoid, paranoid, borderline, antisocial, dependent, schizotypal, histrionic and narcissistic (WHO 1992).

There has been, and is currently, considerable debate regarding how best to provide services for individuals with these conditions, or whether indeed they are treatable at all. It is perhaps true from a disease perspective that such deeply ingrained behavioural patterns, which appear to stand independently of other psychiatric symptoms, may not be amenable to change following a course of medication. However, there is evidence of benefit in the literature of therapies designed specifically for this group, for example, cognitive-behavioural treatment (Linehan *et al.* 1991) and therapeutic communities (Lees *et al.* 1999).

A diagnosis of personality disorder has resulted often in the neglect of the individual by psychiatric services. This is unacceptable although we acknowledge that the individual may be untreatable in the traditional sense of the word. Collaborative, open and honest assessment of the trials of life, triggers for problematic behaviours risk situations, can often provide a good starting point for working with these individuals, upon which alternative strategies can be formulated and advice offered. Clinical experience suggests that an individual with a diagnosis of personality disorder, who consents to such a collaborative enterprise, can derive benefit.

Serious mental illness and common mental health problems

A further distinction between different types of mental disorder is made with reference to 'serious mental illness' (SMI) and 'common mental health problems'. Current mental health policy and practice is influenced significantly by the concept of SMI, the origins of which are many, but we draw attention to two predominant influences from the last decade.

In 1990, White published the third quinquennial national survey of community psychiatric nursing. A key finding was that 80 per cent of people with schizophrenia in England had never been on the caseload of a mental health nurse working in the community. Community psychiatric nurses (CPNs) had tended instead towards providing primary care based liaison services through which they were more likely to encounter patients with neurotic rather than psychotic symptoms.

Alongside this increasing awareness of CPN activity the British media reported a number of high-profile homicides committed by people with a mental illness, which they argued demonstrated the failure of community care. Further, it followed that communities were now at risk from those with serious mental illness (Barker *et al.* 1998). The public concern that such reports generated was allayed by the Department of Health who began to target services towards people with SMI. Thus, the *Health of the Nation: Key Area Handbook* (DH 1994a) identified those with SMI to be the priority target group for services, although it acknowledged that defining this group was problematic. Similarly, the Mental Health Nursing Review Team (DH 1994b) recommended that '. . . the essential focus for the work of mental health nurses lies in working with people with serious or enduring mental illness in secondary and tertiary care . . .' (p. 16).

Early attempts to differentiate SMI from common mental health problems relied heavily on the presence of a psychotic diagnosis as a marker for SMI, for example, McLean and Leibowitz (1989) and Patmore and Weaver (1990). This position has essentially remained the same so that SMI is now synonymous with 'psychoses' and common mental health problems with 'neuroses'.

We make two brief observations regarding these new labels that have entered psychiatric parlance in the last decade. First, they are borne of social fears often fuelled by an ill-informed media. Second, were you (or us) to experience depression to the extent that suicide became a convincing option for you, but you had no psychotic symptomatology, your condition, following McLean and Leibowitz (1989) and Patmore and Weaver (1990), would be considered a common mental health problem rather than a serious one.

While we might understand the basis for these labels their utility in practice is questionable. A nursing profession that sides entirely with the concept of serious mental illness, and its association with psychosis, is narrowing its professional repertoire. Perhaps more importantly, it is overlooking other subgroups within the adult population that will be marginalized by such a narrow definition of SMI (Barker *et al.* 1998).

Prevalence and symptomatology of mental disorders

Prevalence, expressed as a percentage, refers to the number of people with a particular disorder within a given population. Incidence, on the other hand, also expressed as a percentage, refers to the number of new cases that arise within a given population in a given time period. Actual estimates of prevalence and incidence of mental disorders vary from one epidemiological study to the next. Different samples will have been studied and there may be real differences between populations. Also different instruments might have been used, and the results from these might have been interpreted in different ways to define a 'case'.

The NSF for Mental Health (DH 1999) used a variety of sources to present prevalence data including World Health Organization figures, which generate European and other world region estimates, rather than country specific data (though the most recent report (WHO 2001) does provide estimates for Manchester as a marker for UK data). The NSF (DH 1999) also relied on a survey of psychiatric morbidity for adults conducted in the UK in 1994 (Meltzer *et al.* 1995). More recently this survey was repeated (Singleton *et al.* 2001) and it is these data that we have chosen that most accurately represent the prevalence of mental disorders in the UK.

Singleton *et al.* (2001) sampled more than 15,000 private households in England, Wales and Scotland, of which 8,886 took part in the survey, and in each of these households one member completed a battery of instruments. All subjects were between the ages of 16 and 74. The survey gathered symptom data, which were used to describe both the incidence of symptoms among those who did not meet diagnostic criteria, and the prevalence of specific diagnoses where the level of symptoms indicated their presence. ICD-10 diagnoses as presented in Table 1.1 were used for this purpose.

The report provides data for common mental health problems in terms of the weekly prevalence per 1000 adults (Table 1.2). The report also provides data for more severe forms of disorder and substance use in terms of the annual prevalence per 1000 adults (Table 1.3). Notice that Table 1.3 refers to 'probable psychosis' since its confirmation through research interviews can be difficult to accurately discern. 'Probable psychosis' refers to schizophrenia, schizotypal and delusional disorders (F20–29 in Table 1.1).

The mental disorders contained in Tables 1.1, 1.2 and 1.3 can affect a person's mood, thought processes, perceptions and behaviours. Common symptoms associated with these disorders are described below. They are examined in more detail in the chapters to follow, which deal with specific mental disorders.

Table 1.2 Weekly prevalence of common mental disorders

Diagnosis	Weekly prevalence per 1000 adults aged 16–74
Mixed anxiety and depression	88
Generalized anxiety disorder	44
Depression	26
All phobias	18
Obsessive compulsive disorder	11
Panic disorder	7

(Adapted from Singleton *et al.* 2001)

Table 1.3 Annual prevalence of severe mental disorders and substance dependence

Diagnosis	Annual prevalence per 1000 adults aged 16–74
Probable psychosis	5
Alcohol dependence	74
Any drug dependence	37

(Adapted from Singleton *et al.* 2001)

Mood

Anxiety

Anxiety is distinguished from general tension by its accompanying physical sensations (autonomic nervous system arousal), including palpitations, sweating and tremor. Anxiety may occur in response to phobic situations or specific thoughts but can also occur independently of any such trigger (free-floating anxiety), or be linked to a sense that something dreadful is about to occur (anxious foreboding) (Craig 2000). Anxiety may also occur abruptly for short periods during which the person experiences marked fearfulness and may feel they are losing control (panic attacks).

Depression

'Sad', 'gloomy' and 'low spirits' are synonymous with depressed mood. More severe forms of this experience encompass additional features including a reduced emotional response to the ups and downs of life (flattened or blunted affect). The individual may also experience disturbed sleep patterns, loss of appetite and a lack of interest in and engagement with life. More extreme forms of this experience can be accompanied by feelings of hope-lessness, possibly leading to suicidal thoughts. Other terms associated with this experience include *self-deprecation* (loss of confidence in self and a developing sense of worthlessness) and *pathological guilt* (feeling responsible for actions that may be inconsequential to others).

Elation

Individuals who experience elation in the course of a mental health problem may feel euphoric and excited but also irritable and impatient (Craig 2000). Typically, concentration is impaired, there is over-talkativeness, a reduced need for sleep and reckless acts are not uncommon, for example excessive spending sprees. Common to these symptoms is an underlying self-esteem that is exaggerated, and grandiose beliefs, such as having special intelligence, are not uncommon.

Thought processes

Obsessional thoughts and compulsions

A person's thoughts are considered obsessional when they become intrusive, unwanted and no longer amenable to self-control (obsessional ruminations). *Obsessional incompleteness* refers to an overriding desire to ensure every aspect of a task has been correctly executed before the individual can consider it complete. Intrusive thoughts of this type may be accompanied by repetitive, *ritualistic behaviour*. An important feature that distinguishes these types of thought is the person's awareness that they are their own.

Delusions

A delusion is a false impression or belief that we can all be subject to from time to time. In the mental health field additional qualities associated with delusional thought distinguish it as a symptom of mental disorder. The belief is usually held with absolute and compelling conviction, is typically idiosyncratic and resistant to modification through experience or discussion (Craig 2000). Different types of delusion have been classified including *delusions of persecution* and *delusions of reference*. The latter often involves people feeling that news items on the TV, radio or in newspapers have a double meaning and make reference specifically to them.

Thought possession

Some people with mental health problems encounter the sensation that the innermost workings of their mind are amenable to outsiders (Craig 2000). Different sorts of experience have been described including *thought broadcasting* (a person believes that their thoughts are heard aloud by those around them), and *thought insertion* (a loss in the ownership of a person's own thoughts, usually accompanied by a delusional explanation for how thoughts are placed in their mind).

Perceptions

Perception among people who experience mental health problems can become diminished, heightened or distorted (Craig 2000). Hallucinations are a key symptom in this respect, which are defined as false perceptions in so far as there is no adequate external stimulus for the experience. Each of the five human senses can be affected by hallucinations. Thus, hallucinations are typically referred to as *auditory, visual, olfactory, tactile* and *gustatory*.

Behaviour

The behaviour and appearance of people with mental disorders may appear strange or unusual. A lack of self-care and accompanying self-neglect are not uncommon, but neither are they necessarily an indication of mental disorder. The specific patterns and qualities of a person's speech are more useful indicators of a mental disorder. Symptoms may include *pressure of speech* (a rush of words that is difficult to stop), *flight of ideas* (skipping from topic to topic with no logical association), and *poverty of speech* (speaking freely but in such a vague manner that no meaningful information is communicated).

The symptoms associated with the functional psychoses are sometimes also referred to as 'positive' and 'negative'. Brennan explores these terms in detail in Chapter 13.

User perspectives on mental disorders

Thus far, we have proposed a four-quadrant schema for understanding human experience and have described disordered human experience in terms of classification systems, incidence data and symptomatology. Note that these latter terms refer to the upper right quadrant (*objective–self*) of Figure 1.1. They objectify human experience into codified systems of description, including numbers. So, having proposed a four-quadrant integration we have subsequently planted our feet firmly in only one!

Well, this says something of the dominant perspective in contemporary psychiatry. It is not in itself wrong, since human experience is made up of a subjective and objective sense of self and a subjective and objective sense of community. But it is only part of the story, or more precisely, one-quarter. In this final section we begin to redress the balance with reference to the personal accounts of mental health service users and the research they have conducted.

When people who have experienced mental disorders describe the connections that are important to them in the expression of their distress, their needs, and thus the imbalances that have led to their condition, there are striking similarities across individuals and groups. Users value common things such as respect, choice, self-help and advocacy. Their expressed needs include intimacy and privacy, satisfying social and sexual lives, happiness and meaningful activity (Repper 2000). These all stem from left quadrant territory, both *self* and *community*, and we should be grateful for the reminder.

But service users also draw attention to the lower right quadrant where *objective–community* forces can threaten their well-being. Income, housing, benefits and employment are typical examples (Duggan *et al.* 1997). So, what of upper right? Well, mental health service users are actually much more connected to human experience than the professional literature might have us believe. Upper right does not need developing anywhere near as much as the other quadrants, since the objective sciences have that base covered, at least for the time being. And service users readily acknowledge that they have benefited from these *objective–self* sciences. A survey of more than 500 service users, conducted by a research team of service users, concluded that 'while many users suffered from the side effects of psychotropic drugs, most also appreciated the benefits and lessening of symptoms' (Rose 2001: 6). This seems a balanced view.

The evidence points to an integrated understanding of the origins of human experience and a corresponding focus on those areas where care and attention is required (self and community in both subjective and objective terms). This point is made clearly in the service user research introduced above (Rose 2001). Through rigorous methodological procedures, out of respect for the scientific method (upper right), this service user research team designed an interview schedule that could be administered by service users (trained in interview techniques) to describe the perspectives of current mental health service users on community and hospital care. The instrument, which it is hoped will contribute to the formulation of a set of user-defined standards to compliment those already in the NSF (DH 1999), covers all four quadrants.

Personal experiences of self, such as the ability to make choices based on sufficient information (*subjective–self*) are key items in relation to various health care practices, including medication (*objective–self*). Rose's interview method taps social forces that may be experienced as oppressive or liberating, such as the police or user groups (*objective–community*), and also incorporates *subjective–community* interests such as relations with professional staff. A psychotherapist once declared a client's criticism of her service to be a symptom of their psychopathology (Rose 2001). This is a crude analysis in which all experience must be reduced to upper right and stands in sharp contrast to the integrated, four-quadrant, holistic orientation of many service users.

From the evidence to date it would appear that mental health service users do not distinguish one mental health nursing approach or set of skills (model and its treatment implications) as being the correct one or the only one, but recognize the potential value of all, providing no one approach is applied oppressively and providing all are delivered with respect for the person and their choices.

We end this chapter with an insightful piece of literature written by a 'psychiatric-nurse therapist' who experienced a mental disorder during the course of his nursing career (Olson 2002). Tom, his Christian name, takes the reader through the emergence of his distress and the battles that ensued over diagnoses and treatment approaches. Following four separate diagnoses made by four independent practitioners Tom comments that it '. . . was like the story of the blind men who, touching separate parts of an elephant, each reached a different conclusion about what was before them' (p. 437). Tom did not feel as though he was being treated as a person but as bits of a person. Regarding his treatment experience he could conclude only that it '. . . reveal(s) professional ego as an important barrier to coordination of care' (p. 443). All were fighting their own corners, edifying their separate positions, cutting off others, and ultimately, therefore, failing miserably to treat the whole person. The real irony is that they all had something to contribute to Tom's care if only they had contributed unconditionally instead of forcefully pursuing their own agendas.

Conclusion

Nurses are the professional group in closest contact with mental health service users over lengthy periods of illness and wellness, which provides them opportunity to become involved in many areas of a person's life during different stages of health (Repper 2000). We have described various models of mental disorder, each of which taps into different aspects of human experience. These points emphasize the importance of mental health nurses embracing an integrated understanding of human experience, through which all models have something to contribute. This is not to say that we should avoid specializing in interventions derived clearly from one model than the others, for example, behavioural therapy, psychodynamic counselling. Rather, we should acknowledge the necessary but insufficient basis of such specialist knowledge to describe the experience of being human. From this position we will be better placed to provide holistic, integrated care by either broadening our own perspective, or by enjoining with others who possess complimentary specialist knowledge. As we have seen, an important source of complimentary specialist knowledge is the service user, from whom nurses have much to learn if we are to purposefully assist people through their experience of mental disorder, and aid their recovery.

We began this chapter by suggesting that mental illness and mental health are terms of relation that describe the reality of human experience. We have, therefore, given an account of one side of human experience (or at least some shades of its spectrum). To fully appreciate the contribution nurses can make to the well-being of people, we need to understand the concept of mental health, to understand its meaning and the implications this might have for our role. To conclude, we summarize the main points of this chapter below:

- Mental disorders represent shades in the spectrum of human experience, which comprise a *subjective* and *objective* sense of *self* and a *subjective* and *objective* sense of *community*.

- Models of mental disorder describe aetiology and treatment implications in relation to different levels of human functioning: biophysiological organism (disease); the unconscious (psychodynamic); thought processes (cognitive); actions (behavioural); and self in context (social).

- The models can be mapped against a four-quadrant schema of human experience (Figure 1.1), demonstrating their partial, though necessary, contribution to the treatment and care of people who experience mental disorders.

- Mental health nurses need to develop an integrated understanding of mental disorders, to be demonstrated in collaborative partnerships with service users and professional colleagues.

- This chapter represents only part of the story, describing as it does disorder – we must consider the antithesis of this position to fully comprehend human experience, and to realize the full extent of nursing's contribution to mental health care work. To this end we would encourage you to read this chapter in combination with Chapter 2, which considers the concept of health.

Questions for reflection and discussion

1   Reflect on each of the following and consider how much you feel they contribute to your sense of self: genetic endowment; early childhood experiences; learned behaviour or ways of thinking from parents and peers; and social factors.

2   Reflect on a time in your life when you felt distressed (for example losing a loved-one, your job, your self-esteem, or experiencing prolonged periods of stress). Spend a little while familiarizing yourself with the events of that time, what your life looked like and how it felt, and then ask yourself: 'Would others have experienced those events in the same way?' And: 'If not, why not?'

3   Put yourself in the position of a person you have known or nursed who has been diagnosed with a mental disorder. What do you remember or think was their preferred perspective on the nature of their problems and the interventions that they considered most appropriate? Did these differ from the reality of the care they received and, if so, why?

4   Use the schema presented in Figure 1.1 to identify the orientation of the chapters that follow. Are they concerned primarily with the objective or the subjective indicators of health and/or illness at the individual or community level?

5   Before embarking on Chapter 2 think about your own ideas of what mental health is, using the basic schema in Figure 1.1 to explore its likely dimensions.

Annotated bibliography

- Tyrer, P. and Steinberg, D. (1998) *Models for Mental Disorder: Conceptual Models in Psychiatry*. Chichester: John Wiley and Sons. Now in its third edition, this text provides a detailed yet accessible explanation of the main models of mental disorder in contemporary practice. We have adopted Tyrer and Steinberg's five basic model structure in this chapter but have pursued a different path to integration. However, we recommend also Tyrer and Steinberg's approach, which is predicated on levels of functioning rather than, as ours, the components of human experience.
- Gamble, C. and Brennan, G. (eds) (2000) *Working With Serious Mental Illness: A Manual for Clinical Practice*. London: Bailliere Tindall. Though primarily a practice manual as the title suggests, this text devotes a chapter to the stress vulnerability model and a section, comprising eight chapters, to interventions based on a stress vulnerability understanding of serious mental illness.
- *Journal of Psychiatric and Mental Health Nursing* Volumes **5**: 3 and **6**: 4. These volumes are dedicated to the contributions of Hildegard Peplau and Annie Altschul to mental health nursing. These pioneers draw upon interpersonal theories of human experience and psychodynamic principles in their work. Papers in these volumes demonstrate the application of Peplau's and Altschul's ideas to contemporary health care practice.

References

American Psychiatric Association (1994) *Diagnostic and Statistical Manual for Mental Disorders, 4th revision*. Washington: American Psychiatric Association.

Barker, P. (1981) *Basic Family Therapy*. London: Granada.

Barker, P., Keady, J., Croom, S. *et al.* (1998) The concept of serious mental illness: modern myths and grim realities. *Journal of Psychiatric and Mental Health Nursing* **5**: 247–54.

Bates, P. (ed.) (2002) *Working for Inclusion: Making Social Inclusion a Reality for People with Severe Mental Health Problems*. London: Sainsbury Centre for Mental Health.

Brooker, C. and Butterworth, A. (1991) Working with families caring for a relative with schizophrenia: the evolving role of the community psychiatric nurse. *International Journal of Nursing Studies* **28**: 189–200.

Brown, G. and Birley, J. (1968) Crises and life events and the onset of schizophrenia. *Journal of Health and Social Behaviour* **9**: 203–14.

Burnard, P. and Hannigan, B. (2000) Qualitative and quantitative approaches in mental health nursing: moving the debate forward. *Journal of Psychiatric and Mental Health Nursing* **7**: 1–6.

Chadwick, P., Birchwood, M. and Trower, P. (1996) *Cognitive Therapy for Delusions, Voices and Paranoia*. Chichester: John Wiley and Sons.

Craig, T. (2000) Severe mental illness: symptoms, signs and diagnosis, in C. Gamble and G. Brennan (eds) *Working with serious mental illness: a manual for clinical practice*. London: Bailliere Tindall.

Curwen, B., Palmer, S. and Ruddell, P. (2000) *Brief Cognitive Behaviour Therapy*. London: Sage.

Dawson, P. (1997) A reply to Kevin Gournay's 'Schizophrenia: a review of the contemporary literature and implications for mental health nursing theory, practice and education'. *Journal of Psychiatric and Mental Health Nursing* **4**: 1–7.

Dawson, P. (1998) Schizophrenia and genetics: a review and critique for the psychiatric nurse. *Journal of Psychiatric and Mental Health Nursing* **5**: 299–307.

Department of Health (1994a) *The Health of the Nation: Key Area Handbook: Mental Illness*. London: HMSO.

Department of Health (1994b) *Working in Partnership: A collaborative approach to care*. London: HMSO.

Department of Health (1999) *A National Service Framework for Mental Health*. London: The Stationery Office.

Department of Health (2001) *Making It Happen: A Guide to Delivering Mental Health Promotion*. London: DH.

Duggan, M., Ford, R., Hill, R. *et al.* (1997) *Pulling Together: The Future Roles and Training of Mental Health Staff*. London: The Sainsbury Centre for Mental Health.

Duggan, M., Cooper, A. and Foster, J. (2002) *Modernising the Social Model in Mental Health: a Discussion Paper*. London: Training Organization of the Personal Social Services (TOPSS).

Durkheim, E. (1897) *Le Suicide*. Paris: Alcan.

Ellis, A. (1962) *Reason and Emotion in Psychotherapy*. New York: Stuart.

Falloon, I. (1995) *Family Management of Schizophrenia*. Baltimore: Johns Hopkins University Press.

Goater, N., King, M., Cole, E. *et al.* (1999) Ethnicity and outcome of psychosis. *British Journal of Psychiatry* **175**: 34–42.

Gournay, K. (1995) Mental health nurses working purposefully with people with serious and enduring mental illness – an international perspective. *International Journal of Nursing Studies* **32**: 341–52.

Gournay, K. (1996) Schizophrenia: a review of the contemporary literature and implications for mental health nursing theory, practice and education. *Journal of Psychiatric and Mental Health Nursing* **3**: 7–12.

Gournay, K., Denford, L., Parr, A.-M. and Newell, R. (2000) British nurses in behavioural psychotherapy: a 25-year follow up. *Journal of Advanced Nursing* **32**: 1–9.

Hall, D. and Lynch, M. (1998) Violence begins at home: Domestic strife has lifelong effects on children. *British Medical Journal* **316**: 15.

Harrison, G., Owens, D., Holton, A., Nelson, D. and Boot, D. (1989) A prospective study of severe mental disorder in Afro-Caribbean patients. *Psychological Medicine* **19**: 683–96.

Hawton, K., Salkovskis, P., Kirk, J. and Clark, D. (1989) *Cognitive Behaviour Therapy for Psychiatric Problems: A Practical Guide*. Oxford: Oxford University Press.

Hirsch, S. (1988) *Psychiatric Beds and Resources: Factors Influencing Bed Use and Service Planning*. London: Gaskell.

Holmes, T. and Rahe, R. (1967) The social readjustment rating scale. *Journal of Psychosomatic Research* **11**: 213–18.

Keen, T. (1999) Schizophrenia: orthodoxy and heresies. A review of alternative possibilities. *Journal of Psychiatric and Mental Health Nursing* **6**: 415–24.

Kendall, R. (1975) *The Role of Diagnosis in Psychiatry*. Oxford: Blackwell Science Publications.

Kingdon, D. and Turkington, D. (1993) *Cognitive Therapy in Schizophrenia*. New York: Guilford Press.

Lam, D., Kuipers, L. and Leff, J. (1993) Family work with patients suffering from schizophrenia: the impact of training on psychiatric nurses' attitude and knowledge. *Journal of Advanced Nursing* **18**: 233–7.

Lees, J., Manning, N. and Rawlings, B. (1999) *Therapeutic Community Effectiveness. A Systematic International Review of Therapeutic Community Treatment for People with Personality Disorders and Mentally Disordered Offenders. CRD Report 17*. York: NHS Centre for Reviews or Dissemination.

Lewis, G., Croft-Jeffreys, C. and David, A. (1990) Are British psychiatrists racist? *British Journal of Psychiatry* **157**: 410–15.

Liberman, R., Wallace, C., Blackwell, G. *et al.* (1993) Innovations in skills training for the seriously mentally ill: The UCLA Social and Independent Living Skills Modules. *Innovations and Research* **2**: 43–60.

Linehan, M., Armstrong, H., Suarez, A., Allmon, D. and Heard, H. (1991) Cognitive-behavioural treatment of chronically parasuicidal borderline patients. *Archives of General Psychiatry* **48**: 1060–4.

Lloyd, P. and Moodley, P. (1992) Psychotropic medication and ethnicity: an inpatient survey. *Social Psychiatry and Psychiatric Epidemiology* **27**: 95–101.

Marks, I. (1987) *Fears, Phobias and Rituals: Panic, Anxiety and Their Disorders*. Oxford: Oxford University Press.

Marks, I., Bird, J. and Lindley, P. (1978) Behavioural nurse therapists: developments and implications. *Behavioural Psychotherapy* **6**: 25–6.

McLean, E. and Liebowitz, J. (1989) Towards a working definition of the long term mentally ill. *Psychiatric Bulletin* **13**: 251–2.

Meltzer, H., Gill, B., Petticrew, M. and Hinds, K. (1995) *OPCS Surveys of Psychiatric Morbidity in Great Britain, Report 1: the Prevalence of Psychiatric Morbidity among Adults living in Private Households*. London: HMSO.

MIND (1999) *Creating Accepting Communities: Report of the MIND Inquiry into social exclusion and mental health problems*. London: MIND.

Modood, T., Berthoud, R., Lakey, J. *et al.* (1998) *Ethnic Minorities in Britain: Diversity and Disadvantage. The Fourth National Survey of Ethnic Minorities*. London: Policy Studies Institute.

NHS Centre for Reviews and Dissemination (1996) *Ethnicity and Health: Reviews of Literature and Guidance for Purchasers in the Areas of Cardiovascular Disease, Mental Health and Haemoglobinopathies*. York: NHS Centre for Reviews.

Olson, T. (2002) From clinician to client: the lived experience of mental illness. *Issue in Mental Health Nursing* **23**: 435–44.

Owen, S. and Milburn, C. (2001) Implementing research findings into practice: improving and developing services for women with serious and enduring mental health problems. *Journal of Psychiatric and Mental Health Nursing* **8**: 221–31.

Owen, S., Repper, J., Perkins, R. and Robinson, J. (1998) An evaluation of services for women with long-term mental health problems. *Journal of Psychiatric and Mental Health Nursing* **5**: 281–90.

Paterson, B. and Stark, C. (2001) Social policy and mental illness in England in the 1990s: violence, moral panic and critical discourse. *Journal of Psychiatric and Mental Health Nursing* **8**: 257–67.

Patmore, C. and Weaver, J. (1990) *A Survey of Community Mental Health Centres.* London: Good Practice in Mental Health.

Pavlov, I. (1927) *Conditioned Reflexes.* London: Oxford University Press.

Perkins, R. and Rowland, L. (1991) Sex differences in service usage in long-term psychiatric care: are women adequately served? *British Journal of Psychiatry Supplement* **158** (suppl. 10): 75–9.

Provencher, H., Fournier, J.-P. and Dupuis, N. (1997) Schizophrenia: revisited. *Journal of Psychiatric and Mental Health Nursing* **4**: 275–85.

Ramsay, J., Richardson, J., Carter, Y., Davidson, L. and Feder, G. (2002) Should health professionals screen women for domestic violence? Systematic review. *British Medical Journal* **325**: 314–27.

Repper, J. (2000) Adjusting the focus of mental health nursing: Incorporating service users' experiences of recovery. *Journal of Mental Health* **9**: 575–87.

Repper, J. and Perkins, S. (1995) The deserving and undeserving: selectivity and progress in a community care service. *Journal of Mental Health* **4**: 483–98.

Rose, D. (2001) *Users' Voices: The Perspectives of Mental Health Service Users on Community and Hospital Care.* London: SCMH.

Sainsbury Centre for Mental Health (2002) *Breaking the Circles of Fear: A Review of the Relationship Between Mental Health Services and African and Caribbean Communities.* London: SCMH.

Scadding, J. (1967) Diagnosis: the clinician and the computer. *Lancet* **ii**: 877–82.

Singleton, N., Bumpstead, R., O'Brien, M., Lee, A. and Meltzer, H. (2001) *Psychiatric morbidity among adults living in private households.* London: The Stationery Office.

Skinner, B. (1972) *Beyond Freedom and Dignity.* London: Jonathan Cape.

Spector, R. (2001) Is there a racial bias in clinicians' perceptions of the dangerousness of psychiatric patients? A review of the literature. *Journal of Mental Health* **10**: 5–15.

Sturt, E. (1981) Hierarchical patterns in the distribution of psychiatric symptoms. *Psychological Medicine* **11**: 783–94.

Thornicroft, G. (1991) Social deprivation and rates of treated mental disorder, developing statistical models to predict psychiatric service utilisation. *British Journal of Psychiatry* **158**: 475–84.

Thornicroft, G., Davies, S. and Leese, M. (1999) Health service research and forensic psychiatry: A black and white case. *International Review of Psychiatry* **11**: 250–7.

Trower, P, Casey, A. and Dryden, W. (1988) *Cognitive Behavioural Counselling in Action.* London: Sage.

Tyrer, P. and Steinberg, D. (1998) *Models for Mental Disorder: Conceptual Models in Psychiatry* (3rd edn). Chichester: John Wiley and Sons.

Tudor, K. (1996) *Mental Health Promotion: Paradigms and Practice.* London: Routledge.

Ussher, J. (1991) *Women's Madness: Misogyny or Mental Illness*. Hertford: Harvester Wheatsheaf.

Van Horne, J. and McManus, I. (1992) Ventricular enlargement in schizophrenia: a meta analysis of studies of the ventricle:brain ratio. *British Journal of Psychiatry* **160**: 687–97.

White, E. (1990) *The Third Quinquennial National Survey of Community Psychiatric Nursing*. Manchester: University of Manchester.

Whitehead, M. (1992) The Health Divide, in P. Townsend, N. Davidson and M. Whitehead (eds) *Inequalities in Health*. Harmondsworth: Penguin.

Wilber, K. (2000) *Sex, Ecology and Spirituality: The Spirit of Evolution*. Boston: Shambhala.

Wilkin, P. (2001) From medicalization to hybridization: a postcolonial discourse for psychiatric nurses. *Journal of Psychiatric and Mental Health Nursing* **8**: 115–20.

World Health Organization (1992) *International Classification of Disease* – 10th edn. Geneva: WHO.

World Health Organization (2001) *The World Health Report 2001: Mental health; New Understanding, New Hope*. Geneva: WHO.

Zubin, J. and Spring, B. (1977) Vulnerability – A new view of schizophrenia. *Journal of Abnormal Psychology* **86**: 103–26.

2

Mental health promotion[1]

Keith Tudor

Chapter overview

This chapter begins with an examination of key assumptions that underpin contemporary debates about health. Theories and models for understanding health and psychological health are then presented, as is mental health – in terms of concepts, paradigms, elements and empirical research. These considerations allow mental health to be distinguished from mental illness. The *National Service Framework (NSF) for Mental Health* and *Making It Happen* are then critiqued in terms of their respective orientations towards health and illness. The chapter ends with an examination of the role of mental health consultation and, in particular, nursing's contribution to this role.

In summary, this chapter covers:

- health;
- mental health;
- promoting mental health.

Introduction

> 'Health is more difficult to deal with than illness.' (D.W. Winnicott)

It is commonplace that 'health', both as a word and as a concept, is often used to stand for 'illness'. Nowhere is this more true – and detrimental – than in the field of 'mental health'. The ubiquitous term 'people with mental health problems' disguises the actual referent, that is: people diagnosed with a mental illness or personality disorder (or both). Leaving aside the deconstruction of 'mental illness', such definitions by substitution do no favours either for those with a diagnosed mental illness or for those defining and promoting positive mental health. Despite the fact that the distinction between mental health and mental illness – and understanding of that distinction – has been around for, arguably, over 100 years (since the early days of the international mental hygiene movement), policy makers, politicians and practitioners almost wilfully continue to conflate and confuse the two terms. The latest example of this is contained in and indeed represented by the *NSF for Mental Health* (Department of Health (DH) 1999a) and *Making It Happen* (DH 2001) which, while talking the walk (referring to the promotion of mental health in its aim), certainly does not walk the talk (as, within four sentences, it refers to assessing performance of its aim with reference to the National *Psychiatric* Morbidity Survey!).

Taking Winnicott's statement as a challenge to 'deal with' health, the first part of the chapter concentrates on health in its own right, certainly as more than the absence of disease and in a number of ways beyond the medical model. Following this, in the second part of the chapter, the focus shifts to understandings of *mental* health, including a discussion of the relationship between mental health and mental illness and the efficacy of promoting the mental health of the mentally ill. In conclusion mental health promotion theory, policy and practice is summarized and the role of mental health consultation is discussed. Mental *health* is viewed as the concern of all, not some and, therefore, as much the business of mental health nursing as any other discipline or profession. Moreover, just as *mental* health is viewed as criterial to health (an argument referred to in the second part of this chapter), so an understanding of mental health is central to nursing – and, in this, the role of the mental health nurse as consultant, advocate and facilitator is critical.

Health

There are a number of problematic assumptions in contemporary debates about health and health care. Doyal and Pennell (1979), writing about medicine and health, identify three such assumptions:

1   that the determinants of health and illness are predominantly biological;
2   that medicine is assumed to be a science;
3   the belief that scientific medicine 'provides the only viable means for mediating between people and disease' (p. 12) (and, for that matter, health).

In addition, I see two further assumptions which underlie – and undermine – discussions about health and mental health (as distinct from illness):

4   the dualistic split between mind and body;
5   the defining of health in terms of illness.

Despite at least 20 years of critical thinking and practice in health care, these assumptions are alive and kicking and influencing public 'health' policy such as *Our Healthier Nation* (DH 1999b) and the *NSF for Mental Health* (DH 1999a). In the first part of this chapter, responses to these five assumptions frame an exploration of health beyond illness. (A response to a sixth assumption – that government, in this case the British government, its advisers and advisory bodies have the monopoly on the ideology or economics of health – is held over to the second part.)

Health as beyond the biological

The assumption that the determinants of health (and illness) are predominantly biological implies that patterns of health, the prevalence of health (health status), as well as patterns of disease (morbidity) and mortality, all have little to do with the social and economic environment in which they occur. Moreover, solutions to health problems are seen as lying exclusively within the domain of modern medicine. More than 25 years ago, the Lalonde Report (the report in which the term 'health promotion' first appeared) (Lalonde 1975), offered a new perspective on health, arguing that causes of death and disease could be attributed to inadequacies in health care provision and environmental pollution, as well as to lifestyle, behavioural and biophysical characteristics. Following this, a World Health Assembly (meeting in Alma Ata in 1977) incorporated into its declaration a commitment to 'community participation' and, following the *Ottawa Charter* (1985), which among other things, defined health promotion, two further international conferences emphasized the need for 'healthy public policy' (in Adelaide 1988) and for 'supportive environments' (in Sandsvall 1991). Shifting the emphasis from biological determinism to social/environmental factors does not simply shift the blame from the individual to society; rather it acknowledges the impact of social determinants such as poverty and exclusion and helps to focus the hearts and minds of health workers and policy makers on the bigger picture. It also acknowledges that health is for all and concerns all (not only medical practitioners). In his research on *Population Mental Health in Canada*, Stephens (1998) identifies the determinants of mental health (qua *health*) as: demographic characteristics (age, household type, etc.), social conditions, social status (income, activity, education) and working conditions, as well as personal health practices and physical health. This perspective is particularly pertinent in the field of positive mental health as people who promote it are open to the accusation that it is at best irrelevant and at worst self-indulgent in the light of such big issues as poverty, unemployment, homelessness and other forms of social exclusion. However, it is precisely these 'big issues' that have such a deleterious impact on our mental health (and as well as mental illness). Recent policy developments in Britain such as the identification of Action Zones (on health, education and unemployment) and the New Deal for Communities are creating common ground for health and social-care agencies to work together to bring about regeneration and to tackle social exclusion. While the primary focus of these developments is on reducing incidence of mental illness and social exclusion, some initiatives have combined promoting positive mental health (e.g. self esteem and community capacity) by addressing the social determinants of mental ill health (see McCulloch 1999). Postmodernist perspectives on health also contribute to the deconstruction of biology and the biological as well as to the co-construction of health and illness (see Fox 1999).

Medicine as more than science

Following on from this first assumption is a second that assumes medicine as a science:

> the way medicine is presented, and society's acceptance of its claim to authority and resources, rests to a considerable extent on its definition of itself as a natural science . . . and medical progress is said to be based on the use of 'scientific method' which supposedly ensures certain and objective knowledge.
>
> (Doyal and Pennell 1979: 12)

Nowhere is this more true than in psychiatry which has often been viewed as medicine's poor relation (or Cinderella). In response, psychiatry has sought respectability in 'science' – from phrenology to diagnostic manuals of mental disorder. While medical diagnosis has its uses, not the least in providing the relief of a certain kind of knowledge of 'what's wrong', it is also highly problematic; as Steiner puts it: *'alienation is the essence of all psychiatric conditions* . . . everything diagnosed psychiatrically, unless *clearly* organic in origin, is a form of alienation' (1971: 153, original emphasis). Moreover 'objective' medical diagnosis is not the only form of knowledge relevant to a person's illness; what someone knows about themselves and their illness *subjectively* is, arguably, equally if not more relevant to diagnosis, treatment, cure and care. In her seminal work on 'fundamental patterns of knowing' in nursing Carper describes empirical knowledge as: 'knowledge that is systematically organized into general laws and theories for the purpose of describing, explaining and predicting phenomena of special concern to the discipline of nursing' (1978: 14) and goes on to observe that, 'one is almost led to believe that the only valid and reliable knowledge is that which is empirical, factual, objectively descriptive and generalizable' (1978: 16).

Carper suggests that, in addition to *empirical knowing* there are three further ways of knowing, relevant to the nursing task and role – *aesthetics, personal knowing* and *ethical knowing* – which both challenge and ameliorate the dominance of empirical knowledge in medicine and nursing. Although Carper describes these ways of knowing as distinct but interrelated, Johns (1995) argues that, in practice, the aesthetic way of knowing is core, as it is within this way of knowing that reflection on the other ways takes place. In this sense aesthetics may be understood as 'meta' knowledge, with reflection as a meta-skill. Table 2.1 outlines Carper's ways of knowing and applies them both to mental illness and to mental health.

Table 2.1 Ways of knowing, mental illness and mental health (developed from Carper 1978)

Ways of knowing (Carper 1978)	Definition	Application to mental illness	Application to mental health
Empirical knowing	Knowledge that is systematically organized into general laws and theories for the purpose of describing, explaining and predicting phenomena.	Most research in psychiatry and the organization of research in, for example, the *Diagnostic and Statistical Manual of Mental Disorders* (4th revised edn) (*DSMIV-TR*) (American Psychiatric Association 2000).	Research such as Stephens (1998) that defines positive mental health status and considers the determinants of mental health.
Personal knowing	'Concerned with the knowing, encountering, and actualising of the concrete, individual self' (Carper 1978).	Found in accounts of users and survivors of the psychiatric and 'mental health' system; also the (rarer) reflections by professionals on their own response to and relationship with madness.	Reflection on any practitioner's own mental health in terms of, say, coping, stress, self-concept, etc.
Ethical knowing	Involves a process of deliberation and reflection, informed by ethical principles mediated by the practitioner's own values and by 'situational ethics'.	. . . with reference to legislation (i.e. Mental Health Acts), codes and policy as well as relevant professional codes of ethics, practice and conduct (doctors, nurses, social workers, etc.).	. . . with reference to legislation and professional codes relevant to the particular practice under consideration.
Aesthetics	The practitioner's response to a particular situation; it involves a *process* of perceiving, interpreting, envisioning and generating possibilities, responding and reflecting.	e.g. in a 'mental health assessment' (under the *Mental Health Act 1983*), in which the parties to the assessment, at best, perceive, interpret, envision and generate possibilities (based on the principle of the least restrictive alternative), respond and reflect in dialogue with each other.	Reflective – or reflexive – practice as regards any mental health consultation (see Tudor 1996b and below).

Beyond scientific medicine

The third assumption identified by Doyal and Pennell (1979) is the belief that scientific medicine mediates between people and disease, and either that it is the only viable means, or that it is necessarily the best; medicine is seen as good and that the only problem is that there is not enough to go around. Indeed, arguments about resources form the basis of most current political discussion on health care – and, as Doyal and Pennell point out succinctly: 'this assumption, is, of course, dependent on a broader conception of the nature of capitalism – specifically on a belief in its capacity to solve social problems through economic growth' (1979: 13). One of the consequences of this assumption is that the patient (who is expected to wait patiently) is seen as the passive victim of his or her illness, disorder or disease, while the doctor – and, traditionally, to a lesser extent the nurse – are seen as the experts. In the field of mental illness, historically it was far from certain that medicine (scientific or otherwise), would be the principal mediator of madness. Indeed, in Britain, until the nineteenth century, 'madness' was mediated:

1   through the expression of feudal paternalism, by means of trusteeships decided by *the judiciary*;
2   in criminal trials through the defence by an *advocate*;
3   through the domain of *public order legislation* (see Porter 1990).

None of this involved medicine or doctors; indeed, according to Porter (1990), 'mad doctoring' only came of age (on 5 December 1788) when a specialist 'mad doctor', Francis Willis, was called to attend to George III.

In the two centuries since Dr Willis was called to cure the delirium of George III, we have acquired more understanding of madness and the mind, science and medicine, and of the nature of knowledge and theory, authority and expertise. In a present era in which there has been an exponential growth in medical technology that in many ways mediates the relationship with our own bodies, their limitations, breakdown and even failure, there has been a parallel growth of scepticism (even cynicism) with regard to 'scientific medicine' and the doctor as expert. There are a number of factors that support this scepticism or critique:

• the resistance and more recent rise in popularity of medicine and health care complementary to the allopathic medical model;
• the development of public health psychology, community health psychology and critical health psychology;
• the growth and expression of civil rights, as reflected in the consumer movement and, for example in 'patients' charters'. The term 'expert patients' has even appeared as part of the 'Healthy Citizens Programme' promoted by *Our Healthier Nation* (DH 1999b).
• The increasing interest (both in the broader philosophical sphere as well as in health psychology and care) in constructivist, narrative and postmodernist critiques of theory and practice, e.g. viewing illness as metaphor (see Fox 1999).

Sacks (1991, 1995) has documented the refusal of medical and medicalizing definitions of health and illness among his patients; and Fox (1999), in his postmodernist critique of health and illness, questions 'cures' which cut across people's subjectivity, with no acknowledgement of our right to 'otherness'.

Holistic health

The roots of the English word for health, in Old English and Old High German, link it to wholeness and healing: 'etymologically speaking . . . to be healthy is to be whole or holy, which clearly embraces both spiritual and physical features rather than merely the latter' (Graham 1992: 53). The grammar of health, then, is one that implies a holistic or integrative structure to our health and to our understanding of health. Thus, health may be taken as referring to mind (including thoughts, beliefs and feelings), body (including behaviour), and spirit. This common-sense wisdom has prevailed for most of human history; Marks (2002) argues that it can be traced to the earliest period of history around 10,000 BCE. It is only the comparatively recent Cartesian dualism of the seventeenth century that had the effect (if not the intention) to conceptualize a split between the mind and the body, a split which ultimately gave rise and succour to the practice of referring to whole, if ill, person as 'the appendix in Bed 4'. It is a short step from Bed 4 to the back ward and to being referred to – and, perhaps more perniciously, referring to oneself – as '*the* schizophrenic', as if that is all one is. This reductionism of person to symptom and/or behaviour is not only limited and limiting, it is inaccurate and, ultimately, anti-human.

A holistic approach to the person, which 'embraces and affirms complexity, inclusion and diversity and resists reductionism' (Clarkson 1989: 8), also locates the person/organism within their environment. Half a century ago, Lewin (1952) argued that it was impossible to view a person except in the context of their environment or 'environmental field' (hence field theory) – and, of course, the viewer/researcher/doctor/nurse/etc. is also a part of this interactional field: 'only the interplay of organism and environment . . . constitutes the psychological situation, not the organism and environment taken separately' (Perls *et al.* [1951] 1979: 19). In relation to mental health promotion this view is reflected in the notion of mental health as requiring both 'individual resilience' and 'supportive environments' (Joubert and Raeburn 1998) – a notion which proposes a necessary balance in focus between individual and environment, and which offers a challenge to promote the mental health both of individuals (at intrapsychic and interpersonal levels) and of environments (workplace, organization, institution, culture), often through hearts and minds as well as policies and procedures. This interactional view focuses our attention on the health (or otherwise) not only of the subject or figure but also of the other figures in the field and of the environment itself. Thus the health of the doctor and nurse and whether the general practice or hospital is a healthy environment, or similarly the health of the child and the school, become as much the subject for concern and critical enquiry as the health and illness of the patient. Lest holism leads us to some spurious unity, the Zen Buddhist Master, Shunryu Suzuki in the spirit of 'no dualism' offers a reminder of the complexity – and simplicity – of the relationship between mind and body: 'our body and mind are not two, and not one. If you think your body and mind are two, that is wrong; if you think they are one, that is also wrong. Our body and mind are both two *and* one' (1999: 25).

In this sense holistic expansions of the mind/body duality (as above) are but stepping stones to a postmodernist commentary (meta-analysis or meta-text) on health and context, biology and culture (see Fox 1999).

Health beyond the absence of illness

The often quoted World Health Organization's (WHO) definition of health as 'not merely the absence of disease and infirmity' also defines health, somewhat ambitiously, as 'a state of complete physical, mental and social well-being' (1948: 3). There are three implications of this:

1   Health is seen as *a state*, perhaps even a steady state to be achieved, rather than a *process* to be lived and thus something which fluctuates over time – and illness is to be eschewed.

2   The ambition of *complete* health perpetuates a grandiose and perfectionist view of the human condition, one which is implied and exacerbated by the British government's invidious 'league table' mentality in health and education and its consequent 'naming and shaming' of 'failing' institutions. Apart from anything else (such as the psychological reality that no one makes positive changes in response to being shamed), as complete health and perfect hospitals and schools are impossible, this only serves to set up individuals and institutions to fail – failing, that is, in terms of imposed standards, measures and outcomes and a purely external locus of evaluation and control.

3   The WHO identifies 'physical, mental and social' as elements or indeed the parameters of health. This not only misses out the spirit (as in mind-body-spirit) or the spiritual, but also does not adequately acknowledge the multi-faceted nature of health beyond the absence of illness.

There are a number of models that help in the elaboration of health without necessarily referring to illness. Here, in concluding this first part of the chapter, two models are briefly reviewed and applied to health and its promotion. In a paper on the integration of psychotherapies, Groder (1977) identifies, in addition to the affective, behavioural and cognitive dimensions of psychotherapy and human life, the physiological, social systems and the suprapersonal. As a framework this has been found useful, for instance, in designing health education initiatives that, as it were, 'touch all bases' or dimensions and which, therefore, are comprehensive and accessible. One sex education programme, working with young Muslim men, had focused on sexual *behaviour* and was foundering: the young men were embarrassed at the presence of plastic models of penises and the workers felt stuck (rather like the unsuccessful attempts to roll on the condoms). A consultant intro- duced the male workers involved to Groder's framework and discussed the efficacy of discussing values and faith (the *suprapersonal* or *spiritual* dimension) as well as the young men's culture (social systems) before further behavioural interventions. The workers took this back to their work, put the penises away, and later reported lively and useful discussions with the young men about religion, faith, morality, sexuality, culture and racism. (Other specific initiatives that reflect Groder's other dimensions are summarized in Tudor 1996b.)

Although any such dimensional model is open to addition, it is also open to the criticism (ironically) that it appears somewhat one-dimensional and fixed. Another model, based on existential philosophy and psychology, provides a sense of the more dynamic relationship we have with our health and, indeed, our existence:

> the existential approach considers human nature to be open-minded, flexible and capable of an enormous range of experience. The person is in a constant state of becoming . . . this impermanence and uncertainty give rise to a deep sense of anxiety (Angst), in response to the realization of one's insignificance, and simultaneous responsibility to have to create something in the place of that emptiness. Everything passes and nothing lasts.
>
> (van Deurzen-Smith 1996: 169)

Existentialism identifies four basic dimensions to human existence (see Table 2.2) in each and all of which we struggle with the givens of the past and the possibilities for the present and future, and with the meaning of our lives. Table 2.2 applies this conceptual framework to health. Although existential philosophy and psychology do not favour any one dimension, authors and practitioners in the field of health, mental health and its promotion may and do. French and Adams, for instance, assert that: 'the most significant determinant of health is social and economic circumstance' (1986: 73) (a position which leads them to place a collective action model of health education at the top of their hierarchy of health education models).

In an important study on 'emotional labour' in a hospice, James found that: 'the social, spiritual, emotional and physical care encompasses elements of care which are usually obscured in medical settings . . . and require management and attention in the same way that physical symptoms do' (1989: 20).

Mental health

In this part of the chapter some concepts of mental health (*qua* health) are introduced and discussed; then, having differentiated mental health from mental illness, the relationship between the two is explored; finally current social policy concerning mental health promotion is examined – and found wanting. Discussing mental health is, at least for this author, strategic: given

Table 2.2 Existential dimensions of human existence applied to health

Dimensions of human existence	Definition	Struggles/existential crises	Application to health
Physical (*Umwelt*)	How we relate to our environment and the givens of the natural world, including our body, concrete surroundings, climate and weather, objects and material possessions.	Between the search for dominion and domination over the elements and natural law, and the need to accept the limitations of natural boundaries such as age, ability and fertility.	How we relate to our body, the age, size and shape we are; to what extent we accept who and how we are, or rail against this. Health issues include the acceptance of such limitations or the application of medical technology to ameliorate the limitations of, for instance, disability, infertility and old age.
Social (*Mitwelt*)	How we relate to others and interact with the public world, including understandings in terms of class, gender, race, sexuality, etc.	Between acceptance and rejection, belonging and not belonging and isolation, success and failure.	How our health is affected by our status and wealth as well as class, gender, etc. Health issues focus on social health, health status, resources and planning, systems of care, as well as accessibility to services and on health and community (see Money 1993).
Psychological (*Eigenwelt*)	How we relate to ourselves and our personal (intrapsychic) world: our temperament and personality, our past and possibilities.	Between what are perceived as personal strengths and weaknesses, between a sense of identity and of being substantial and states of disintegration and confusion.	How we relate to and understand our 'internal life', our personal development and crises. If not somatized (physical) or acted out (social), health issues are expressed through some form of reflection, e.g. meditation, talking and/or psychotherapy.
Spiritual (*Ueberwelt*)	How we relate to the unknown, and make meaning of it, through ideology, philosophy, religion, etc.	Between purpose and absurdity, hope and despair, being and nothingness.	How/whether we make time for our spiritual health, for instance, through some regular meditative, contemplative or reflective practice. Health issues include how we understand (and make meaning of) some of the struggles and contradictions of our physical, social and psychological existence and worlds.

a holistic appreciation of health, it would be more accurate and useful if our understanding and discourse included all the elements or parameters discussed earlier (mind, body, spirit, etc.); indeed, in training workshops on this subject I am increasingly using the more generic term 'health'. Nevertheless, at present, the 'mental' in health needs elaboration and 'mental health' needs to be distinguished from 'mental illness' if it is not to be subsumed beneath the conflated term 'mental health' or the ubiquitous 'mental health problems' – and thereby confused, ignored, misinterpreted and misunderstood. There is also an argument, advanced by Neumann *et al.* (1989), that our mind or psyche, as the agent of all health-relevant interactions, is at the centre of all dimensions of mental health and thereby criterial to health. Similarly, in his work on multiple intelligences, Gardner (1993) suggests that the personal intelligences (the *inter*personal and the *intra*personal), which amount to information-processing capacities, and the combination or fusion of which provides a sense of self, are in effect the intelligences with which we reflect on the other intelligences (linguistic, musical, logical-mathematical, spatial, and bodily-kinesthetic).

Mental health – concepts, paradigms, elements and research

There are, no doubt, as many definitions of mental health as there are readers of this book. Although some authors offer definitions of mental health, they are inevitably subjective, partial and, at worst, simplistic – *Making It Happen* defines mental health as 'thinking, feeling and physical health and well-being' and the relationship between the three described and defined by three double-headed arrows! More useful than any one definition is to consider the elements of mental health common to such definitions – hence the importance of *concepts* of mental health. This approach to the subject was first adopted by Marie Jahoda in 1958 who, in a report to a United States Joint Commission on Mental Illness and Mental Health (readers will note the distinction explicit in its title) identified six major categories of concepts:

- mental health as indicated by the *attitudes of an individual towards themselves*;
- mental health as expressed in the individual's style and degree of *growth, development or self-actualisation*;
- mental health as *integration* of the above (that is, the individual's ability to integrate developing and different aspects of themselves over time).
- mental health based on the individual's relation to reality in terms of:
  - *autonomy*;
  - *perception of reality*;
  - *environmental mastery* (Jahoda 1958).

While these are categories of concepts, each one of which represents a literature in itself (which, in the last four decades has obviously expanded with the growth of interest in self-development and popular psychology), nevertheless Jahoda's categories may be adopted by professionals and clients as the basis of a genuine mental *health* assessment. Drawing on an appreciation of the interpersonal field and the significance of the environment or context, mental health may be viewed as relevant at four levels – the personal, the interpersonal, the institutional and the cultural – first identified by Jones (1972) as ones in which racism is expressed; and, in relation to mental health, as with racism, all four levels interact. Applying Jahoda's categories to these levels offers practitioners, workshop participants (and, of course, the reader) a comprehensive and practical frame with which to assess mental health – for themselves, for and with others, and as regards the institution or workplace as well as the broader culture or sub-culture. Table 2.3 lays out this framework with some examples to stimulate the reader to apply their own and to fill in the gaps.

Drawing on the work of Kuhn (1970) and Burrell and Morgan (1979), I followed in this tradition of conceptualizing mental health, developing a conceptual framework of mental health through the application of paradigm analysis to the different and differing definitions of mental health and its promotion. Putting together two dimensions as axes – one, concerning assumptions about the nature of science (a subjective–objective dimension), the other concerning assumptions about the nature of society (a regulation–radical change dimension), Burrell and Morgan defined four distinct sociological paradigms (Figure 2.1).

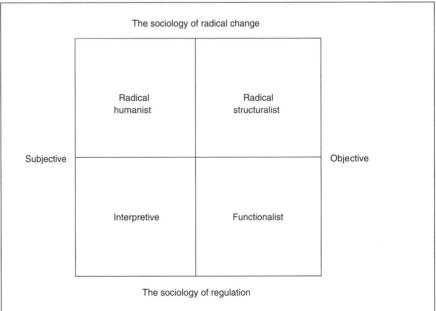

Figure 2.1 Four paradigms for the analysis of social theory (Burrell and Morgan 1979)

Burrell and Morgan make a number of points about the nature and use of paradigm analysis:

1   That although each paradigm contains a variety of viewpoints, there is essential unity within the paradigm, defined by its external boundaries. Thus, the 'essential unity' of notions of mental health within the interpretive paradigm is defined by the boundaries of and adherence to subjective knowledge and social regulation. In this paradigm mental health is viewed in interpretive and relational terms (e.g. Neumann *et al.* 1989) with a focus on the regulation of the individual to conform to a harmonious and integrated sense of self and society.

2   That 'all social theorists can be located within the context of these four paradigms according to the meta-theoretical assumptions reflected in their work' (Burrell and Morgan 1979: 24). Thus when Preston (1943) talks about mental health as consisting of 'the ability to live . . . happily . . . productively . . . without being a nuisance' (p. 112), he is clearly reflecting a view of society that is concerned with social regulation, and representing a view of mental health which claims a certain certainty and 'objectivity' – and thus, in terms of our analysis, is located within the functionalist paradigm. This is confirmed by an appreciation of the wider historical context of the mental hygiene movement that predominantly portrayed a conformist and functional view of health and productivity: 'a healthy worker is a productive worker'.

3   That, by definition, the four paradigms are mutually exclusive: 'a synthesis is not possible' (ibid. p. 25). Paradigm analysis thus describes the conceptual and theoretical assumptions underpinning differences which lead to – and are often demonstrated through – differences in practice and action such as that of the consultant psychiatrist who refused to sit on the same conference platform as representatives of the psychiatric user movement.

Paradigm analysis has thus proved useful in understanding and exploring differences in definition, policy and practice. Caplan (1986) applied this analysis to health education theory – and in doing so, offers a paradigmatic way out of the often futile 'health promotion *versus* health education' debate: theory and practice in both is based on underlying assumptions which may be analysed and located within the four paradigms. Developing Caplan's ideas, the present author subsequently applied it to the field of mental heath and community mental health promotion (Tudor 1996b), and in doing so identified mental-illness prevention with its focus on identifying vulnerability and causative factors and 'targeting' as little to do with mental health promotion.

In elaborating this analysis, as a result of an extensive literature review and in the spirit of Jahoda's work, I identified eight elements (two representing each paradigm: the functionalist, interpretive, radical humanist and radical structuralist, respectively), each of which may be viewed as on a continuum of health–ill-health (Box 2.1).

Table 2.3 Jahoda's concepts of mental health applied to levels of human experience and context

Personal	Interpersonal	Institutional	Cultural
The attitudes of an individual towards themselves, e.g. self-concept, self-esteem	The attitude of individuals towards each other including communication and social support, both positive – Birtchnell (1993) describes mental health as positive relating – and negative, such as bullying and harassment; hence the importance of emotional literacy	The attitude of the institution towards itself, e.g. the 'self'-concept of the organization	The attitude of the culture or sub-culture towards itself and other groups
Personal growth, development and actualization	Growth, development and actualization with others expressed in group and cooperative initiatives	Growth, development and actualization of the institution/organization including initiatives which promote 'workplace well-being'	Growth, development and actualization of the culture perhaps most explicitly expressed in *The Possible Scot* (Stewart 1998)
Personal integration (of the above) through forms of personal reflection (therapy, non-managerial supervision, etc.), sometimes referred to as coherence and measurable as such (see Antonovsky 1993)	Interpersonal integration (of the above) through forms of reflection with others, e.g. group therapy, group supervision, 'circle time' in school or 'check in' times at work	Institutional integration (of the above) through institutional forms of reflection such as reflective and consultative 'review days' or 'mental health away-days'	Cultural integration (of the above) through initiatives involving cultural groupings and, at a national level, policies and even legislation

	Personal	Interpersonal	Institutional	Cultural
Autonomy	Personal autonomy	Interpersonal autonomy although viewed by some as an apparent contradiction, the arena for discussion between two or more people (say, a couple or a family) and concerned with everyone achieving autonomy in the context of relationships	Institutional autonomy – the extent to which an institution is autonomous – in the context of other institutions, legislations, etc.	Cultural autonomy often expressed through the struggle for and the achievement of cultural and/or regional or national independence
Perceptions of reality	The individual's perception of reality – the nature and extent of an individual's relationship with consensual reality, as well as how they manage their uniqueness and 'otherness'	Interpersonal perceptions of reality – the business of much interpersonal communication	Institutional perceptions of reality	Cultural perceptions of reality – the arena of cultural and intercultural studies and intergroup relations (see Tudor 1999)
Environmental mastery	The individual's environmental mastery – the nature and extent of the individual's mastery of their environment	Interpersonal environmental mastery	The environmental mastery of the institution, e.g. the health promoting hospital and the health promoting school (Weare 1996, 2000)	The environmental mastery of the culture expressed in initiatives such as the WHO's 'Healthy Cities' project (see Kickbush 1989) and in health and community (Money 1993)

These elements do not stand alone as defining mental health; they are representative of the literature and of the four paradigms. McDonald and O'Hara (1998) also identify elements of mental health, mapping ten, comprising five elements each of mental health promotion and demotion (see Box 2.2).

McDonald and O'Hara map these elements on three levels, a mapping that acknowledges (at least conceptually) the relevance of the individual (micro level), groupings (meso level) and wider, social systems (macro) in terms of taking action on promoting mental health. However, it is not exactly clear in McDonald and O'Hara's model what the relationship between promotion and demotion is. Thus, for instance, emotional abuse is not the opposite of self-esteem or the only element that demotes self-esteem; also, identifying stress as demoting mental health does not account for positive stress (or 'eustress') (see Seyle 1956; Antonovsky 1979, 1987). Finally, the interpersonal aspect of mental health is almost completely missing from this model.

Undoubtedly the most impressive piece of empirical research on mental health is Stephens's (1998) work on population health in Canada. Prepared for the Mental Health Promotion Unit, Health Canada which, under the directorship of Natacha Joubert, led the field in its advocacy and resourcing of positive mental health promotion, the report is clear in the distinction between mental health and mental illness. From his survey of data and previous research Stephens presents evidence that considers mental health

---

Box 2.1 Eight elements of mental health (Tudor 1996b)

Health _____ Ill-health

Coping
Tension and stress management
Self-concept and identity
Self-esteem
Self-development
Autonomy
Change
Social support

Box 2.2 Ten elements of mental health promotion and demotion (McDonald and O'Hara 1998)

Mental health promotion	*Mental health demotion*
Environmental quality	Environmental deprivation
Self-esteem	Emotional abuse
Emotional processing	Emotional negligence
Self-management skills	Stress
Social participation	Social exclusion

status on the 'positive dimension' in terms of happiness, self-esteem, mastery, sense of coherence and work satisfaction, as well as the negative (in relation to depression, distress, child emotional disorders, cognitive problems, hospitalized disorders and suicide). The whole report is set in the context of socioeconomic restructuring and health care reform in Canada. Stephens distinguishes between *indicators* of mental health status (as above) and its *determinants* (demographic characteristics, social conditions, social status, working conditions, personal health practices and physical health). While the conclusion is that superficially the mental health status of Canadians appears to be reasonably good – three quarters of the population describe themselves as usually happy and interested in life and 91 per cent report some degree of job satisfaction – Stephens cautions that: 'comparisons among population groups reveal that both positive and negative mental health are far from evenly distributed in the population: there are sharp differences according to an individual's household type and age, and, to a lesser extent, province of residence and gender' (1998: 40) (see also Stephens *et al.* 1999).

From the discussion in this section, a number of points may be made:

1 Particular definitions of mental health are useful, especially for the individual concerned.

2 In order to grasp and, indeed, to develop the field of mental health, it is necessary to think in terms of concepts or even categories of concepts of mental health.

3 All concepts and elements of mental health may – arguably, must – be viewed in *context*. One contextual frame has been presented and applied to concepts of mental health.

4 In order to understand different and differing (competing) definitions of mental health, a meta-theoretical framework is essential with which to analyse the underlying assumptions of particular definitions and their implications for policy and practice. This may, of course, be applied to any and all empirical research in the field of mental health.

5 In terms of forms of knowledge, there are differences between a definition, an element, a concept, a category, research, a model, a theory and a paradigm.

Mental health and mental illness

This chapter has argued for the separation of mental health from mental illness. At present most policy and practice is based on the conflation of the two under the one referent 'mental health'. In effect this conceptualizes the two on one continuum which I represent as a slide (as that is what people seem to fear) from mental health into mental illness (Figure 2.2).

What this means in practice is that people neither talk about mental health (*qua* health) as they think others are assuming that they are referring to mental illness; nor do they discuss mental illnesses, preferring instead to

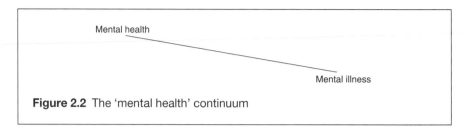

Figure 2.2 The 'mental health' continuum

refer to them with the anodyne phrase 'people with mental health problems'. Merely substituting the term 'mental illness' with this libertarian nomenclature does nothing to challenge the power of the medical/psychiatric model in this field, or to advance a critique of diagnosis, or to change the stigmatizing effect of mental illnesses and the general public's attitude to them – exacerbated by the then British home secretary, Jack Straw, who consistently conflated 'personality disorders' with dangerousness – with serious (and dangerous) consequences for proposed changes to future Mental Health Acts, currently under review (see http://www.DH.gov.uk/mentalhealth/summary.htm and http://www.DH.gov.uk/hspch/visped.htm Proposing a conceptual separation between the two terms may be represented by *two continua*, first advanced by the Canadian Minister of National Health and Welfare (MNHW) in 1988.

There are a number of implications – and advantages – to this formulation:

- Conceptual: As we know from our own experience that we can be ill and well at the same time (having a cold and feeling good, being physically ill and mentally healthy, etc.) and, as according to Euclidian physics, we cannot be in two places at once, so we need the concept of two continua to explain this aspect of our human experience.

- Philosophical: By separating the two fields, the two continua concept opens up the possibility of dialogue between health and illness (which, in its one-dimensional approach, the one continuum concept avoids). From this we can then engage in the debates advocated, albeit from their different perspectives, by Fox (1999) and Suzuki (1999). In considering the relationship between the two, Duff (1993) reminds us of the value of illness to health: 'illness is to health what dreams are to waking life – the reminder of what is forgotten, the bigger picture working toward resolution' (p. 33). Illness as

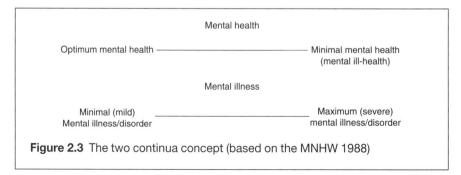

Figure 2.3 The two continua concept (based on the MNHW 1988)

metaphor, the 'healing crisis' familiar to complementary health practitioners, the significance of subjectivity and the concept of *arché-health* (Fox 1999) – 'the condition of possibility for health and illness (p. 10) – are all examples of the complex interrelationship between illness and health.

- Practical: It is only possible to promote the mental health of the mentally ill (as *The Health of the Nation* (DH 1992) first proposed) if we advance the two continua concept (else they are left languishing at the ill end of the one continuum, with no possibility of health). Some forms of occupational therapy, self-development courses, a women's consciousness-raising group, patients' meetings, all within the psychiatric setting, and involving users in their diagnosis and treatment and in the planning of services – are all examples of mental health promotion of the mentally ill and all depend on the view that, while having a diagnosed mental illness or disorder, they also have mental health which can be promoted and enhanced. This approach also addresses the critical comment the Standing Nursing and Midwifery Advisory Committee (1999) made in a report on mental health nursing, admitting that 'users have no real role in designing and implementing professional education and training'.

- Clinical: The two continua concept is congruent with the multi-axial diagnostic approach taken by the *Diagnostic and Statistical Manual of Mental Disorders-IV-TR* (American Psychiatric Association 2000) (an approach adopted in the revision of its third edition in 1987). This multi-axial system proposes five axes or continua which in effect describe a holistic approach to diagnosis:

Axis I:	Mental disorders
Axis II:	Development disorders
	Personality disorders
Axis III:	Physical disorders and symptoms
Axis IV:	Severity of psychosocial stressors
Axis V:	Global assessment of functioning

It is a short logical step to propose a sixth axis on mental health and, even more radically, to propose in addition, a dialogic approach to each axis, thus:

Axis I:	Mental disorders _____	Mental 'order' or integration
Axis II:	Development disorders _____	Healthy development
	Personality disorders _____	Personality process (based on a process conception of personality (see, for instance, Rogers 1951)
Axis III:	Physical disorders and symptoms _____	Physical health
Axis IV:	Severity of psychosocial stressors	
Axis V:	Global assessment of functioning	
Axis VI:	Mental health	

Indeed this could almost define the role of the mental health nurse in mental illness diagnosis, treatment and care *and* in mental health care and promotion.

- Pragmatic – the two continua concept can be (and has been) viewed as pragmatic: it claims mental *health* for all while not necessarily challenging the authority or territory of psychiatrists or mental 'health' professionals. In this sense the concept may be welcomed by already overworked practitioners in this field with some relief that they do not have to 'do' or 'take on' mental health promotion.

- Political – on the other hand, claiming mental *health* for all may also be viewed as highly political, as the logic of promoting the mental health of the mentally ill may well involve other (non-psychiatric/mental 'health') professionals and lay people, as it were, breaking into the asylum. At one point in the 'Italian experience' of mental health reform, psychiatric patients and staff in Trieste built a wooden horse (called Marco) which, in the same way that its Ancient Greek counterpart was taken into the city of Troy (only later to reveal its contents), was also paraded around the streets of the city (see Tudor 1990/91). The approach to mental health promotion advocated in this chapter and other similar work might well be viewed as a subversive 'wooden horse': this time putting sanity into the mental hospital and, indeed, seeing sanity in and alongside madness.

'Not making it happen': The failure of mental health policy

A further problematic assumption (in addition to those identified in the first part of this chapter) concerns the monopoly the government and its agents have or claim on health policy. This involves a certain ideology, enacted through legislation and policies such as *The Health of the Nation* (DH 1992) and *Our Healthier Nation* (DH 1999b) and backed up with certain economic resources, although not a planned economy of health – or illness.

Elsewhere (Tudor 1996b) I offered a critique of *The Health of the Nation* and other health policies of the early 1990s in so far as it and they concerned health and specifically mental health. From the wealth of paper generated by this legislation and related documents (such as the key area handbooks 1993) only two strands emerge which support mental health and its promotion:

1 the aim to improve significantly the health and social functioning of mentally ill people (*The Health of the Nation*); and

2 the development of good practice to improve mental health in the NHS and local authority workplace (*Key Area Handbook on Mental Illness*, DH 1993).

Despite extensive criticism of this previous health policy, the politicians, civil servants and advisers changed little: *Our Healthier Nation* (*OHN*) suffers from the same confusions and deficiencies as previous policies.

Alongside cancer, coronary heart disease and stroke, 'mental health' (predominantly meaning mental illness) is one of four national targets for 2010 identified in *OHN*. From its subsections (modernizing mental health services, the NHS plan, the review of the Mental Health Act, etc.) it is clear that 'mental health' refers to mental illness. As part of its strategy to modernize mental health services the government has, with the help of an 'expert reference group', chaired by a psychiatrist, developed a *NSF for Mental Health* (DH 1999a). The framework:

- sets national standards for both health and social care, and establishes performance indicators to measure the progress made by services, ensuring that they meet all basic criteria;

- addresses the range of mental health service provision, from primary care, where the majority of mental health problems can be managed, through to specialist mental health services;

- will help to ensure that people with mental health problems receive the service they need, regardless of who they are or where they live. (DH 1999a)

This is clearly about 'people with mental health problems', i.e. people with a mental illness. The framework then sets five standards, the first of which covers mental health promotion: 'health and social services should: promote mental health for all, working with individuals and communities; combat discrimination against individuals and groups with mental health problems, and promote their social inclusion' (DH 1999a). In some ways this is positive as the first clause names 'mental health for all', although it is still somewhat confusing that the framework uses the same term in the second clause when clearly referring to people with mental illness. More problematic is the separation of the two clauses: it is not clear whether combating discrimination (of the mentally ill) forms part of mental health promotion or whether it is viewed as part of the government's commitment to social inclusion, separate from its understanding of mental health. The subject becomes clearer from the rationale which follows the aim and standard of the framework which refers to depression (twice), mental disorder (three times) and the ubiquitous 'mental health problems' (four times) – terms used interchangeably. Moreover, given that this aim was outlined in *The Health of the Nation*, one might be forgiven for questioning why it took seven years for the government to produce a document with the same conflation and confusion of terms.

In order to support local services in a mental health promotion strategy, the DH commissioned the mental health charity Mentality (the mental health interest of the defunct Health Education Authority (HEA) under a new name) to prepare a mental health promotion framework document which was published as *Making It Happen* (DH 2001). From the perspective advanced in this chapter this is a profoundly disappointing document. Throughout, it confuses mental health and mental illness: the lack of clarity in the framework concerning mental health promotion and combating discrimination is echoed throughout *Making It Happen*. Its definition of mental health (p. 16) is simplistic in the extreme. It refers only to one model of mental health promotion in the now substantial literature on the subject, and invites no critical reflection on the field. It is completely uncritical of the government – on public mental health it simply asserts that 'standard one of the National Service Framework presents a significant opportunity for further developing mental health promotion work' (DH 2001: 16). It is contradictory: at one point it affirms that 'reflective practice, the ability and willingness to think critically, is at the core of developing a robust and inclusive evidence base' (p. 93), yet on the next page it summarizes the framework's 'grades of evidence' which do not include any reference to reflective, let alone critical practice – and does so without comment or irony! It is also uneven as some of it is about mental *health*; some sections are well-researched, e.g. S3.2 on the relationship between physical health and mental health (i.e. illness); and some of the examples of interventions are reflective of mental health promotion. It is nonetheless disappointing. However, given it provenance, this is not surprising. The HEA had a reputation of marginalizing and excluding critical perspectives, and of capitulating to its political paymasters – on one occasion (in)famously, and at great expense, shredding a sex education booklet aimed at young people because Margaret Thatcher did not approve of the language it contained! – and Mentality appears to have inherited the HEA's conservatism. *Making It Happen* is the latest in a line of lost opportunities in ten years of public health policy that has failed to develop and advance mental health promotion as a reflective and critical practice, capable of transforming levels of emotional literacy in the population, institutions and in the culture, and of creating a real sense of social inclusion, participation and civic well-being. As Campbell (2000) puts it in a rare contribution on mental health promotion from the perspective of a 'community mental patient': 'the current contract available to people with a mental illness diagnosis – both as citizens and service users – appears to be linked to a vision of essentially anti-social contribution and the need for compliance' (2000: 96).

For this sense of transformation, we need to look 'beyond' the *NSF for Mental Health* and to develop the art and science of mental health nursing.

Promoting mental health

In this third and concluding part, mental health promotion beyond the *NSF for Mental Health* is envisioned, and the mental health nurse as consultant, facilitator and advocate is discussed.

Beyond the framework

From the review of recent health policy (above), it is clear (at least to this author and practitioner) that in order to promote positive mental health we need to look elsewhere for inspiration in order to advance theory, policy and practice.

Theory

Craig (1987) talks about 'the unavoidability of theory'. All action is based on – or may be traced back to – some idea or theory. A simple exercise makes this point (Box 2.3).

Box 2.3 Identifying personal theory[2]

Think about a piece of work you did or an interaction you had with a client about which you were really satisfied ('a job well done'). Write down a simple statement that summarizes your feeling about it. Working with someone else, tell them your simple statement. They, in turn, ask you, 'Why did you do that?' or 'What was your thinking about doing what you did?' You answer and they ask you again, 'What was your thinking about *that*?' and so on until you come to a natural conclusion. This 'laddering up' exercise often uncovers the personal theory behind particular actions and interactions.

Theory can be hugely complex (and off-putting) and incredibly simple (and accessible). The personal theory behind the theory advanced in this chapter, as the reader will by now be aware, favours subjectivity over objectivity. This is because I value personal, subjective forms of knowledge, fluidity over fixity and rigidity, multiplicity over singularity, and accessibility and equality – and therefore find, for example, Carper's (1978) ways of knowing liberating. Beyond a particular theory and application of that theory, paradigm analysis offers a meta-theoretical framework with which to understand differences, based on underlying assumptions.

Policy

It has already been noted that in the field of health promotion from the Ottawa Charter onwards and in the field of policy and research in mental health promotion, Canada, and specifically Health Canada, has led the way. New Zealand also has a comparable track record, aided by the work of the psychologist, community development activist and academic John Raeburn (see Raeburn and Rootman 1998). For thinking about genuinely positive mental health policies in Britain we have to go north of the border to Scotland where, despite the fact that *Our National Health* (NHS Scotland 2001) is as disappointing in relation to mental health as its English and Welsh counterpart, the Scottish Council Foundation (SCF) has published *The Possible Scot* (Stewart 1998). This document, published by the SCF, which was launched in 1987 with a mission to promote independent thinking in public policy, is, from its inspiring title onwards, innovative in a number of ways. It argues (among other matters):

- that *possible Scots* should be involved in decision making at all levels;

- that reaching one's potential is not the preserve of the affluent but is the birthright of all;

- that health services should not dominate the health policy agenda – and that the health of the Scottish people would be best served by abandoning health policy as a separate entity and embracing 'holistic government';

- that the dimensions of health can be measured both subjectively and objectively; and

- that if the determinants of health are multiple and interactive, then policy making must be holistic rather than fragmented – holistic government is defined as 'incorporating incentives for cross-departmental and cross-tier working and for cooperation with non-governmental actors' (Stewart 1998: 15)

It is perhaps no accident that *participation* – a central plank of 'people-centred health promotion' (Raeburn and Rootman 1998) – is a feature of *The Possible Scot*, set in the context of the aspiration for a more participative political system since devolution. In the section on life skills for the young, citing Gardner's (1993) theory of multiple intelligences and Goleman's (1996) work on 'emotional intelligence', it argues for a shift of focus in education 'from content and recall to processes and skills' (Stewart 1998: 25). The SCF has gone on to apply the same principles in a subsequent publication *The Possible Human: America's Approach* (SCF 2002). The content, style and tone of both publications are, in contrast to the UK government's policies (discussed above), exciting, innovative, accessible and inclusive. Policy is also strategic. Elizabeth Morris, Principal of the School of Emotional Literacy, makes a similar point in describing the programmes that the school promotes: 'we have found time and time again that for emotional literacy to have any significant impact on pupils it needs to start at a strategic level . . . it has to be written into the policy documents and driven from there' (personal communication, 9 September 2002).

Practice

As mental health promotion is a disputed concept, its practice is not unproblematic. An analysis of three successive annual conferences on mental health promotion revealed that only just over a third (37 per cent) of all presentations were directly concerned with mental health – and by no means were all of these concerned with practice (see Tudor 1996b). Nevertheless, there are examples of good practice in the literature (see Tudor 1996b; McCulloch and Boxer 1997; Raeburn and Rootman 1998; see also www.antidote.org.uk and www.schoolofemotional-literacy.com); some examples in the conference papers from the Annual (now European) Conference on the Promotion of Mental Health (various editors, published by

Ashgate, 1992–present); and some in *Making It Happen* (DH 2001). More important, however, is the practice generated by the practitioner and the client/s working together. As has been noted, the *Key Area Handbook on Mental Illness* (DH 1993) elaborating *The Health of the Nation* (DH 1992) advocated the development of good practice to improve mental health in the NHS and local authority workplace. In some ways this may be viewed as a cascade approach to promoting mental health at work: facilitating the mental health of carers in their working environment so that they can go out and facilitate others. Of course, it does not always work like this. The NHS and local authorities are not necessarily the most benevolent or forward-thinking of employers, and carers for their part are notoriously diffident about looking after themselves let alone putting themselves first. One might argue that if, as carers, we cannot look after our own health needs and interests, then who are we to tell others how to do it? The irony of practitioners charged with the task of mental health promotion who are themselves overworked, under-resourced and stressed must not be lost. Elsewhere I have applied a similar analysis to mental health promotion at work (Tudor 1996a).

Undoubtedly the single greatest change will come from the extension of the employers' duty of care under health and safety legislation to include *health* and the promotion of positive workplace health and mental health or well-being; and it is possible that European legislation may enable such extensional responsibilities and thinking. In this context it is perhaps not surprising that in recent years there has been increasing interest in the balance between work and the rest of life, sometimes referred to as the work–life balance. There is a National Work–Life Forum (website: www.worklifeforum.com) which, in conjunction with The Industrial Society (now The Work Foundation), produced a *Work–Life Manual* (McCarraher and Daniels 2000) that encourages innovative work organization (flexitime, compressed working week, etc.), leave provision, and employee development and support (see also McCarraher and Daniels 2002).

Mental health nursing – consultation, facilitation, advocacy

Mental health nurses need grounding and information in order to question practice, to contribute to decision making in multi-disciplinary teams, and to draw on research-based knowledge in the delivery of care and the development of mental health services. It is hoped that much of this chapter contributes to meeting such needs. Thus, how 'grounded' nurses are depends on themselves at a personal level; in relationships at work with patients, colleagues, supervisors and managers; in their sense of themselves within the institution/organization and, more broadly, within the culture (see Table 2.2). Information with which both to question and to contribute to practice comes partly from individual resilience (coherence and personal integration) and partly from supportive environments, both physical and intellectual (of which this chapter hopefully forms a part). There are many forms of research-based knowledge from the objective to the subjective (see Burrell and Morgan 1979 and p. 46) and simply knowing this may support the practitioner to question the hegemony of certain forms and frames of knowledge, research and 'evidence', as in 'evidence-based research', which usually refers to 'objective' empirical evidence. In advancing this kind of reflective and critical practice in action, the practitioner, in this case the mental health nurse, may – even must – become consultant, facilitator and advocate.

The term 'mental health consultation' dates back some 30 years to the work of Gerald Caplan who viewed it as 'one of the essential ingredients of an organized program of community mental health' (1964: 35). Caplan's views on mental health consultation are set out in his own work (and summarized and discussed in Tudor 1996b); nevertheless several points are worth making here:

- the relationship between the two professionals involved (i.e. consultant and consultee) is 'coordinate', i.e. non-hierarchical in terms of management authority;
- the consultant has no administrative or coercive responsibility as regards the client; and
- the consultant has no liability for outcome.

While there are many different personal styles of consultancy, the term facilitation (meaning rendering easier, helping forward) implies a certain philosophy about the role of the consultant/nurse/etc. and their relationship to the client (whether an individual, group or organization). Rogers (1983) describes the best facilitator in the words of the Chinese philosopher Lao Tse and author of the *Tao Te Ching*:

> A leader is best
> When people barely know he exists,
> Not so good when people obey and acclaim him,
> Worst when they despise him.
> But of a good leader, who talks little,
> When his work is done, his aim fulfilled,
> They will say 'We did this ourselves'.

If a facilitator is, at best, self-effacing, the good advocate is often 'in your face'. Commonly defined as someone who is called in as a witness, one who pleads or speaks for, or who intercedes on behalf of someone else, advocacy also carries a sense of argument and recommendation. Both fields – of mental health and mental illness – need advocates who have the personal resilience to stand up for themselves and the people for and with whom they are advocating, as well as (ideally) the supportive environments, networks and groups in which to operate. The emphasis in recent years, again in both fields, on participation and on citizenship is significant. Campbell (2000) argues that it is more important, for instance, for mental illness service users to be talking and acting in terms of rights and citizenship than in tinkering with the review of the Mental Health Act. He goes on to observe increased activity among 'mental health' service users in the consortium *Rights Now* since the passing of the Disability Discrimination Act 1995 (which for the first time included people with a mental illness diagnosis). Within mental *health*, alongside the notion of healthy environments, schools, hospitals, communities and cities, the concept of 'civic well-being' (Stewart 1998) is developing. Consultation, and to a lesser extent, facilitation, implies that the practitioner has been approached by someone to act as a consultant or facilitator; the advocate generally needs no invitation! As mental health is for all then it is the business of all and in this the mental health nurse, with the help of education and training, can and must play their part.

Conclusion

In summary, the main points of this chapter are:

- Health and illness are integral parts of the human condition, the relationship between the two being complex and understood from a number of different and differing perspectives.
- In order to develop a dialogue and discourse about health between health and illness it is necessary to separate the two and to develop perspectives on positive, holistic health.
- Similarly, it is helpful, if only strategically, to separate mental health from health, and to distinguish it from mental illness and to develop concepts of positive mental health or well-being.
- Current government health policy in Britain is largely limited and unhelpful in advancing understanding of positive mental *health* and its promotion.
- The mental health nurse is in as good a position as any to promote mental health in the general population as well as in those diagnosed as mentally ill.
- Reflective practitioners need to view themselves as mental *health* consultants and to develop as consultants, facilitators and advocates.

Notes

1   The author wishes to thank Fiona Begbie, Natacha Joubert, Elizabeth Morris and John Raeburn for their support and their comments on earlier drafts of this chapter.
2   I am grateful to Adrienne Lee for introducing me to a similar exercise.

Questions for self-reflection and discussion

1 In what ways is health more than the absence of illness?
2 Distinguish the 'mental' in mental health.
3 Do you (the reader) have a sense of your own health and mental health – and, in what ways do you identify, maintain, develop and promote it?
4 'Mental health for all' – how is this reflected in common interests and difficulties in the fields of health, education and social work?
5 How do you view the role of the mental health nurse in promoting mental health?

Annotated bibliography

- Tudor, K. (1996b) *Mental Health Promotion: Paradigms and Practice.* London: Routledge. The first book published on the subject (and winner of the Bruce Burns Annual Mental Health Promotion Award), it offers, according to George Albee's preface, 'a detailed critical analysis of the underlying assumptions, concepts and models of mental health – and mental illness – and especially of community-based interventions'. It defines the field – through a review of mental health, health promotion, mental health promotion, community and community mental health promotion – develops the field through discussions of mental health policy, assessment, consultation, education and training – and concludes with a chapter on breaking out of the field. It details a paradigm analysis of the field of mental health and its promotion.
- McCulloch, G.F. and Boxer, J. (1997) *Mental Health Promotion: Policy, Practice and Partnerships.* London: Bailliere Tindall. This book provides a critical overview of the environment of service provision and planning, and the impact of research and education on the development of good practice in mental health care. With a strong emphasis on the political and policy context, on anti-oppressive practice and on the user focus, it provides a comprehensive and practice-focused introduction to what is viewed as the challenging area of mental health promotion.

References

American Psychiatric Association (2000) *Diagnostic and Statistical Manual of Mental Disorders IV-TR* (4th edn text rev.). Washington, DC: APA.
Antonovsky, A. (1979) *Health, Stress and Coping: New Perspectives on Mental and Physical Well-being.* San Francisco, CA: Jossey-Bass.

Antonovsky, A. (1987) The salutogenetic perspective: Toward a new view of health and illness. *Advances* **4**: 47.

Antonovsky, A. (1993) The structure and properties of the sense of coherence scale. *Social Science and Medicine* **36**: 725–33.

Birtchnell, J. (1993) *How Humans Relate: A New Interpersonal Theory*. Westport, CT: Praeger.

Burrell, G. and Morgan, G. (1979) *Sociological Paradigms and Organizational Analysis*. London: Heinemann.

Campbell, P. (2000) Surviving social inclusion, in C. Newnes, G. Holmes and C. Dunn (eds) *This is Madness too*. Llangarron: PCCS Books (pp. 93–102).

Caplan, G. (1964) *Principles of Preventative Psychiatry*. New York: Basic Books.

Caplan, R. (1986) *The Implications of Socio-theoretical Constructs for the Evaluation of Health Education Theory*. Unpublished MSc dissertation, King's College, University of London.

Carper, B. (1978) Fundamental ways of knowing in nursing. *Advances in Nursing Science* **1**(1): 13–23.

Clarkson, P. (1989) *Gestalt Counselling in Action*. London: Sage.

Craig, I. (1987) The psychodynamics of theory. *Free Associations* **10**: 32–56.

Department of Health (1992) *The Health of the Nation*. London: DH.

Department of Health (1993) *The Health of the Nation: Key Area Handbook Mental Illness*. London: DH.

Department of Health (1999a) *National Service Framework for Mental Health*. London: DH.

Department of Health (1999b) *Our Healthier Nation*. London: DH.

Department of Health (2001) *Making it Happen*. London: DH.

Doyal, L. and Pennell, I. (1979) *The Political Economy of Health*. London: Pluto.

Duff, K. (1993) *The Alchemy of Illness*. London: Virago.

Fox, N.J. (1999) *Beyond Health: Postmodernism and Embodiment*. London: Free Association Books.

French, J. and Adams, L. (1986) From analysis to synthesis. Theories of health education. *Health Education Journal* **45**: 71–4.

Gardner, H. (1993) *Frames of Mind: the Theory of Multiple Intelligences* (2nd edn). London: Fontana Press.

Goleman, D. (1996) *Emotional Intelligence: Why it can matter more than IQ*. London: Bloomsbury.

Graham, H. (1992) Imaginative assessment of personal health needs, in D.R. Trent (ed.) *Promotion of Mental Health, Vol. 1*. Aldershot: Avebury (pp. 53–62).

Groder, M. (1977) Asklepieion: An integration of psychotherapies, in G. Barnes (ed.) *TA after Eric Berne*. New York: Harper & Row (pp. 134–7).

Jahoda, M. (1958) *Current Concepts of Positive Mental Health*. New York: Basic Books.

James, N. (1989) Emotional labour: skill and work in the social regulation of feelings. *Sociological Review* **37**: 15–42.

Johns, C. (1995) Framing learning through reflection within Carper's fundamental ways of knowing in nursing. *Journal of Advanced Nursing* **22**(2): 226–34.

Jones, J.M. (1972) *Prejudice and Racism*. Reading, MA: Addison-Wesley.

Joubert, N. and Raeburn, J. (1998) Mental health promotion: People, power and passion. *International Journal of Mental Health Promotion* **1**: 15–22.

Kickbush, I. (1989) Healthy cities: A working project and a growing movement. *Health Promotion* **4**: 77–89.

Kuhn, T. (1970) *The Structure of Scientific Revolutions* (2nd edn). Chicago, IL: University of Chicago Press.

Lalonde, M. (1975) *A New Perspective on the Health of Canadians*. Ottawa: Information Canada.

Lewin, K. (1952) *Field Theory in Social Science*. London: Tavistock.

Marks, D.F. (ed.) (2002) *The Health Psychology Reader*. London: Sage.

McCarraher, L. and Daniels, L. (2000) *The Work–Life Manual*. London: The Industrial Society.

McCarraher, L. and Daniels, L. (2002) *The Book of Balanced Living*. London: The Work Foundation.

McCulloch, G. (1999) Strategic approaches in Sheffield. *Regeneration and Mental Health*. Briefing No. 1, p. 5.

McCulloch, G.F. and Boxer, J. (1997) *Mental Health Promotion: Policy, Practice and Partnerships*, London: Bailliere Tindall.

McDonald, G. and O'Hara, K. (1998) *Ten Elements of Mental Health, its Promotion and Demotion: Implications for Practice*. London: Society of Health Promotion Specialists.

Minister of National Health and Welfare (1988) *Mental Health for Canadians*. Ottawa: MNHW.

Money, M. (1993) *Health and Community*. Dartington: Green Books.

NHS Scotland (2001) *Our National Health: A Plan for Action, a Plan for Change*. Edinburgh: Scottish Executive.

Neumann, J., Schroeder, H. and Voss, P. (1989) Mental health and well-being in the context of the health promotion concept, in J. Neumann, H. Schroeder and P. Voss (eds) *Mental Health Within the Health Promotion Concept*. Dresden: German Hygiene Museum/Copenhagen: WHO (pp. 3–17).

Perls, F.S., Hefferline, R.F. and Goodman, P. ([1951] 1979) *Gestalt Therapy: Excitement and Growth in the Human Personality*. Harmondsworth: Penguin.

Porter, R. (1990) *Mind-forg'd Manacles*. London: Penguin.

Preston, G.H. (1943) *The Substance of Mental Health*. New York: Farrar & Rinehart.

Raeburn, J. and Rootman, I. (1998) *People-centred Health Promotion*. Chichester: Wiley.

Rogers, C.R. (1951) *Client-centered Therapy*. London: Constable.

Rogers, C.R. (1983) *Freedom to Learn for the 80s*. Columbus, OH: Charles E. Merrill.

Sacks, O. (1991) *Awakenings*. London: Picador.

Sacks, O. (1995) *An Anthropologist on Mars: Seven Paradoxical Tales*. London: Picador.

Scottish Council Foundation (2002) *The Possible Human: America's Approach*. Edinburgh: Scottish Council Foundation.

Seyle, H. (1956) *The Stress of Life*. New York: McGraw-Hill.

Standing Nursing and Midwifery Advisory Committee (1999) *Mental Health Nursing: Addressing Acute Concerns*. London: DH.

Steiner, C. (1971) Radical psychiatry: Principles, in J. Agel (ed.) *The Radical Therapist*. New York: Ballantine Books (pp. 3–7).

Stephens, T. (1998) *Population Mental Health in Canada*. Toronto: Mental Health Promotion Unit, Health Canada.

Stephens, T., Dulberg, C. and Joubert, N. (1999) Mental health of the Canadian population: A comprehensive analysis. *Chronic Diseases in Canada* **20**(3): 18–126.

Stewart, S. (ed.) (1998) *The Possible Scot: Making Healthy Public Policy*. Edinburgh: Scottish Council Foundation.

Suzuki, S. (1999). *Zen Mind, Beginner's Mind* (revd edn). New York: Weatherhill.

Tudor, K. (1990/91) One step back, two steps forwards: Community care and mental health. *Critical Social Policy* **30**: 5–22.

Tudor, K. (1996a) Mental health promotion at work, in D.R. Trent and C.A. Reed (eds) *Promotion of Mental Health, Vol 5*. Aldershot: Avebury (pp. 127–43).

Tudor, K. (1996b) *Mental Health Promotion: Paradigms and Practice*. London: Routledge.

Tudor, K. (1999) *Group Counselling*. London: Sage.

van Deurzen-Smith, E. (1996) Existential therapy, in W. Dryden (ed.) *Handbook of Individual Therapy*. London: Sage (pp. 166–93).

Weare, K. (1996) Mental health in the school system: 'The health promoting school' idea, in D.R. Trent and C.A. Reed (eds) *Promotion of Mental Health, Vol. 5, 1995*. Aldershot: Avebury (pp. 161–70).

Weare, K. (2000) *Promoting Mental, Emotional and Social Health: A Whole School Approach*. London: Routledge.

World Health Organization (1948) *Constitution of the World Health Organization*. New York: WHO.

3

Mental health nursing: origins and orientations

Ian Norman and Iain Ryrie

Chapter overview

This chapter seeks to provide a historical perspective on the practice of mental health nursing upon which nurses and other mental health care workers of the future must build. The first part traces the origins of mental health nursing from the eighteenth century to the present day and outlines recent influences on its development. The strength of the old mental hospitals lay in their structure. This structure did not allow mental health nursing to grow and develop, because it did not provide nurses with opportunities for independent thinking and action. But it did provide them with a sense of security and a common shared identity based on a clear sense of their place within the hospital structure, without need to define the nursing role and remit, or the underpinning values or knowledge base of the discipline. Closure of the old hospitals and the development of community-based mental health services meant that these things were to change. Nurses were required to reconsider their roles and responsibilities, their place within multi-disciplinary clinical teams and their relations with mental health service users.

UK government reviews of mental health nursing *Psychiatric Nursing: Today and Tomorrow* published in 1968 (Standing Mental Health and Standing Nursing Advisory Committees 1968) and *Working in Partnership* published in 1994 (Mental Health Nursing Review Team 1994) provided some touchstones for the specialty at times of great change. *Working in Partnership*, in particular, reaffirmed that the work of mental health nurses rests fundamentally on their relationships with service users. In this it reflected strongly the considerable influence on mental health nursing of Peplau's emphasis on phases in the development of the nurse–patient relationship expressed first in her book, *Interpersonal Relations in Nursing* (Peplau 1952). But, almost a decade after the publication of *Working in Partnership*, the dominant influence of the evidence-based health care movement threatens mental health nursing in the interpersonal relations tradition. Today's mental health nurses differ in their view of the proper focus of nursing care, and the discipline appears more fragmented than in the past.

The second part of this chapter traces the origins of this fragmentation of mental health nursing as an academic and practice discipline. We single out the work of Annie Altschul and Phil Barker as being particularly influential in the dissemination and development of Peplau's interpersonal relations approach to mental health nursing in the UK, and set out the main elements of the contrasting evidence-based health care approach. This approach has a long history but owes much to the development of evidence-based medicine, a term first coined by Gordon Guyatt's group at McMaster University Medical School in Canada in 1992 (Sackett *et al.* 2000). Represented as in conflict we argue for coexistence of both the interpersonal relations and the evidence-based health care orientations to mental health nursing, and that both are needed to help service users on their diverse roads to recovery.

In summary this chapter covers:

- the origins of mental health nursing in the eighteenth and nineteenth centuries;

- twentieth-century developments, in particular the impact on mental health nursing of the decline of the old mental hospitals and the development of a community-based service;

- the development of community-based nursing;

- *Working in Partnership*, the UK government's review of mental health nursing published in 1994;

- Contemporary orientations to mental health nursing:
  - interpersonal relations – Peplau and her legacy;
  - the evidence-based practice movement.

Over the past two decades nurses in the UK have chosen to call themselves 'mental health nurses', rather than 'psychiatric nurses', a well-established term which reflected the registered qualification of 'mental nurse'. In part this change in terminology would appear to reflect a desire by nurses to establish their profession as distinct from the discipline of psychiatry and also to find a more positive identity as people who can help people who are mentally ill become mentally healthy. However, the terms psychiatric nurse and mental health nurse also highlight rather different aspects of the nurse's role. 'Psychiatric nursing', for many nurses, implies crisis resolution work with people who are at risk to themselves or to others. In contrast, 'mental health nursing' implies developmental work with people who are no longer in a state of crisis and who need help to regain their mental health and so control over their lives. While we recognize this distinction, both these aspects of work are integral to mental health nursing as a practice discipline and we prefer to integrate both elements, rather than apply different labels to them.

We use both the terms 'patient' and 'service user' to refer to those people in receipt of mental health nursing care and vary these according to the context of care described; for example, whereas service user is the term preferred currently by many mental health nurses, those in receipt of care in the old mental hospitals are referred to more appropriately as patients.

Origins

Eighteenth and nineteenth centuries

Throughout the ages people with mental disorder have been the recipients of various forms of care and control. From the twelfth century, the asylum provided a setting for such care, although the importance of the asylum system grew from the late seventeenth century under the influence of the intellectual tradition of the Enlightenment. Notable pioneers were Philippe Pinel in France and the Quaker, William Tuke, in England who, almost simultaneously, but independently, introduced reforms that unchained the lunatics, and turned the asylums into havens for the insane.

Tuke founded the Retreat at York in 1792 on principles of 'moral treatment'. Chapman (1992) tells us that Tuke believed madness and deranged behaviour to stem from the mode of service provision in eighteenth-century 'madhouses' where 'lunatics' suffered degradation, repression and cruelty. Scull (1981) wrote about care of mentally ill people before the nineteenth century as being a way of solving society's difficulty in knowing how to handle socially disadvantaged groups. Tuke replaced physical constraints with moral constraints based on reason supported by purposeful work and social and educational activities in a normal domestic environment. The 'moral therapists' challenged medical dominance in the treatment of the insane, arguing that medicine had abused care, and medical treatment was unnecessary in moral therapy because carers were selected for their attitude and personality. The moralists considered the newly industrialized society to be the source of mental instability and that cure could be found in calm, productive, non-competitive communities (Scull 1981). The asylum attendants in the Retreat and other similar communities were the first official care agents, and are often regarded as the predecessors of the mental health nurse.

The moral therapy movement marked the start of changing social attitudes towards the insane, which by the first half of the nineteenth century were influenced by a growing social conscience based on a common ethical principle, a belief that the community had a responsibility to the weak (Jones 1960). This found expression in the Lunatics Act (1845), which was a major achievement of the work of the Earl of Shaftesbury as was the construction of a number of Victorian asylums, some of which are still in use today. Changing attitudes to the insane had implications for the role of lunatic attendants who, by the mid-nineteenth century, were expected to set a positive example to patients and to offer them guidance rather than simply be custodians. But, it was difficult to recruit attendants of the right type. Connolly (1992) quotes Dr Browne who, writing in 1897 of male attendants, described them as 'the unemployable of other professions . . . if they possess physical strength and a tolerable reputation for sobriety, it is enough; and the latter is frequently dispensed with' (Dr Browne, cited by Connolly 1992: 7). According to Connolly (1992) women attendants of the right type were easier to recruit than men because nursing was widely perceived to be in women's nature.

These recruitment problems are not surprising when one considers working conditions of the time, which were very poor. Records from Springfield Hospital in Tooting, London (then the Surrey Lunatic Asylum) referred to by Connolly (1992), show that in 1842 attendants worked from 6.00 a.m. until 9.00 p.m., and slept in rooms adjacent to the wards. There were nine male and nine female attendants for 350 patients. In a report to Visiting Justices that year, attendants were described as 'the instruments for carrying into effect every remedial measure', the work requiring 'firmness and self control blended with humanity and forbearance' and involving 'many menial offices'. For this male attendants working in the Surrey Asylum received between £25 and £30 per year. This compared well with the national average salary of male attendants, which was £26 per year. But attendants were among the lowest paid people in the country, and female attendants were paid substantially less than their male counterparts – between £12 and £16 per year on average.

Given the developing role of the asylum attendant beyond a purely custodial function, a number of medical superintendents became convinced of the need for some sort of education and training for attendants. The first course of lectures for attendants was probably given by Alexander Morrison the Surrey Lunatic Asylum's Medical Superintendent in 1843. This course served as a stimulus for the spread of similar courses of instruction, which culminated in publication of the Handbook for Instruction of Attendants on the Insane, by the Royal Medico-Psychological Association (RMPA) – the Red Handbook – which became a standard text. By 1889 100 hospitals offered programmes of instruction based on the Red Handbook and in 1890 the RMPA established the first register for attendants, who had completed successfully a two-year training programme (Walk 1961). Thus, mental health nursing as a practice discipline represented by qualification and register is only 114 years old.

In spite of these positive developments it would be incorrect to interpret the history of mental health nursing as one of progressive improvement in the conditions for patients and their carers in the asylums. Moral treatment, which had heralded positive changes in social attitudes to the insane and the notion of attendants as therapeutic agents, lasted only 50 years in Great Britain (Chapman 1992) because a growing number of patients gradually outstripped the human resource to provide moral treatment to an adequate standard. By the mid-nineteenth century asylums were being built for thousands at a time to, in effect, warehouse madness. These institutions quickly became overcrowded: for example, by 1909 the number of patients in the Surrey Asylum, built originally for 350, had risen to 1235 (Connolly 1992). Bureaucratic organization of patients' lives based on rigid doctor, nurse, patient hierarchies became the norm and attendants were once again relied upon for strength and intimidation, rather than friendliness and common sense (Jones 1960).

The beginning of the nineteenth century also marked the start of a shifting and often uneasy relationship between mental health and general nursing, which continues to the present day. The British Nursing Association (later the Royal British Nursing Association (RBNA)) founded for general nurses in 1887 refused entry to the nursing register to graduates of the Royal Medico-Psychological Association (RMPA) register for attendants. Mrs Bedford-Fenwick, the RBNA President, set out the reasons for this in 1895 when she pointed to the narrow training received by asylum attendants and concerns about the possible effects of admission on nurses' social status:

> No person can be considered trained who has only worked in hospitals and asylums for the insane . . . considering the present class of persons known as male attendants, one can hardly believe that their admission will tend to raise the status of the Association.
>
> (Adams 1969: 13, cited by Connolly 1992: 9)

The College of Nursing (eventually to become the Royal College), which was established in 1916, maintained the stance taken by the RBNA by continuing to refuse admission to registered attendants. However, the later established General Nursing Council (GNC) started its own course and examination for attendants, thereby introducing an alternative qualification.

Connolly points out that the drive for equal status with general nursing was spearheaded by medical superintendents and senior attendants, and was of little concern to rank and file asylum attendants who, through the National Asylum Workers' Union, were concerned to improve conditions of service and pay, but were not concerned with status or professionalism for many years. Moreover, qualifications, whether registration with the RMPA or the later GNC, carried little weight. Neither was needed to obtain a senior position in an asylum and many asylum matrons had general nursing training only and no experience of asylum work.

Twentieth century

The first half of the twentieth century was marked by renewed optimism in psychiatry. In the inter-war period nomenclature changed, asylums became mental hospitals and male and female attendants became nurses, and the management of mental health was incorporated into the National Health Service (NHS), so providing free care as a right of citizenship. However, mental hospitals remained overcrowded, particularly during both world wars when many staff members were enlisted in the forces or redeployed, so that patients had to be redistributed. Thus the main role of the mental nurses during the first half of the twentieth century remained containment and management of large numbers of patients in overcrowded conditions.

During the early twentieth century allegations of malpractice rose sharply with nurses being the main target for criticism. Such allegations led to calls for a Royal Commission into Lunacy Laws which was established in 1926 and led in turn to the Mental Treatment Act (1930) which introduced categories of 'voluntary' and 'temporary' patients which avoided the pessimistic experience of certification for some patients. The category of 'voluntary patient' was extended and by 1957 this group constituted 75 per cent of admissions. However, admission procedures and rights of patients remained unchanged until the Mental Health Act (1959), which, Connolly (1992) points out, marked the end of the power of magistrates over the asylum system and regain of control by mental health professionals.

During the 1930s many men from depressed areas of the country entered mental health nursing. Ideal entry requirements for nurses from this period into the 1950s were that they should be physically fit, able to take part in organized games or play a musical instrument – criteria that contributed to active sporting and community activities within and between asylums, but did little to improve standards of patient care (Jones 1960). While mental nurses were expected to show kindness and forbearance towards patients and set them a good example, asylum regulations in the early twentieth century governing the conduct of staff were strict and gave little opportunity for the exercise of responsibility or common sense – as envisaged by advocates of moral treatment so many years before. For example, Connolly (1992) cites regulations from Springfield Mental Hospital (formerly the Surrey Asylum) in 1926 which shows that patients had to be counted in and out of the wards and gardens, specified that five rounds be made of the Female Division and six of the Male Division during each period of night duty, and that attendants who were judged negligent, resulting in patients escaping, were required to pay a portion of the expense incurred in recapturing them.

Drawing upon archival evidence and interviews with nurses employed at Springfield Hospital during the postwar years, Connolly provides a picture of mental health nurses' lives and work in a typical mental hospital in the first part of the twentieth century. In the years immediately following the Second World War he reports that

> all the wards at Springfield Hospital were locked, apart from a few geriatric wards. The gardens were also locked and the hospital as a whole was surrounded by fences. The main block was strictly segregated – male staff and male patients on one side, female staff and female patients on the other. Only maintenance staff and doctors regularly saw both sides. The wards themselves were furnished with hard wooden chairs and long workhouse tables, and there were no curtains between the beds.
>
> (Connolly 1992: 11)

From Connolly's account mental nurses of the time, with their general nursing counterparts, were much preoccupied by cleanliness and orderliness to the extent that beds would be lined up with pieces of string to ensure regularity. Task allocation was the dominant form of work organization and time periods were set aside for these tasks to be accomplished – such as bed making, and mealtimes when staff and patients would eat together in the wards. Nursing work was varied, with an emphasis on organizing patients' work: in the wards (for example, cleaning and maintaining the wards, cleaning or feeding other patients), on the farm, in the hospital grounds (for example, rolling the cricket pitch) or in the laundry or tailor's shop where they would make and maintain clothing and bedding. In spite of the emphasis on constructive activity for patients there was little emphasis on preparing patients for return to the world outside hospital.

Psychiatric hospitals in decline

The community had long been considered a brutalizing environment for people with mental health problems (Wing 1990), but in the 1960s a number of factors combined to make it an increasingly attractive care location for local authorities and the government. These factors included:

- gross overcrowding of hospitals, the population of which had reached 150,000 by the mid-1950s, which was more than the buildings could satisfactorily accommodate;
- crumbling building stock which would have required a great deal of money to repair and most of which were unsuitably located to serve the major centres of population;
- escalating NHS labour costs, particularly in the 1960s when the Confederation of Health Service Employees (COHSE), by now the major union for mental health nurses, were awarded major pay increases of 12 per cent in 1959, 14 per cent in 1962 and 5 per cent in 1963 (Nolan and Hooper 2000);
- the majority view that new drugs offered a genuine opportunity for the control of symptoms and, in some cases, cure; and
- the Mental Health Act (1959), which placed a strong emphasis on community involvement in psychiatric care services.

The shift away from the old hospitals to a community-based service was accelerated by other factors, in particular the diminishing power-base of the physician superintendents in the hospitals, which was undermined by new consultant psychiatrists created within the new NHS. The power-base of the consultant psychiatrists was strengthened by the transfer of services such as radiography, pathology and surgery, formerly provided within the mental hospitals to purpose-built general hospitals. Moreover, the consultants were empowered by new drugs on the market, and were free to select their own treatments independent of the physician superintendent's views. As the power of the consultant psychiatrists increased, so the power of the physician superintendents declined until in 1960 the post was declared obsolete.

With the demise of physician superintendents, and the change in the philosophy of psychiatric care away from manual labour as therapy towards therapeutic relationships and environments, the psychiatric hospitals began to change. Wards were unlocked, military-type uniforms (brass buttons, peaked caps) for male nurses were abandoned in favour of white coats, hospital farms which had once provided employment and income were run down and sold off, and ancillary staff were employed to carry out the manual tasks once carried out by nurses and patients.

Many nurses were resistant to such changes, concerned that an attack on the psychiatric hospital would threaten their economic security and prospects. However, others embraced the changes and the more able, ambitious and innovative nurses left the old hospitals to work in new psychiatric units established in the 1960s and 1970s in district general hospitals. Loss of the most able nurses and medical staff left those who remained increasingly vulnerable to the mounting tide of criticism of psychiatry in general and the old mental hospitals in particular.

The influence of the anti-psychiatry movement was, in the 1960s, at its peak. Leading figures in the movement – Laing, Szasz, Sedgewick and Foucault – came from very different philosophical and political positions but were united in their mistrust and scepticism of orthodox psychiatry and challenged it to re-examine its *history, origins, claims and achievements* (Nolan 1993: 1). Anti-psychiatrists saw psychiatry as performing a role of social control and so could not claim to be a branch of medicine or a respectable science. The anti-psychiatrists were criticized for underestimating the effectiveness of modern psychiatry in diagnosing and treating mental illness and for overestimating its control function (Chapman 1992). However, their ideas were influential in drawing attention to the coercive aspects of psychiatry in which nurses were perceived to be front-line agents of social control.

Criticism from the anti-psychiatrists was supported by growing evidence about the effects of institutional life on patients. The structure and organization of traditional hospitals was gradually seen to be pathogenic as the new therapeutic regimes at the Cassel, Claybury and Fulbourne hospitals demonstrated the benefits of an 'open-door policy' (Nolan 1993) and a partnership approach to care between staff and patients (Chapman 1992).

Goffman's *Asylums* (1961) is a landmark in the history of care of the mentally ill and of the anti-psychiatry movement. His attack on the 'total institution' in the USA, with its emphasis on block treatment, denial of individuality and social distance between staff and patients, caused the USA and the UK to rethink institutional care (Nolan 1993). Other critics in Britain were also condemning conditions in mental hospitals at the time (Barton 1959; Townsend 1962). Nurses who ran the hospitals felt powerless to respond because they had no decision-making power (Nolan 1993).

The final blow to the mental hospital system came from a series of psychiatric hospital scandals and public inquiries in the 1960s and 1970s that exposed professional neglect and suffering of mentally ill patients, and that seriously weakened psychiatric nursing. In 1961 Enoch Powell, the then Minister of Health, declared that mental hospitals must close and the development of community care for the mentally ill remained a policy of

successive governments. Throughout the 1960s and 1970s only limited progress was made in moving patients from the larger hospitals into community
settings, and community care itself lacked conceptual clarity. Although
overcrowding and the resident population of large psychiatric hospitals had
gradually decreased, by 1975, none had closed. Twenty-seven years after his
announcement in 1961 that hospitals must close, Enoch Powell reflected on
the entrenched bureaucracies of the psychiatric hospitals that prevented
even modest changes, let alone closure, being contemplated (Powell 1988,
cited in Nolan 1993).

Nevertheless, the government's White Paper, *Better Services for the
Mentally Ill* (DHSS 1975), claimed that the government's policy was working. The development of local services with a shift away from hospital provision towards community-based social services care was still the target
although the White Paper declared also that the hospital would remain the
centre for mental health care services for the foreseeable future; that is,
until adequate community care facilities were in place to prevent 'revolving
door' patients, that is, those who needed supervision of their medication,
followed by a rapid return to the community, perhaps precipitating readmis-
sion. *Better Services for the Mentally Ill* set the tone for the future community-based care of people with mental illness and continues to provide a
useful reference point from which current mental health care services can be
judged.

Development of community mental health nursing

Closure of the large mental hospitals and their replacement by smaller units
attached to local district hospitals, and the development of day hospitals
and community-care facilities had a marked impact on the practice of
mental health nursing from the 1960s. May and Moore (1963) describe the
work of two (later four) nurses seconded from Warlingham Park Hospital in
1954 to visit patients discharged from hospital and now living in Croydon.
These 'outpatient' nurses saw ex-patients suffering from schizophrenia and
depression, and their duties were to:

- monitor their compliance with medication and attendance at outpatient
  clinics;
- assess and monitor their mental state;
- monitor difficulties in their personal habits and seek to improve these and;
- reassure relatives.

Their role was clinical and investigation and reporting patients' family and
social circumstances was not expected; this was the remit of the psychiatric
social worker. Each nurse was responsible for a ward of patients. They
attended a weekly ward round, and also outpatient clinics and evening
aftercare groups.

McNamee (1993) reports that Moorhaven Hospital established what
was known as a 'Nursing After-Care' service in 1957. This differed from the

Warlingham Park Hospital service in that it involved nurses working both in the wards as well as with patients who had been discharged. It is ironic that more than 40 years later this flexible model of working which offers one approach to bridging the gap between inpatient and community care is rarely seen in practice. Moorhaven Hospital community psychiatric nurses (CPNs) were expected to build relationships with their patients and to use this as a medium for care delivery and for helping patients to cope with the effects of their illness. Thus, the nurse was envisaged as a therapeutic agent, a role that served also to enhance the status of nursing at the time.

The CPN role continued to develop. According to Hunter (1974) their functions in the 1960s included:

- providing practical assistance to patients and their families (for example, help bathing and shaving patients);
- giving advice particularly to patients' families on medication, monitoring its side effects and cooperating with general practitioners and psychiatrists to reduce these;
- acting as a link between the ward and community and facilitating admission in the event of relapse;
- ensuring continuity of care for designated groups of patients (including those with schizophrenia, recurrent depression and organic psychosis);
- supervising patients in outpatient clinics;
- assisting in running social clubs and work groups; and
- assisting patients to gain employment and accommodation on discharge from hospital.

The CPN role expanded to assume social and rehabilitative functions particularly from the 1970s following the Local Authority Social Services Act (1970), which abolished specialist social workers for people with mental health problems. CPNs began to offer crisis intervention, group work, psychotherapy and behaviour therapy (Hunter 1974). However, in the 1960s and 1970s CPNs worked primarily within hospital treatment teams, received all referrals from hospital consultants and carried out care programmes that were medically oriented.

A change of emphasis away from medical domination towards a more autonomous social model of care followed attachment of CPNs to general practice in Oxford and elsewhere in the 1970s. These CPNs accepted referrals from many sources (open referral system), including each other, and developed into far more independent practitioners responsible for patient assessment, and also planning and implementing an appropriate care package. Later, though, attachment of CPNs to primary-care teams was criticized (for example, White 1990b; Gournay and Brooking 1994) for deflecting the attention of nurses towards the so-called 'worried well' and away from the needs of people with serious mental illness who are a government priority for mental health care. Thus the trend has been towards CPNs operating in secondary mental health services based in community mental health teams.

In the early 1970s, and particularly following the White Paper, *Better Services for the Mentally Ill* (DHSS 1975), there was a growing lobby for specialist community training for mental health nurses. The Joint Board of Clinical Nursing Studies (JBCNS) established a committee to examine requirements for an approved community psychiatric nurse (CPN) course that did not overlap with the requirements for district nurses or health visitors. It was agreed that a separate course was needed to produce highly trained nurses who could meet the specific needs of mentally ill people. In 1974 the JBCNS published the *Outline Curriculum in Community Psychiatric Nursing for Registered Nurses* (JBCNS 1974). This 36–39 week course was designed to prepare Registered Mental Nurses (RMNs) to work in multi-professional environments and to give both rehabilitative and therapeutic care in the community. A major element of the course was community placement, particularly with the community psychiatric service, which the student would join following qualification (White 1990a).

The first CPN course was started by Chiswick College in 1973 (White 1990a) and, by the end of the 1970s, CPNs had achieved independent recognition and other colleges and polytechnics were running courses. CPNs worked from general practice clinics or accepted referrals from other agencies, and developed specialist skills to assist and work with care groups and organizations (Simmons and Brooker 1990).

Increased specialization of CPNs and other mental health nurses from the 1970s mirrored and was sometimes forced by increased specialization by their medical colleagues. An important example was the development of training for nurses in behaviour therapy by Isaac Marks at the Maudsley Hospital from 1972 (Simmons and Brooker 1986). This led to the English National Board (ENB) course 650 – 'Short-term Adult Behavioural Psycho-therapy', which was the first of a series of post-registration courses to provide community mental health nurses with specialist skills and a specific therapeutic orientation. A more recent example is the Thorn Programme developed and disseminated from the Institute of Psychiatry, King's College London, and the University of Manchester, which trains mental health nurses and other professionals to deliver research-based care and treatment programmes to people suffering from severe and enduring mental illness (Gournay 1997).

UK government reviews of mental health nursing

A major review of psychiatric nursing *Psychiatric Nursing: Today and Tomorrow* published in 1968 by the then Ministry of Health (Standing Mental Health and Standing Nursing Advisory Committees 1968), focused particularly on inpatient psychiatric nursing, which was the dominant setting for care in that period. This report highlighted the importance of the personal relationship between the nurse and patient as central to the nurse's role. Among other recommendations it identified the need for psychiatric nurses to develop skills in psychotherapy, a view which resonated with Peplau's (1952) interpersonal relations approach to mental health nursing, which was promoted by opinion leaders of the time, such as Altschul (of whom more later). Altschul had endorsed interpersonal skill development for mental health nurses several years previously (Altschul 1964) and had demonstrated its absence in her study of nurse–patient interaction published in 1972 as *Patient–Nurse Interaction in Psychiatric Acute Wards* (Altschul 1972).

A further 26 years were to pass before the next government review of mental health nursing, by which time the context of mental health nursing was much changed. The Thatcher years (1979–90), the *NHS and Community Care Act* (1990), and the development of the internal market in health care with purchaser and provider roles had led to a very different care environment. Marked advances in medical science had led to new drugs (for example, Prozac) and a growing confidence in some psychological therapies (for example, cognitive behaviour therapy), and patients' expectations for care and treatment had risen. In addition there had been major changes in nurse education, consequent upon Project 2000 (UKCC 1986) which had moved education from hospital-based training schools into higher education, and gradual acceptance that nursing should be a research-based profession, leading more nurses to question their existing practice and seek clarification of their role. In the light of these changes, by the 1990s it seemed to many that the review of mental health nursing was both timely and necessary.

Much lobbying behind the scenes (Smith 1994) led to the review which was announced by the Department of Health in 1992 under the chairmanship of Professor Tony Butterworth. The Review Team presented its report entitled *Working in Partnership: a Collaborative Approach to Care* two years later (Mental Health Nursing (MHN) Review Team 1994). The terms of reference for the review were 'to identify the future requirements for skilled nursing care in the services for people with mental illness' (MHN Review Team 1994: vi), which the Review Team interpreted as setting out 'the future role and function of mental health nurses and their potential contribution in a wide variety of settings' (MHN Review Team 1994: 6). Evidence was collected, using a range of methods (both oral and written evidence, consultative conferences and expert advice) from a range of stakeholders involved in organizing, using and purchasing psychiatric care in a range of care settings – rural and urban, hospital and community, general and specialist services and regional centres of excellence.

The strongest message of the report was that the relationship between the nurse and service user is at the heart of nursing practice. The report states, 'This review starts from a belief that the work of mental health nurses rests on their relationship with people who use mental health services. This relationship should have value to both parties' (MHN Review Team 1994: 9). As reflected in the title, partnership between nurses and their patients that is based on trust and mutual respect is seen to lead to care that is meaningful and important to those who receive it.

Working in Partnership made 42 recommendations grouped under the following headings: the relationship between nurses and people who use services, the practice of mental health nurses, delivery of services, challenging issues and research and education. The review identified a central role for mental health nurses in the provision of mental health services. Among its recommendations was that nurses should: act as keyworkers, become involved in supervised discharge, and take the lead as providers of information to service-users. The report urged increased opportunities for patients to become involved in their care in partnership with nurses and for nurses to focus their work on the care of people with serious and enduring mental illness. The focus of mental health nurses on this group has strengthened over the past decade and this recommendation is perhaps the most enduring contribution of the report to mental health nursing policy.

The Review Team supported the change in title from 'psychiatric nurse' to 'mental health nurse', on the grounds that this represents the broadening scope of contemporary practice and endorsed continuation of the specialist pre-registration branch of mental health nursing, rather than the creation of a generic nurse and conversion of mental health nursing into a post-registration specialty. The report made recommendations also about the quality and nature of services for patients, including: questioning the value psychiatric units attached to district general hospitals, supporting choice for patients in single-sex accommodation, and gender of key workers. In addition it urged the development of clinical supervision, a focus on the professional training needs of nursing staff still based in the old mental hospitals and increased opportunities for nurses to contribute to and to access up-to-date research-based information upon which to base their practice.

Almost a decade has passed since the publication of *Working in Partnership*, but in the intervening years its impact on mental health nursing is difficult to gauge. Its recommendations were not prioritized or costed and the report itself appears to have received only a lukewarm reception from the government of the day, probably because of its potential cost implications. Writing at the time, Butterworth (1994) points out that it was 'regrettable' that the executive letter that accompanies the report from the then Chief Executive of the National Health Service Management Executive, 'was warm rather than commanding' (Butterworth 1994: 42). Thus, mental health service providers and purchasers of the time were not obliged to respond to its recommendations.

Smith (1994), in a critique published shortly after *Working in Partnership* was released, criticizes the Review Team for interpreting their brief so widely, a course of action which she considers brave but foolish: 'Brave because they (the Review Team) believed that mental health nursing required a wide-ranging overview; foolish because to pursue a course of action outside their remit was to beg an indifferent response and perhaps to consign the report to the shelf' (Smith 1994: 182).

Smith is critical, in particular, of the report's limited attention to defining the skills of the mental health nurse, which, in spite of being central to its terms of reference, are listed in an annexe, 'as if an afterthought rather than the key task of the Report' (1994: 181). With the benefit of hindsight Smith's criticism seems valid. Under the growing influence of the evidence-based practice movement (discussed below), which emphasizes the importance of good technique, there have been several influential attempts to define the core skills and competencies of nurses and other mental health workers, by the Sainsbury Centre, in particular; for example, the core skills, knowledge and attitudes required by mental health staff working with people with severe mental illness (SCMH 1997) and, more recently, capabilities of the mental health workforce (SCMH 2000; SCMH and NHSE 2001). The *Working in Partnership* review offered nurses an opportunity to focus clearly on their skills before others did, but this opportunity was missed.

Working in Partnership contained little that was new, and much of it endorsed conventional wisdom of the time. But it was valued by mental nurses for clarifying their roles at a time of great change in the development of mental health services, and for shoring up the boundaries of the specialty by rejecting generic pre-registration education which would, many feared, dilute mental health nurses' unique identity and contribution to care (Norman 1998). However, it paid too little attention to psychological and other interventions of proven effectiveness delivered by nurses to patients, and the skills required to do this. Although *Working in Partnership* acknowledges the importance of mental health nursing being research based, in the 1990s the specialty had yet to feel the impact of the evidence-based health care movement, which some nurses now perceive to threaten mental health nursing in the interpersonal relations tradition.

Orientations

In this section we trace the origins of two contrasting orientations to mental health nursing to the influential ideas of Hilda Peplau and the rise and rise of evidence-based health care.

Nursing in the interpersonal relations tradition: Peplau and her legacy

The interpersonal relations orientation of mental health nursing can be traced directly to Hildegard (Hilda) Peplau who was a major figure in mental health nursing from the early 1950s until her death at the age of 89 in 1999. Described by some of her admirers as the 'mother of psychiatric nursing' (Barker 1999: 175) Peplau was the first to coin the term 'nurse–patient relationship' and her book *Interpersonal Relations in Nursing* (1952) became a classic and is still widely read, having been reprinted in London in 1988.

Born in Reading, Pennsylvania in 1909 Peplau graduated as a nurse from Pottsdown, Pennsylvania School of Nursing in 1931. After a varied career as a general nurse Peplau became fascinated by psychiatry and took a BA degree in interpersonal psychology from Bennington College in Vermont in 1943. At Bennington College Peplau studied with Erich Fromm, the foremost post-Freudian analyst of his day; and during this period worked on children's wards in Bellvue Hospital in New York, and also at Chestnut Lodge, a private psychiatric hospital in Rockville, Maryland. It was at Chestnut Lodge that Peplau came into contact with Harry Stack Sullivan, a psychiatrist, who was developing an interpersonal theory of psychiatric illness (Sullivan 1947). For Sullivan psychiatry was not concerned simply with the study of mentally ill people or group processes, but was a broader enterprise concerned with 'the study of what goes on between two or more people, all but one of whom may be completely illusory' (Peplau 1987: 202).

Peplau's major contribution in *Interpersonal Relations in Nursing* was to apply and so develop Sullivan's theoretical perspective to the interpersonal world of the nurse and patient. For Peplau (1987) mental health nursing is an important, therapeutic, interpersonal process characterized by three overlapping and interlocking phases in the nurse–patient relationship – orientation, working and termination. Her study of interpersonal relations revealed for Peplau various roles for the nurse; as, for example, a resource person, teacher, surrogate parent and leader. Later she was to describe these as 'sub-roles' and the role of counsellor or psychotherapist as the heart of psychiatric nursing. Through the medium of their relationships with patients nurses strive to create conditions that aim to promote health and develop patients' ability to engage with those around them.

In 1954 Peplau established the first graduate-level programme for clinical nurse specialists in psychiatric nursing and led this programme until her formal retirement in 1974. During this period, and thereafter, she developed her ideas on interpersonal relations in conference papers and publications (for example Peplau 1987, 1994).

Peplau's influence on UK mental health nursing

Peplau's ideas took a long time to influence academic psychiatric nursing in the UK and it was not until the late 1970s and early 1980s that they gained a secure foothold. A number of mental health nurses contributed to the diffusion of Peplau's ideas in the UK, but we single out two as being particularly influential: Annie Altschul and Phil Barker.

Altschul

Annie Altschul was immediately aware of the importance of *Interpersonal Relations in Nursing* in providing a framework for psychiatric nursing practice, and promoted it. In 1958 Altschul won a Commonwealth Scholarship to study psychiatric nurse education in the USA, in particular psychiatric

nurse training for general nursing students. During her trip she was introduced to a nursing curriculum that focused on helping nurses to establish
relationships with patients, to use these relationships to move forward
patients' recovery and rehabilitation, and terminate these relationships at an
appropriate time. Nolan (1999) explains that while this approach presented
practical difficulties, such as several nurses being attached to one patient at
the same time, Altschul became convinced that this was the way forward for
mental health nursing in the UK. Such relationships she believed evolved
over time and were fostered by good mentoring, supervision and support of
students, and also by nurses being accountable for their actions. Over the
next four decades Altschul was well placed to promote her ideas, first as
Principal Tutor at the Maudsley Hospital in London and from 1964 at the
University of Edinburgh where in 1976 she became the first psychiatric
nurse to hold a Chair in Nursing in the UK. She was Emeritus Professor of
Nursing at the University of Edinburgh until her death.

Altschul's main contribution to the psychiatric nursing research literature, published in 1972 as *Patient-nurse Interaction*, is her study towards an
MPhil degree of how therapeutic relationships between nurses and patients
could be established and developed in an inpatient ward. Data collection
involved Altschul observing and timing didactic nurse–patient interactions
in acute psychiatric wards in the Royal Edinburgh Hospital. For interactions
of five minutes' duration or more Altschul asked the nurse what had taken
place, on the assumption that these more lengthy interactions were those
when a special therapeutic relationship is most likely to develop between
nurse and patient, or that interaction would be underpinned by therapeutic
principles or intent.

Altschul's study looked for evidence of therapeutic principles underpinning interactions between nurses and patients, but in this she was to be
disappointed. She found that nurses in her study did 'not have any identifiable perspective to guide them in their interactions with patients' and the
nurses themselves saw mental health nursing as "just common sense" '
(Altschul 1972: 192). She concludes that the relationship between the nurse
and the patient was 'irrelevant to psychiatric treatment' (1972: 193). In spite
of this, most patients described their relationship with the nurses as helpful;
although this finding must be considered in the light of patients' reluctance to
criticize nurses, particularly when they are hospitalized and feel vulnerable.

Altschul does not explain clearly the criteria she used for rating interactions for therapeutic content, or her cut-off point of five minutes, rather
than four or three. But, a more fundamental limitation of her study, as
Macilwaine (1983) points out, is her assumption that the nurses she
studied should have based their practice according to theoretical principles,
specifically those relevant to forming personal relationships with patients.
Although Peplau's writings were popular in the USA, nurse training in
the UK in the 1960s did not emphasize nurse–patient relationships. Thus,
Altschul's finding that nurses regarded their practice as just common
sense could have been confidently predicted. Altschul's study is important,
nevertheless, because it was the first British clinical study of mental health

nursing carried out by a nurse. Moreover, published only four years after the government's 1968 review of mental health nursing, *Psychiatric Nursing Today and Tomorrow* (Standing Mental Health and Standing Nursing Advisory Committees 1968), it proved a great impetus to UK mental health nurse education being oriented towards providing nurses with knowledge and skills to form relationships with patients and use these therapeutically. *Patient-nurse Interaction* established Altschul's commitment to the study of therapeutic relationships in psychiatric nursing. It also influenced the work of subsequent researchers (for example, Towell 1975; Cormack 1983) and the direction of, in particular, pre-registration nurse education in the UK in the late 1970s and 1980s, which emphasized the acquisition of interpersonal skills (see, for example, ENB and WNB 1982).

An interesting footnote is that towards the end of her life Altschul was to revise her position on the central position of the nurse–patient relationship to nursing practice. Reflecting on her professional life in 1999 Altschul (1999) writes that although her observations of nurse education in the USA in 1958 convinced her that focusing nurse training around the concept of the therapeutic relationship offered substantial benefits for the nurses, she was 'much less convinced that the patients benefited'. She notes that nursing students of the time who had been well taught to establish and use their relationships with patients constructively, considered that psychiatric nursing could only be conducted under circumstances where it would be possible for nurses to have a well-defined caseload of patients with whom they could have time restricted, intensive one-to-one relationships. In the USA in the late 1950s this could be achieved only if nurses were based in private practice. Altschul reports that she was unconvinced at the time, but had changed her mind. The distinctive contribution of nurses to patient care is often attributed to their continuous presence with patients, in contrast with the sporadic appearance of others such as the psychiatrist, psychologist or occupational therapist. Altschul's position in 1999 appears to be that a continuing presence between the nurse and patient, as occurs in inpatient care, is not conducive to the development and constructive use of therapeutic relationships, since giving attention to a ward of patients is too draining for nurses and relationships with several nurses, simultaneously, is too demanding for inpatients.

Barker

The continuing development of the interpersonal relations orientation within UK mental health nursing literature and practice is well illustrated by the work of Philip (Phil) Barker, formerly Professor of Psychiatric Nursing Practice at the University of Newcastle-upon-Tyne. Barker has written extensively on a range of issues, which include people in psychosis, suicidal depression, nursing assessment and the role of the psychiatric nurse. It is his views on the latter with which we are concerned here.

Unlike Peplau whose *Interprofessional Relations in Nursing* set the agenda for most of her subsequent work, Barker's views on the role and focus of the psychiatric nurse have emerged over time from a series of published papers some of the more important we refer to in the annotated reading list which follows this chapter. His views on the proper focus of psychiatric nursing owe much to his long interest and study of Oriental philosophy and to the influence of writers such as Ed Podvol (also influenced by Buddhism), psychiatrists such as Szasz, his long friendship with Peplau and Altschul, and also first-hand accounts of mental disorder from service users.

One of Barker's recent initiatives is the development, testing and dissemination of the Tidal Model (Barker 2003) which was introduced into practice at Newcastle City Health Trust in the UK in May 2000, supported by a multi-media training programme for nurses (Barker 2003) and an action-research project to follow its development. Barker's Tidal Model website in late 2003 (Barker 2003) reports that over 70 different Tidal Model projects have been established in the UK, Ireland, New Zealand, Canada and Australia in a wide range of therapeutic settings suggesting that the model might be applied to address people's human needs, irrespective of their clinical diagnosis.

The Tidal Model, which draws on nautical metaphors, is based upon four closely related ideas (Barker 2003):

* Life for us all is a journey on an 'ocean of experience'. Psychiatric crises are one thing among many that disrupt people's 'life journey'. The ultimate aim of mental health care is to return people to that ocean (within the community) to continue their voyage.

* Empowerment is the primary goal of the caring process, so that people are able to take greater control over their lives. This reflects Barker's concept of nursing, developed several years previously, as a social process for facilitating human growth and development, or what he terms 'trephotaxis'.

* Change is a constant feature of the life journey, although we may be unaware of it. One aim of interventions within the Tidal Model is to raise people's awareness of the small changes that occur that, ultimately, will have a large effect on their lives.

* Effective nursing occurs when 'the nurse and the person are united (albeit temporarily) like dancers in a dance', when it is difficult or impossible 'to tell the dancers from the dance'. 'Nursing is something, which involves caring with people, rather than for them or even just about them' (Barker 2003).

The interpersonal relations tradition and recovery

The interpersonal relations approach to mental health nursing practice, particularly as expressed by Barker's Tidal Model seems to have common ground with the emerging literature on recovery, which is discussed in detail by Perkins and Repper in Chapter 5 and drawn upon by us in Chapter 30. Recovery has been used traditionally within the medical literature to refer to clinical recovery, that is reduction of symptoms. However, over the past 15 years a more personalized, subjective definition of recovery and an approach to caring for persons with mental distress has been emerging in the mental health care literature, particularly from the writings of service users. Recovery as described by service users emphasizes aspects of the recovery process other than clinical recovery, in particular improved social circumstances (for example having friends, paid employment, a reasonable standard of living) and positive changes in self-concept (for example rekindling of hope, active coping, a renewed sense of self). This personal dimension of recovery is illustrated clearly in Anthony's (1993) description of recovery as:

> a deeply personal, unique process of changing one's attitudes, values, feelings, goals, skills and/or roles. It is a way of living a satisfying, hopeful and contributing life, even with limitations caused by the illness. Recovery involves the development of new meaning and purpose in one's life as one grows beyond the catastrophic effects of mental illness.
> (Anthony 1993: 12)

Although these personal and social dimensions of recovery are relatively new arrivals in the mental health care literature, actions by nurses, which can contribute to the personal and social recovery of people in distress can be seen clearly in the well-established interpersonal relations tradition of mental health nursing.

Supporting and facilitating recovery which highlights two areas of work for mental health nurses: helping people with mental illness adapt and respond positively to the challenges that face them; and tackling social disability, that is the ways in which a person in distress is disabled by the expectations of those around them (Repper 2000). The first area highlights mental health nursing as an interpersonal process, one in which the nurse–patient (person in distress) relationship is central and in itself therapeutic. The nurse needs to become the person's trusted 'ally', supporting them through the good and bad times in their illness and providing them with practical help. Nurses need to:

1   believe in the person's capacity to recover, however severe their problems;

2   be honest, clear and informative in their interactions with them;

3   be genuinely interested in and take account of their viewpoint and feelings; and

4   draw on this information in ways that will help them.

The second area of work involves nurses helping people to negotiate the hostile world around them and to fulfil their roles, relationships and activities, and access the facilities they need to rebuild their lives. In this the nurse's relationship with the person remains central, since the nurse may accompany the person to social gatherings (the pub, the church) to encourage and support them and give them the confidence to interact with others and to manage rejection. As Repper points out such activities may also change public attitudes to mental illness in a positive direction, since such attitudes are more amenable to personal acquaintance with a person who has found ways to cope with mental health problems than to public education, for example (Repper and Brooker 1996, 1997; Repper *et al.* 1997).

Evidence-based health care

The view that mental health nursing practice should be evidence based has emerged strongly over the past 15 years and is supported strongly by government policy documents on mental health services both in the UK and other developed countries. The evidence-based practice movement reflects increasing confidence in scientifically proven methods for treating mental illness. It reflects too certain assumptions about mental health services currently, notably that they either do not provide evidence-based practices, or lack fidelity to evidence-based procedures, and that given resource constraints, patients have a right to treatments with proven efficacy.

Evidence-based health care has a long history dating back, say some authorities, to post-revolutionary Paris, when physicians like Pierre Louis rejected the wisdom of authorities that venesection was good for cholera, and sought answers in the systematic observation of patients (Rangachari 1997). However, it was in 1992 that the term 'evidence-based medicine' was coined by a group led by Gordon Guyatt at McMaster University Medical School in Canada. The term has spread globally since, and 'medicine' has been replaced by 'health care' as other health care professionals, including mental health nurses, have adopted its principles.

Evidence-based medicine (health care) is defined by Sackett *et al.* (2000) as the integration of three main elements:

- Best research evidence, i.e. clinically relevant research often in the basic medical sciences but, in particular, clinical research into the accuracy of diagnostic tests, the predictive power of prognostic markers and the efficacy and safety of preventive, therapeutic and rehabilitative treatments (interventions).

- Clinical expertise, i.e. effective use of clinical skills to assess the risks and benefits of particular interventions for individual patients, given their diagnosis, general state of health.

- Patient values, i.e. taking into account in making clinical decisions, patients' particular concerns, expectations and values.

Critics of evidence-based health care tend to emphasize the first two of Sackett's elements, but pay little attention to the third, which demonstrates that evidence-based health care is not incompatible with a patient-centred approach. Indeed Sackett *et al.* (2000) point out that when these three elements are integrated in clinical decision making, the outcome will be a therapeutic alliance between the clinician and the health care professional, which will optimize the patient's clinical outcomes and quality of life.

But why the sudden interest in evidence-based health care? Sackett *et al.*'s (2000) comments in relation to evidence-based medicine apply to evidence-based health care more generally. Sackett and colleagues point to the realization that:

- busy health care professionals need on-the-spot valid information about diagnosis, prognosis, therapy, prevention and care but can set aside very little time for general reading or study; moreover

- traditional sources of this information are inadequate because they are out of date (for example, textbooks), wrong (for example, views of 'experts'), ineffective (for example, didactic continuing professional education), or overwhelming in their volume and diversity (for example, health care journals).

As a result there is an increasing disparity between health care professionals' skills and clinical judgement, which tend to improve over time, and their knowledge base and clinical performance, which decline. Until recently these problems were insurmountable for busy health care professionals, but now several recent developments have enabled this state of affairs to be tackled. The most important of these are:

- The development of strategies for tracking down and appraising the validity and relevance of evidence. Steps in this process include:

  1 translating information needs into answerable clinical questions;

  2 tracking down the best evidence with which to answer that question;

  3 appraising that evidence for its validity, impact (effect size) and applicability to clinical practice;

  4 integrating this critical appraisal with knowledge of a patient's unique personal circumstances; and

  5 evaluating how steps 1–4 were carried out, and identifying how they might be carried out more efficiently and effectively next time.

  Steps 1–3, in particular, are the focus of a growing number of evidence-based decision making in health care courses and manuals (for example, Greenhalgh and Donald 2000; Sackett *et al.* 2000) that are available.

- The development of systematic reviews and concise summaries of the effects of health care, many of which have been conducted by groups operating under the umbrella of the Cochrane Collaboration.

- The expansion of evidence-based journals of secondary publications (for example, *Evidence-Based Nursing, Evidence Based Mental Health*) that publish around 2 per cent of clinical papers that are considered to offer valid evidence to guide clinical practice.

- The development of information technology, which enables almost immediate access to evidence-based journals and systematic reviews.

- Increasing emphasis on lifelong learning and better understanding of strategies, which are effective in this and for improving clinical performance; much work in this field has been undertaken by the Cochrane Effective Practice and Organization of Care Group (EPOC).

The methods of evidence-based health care are developed most fully in relation to questions of treatment effectiveness. So, for example, there is a well-established hierarchy of evidence which identifies various types and grades of evidence which relate in turn to the robustness of the evidence source, and so how much it can be trusted to provide a valid answer to questions treatment of effectiveness. The hierarchy of evidence used by the authors of the *NSF for Mental Health* (DH 1999), is shown in Box 3.1.

Box 3.1 Levels of evidence

Type 1 evidence: at least one good systematic review, including at least one randomized controlled trial.

Type 2 evidence: at least one good randomized controlled trial.

Type 3 evidence: at least one well-designed intervention study without randomization.

Type 4 evidence: at least one well-designed observational study.

Type 5 evidence: expert opinion, including the opinion of service users and carers.

(After *NSF for Mental Health*, DH 1999: 6)

In this hierarchy the randomized controlled trial (RCT) (Type 2 evidence) is considered to offer the highest level of research evidence to answer effectiveness questions, apart from the well-conducted systematic review, which must include at least one RCT (Type 1 evidence). However, by definition, the concerns of evidence-based health care must go beyond the clinical trial because the search is for the best available evidence to answer a clinical question. In the hierarchy readers will note that expert opinion, *including the opinions of service users and carers* is at the bottom of the pile (Type 5 evidence); evidence from this source is to be trusted only in the absence of anything better! This should not always be the case for mental health nurses, however, as we argue later in this chapter.

A leading UK mental health nurse in the evidence-based practice tradition is Kevin Gournay, Professor of Psychiatric Nursing at the Institute of Psychiatry, King's College London, and a contributor to this book (cf. Chapter 15). Gournay rejects discrete nursing activities in favour of multi-disciplinary approaches to care and treatment. His primary focus is not nurses' relationships with patients, but on 'extending' nurses' roles (to incorporate the roles occupied previously by doctors and psychologists, for example) so that they can contribute fully to delivering evidence-based interventions to patients with recognized mental illness.

Gournay recommends more RCTs to test the efficacy of interventions in which nurses are involved – and has contributed substantially to the research literature in this respect, in collaboration with psychiatrists and psychologists, in particular; for example evaluations of nurses as counsellors (Gournay and Brooking 1994) and the Thorn Programme, a training course for nurses and other health care professionals in the care of people with severe and enduring mental illness (Gournay 1997). Today, Gournay and other nurses in the evidence-based tradition are, we perceive, more ready than previously to recognize the practical limitations of the RCT in the complex field of mental health services. As a result they are more inclined to see the RCT as perhaps the most important, but as only one of several research methods, which can be used to understand nurses' work with patients. Other research designs valued within the evidence-based tradition include epidemiological studies to assess the health needs of populations and also qualitative research methods to examine the nature and experience of mental health nursing interventions. However, in Gournay's view, qualitative studies are best carried out in combination with quantitative research studies and vice versa; a view with which some qualitative researchers would take issue.

In mental health care today the research evidence supports a relatively small set of interventions. Drake *et al.* (2001) identifies these as: prescription of medications within prescribed parameters, education designed to help patients and carers to manage their illness, assertive community treatment, family psycho-education, supported employment and integrated treatment for patients with co-occurring substance use disorders. Although traditional outcomes, such as adherence to treatment, relapse or rehospitalization prevention, are important – consumer-oriented outcomes such as independence, employment, satisfying relationships and good quality of life (the social dimensions of recovery) are recognized as important too. So described, evidence-based practice seems unassailable. Who could object to promoting treatments that are proved to work (however defined) as opposed to ones that do not?

But nurses within the interpersonal relations tradition are unconvinced. Barker (2003) challenges the assumption of evidence-based health care that nurses need to learn new skills and approaches to care that are tried and tested. He writes:

> Many nurses are encouraged to believe that they need to develop 'new' skills or learn 'new' therapeutic models, in order to become effective in mental health care. The Tidal Model challenges such assumptions . . . Nursing originally meant to offer nourishment. Nothing has changed across the centuries. Today, people in mental distress need the nourishment that nursing can offer. They need the human support that will help them deal more effectively with the tidal forces that have rocked their lives. They need help to gain the confidence to get back in the boat and push off, from the shore, to begin again the journey on their ocean of experience.
>
> (Barker 2003, http://www.tidalmodel.co.uk)

Other mental health nurse researchers in the interpersonal relations tradition are critical of the RCT which they regard as an inappropriate research method for mental health nursing, because it fails, as they say, to recognize the importance of individual experience, which is crucial to the proper focus of mental health nursing. This argument, as expressed by Rolfe (1996) for example, proposes that unlike medicine and psychology, mental health nurses should not be concerned with putting people into diagnostic categories, providing treatment appropriate to that diagnosis and assessing the effectiveness of this through a well-conducted RCT. Mental health nurses should be concerned with differences between people, rather than similarities between them. The focus of mental health nursing should be on individual presentation of a particular problem, rather than providing *general* interventions to meet *general* problems experienced by people who happen to be in a particular diagnostic category. This is because problems experienced by a group of people generally (for example poor attention span in schizophrenia) is only an approximate guide to the problems experienced by the individual; reduced concentration span might not *be* a problem to the person at all. For Rolfe, the approach to mental health nursing advocated by supporters of evidence-based health care and the RCT runs the danger of swallowing up the specific needs of particular individuals 'in a general solution to a perceived common problem' (Rolfe 1996: 333).

In response to an article by Gournay advocating the RCT for mental health nursing research Rolfe says, 'Gournay's assertion that we should employ "the rigor of RCTs" is inappropriate and misleading, as are the findings from such studies (see for example, Gournay and Brooking 1994)' . . . Rolfe concludes. 'The proper focus of nursing is the therapeutic relationship, and we (mental health nurses) must demonstrate on our own terms and not on the terms of medicine that this focus is effective' (Rolfe 1996: 333).

We do not share Rolfe's aversion to the well-conducted RCT, which is the ideal study design to answer questions of treatment effectiveness for groups of people in well-defined categories. It presents practical problems in the complex world of mental health nursing interventions and services and is probably not the best choice of research method to investigate therapeutic relationships. But therapeutic relationships are not, in our view, the only proper focus for mental health nurses. As the title of this book suggests, mental health nursing is a science as well as an art. The art of nursing is concerned with therapeutic relationships, with a person's internal world and sense of self (with the left-hand quadrants of the schema we introduced in Chapter 2 to integrate models of mental disorder – see Figure 2.1). The science of nursing, in contrast, is concerned with a person's biophysiological profile and their observable behaviour (with the right-hand quadrants of our schema). Nurses must be concerned with change in all four quadrants in response to pharmacological and psychosocial interventions (covered in Chapters 10 and 11), or different forms of care organization – such as assertive community treatment (covered in Chapters 22 and 29).

Notwithstanding the contribution of clinical trials to the knowledge base of mental health nursing, it is also true however, that in their daily work with individual service users evidence from the upper end of the hierarchy of evidence shown in Box 3.1, is of greatest practical value to nurses in the absence of detailed knowledge of the service user as a person – at first assessment or in early stages of a mental illness, for example. In such cases an important question for the nurse in planning care is, 'How far is this individual similar to the sample of individuals for whom this or that treatment intervention has been found to be effective, as demonstrated by the most valid research evidence available?' As the nurse gathers detailed knowledge of the service user as a person, however, sources of high quality evidence become much less useful for individualized care planning. In such cases the important question is, 'What treatment interventions have worked best for this individual in the past, when they have been in a similar situation and/or have behaved in similar ways?' Evidence from clinical trials cannot answer this question. The best source of evidence is often found at the bottom of the hierarchy, in Type 5 evidence (expert opinion), the experts in such cases being service users and their carers whose knowledge of what works best for this person and when, trumps evidence produced by any number of trials.

In summary, evidence-based health care is a movement with a long history whose time has now come. Its assumption that the well-conducted randomized controlled trial (RCT) is the gold standard for determining outcome and should be the ultimate test for any health care intervention, including interventions in mental health nursing, is held by many nurses and the majority of researchers in allied disciplines (such as psychology and psychiatry), and (importantly) by those responsible for funding projects and making public policy. While the hierarchy of evidence adopted by the *NSF for Mental Health* is valuable to mental health nurses who seek to appraise the evidence base of their own practice, there are circumstances when nurses would do best to turn the hierarchy on its head and give most weight to the expert opinions of service users and their carers.

Conclusion

A historical perspective shows that mental health nursing has and continues to be shaped by responses to the challenges presented by people with mental disorder that arise in each succeeding era. It arose under the patronage of the medical profession at a time when philanthropy was fashionable, and its development has been linked closely with developments in psychiatric medicine. A historical perspective shows too that early developments of the nurse's role as a therapeutic agent, as envisaged by advocates of moral treatment, was undermined by social forces which meant that by the early twentieth century asylums became warehouses for madness, and dumping grounds for socially disadvantaged people who were difficult to manage. Hence, nurses became an essential element in a bureaucratic system for organizing patients' lives, a role that involved operating within rigid doctor/ nurse/patient hierarchies to contain large numbers of people in often overcrowded conditions. Nurses throughout this period were, for the most part, poorly educated, undervalued and very poorly paid. They led routinized working lives that were compensated to some extent by an active community life within the hospitals based on sports and social activities. However, in spite of the regulation and impersonal procedures that characterized patient care in the old hospitals, accounts from nurses working in the postwar period paint a sense of common purpose between nurses and patients in communities that were self-contained and virtually self-supporting (Nolan and Hooper 2000).

The strength of the old mental hospitals lay in their structure. This structure did not allow mental health nursing to grow and develop, because it did not provide opportunities for independent thinking and action. But it did provide nurses with a sense of security and a common shared identity based on a clear sense of their place within the hospital structure without a need to define the nursing role and remit, or the underpinning values or knowledge-base of the discipline.

The decline and closure of the psychiatric hospitals in the 1960s and 1970s and their replacement by smaller units attached to local district hospitals, day hospitals and community care facilities marked a sea of change for psychiatric nursing practice which became community based. Community psychiatric nursing services, which were initially hospital based and medically oriented, developed over the years to encompass broader social approaches to mental health care. Mental nurses themselves became increasingly specialized and, particularly those working in primary care teams, enjoyed relative autonomy from the psychiatrists. Nolan and Hooper (2000) argue that the breakdown of the old hospitals, the supportive infra-structure they provided and the development of community-based mental health care faced mental health nursing with a crisis of identify from which it has yet to recover.

Two UK government reviews of mental health nursing, the first published in 1968 and the second in 1994, set out the roles and responsibilities of mental health nurses, and in so doing clarified the identity of the discipline at times of great change in society and in mental health services. Both reports, in particular *Working in Partnership*, affirmed that the work of the mental health nurse rests fundamentally on their relationships with patients, so reflecting the major influence of Peplau's ideas, which had become well known in the UK under the influence of Altschul and others during the 1970s and 1980s, and revisions of the pre-registration mental health nursing curriculum (for example ENB and WNB 1982) to emphasize teaching of interpersonal skills. With the benefit of hindsight it is clear that the report paid too little attention to psychological and other interventions of proven effectiveness delivered by nurses to patients, and the skills required to do this. However, it played an important role in re-directing the focus of mental health nurses to the care of people with severe and enduring mental illness, a focus which continues today.

In our distinction between the interpersonal relations and evidence-based practice orientations in mental health nursing we see a long-running debate between those who emphasize the 'art' of mental health nursing and those who emphasize the 'science'. This distinction reflects all left-hand quadrants (artists) and all right-hand quadrants (scientists) in the schema used to integrate models of mental disorder introduced in Chapter 2 (Figure 2.1). The debate between artists and scientists is not unique to nursing, but is present in all practice disciplines. It reflects differing research traditions (phenomenological v. scientific) and differing views about what passes as knowledge (Repper 2000).

The artists, much influenced by Peplau's (1952) emphasis on the nurse–patient relationship, are concerned primarily with understanding 'the process of nursing as a discrete activity based on a relationship between the nurse and the individual person in distress. In contrast the scientists are concerned primarily with specific interventions or treatments for patients with diagnosed mental illness' (Repper 2000: 576).

For most artists mental health nursing has a distinct and unique identity, which has a clear value base and is readily identifiable in any context. By contrast scientists see nursing as a 'function' that contributes to and is shaped by a multi-disciplinary mental health service. Artists go to great pains to clarify nursing values, roles and activities; to make explicit the particular contribution of nursing to the care of people in emotional distress. Scientists are little concerned with such questions – for them, nurses are there to deliver tried and tested interventions to mentally ill patients. A good relationship between the nurse and patient is taken for granted by scientists. It is important, because without this the patient is unlikely to take advice, but this relationship is simply one aspect of the treatment approach and is not a priority for study in its own right. Artists may formulate or draw upon normative models of nursing (Peplau's interpersonal relations 'model' or Barker's 'Tidal Model', for instance) that set out ways in which nurses should work with distressed people. For scientists normative models of nursing are to be discouraged because in distinguishing nursing from other care approaches they reinforce a tribal mentality and so can lead to a fragmented and poorly coordinated care approach (Gournay 1997).

The distinction between artists and scientists is not so clear cut as our description suggests. Practising mental health nurses in the UK today are influenced by both traditions discussed in this chapter and most tread a middle path; this book, as the title indicates, is written primarily for them. However, the traditions do influence the direction of mental health nursing as a practice discipline. The evidence-based health care tradition has spawned within nursing a group of expert practitioners, who have the capacity and aspiration to take over many of the functions associated traditionally with psychiatric medicine. Barker (2000) foresees that it is a only a matter of time before this group of nurses takes over most of the functions of medicine, and also social work and psychology, following the lead taken by North American Advanced Nurse Practitioners. Soon they will have powers of admission and discharge, prescribing drugs and of detaining people under the Mental Health Act.

In turn, the interpersonal relations tradition has spawned nurses who reject psychiatric 'scientism', and who seek to develop instead what Barker and Whitehill (1997) refer to as 'a craft of caring' aimed at producing human beings who are able to meet the immediate personal needs of other human beings who use mental health services. This group of nurses, much influenced by Peplau's emphasis on the nurse–patient relationship and the emerging literature on 'recovery', have forged close links with service users (for example, Coleman and Smith 1997), and may in future break the professional boundary of nursing to evolve into mental health workers who offer health care alternatives, perhaps informed by the personal experience of being a mental health service user themselves (Barker 2000).

An important question is whether these different care traditions to mental health nursing care can coexist. More specifically, can mental health nursing in the evidence based health care tradition, which emphasizes external scientific reality, accommodate the more subjective, personalized approach to nursing care in the interpersonal relations tradition? Opinions are mixed. Gournay (2000) calls for nursing to get in step with mainstream (evidence-based) psychiatric research and practice; sentiments that highlight Barker's fear that mental health nursing 'looks set to narrow its focus abandoning some of its traditional values in the hope of gaining a public vote of confidence' (Barker 2000: 618). In contrast Barker (2000) calls for the discipline to respect diversity and value difference in its ranks, so recognizing that different sorts of mental health service user need different sorts of services at different times.

But how might this work out in practice? One solution is suggested by Frese *et al.*'s (2001) attempt to integrate evidence-based practices and the recovery model of mental health services, which rests upon the ability of the patient to make rational decisions. Thus it might be that for persons who do not have the capacity to make decisions a paternalistic, externally reasoned evidence-based treatment approach is quite appropriate, and in their best interest. Leaving treatment decisions to those who are unable to make them rationally is tantamount to abandonment. However, as these patients benefit from these treatments, they become 'persons' who must be afforded a larger role in selecting treatments and services for themselves. In these circumstances a close relationship with nurses who support them to make such decisions and to, once again, take control of their lives may be crucial to their recovery. Thus patients need tried and tested interventions within the evidence-based health care tradition, so that they can become well enough to benefit fully from the interpersonal relations approach, the traditional strength of mental health nursing.

To conclude we summarize the main points of this chapter below:

- A historical perspective shows that the practice discipline of mental health nursing arose under the patronage of the medical profession and its development has been linked closely with developments in psychiatric medicine.

- The origins of the much discussed therapeutic nurse–patient relationship can be traced to 'moral treatment', which was, however, undermined by asylums becoming dumping grounds for socially disadvantaged people who were difficult to manage.

- The breakdown of the asylum system heralded a period of insecurity but also of opportunity for nursing to grow and develop new ways of working with people with mental health problems in the community.

- UK government reviews of mental health nursing conducted in 1968 and 1994 sought to clarify the identity and remit of mental health nursing at times of great change. The 1994 review, in particular, reaffirmed that the work of the mental health nurse rests fundamentally on their relationship with patients and redirected the role of nurses towards working with people with severe and enduring mental illness.

- We identify two contemporary orientations to UK mental health nursing: the interpersonal relations approach (the artists) and the evidence-based practice approach (the scientists). Represented as in conflict we argue that both artists and scientists are valuable to mental health service users on their road to recovery.

Questions for reflection and discussion

1 Consider the role and responsibilities of mental health nurses today compared with those of their forebears working in mental hospitals in the 1950s and 1960s.

2 How far are you convinced by the attempt to integrate the evidence-based health care and interpersonal relations traditions in mental health nursing set out in the final section of this chapter? Are there better solutions to integration, or are the two traditions irreconcilable?

Annotated bibliography

- Nolan, P.A. (1993) *A History of Mental Health Nursing*. London: Chapman & Hall. Probably the most authoritative and comprehensive history of UK mental health nursing yet written.
- *Journal of Psychiatric and Mental Health Nursing*, volumes 5(3) and 6(4). These issues are devoted to a consideration of the contribution of Hilda Peplau and Annie Altschul to mental health nursing.
- Peplau, H. (1952) *Interpersonal Relations in Nursing*. New York: G.P. Putman. Peplau was the first to coin the term 'nurse–patient

relationship' and her 1952 book was to become a classic. Contemporary ideas about the nurse–patient relationship owe a debt to Peplau's pioneering work. To her supporters Peplau presents an empirically precise theory of nursing that can be verified and developed through further research. To her critics Peplau's theory of nursing, based upon psychodynamic principles, bears little relation to the work that nurses carry out, contains few operational (empirically testable) definitions and fewer tests of validity. Read Peplau's classic text and judge for yourself.

- Barker's ideas on the proper focus of mental health nursing are set out in a series of published papers (some of the more important of which are cited below) and also on his The Tidal Model website (http://www.tidalmodel.co.uk).

  - Barker, P. (1989) Reflections on the philosophy of caring in mental health. *International Journal of Nursing Studies* **26**(2): 131–41.
  - Barker, P.J., Reynolds, W. and Stevenson, C. (1997) The human science basis of psychiatric nursing theory and practice. *Journal of Advanced Nursing* **25**(4): 660–7.
  - Barker, P., Jackson, S. and Stevenson, C. (1999) What are psychiatric nurses needed for? Developing a theory of essential nursing practice. *Journal of Psychiatric and Mental Health Nursing* **6**(4): 275–82.
  - Barker, P. (1999) *The Philosophy and Practice of Psychiatric Nursing.* Edinburgh: Churchill Livingstone.
  - Barker, P.J. (2000) Reflections on a caring as a virtue ethic within an evidence-based culture. *International Journal of Nursing Studies* **37**(4): 329–36.

- Follow the debate concerning the proper focus of nursing conducted primarily in a series of commentaries in the *Journal of Psychiatric and Mental Health Nursing*. We list some of the more important contributions below:

  - Gournay, K. (1995) What to do with nursing models. *Journal of Psychiatric and Mental Health Nursing* **2**: 352–27.
  - Barker, P.J. and Reynolds, B. (1996) Rediscovering the proper focus of nursing: a critique of Gournay's position on nursing theory and models. *Journal of Psychiatric and Mental Health Nursing* **3**: 75–80.
  - Rolfe, G. (1996) What to do with psychiatric nursing. *Journal of Psychiatric and Mental Health Nursing* **3**: 331–3.
  - Coleman, M. and Jenkins, E. (1998) Developments in mental health nursing: a critical voice. *Journal of Psychiatric and Mental Health Nursing* **5**: 355–9.
  - Clarke, L. (1999) *Challenging Ideas in Psychiatric Nursing.* London: Routledge.
  - Grant, A. (2001) Psychiatric nursing and organizational power. *Journal of Psychiatric and Mental Health Nursing* **8**: 173–88.

- Norman, I.J. (1998) The changing emphasis of mental health and learning disability nurse education in the UK and ideal models of its future development. *Journal of Psychiatric and Mental Health Nursing*

5(1): 41–51. Developments in nurse education have exerted an important influence on mental health nursing as a practice discipline, but are not covered in this chapter. This paper considers the relationship between mental health and general nursing from a historical perspective and presents alternative models of pre-registration education, which reflect contrasting views of the nature of mental health nursing as a practice discipline.

References

Altschul, A. (1964) Group dynamics and nursing care. *International Journal of Nursing Studies* **1**: 151–8.

Altschul, A.T. (1972) *Patient–Nurse Interaction: A Study of Interaction Patterns in Acute Psychiatric Wards.* Edinburgh: Churchill Livingstone.

Altschul, A.T. (1999) Editorial. *Journal of Psychiatric and Mental Health Nursing* **6**(4): 261–3.

Anthony, W.A. (1993) Recovery from mental illness: the guiding vision of the mental health service system in the 1990s. *Psychosocial Rehabilitation Journal* **16**(4): 11–24.

Barker, P. (1999) Hildegard E. Peplau: the mother of psychiatric nursing: obituary. *Journal of Psychiatric and Mental Health Nursing* **6**: 175–6.

Barker, P. (2000) Commentaries and reflections on mental health nursing in the UK at the dawn of the new millennium: commentary 1. *Journal of Mental Health* **9**: 617–19.

Barker, P. (2003) *The Tidal Model.* http://www.tidalmodel.co.uk

Barker, P. and Whitehill, I. (1997) The craft of care: towards collaborative caring in psychiatric nursing, in S. Tilley (ed.) *The Mental Health Nurse: Views of Education and Practice.* Oxford: Blackwell.

Barton, R. (1959) *Institutional Neurosis.* Bristol: Wright.

Butterworth, T. (1994) Working in partnership: a collaborative approach to care. The review of mental health nursing. *Journal of Psychiatric and Mental Health Nursing* **1**: 41–4.

Chapman, G. (1992) Nursing in therapeutic communities, in J.I. Brooking, S.A.H. Ritter and B.L. Thomas (eds) *A Textbook of Psychiatric and Mental Health Nursing.* Edinburgh: Churchill Livingstone.

Coleman, R. and Smith, M. (1997) *Working with Voices: Victim to Victor.* Newton-le-Willows: Handsell Publications.

Connolly, M.J. (1992) History, in J. Brooking, S. Ritter and B. Thomas, *A Textbook of Psychiatric and Mental Health Nursing.* Edinburgh: Churchill Livingstone.

Cormack, D. (1983) *Psychiatric Nursing Described.* Edinburgh: Churchill Livingstone.

Department of Health (DH) (1999) *A National Service Framework for Mental Health.* London: DH.

Department of Health and Social Security (1975) *Better Services for the Mentally Ill.* London: HMSO.

Drake, R.E., Goldman, H.H., Leff, H.S. *et al.* (2001) Implementing evidence-based practices in routine mental health service settings. *Psychiatric Services* **52**: 45–50.

English and Welsh National Boards for Nursing, Midwifery and Health Visiting (1982) *Syllabus of Training: Professional Register – Part 3 Registered Mental Nurse*. London: ENB.

Frese, F.J., Stanley, J., Kress, K. and Vogel-Scibilia, S. (2001) Integrating evidence-based practices and the recovery model. *Psychiatric Services* **52**: 1462–8.

Goffman, E. (1961) *Asylums: Essays on the Social Situation of Mental Patients and Other Inmates*. Harmondsworth: Penguin.

Gournay, K. (1997) Responses to: 'What to do with nursing models' – a reply from Gournay. *Journal of Psychiatric and Mental Health Nursing* **4**: 227–31.

Gournay, K. (2000) Commentaries and reflections on mental health nursing in the UK at the dawn of the new millennium: commentary 2. *Journal of Mental Health* **9**: 621–3.

Gournay, K. and Brooking, J. (1994) Community psychiatric nurses in primary healthcare. *British Journal of Psychiatry* **165**: 231–8.

Greenhalgh, T. and Donald, A. (2000) *Evidence Based Health Care Workbook*. London: British Medical Journal Publications.

Hunter, P. (1974) Community psychiatric nursing: a literature review. *International Journal of Nursing Studies* **11**: 223.

Joint Board of Clinical Nursing Studies (1974) *Outline Curriculum in Community Psychiatric Nursing for Registered Nurses*.

Jones, K. (1960) *Mental Health and Social Policy 1945–59*. London: Routledge & Kegan Paul.

Macilwaine, H. (1983) The communication patterns of female neurotic patients with nursing staff in psychiatric units of general hospitals, in J. Wilson-Barnett (ed.) *Nursing Research: Ten Studies in Patient Care*. Chichester: John Wiley and Sons.

May, A.R. and Moore, S. (1963) The mental nurse in the community. *Lancet* **1**, 213–14.

McNamee, G. (1993) A changing profession: the role of nursing in home care, in P. Weller and M. Muijen, *Dimensions of Community Mental Health Care*. London: W.B. Saunders & Co. Ltd.

Mental Health Nursing Review Team (1994) *Working in Partnership*. London: Department of Health.

NHS and Community Care Act (1990). London: HMSO.

Nolan, P. (1993) *A History of Mental Health Nursing*. London: Chapman & Hall.

Nolan, P. (1999) Annie Altschul's legacy to 20th century British mental health nursing. *Journal of Psychiatric and Mental Health Nursing* **6**(4): 267–72.

Nolan, P. and Hooper, B. (2000) Revisiting mental health nursing in the 1960s. *Journal of Mental Health* **9**(6): 563–74.

Norman, I.J. (1998) Priorities for mental health and learning disability nurse education in the UK: a case study. *Journal of Clinical Nursing* **7**: 433–41.

Peplau, H. (1952) *Interpersonal Relations in Nursing*. New York: G.P. Putman.

Peplau, H. (1987) Interpersonal constructs in nursing practice. *Nursing Education Today* **7**: 201–8.

Peplau, H.E. (1994) Psychiatric mental health nursing: challenge and change. *Journal of Psychiatric and Mental Health Nursing*. **1**(1): 3–8.

Powell, J.E. (1988) My Years as Health Minister. *The Spectator*, 20 February, pp. 8–10.

Rangachari, P.K. (1997) Evidence-based medicine: old French wine with a new Canadian label. *Journal of the Royal Society of Medicine* **90**: 280–4.

Repper, J. (2000) Adjusting the focus of mental health nursing: incorporating service users' experiences of recovery. *Journal of Mental Health* **9**(6): 575–88.

Repper, J. and Brooker, C. (1996) Attitudes towards community facilities for people with serious mental health problems. *Health and Social Care in the Community* **4**: 290–399.

Repper, J. and Brooker, C. (1997) Difficulties in the measurement of outcomes in people who have serious mental health problems. *Journal of Advanced Nursing* **27**: 75–82.

Repper, J., Sayce, L., Strong, S., Wilmott, J. and Haines, M. (1997) Tall stories from the backyard. *National Survey of Local NIMBY Opposition to Community Mental Health Facilities*. London: MIND Publications.

Rolfe, G. (1996) What to do with psychiatric nursing. *Journal of Psychiatric and Mental Health Nursing* **3**: 331–3.

Sackett, D.L., Straus, S.E., Richardson, W.S., Rosenberg, W. and Haynes, R.B. (2000) *Evidence-based medicine* (2nd edn). Edinburgh: Churchill Livingstone.

Sainsbury Centre for Mental Health and NHSE North West Education Directorate (2001) *The Capable Practitioner: Report on Expert Panels for the Workforce Action Team NSF*. London: SCMH.

Sainsbury Centre for Mental Health (1997) *Pulling Together: The Future Roles and Training of Mental Health Staff*. London: SCMH.

Sainsbury Centre for Mental Health (2000) *The Capable Practitioner: A Framework and List of the Practitioner Capabilities Required to Implement the NSF for Mental Health*. Interim Report commissioned by the NSF Workforce Action Team. London: SCMH.

Scull, A. (1981) *Madhouses, Mad-doctors and Madmen*. London: Athlone.

Simmons, S. and Brooker, C. (1986) *Community Psychiatric Nursing: A Social Perspective*. London: Heinemann Nursing.

Simmons, S. and Brooker, C. (1990) *Community Psychiatric Nursing: A Social Perspective*. Oxford: Butterworth-Heinemann.

Smith, L.N. (1994) A review of the *Report on Mental Health Nursing in England: Working in Partnership*. *Journal of Psychiatric and Mental Health Nursing* **1**: 179–84.

Standing Mental Health and Standing Nursing Advisory Committees (1968) *Psychiatric Nursing Today and Tomorrow*. London: Ministry of Health – Central Health Services Council.

Sullivan, H.S. (1947) *Conceptions of Modern Psychiatry*. Washington, DC: William A. White Psychiatric Foundation.

Towell, D. (1975) *Understanding Psychiatric Nursing: A Sociological Analysis of Modern Psychiatric Nursing Practice*. London: Royal College of Nursing.

Townsend, P. (1962) *The Last Refuge: A Survey of Residential Institutions and Homes for the Aged in England and Wales*. London: Routledge & Kegan Paul.

United Kingdom Central Council for Nursing, Midwifery and Health Visiting (1986) *Project 2000: A New Preparation for Practice*. London: UKCC.

Walk, A. (1961) The history of mental nursing. *Journal of Mental Science* **107**: 466.

White, E. (1990a) The historical development of the educational preparation of CPNs, in C. Brooker (ed.) *Community Psychiatric Nursing: A Research Perspective*. London: Chapman Hall.

White, E. (1990b) *The Third Quinquennial National Survey of Community Psychiatric Nursing*. Manchester, UK: University of Manchester.

Wing, J.K. (1990) The function of asylum. *British Journal of Psychiatry* **157**: 822–7.

4

The policy and service context for mental health nursing

Richard Ford

Chapter overview

In this chapter we examine the prevalence of mental health problems and their association with socio-demographic, social and economic factors. The history of mental health service development is charted over the last 50 years and we describe current mental health service provision, and the associated roles of mental health nurses. Current mental health policy, including the *National Service Framework (NSF) for Mental Health* (DH 1999b) is examined, as is the *Capable Practitioner* framework (Lindley *et al.* 2001) for contemporary practice. We conclude by forecasting the impact of current developments on the mental health nursing roles of the future.

This chapter covers:

- mental health and mental illness;
- principles of mental health care;
- a brief history of mental health service provision since 1950;
- current services and workforce;
- current mental health policy;
- the capable practitioner;
- future practice.

We are all affected by mental health problems, although this is seldom acknowledged. Stigma, fear and ignorance may blind us to the facts. In any one year 25 per cent of us will have a recognizable mental health problem (Singleton *et al.* 2001). Nurses, like any other professional group, are not immune. All of us have either suffered from a mental health problem or been affected by the mental ill health of a close family member, friend or colleague. Mental ill health is not something that happens to other people.

Mental health and mental illness

Mental health services and the professional staff working within them are not just concerned about mental ill health. We also have a direct interest in promoting positive mental health and well-being as individuals and in our family, workplace and community (cf. Chapter 2).

Mental ill health is commonly defined by disease categories. Some authors do not see any relevance in this approach and see mental illness as a myth (Szasz 1961). They argue that the medical disease model has become an arm of the social control of 'deviant' behaviour. What psychiatrists see as the symptoms of mental illness they see as individual responses to stressful contexts. The use of psychiatric labels becomes institutional psychiatry that controls, stigmatizes and discriminates against people whose thoughts and actions are seen as outside of the bounds of 'normal' (see, for example, Goffman 1961; Laing 1990). It should be noted that this stigmatization and control process can happen regardless of the validity of the diagnosis – this is the difference between classifying someone as suffering from schizophrenia in order to understand and respond to them as an individual and labelling where the label becomes the person. Most commentators would at least partially accept Goffman's observations about labelling.

Most current commentators, however, see at least limited relevance in disease categories, although they would not agree with a strict medical model of a diagnosis giving rise, on its own, to a specific treatment or intervention. The most generally accepted model in mental health care is that medical diagnosis provides part of a complex bio-psychosocial presentation of need. For example the 'stress-vulnerability' model of schizophrenia lies behind most contemporary therapeutic approaches to care for people with severe mental health problems (see, for example, Birchwood and Tarrier 1992; Norman and Malla 1993). It is, therefore, helpful to have an understanding of the epidemiology of mental ill health and of the equally important psychological and social factors that impact on mental health and illness.

The facts are that (Sainsbury Centre for Mental Health 1998; Bird 1999; Singleton *et al.* 2001):

- One in four will experience some kind of mental health problem in the course of a year. 10–25 per cent of the population present with mental health problems, usually in primary care. Within this figure, 2–4 per cent have a severe mental illness. Only 0.3–1.5 per cent of the population have severe and enduring mental health problems.

- Neuroses are the most common form of mental health problem. The Office for National Statistics (ONS) survey in 2000 (Singleton *et al.* 2001) reported that 1 in 6 adults were assessed as having a neurotic disorder in the week before interview. Somewhere between 1 in 4 and 1 in 6 people will have serious depression at some stage in their lives. Clinical depression is second only to coronary heart disease in terms of international health burden. One in 10 people will have a disabling anxiety disorder at some stage in their lives. This may be a general anxiety mental health problem or a more specific phobia or obsessive compulsive disorder. Most neuroses last under one year, although there is a strong chance of recurrence. The ONS survey found that prevalence rates for all neurotic disorders, except for panic, were higher among women than men. The highest prevalence rates were for people aged 40–54 and lowest for those over the age of 65. There were few differences between the 1993 and 2000 ONS surveys.

- Psychoses are less common. One in 100 people will suffer from manic depression and 1 in 100 from schizophrenia at some stage in their lives. A quarter of people recover completely after a psychosis. Most people have multiple 'acute' episodes. An estimated 10–15 per cent of people with schizophrenia develop severe long-term disabilities. Again the ONS surveys of 1993 and 2000 show few changes over time in prevalence rates.

- Eating disorders are often not recognized or reported and studies may under-estimate prevalence. Anorexia nervosa affects 1 per cent of women aged 15–30. Half of these cases occur before the age of 20 and women outnumber men by 12 to 1. Bulimia nervosa affects 1–2 per cent of adult women.

- For the first time the 2000 ONS survey investigated the prevalence of personality disorder. Overall, 1 in 25 adults were assessed as having a disorder. The most common was obsessive-compulsive personality disorder with avoidant, schizoid, paranoid, borderline and anti-social disorders each having a prevalence of less than 1 per cent. Slightly more men than women were considered to have a personality disorder.

- Problems with drinking alcohol are common. The ONS 2000 survey revealed a prevalence of 38 per cent of men and 15 per cent of women as having a hazardous pattern of drinking during the year before interview. This prevalence decreased markedly with increasing age. Alcohol dependence was assessed as affecting 12 per cent of men and 3 per cent of women.

- Overall, 13 per cent of men and 8 per cent of women reported using illegal drugs in the ONS 2000 survey. Cannabis was the most commonly used drug (10 per cent) with amphetamines, cocaine and ecstasy each used by 2 per cent of adults aged 16–74. As with alcohol use, prevalence of illegal drug use declines sharply with increasing age. The ONS 2000 survey assessed dependence using a low threshold and found 4 per cent of the population to be dependent on one or more illegal drugs (6 per cent for men, 2 per cent for women). This is double the figure reported in the 1993 survey.

- Mental health problems in children and young people are also common. Studies have shown that 10 per cent of children and young people require specialist help. Anxiety, depression and hyperactivity and conduct disorder are the most common mental health problems. Estimates of prevalence vary widely because of different definitions and the high level of hidden morbidity.

- Common mental health problems affect older people but may go unrecognized or untreated. Dementia affects 1 per cent of people aged 60–65, 5 per cent of those over 65 and perhaps as many as 20 per cent of those aged over 80. One in 1000 people under 65 have Alzheimer's disease (a form of dementia).

Mental health problems do not affect all groups of people equally. Many factors are associated with mental health problems. It must however be remembered that association is not the same as causality. For example social isolation may both lead to mental health problems and be a psychological and social response to mental health problems. Epidemiological studies have found the following:

- **Isolation**: people with a neurosis and more markedly people with a psychosis are more likely than the general population to be separated or divorced and live in a one-person family unit.

- **Social class**: people with a probable psychosis are more likely to be defined as being in social classes IV or V.

- **Unemployment**: 39 per cent of people with a neurosis and 70 per cent with a psychosis were found to be economically inactive compared to 28 per cent with no disorder.

- **Social deprivation**: there are clear associations between social deprivation (e.g. poor housing/homelessness, employment and education) and mental illness morbidity. The Department of Health's psychiatric needs index shows a four-fold variation in need between the most affluent local authorities and the most deprived. Many authors argue that the variation in need is even greater for the most severe mental health problems. It is thought that the need for assertive outreach style services for people with the most severe difficulties varies from 12 to 200 people per 100,000 people aged 16 to 64 (Sainsbury Centre for Mental Health 1998).

- **Physical ill health**: 57 per cent of people with a neurosis and 62 per cent with a psychosis reported having a physical complaint, compared to 38 per cent of those with no mental health problem.

- **Black and minority ethnic communities**: Asian and African-Caribbean people are less likely to have mental health difficulties recognized by their GP. The prevalence of schizophrenia among Black African and African-Caribbean people is a much contested area of research. Whatever the underlying reasons it is clear that these Black communities are considerably over-represented in secure settings and detentions under the Mental Health Act 1983. Many authors have argued that the cause is institutional racism, although this is seldom seen as the only factor and interventions coming too late in the development of problems is a major issue. Mental health services are also considered to fail in meeting the needs of these communities (Soni Raleigh 1995). More positive ways of responding have been proposed (Sainsbury Centre for Mental Health 2002).

- **Suicide**: about 5000 people a year in England take their own lives. The government's *National Suicide Prevention Strategy* (Department of Health 2002) reports that on average somebody dies from suicide every two hours. It is the commonest form of death in men under 35 and is the main cause of premature death in people with mental illness. The majority of suicides occur in young adult men. Suicide rates are low among Asian men and older people but high in young Asian women. Suicide is far more common in social class V than any other social class. The most common means of suicide are hanging and poisoning with analgesic or psychotropic prescribed drugs.

- **Criminal justice system**: all forms of contact with the police, courts, prison and probation system are associated with high prevalence rates of mental health problems. For example, 56 per cent of sentenced women and 37 per cent of sentenced men are considered to have a psychiatric disorder. The prevalence of mental health problems is higher for remand prisoners.

Principles of mental health care

The mental health user and survivor movement has grown substantially over the last decade. There are now hundreds of groups across the UK. In particular they have been able to influence the implementation of the *NSF for Mental Health* (DH 1999b). Demands for user-focused care have not just come from user organizations. Bracken and Thomas (2001), two psychiatrists, have put forward a cogent argument for a postmodern form of post-psychiatry, which embraces users and survivors as taking the centre stage. It is the NSF that sets out the principles for contemporary mental health care in England. There is little dispute about these principles (Table 4.1) although the extent that they have been put into practice is variable. For example *Users' Voices* (Rose 2001) found that a majority of users did not receive all the information they required and did not know if they had a care plan or a key worker in line with the Care Programme Approach (CPA). It is now clear that people who use public services, including mental health services, must be enabled to become 'capable users'. A capable user is well informed about mental health and mental health services, is at the centre of their care, working in partnership with staff, and can exercise choice.

Table 4.1 National Service Framework for Mental Health Guiding Values and Principles (DH 1999b)

People with mental health problems can expect that services will:

- involve service users and their carers in planning and delivering care;
- deliver high quality treatment and care which is known to be effective and acceptable;
- be well suited to those who use them and non-discriminatory;
- be accessible so that help can be obtained when and where it is needed;
- promote their safety and that of carers, staff and the wider public;
- offer choices which promote independence;
- be well coordinated between staff and agencies;
- deliver continuity of care for as long as this is needed;
- empower and support staff;
- be properly accountable to the public, service users and carers.

A brief history of mental health service provision since 1950

Until the 1960s/1970s mental health care was organized around the old asylums, which were built mainly in the period 1840–1920. From the end of the 1950s onwards, the asylum population started to decline significantly because of the introduction of new medication, and changes in care and philosophy. This process became recognized by the government and it was Enoch Powell, then Health Minister, who announced that the asylums would decline in his famous 'water tower' speech. This policy is now in the final stages of implementation and most of the old long-stay beds have disappeared.

As the total number of psychiatric beds for people of all ages declined from about 140,000 in the early 1950s to fewer than 30,000 at the time of writing, the utilization of acute beds became much more intensive. This increase in the intensity of use has been due not just to the loss of beds, but also to an increase in demand (McCulloch *et al.* 2000).

In parallel with the reduction in bed numbers, the level of community provision for people with mental health problems has increased steadily. However, most community mental health teams are far too heavily loaded to deliver comprehensive care packages. More specialized community teams, such as assertive outreach and crisis intervention teams have been slower to develop, but the *NSF for Mental Health* (DH 1999b) and *NHS Plan* (DH 2000) have stimulated such developments, and assertive outreach in particular – a system of intensive support for people with severe mental health problems who have difficulty in engaging with other services – is developing rapidly.

The development of services on the ground has been reflected by the development of national policy. In the 1970s the replacement model for the old asylums was seen to consist of acute psychiatric units in district general hospitals, coupled with multi-disciplinary community mental health teams. This vision has since been elaborated within the NSF to include a comprehensive system of care embracing:

- inpatient care;
- crisis care;
- assertive outreach;
- community teams;
- 24-hour nursed care;
- residential care;
- supported housing;
- daytime activities;
- social support.

The *NHS Plan* set specific targets for the introduction of intensive community teams such as assertive outreach. The protection of the public has become an increasing part of the mental health policy agenda and has led to difficulties for staff in terms of paperwork and in knowing whether their function is to care for individuals or to protect others.

Current services and workforce

Although the UK has a national health service, mental health care is delivered by a large number of relatively autonomous NHS trusts, local authority social services departments, and independent for profit and voluntary sector organizations. To add to this complex organizational picture, health services are commissioned by local NHS primary care trusts and social care services are commissioned by social services departments, either from their own in-house providers or from independent sector agencies (these are the English organizational arrangements – Scotland, Wales and Northern Ireland have different structures). An overview is provided by the 28 strategic health authorities, which represents the local headquarters for the NHS. It is, therefore, not easy to establish what services are being provided by which groups of staff. In this section we have attempted to estimate numbers based on a range of returns made by local services to central government in England.

In 2000/1 the NHS in England spent £3,392 million on hospital and community mental health care for people of all ages. This figure does not include primary mental health care. In the same period local authority social services departments spent £601 million on mental health care for adults aged 16–65. It is not possible to determine social services expenditure on younger or older people. These figures represent approximately 11 per cent of NHS expenditure on hospital and community services and 5 per cent of social services overall expenditure.

Inpatient services (including acute, forensic, secure, intensive care, long stay and rehabilitation) still dominate NHS mental health expenditure. In 2000/1 they accounted for 60 per cent of funding. During the same period there were about 20,000 places for adults aged 16–65 and 138,000 admissions per annum. Many admissions involve involuntary detention under the Mental Health Act. During 2000/1 there were 25,000 detentions under the Act (some people may be detained more than once during a year).

Department of Health returns indicate that on 30 September 2001 there were 36,970 whole-time equivalent qualified nursing posts in the mental health field (14 per cent of all qualified nursing posts). Most nurses continue to work in hospital or residential settings. Figure 4.1 shows that 69 per cent of mental health nurses work in an institutional location. An increasing number of nurses work in community teams and a small number (2 per cent) work as more specialist psychological therapists (Figure 4.1).

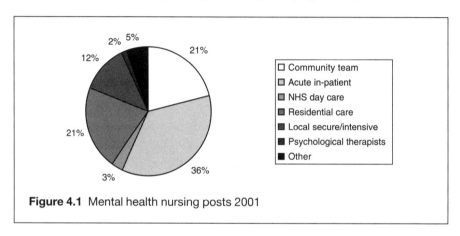

Figure 4.1 Mental health nursing posts 2001

Community services have continued to expand. In October 2001 service mapping returns to the University of Durham, acting on behalf of the Department of Health, showed there were 931 community mental health teams for adults of working age across England (Glover and Barnes 2002). In addition, there were 180 assertive outreach, 52 crisis resolution, and 16 early intervention in psychosis teams. These teams employ in excess of 5000 staff from a variety of professions. Increasingly they employ staff from non-traditional backgrounds such as support workers; although it is difficult to obtain figures.

Current mental health policy

The White Paper, *Modernising Mental Health Services* (DH 1998a) was the first comprehensive statement from the government about the future direction of mental health policy since *Better Services for the Mentally Ill* in the 1970s (Department of Health and Social Security (DHSS) 1975). *Modernising Mental Health Services* emphasizes three key aims of the government's vision for mental health:

- safe services: to protect the public and provide effective care for those with mental illness at the time they need it;

- sound services: to ensure that patients and service users have access to the full range of services that they need;
- supportive services: working with patients and service users, their families and carers to build healthier communities.

It also laid down the principles for modernization, which will be implemented through the *NSF for Mental Health* (DH 1999b). The modernization agenda will be delivered through a number of mechanisms including:

- *Additional investment in mental health services.* There will be an additional £300 million each year for mental health services for working-age adults coming on stream in 2002/3 and targeted mainly on the development of specialist community teams. However, this money has not been ring-fenced to be spent on mental health and there is a history of such growth monies being spent elsewhere.
- *Legal framework.* In July 1998, ministers announced a root and branch review of the Mental Health Act to ensure that the legislative framework supports modern mental health care. An independent expert group prepared initial proposals for consultation early in 1999 and following a Green Paper, a White Paper was published at the end of 2000. In 2002 a draft bill was published for further consultation.
- *Organizational framework.* The new policy environment emphasizes the need for integrated and multi-agency partnerships in care and requires more coherent and effective management of the interfaces and boundaries of services and functions. Specific arrangements will need to be made to ensure effective commissioning, leadership and delivery of mental health services. There will need to be a 'joined-up approach' to ensure that mental health policy and services are congruent with the proposals of a range of government policies, particularly the new strategy for public health published in *Saving Lives: Our Healthier Nation* (DH 1999a) which established mental health as a national public health priority; the 1999 Health Act which introduced new flexibilities across health and local government functions, and the Health and Social Care Act 2001 which introduced care trusts covering both health and social care.

The national service frameworks

The *NSF for Mental Health* (DH 1999b) was the first national service framework, and seeks to implement the government's agenda to drive up quality and reduce unacceptable variations in health and social services. The government's strategy for delivering core standards for the NHS is now in place and these are:

- set by the National Institute for Clinical Excellence, Social Care Institute for Excellence and national service frameworks;
- delivered by clinical governance, underpinned by professional self-regulation and lifelong learning;

- monitored by the Commission for Health care Audit and Inspection and the Commission for Social Care Inspection.

The *NSF for Mental Health* (DH 1999b) addresses the mental health needs of adults of working age. It sets out national standards and national service models, specifies approaches to implementation at national and local levels, and sets a series of milestones and performance indicators to assure progress. It also identifies an organizational framework for providing integrated services and for commissioning across the spectrum of care.

The *NSF for Mental Health* sets standards in seven areas, each based on the evidence and knowledge base available and supported by service models and examples of good practice. These are set out in Table 4.2.

Table 4.2 The National Service Framework for Mental Health standards (DH 1999b)

Standard 1 aims to ensure health and social services promote mental health and reduce the discrimination and social exclusion associated with mental health problems.

Health and social services should:
- promote mental health for all, working with individuals and communities;
- combat discrimination against individuals and groups with mental health problems, and promote their social inclusion.

Standards 2 and **3** aim to deliver better primary mental health care, and to ensure consistent advice and help for people with mental health needs, including primary care services for individuals with severe mental illness.

2 Any service user who contacts their primary health care team with a common mental health problem should:
- have their mental health needs identified and assessed;
- be offered effective treatments, including referral to specialist services for further assessment, treatment and care if they require it.

3 Any individual with a common mental health problem should:
- be able to make contact round the clock with the local services necessary to meet their needs and receive adequate care;
- be able to use NHS Direct, as it develops, for first-level advice and referral on to specialist helplines or to local services.

Standards 4 and **5** aim to ensure: that each person with severe mental illness receives the range of mental health services they need; that crises are anticipated or prevented where possible; prompt and effective help if a crisis does occur; timely access to an appropriate and safe mental health place or hospital bed, including a secure bed, as close to home as possible.

4 All mental health service users on CPA should:
- receive care which optimizes engagement, anticipates or prevents a crisis, and reduces risk;
- have a copy of a written care plan which:
  - includes the action to be taken in a crisis by the service user, their carer and their care coordinator,

- advises their GP how they should respond if the service user needs additional help,
- is regularly reviewed by their care coordinator,
- is able to access services 24 hours a day, 365 days a year.

(*Note*: Standard 4 reinforced the Care Programme Approach (CPA) which was first introduced in 1990.)

5 Each service user who is assessed as requiring a period of care away from their home should have:

- timely access to an appropriate hospital bed or place which is:
    - in the least restrictive environment consistent with the need to protect them and the public,
    - as close to home as possible;
- a copy of a written care plan agreed on discharge which sets out the care and rehabilitation to be provided, identifies the care coordinator, and specifies the action to be taken in a crisis.

Standard 6 aims to ensure health and social services assess the needs of carers who provide regular and substantial care for those with severe mental illness, and provide care to meet their needs.

6 All individuals who provide regular and substantial care for a person on CPA should:

- have an assessment of their caring, physical and mental health needs, repeated on at least an annual basis;
- have their own written care plan which is given to them and implemented in discussion with them.

Standard 7 aims to ensure that health and social services play their full part in the achievement of the target in *Saving Lives: Our Healthier Nation* to reduce the suicide rate by at least one fifth by 2010.

Local health and social care communities should prevent suicides by:

- promoting mental health for all, working with individuals and communities (Standard One);
- delivering high quality primary mental health care (Standard Two);
- ensuring that anyone with a mental health problem can contact local services via the primary care team, a helpline or an A&E department (Standard Three);
- ensuring that individuals with severe and enduring mental illness have a care plan which meets their specific needs, including access to services around the clock (Standard Four);
- providing safe hospital accommodation for individuals who need it (Standard Five);
- enabling individuals caring for someone with severe mental illness to receive the support which they need to continue to care (Standard Six);

and in addition:

- support local prison staff in preventing suicides among prisoners;
- ensure that staff are competent to assess the risk of suicide among individuals at greatest risk;
- develop local systems for suicide audit to learn lessons and take any necessary action.

For the first time government policy on mental health is accompanied by an explicit standards-based implementation framework. In time this may do much to overcome the patchiness and fluctuating quality of mental health care overall. It also specifies what is required from all those working in mental health services at various levels to deliver effective mental health services. This carries with it a clear requirement that training and professional development is oriented towards the implementation of the strategy and the achievement of the standards.

Each local health and social care community was required to prepare for implementing the NSF by establishing a local implementation team, which would then produce a local implementation plan.

The NHS Plan

The NHS Plan (DH 2000) added significantly to the specific proposals set out in the NSF and detailed the specific service components required. All of these have major implications for the workforce, and they are summarized in Table 4.3.

The NHS Plan, like the *NSF for Mental Health*, recognized that implementation will only succeed if staff are available in the right numbers, and are well trained and motivated. The Plan considerably raised the demand for staff implied in the *NSF for Mental Health*. In addition to the NSF another 3300 staff, 435 community teams, about 100 day centres and 200 secure beds were promised. In combination this implies that an additional 8000 staff are required: a 12 per cent addition to the workforce, and many of them requiring new or specific specialist skills on top of basic training.

Mental health policy implementation guide

The flurry of policy guidance did not end with the *NHS Plan*. The original strategy gave the overall framework, the *NSF for Mental Health* put into place national standards, and the *NHS Plan* then detailed some of the service models. This has since been reinforced by detailed policy guides on:

- effective care coordination;
- mental health promotion;
- workforce action team report;
- choosing talking therapies;
- assertive outreach;
- crisis resolution;
- early intervention in psychosis;
- acute inpatient care and psychiatric intensive care;
- community mental health teams;

Table 4.3 Mental health clinical priorities in the NHS Plan

• Money for the National Service Framework (2003/4)	£300 million

Primary care

• Help for GPs on common mental health problems (2004)	1000 new graduate primary care mental health workers to help 300,000 people
• Help for primary care teams, NHS Direct and A&E departments for people who need immediate help (2004)	500 community mental health staff to help 500,000 people

Community services

• Treatment and support for young people and their families (2004)	50 early intervention teams to help all young people who experience first episode of psychosis – around 7500 a year
• Crisis resolution (2004)	335 teams, treating around 100,000 people a year and reducing pressure on acute inpatient units by 30 per cent
• Assertive outreach (2003)	50 teams, in addition to the target of 170 for April 2001, helping 20,000 people
• Services for women (2004)	Women-only day centres in every health authority

Carers

• Respite care (2004)	700 more staff to increase breaks for carers, helping about 165,000 carers

High secure hospitals

• Reduction in places (2004)	Move 400 patients to more appropriate accommodation
• Long-term secure care (2004)	200 extra beds
• After discharge support (2004)	400 more community staff to provide intensive support

Prisons

• Better health screening and support for prisoners (2004)	300 more staff to identify and provide treatment. Everyone with severe mental illness will receive treatment and none should leave prison without a care plan and a care coordinator.

Personality disorders

• Secure accommodation and rehabilitation (2004)	140 new secure places, 75 specialist rehabilitation, hostel places and almost 400 extra staff for people with severe personality disorder who pose a high risk to the public.

- dual diagnosis (coexisting mental health and substance misuse problems);
- suicide prevention strategy;
- primary mental health care;
- mental health needs and care for people from black and minority ethnic communities;
- personality disorder.

(all available from www.nimhe.org.uk). The National Treatment Agency also has guidance on service models (www.nta.nhs.gov.uk).

National service framework for older people

There is little in the way of health and social-care policy that specifically addresses the needs of older people with mental health problems. However, the *National Service Framework for Older People* (*NSFOP*) (DH 2001a) has eight standards with one specific standard for mental health care: **Standard Seven** covers the promotion of good mental health in older people and the treatment and support of older people with dementia and depression (cf. Chapter 19).

> 7   Older people who have mental health problems have access to integrated mental health services, provided by the NHS and councils to ensure effective diagnosis, treatment and support, for them and for their carers.

This standard is broad. The *NSFOP* also refers to key interventions under Standard 7. It points out that improving prevention, care and treatment depend on promoting good mental health, the early recognition and management of mental health problems in primary care with the support of specialist old age mental health teams, and access to specialist care. In this way the structure of the *NSFOP* is similar to that for working-age adults. The emphasis is on mental health promotion and supporting primary care and only where necessary providing direct care within specialist services. The *NSFOP*, like the *NSF*, puts an emphasis on comprehensive, multidisciplinary, accessible, responsive, accountable and systematic services.

The other standards of the *NSFOP* also apply to older people's mental health services. Particular note should be given to: **Standard One** which aims to ensure that older people are never unfairly discriminated against in accessing NHS or social care services as a result of their age.

> 1   NHS services will be provided, regardless of age, on the basis of clinical need alone. Social care services will not use age in their eligibility criteria or policies, to restrict access to available services.

Standard Two which aims to ensure that older people are treated as individuals and that they receive appropriate and timely packages of care which meet their needs as individuals, regardless of health and social services boundaries.

2   NHS and social services treat older people as individuals and enable them to make choices about their own care. This is achieved through the single assessment process, integrating commissioning arrangements and integrated provision of services, including community equipment and continence services.

Although Standard 2 of the *NSFOP* is clear about the organizational model of integrated commissioning and provision there is no further guidance on the service models. On the one hand this gives services greater freedom to develop models that are responsive to local need. Where resources and expertise are limited poor models may develop, for example where one ward attempts to meet the needs of people with dementia and those with functional mental illness within the same setting.

Child and adolescent mental health services

The *Handbook on Child and Adolescent Mental Health* (1995) remains the last significant statement by the UK government on Child and Adolescent Mental Health Services (CAMHS), and it was closely related to and based on parallel work by the Health Advisory Service, which has been widely accepted as influential in shaping the development of CAMHS (cf. Chapter 18). At the time of writing, this handbook was out of print and further guidance was expected. It will remain to be seen how much the pending NSF on children and associated policy work will change the position. The 1995 guidance placed strong emphasis on building up core CAMHS services within each area and argued that CAMHS must be:

- planned on a multi-agency basis;
- provided on a multi-disciplinary basis;
- seen as a fundamental part of both overall mental health services and wider children's services.

The guidance provided a structure for CAMHS based around four tiers, Tier 1 being for the least severe problems. Many services are provided at Tier 1 by general practitioners, health visitors and other primary care staff, teachers, social workers and voluntary agencies. At Tier 2, professionals tend to work on their own. At Tier 3, specialists from various disciplines work together in teams. Tier 4 comprises highly specialized services, such as inpatient facilities (Audit Commission 1999). It set out a basic action plan for the concerned agencies, which, of course, include education authorities as well as health and social care agencies, to build up CAMHS.

At present CAMHS provision remains patchy with children in parts of inner London and close to other centres of excellence having access to a range of services, while in some areas specialist staff are few and far between and may offer a very limited range of interventions. It has been estimated that there is a seven-fold variation across the country in the level of expenditure by health authorities (Audit Commission 1999). CAMHS services employ a variety of therapy staff, psychologists, psychiatrists, teachers, social workers and nurses (26 per cent of all staff on average). These services, working at Tiers 2 to 4 spend only 1 per cent of their time supporting Tier 1 services where the majority of children and adolescents attend. Services at Tier 1 find it difficult to access specialist CAMHS. Confusion surrounds responsibility for meeting the needs of young people aged 16–18. Should they receive care and treatment from CAMHS or adult services? Similar problems exist for young people with ongoing needs who have to move from CAMHS to adult services as they get older. For people with severe psychosis the new Early Intervention in Psychosis (funded by the NHS Plan) services should help. On a more positive note many of these difficulties around funding, capacity and access are acknowledged and CAMHS services look set to become a renewed policy priority.

Effectiveness: a service that achieves its aims

A modern effective mental health service will be orientated towards the needs of users and underpinned with:

- high levels of expertise;
- correct targeting;
- timely and accessible delivery;
- evaluation and review, supporting both internal and external continuous quality improvement.

It is acknowledged that achieving quality in mental health care is not just about clinical effectiveness, but about improving health and social outcomes for people who use the service. Aspirations to improve services and deliver a sustained quality service have not, in the past, had systems and structures to enable them to succeed. A range of new structures and systems has been established to ensure that quality is continually improved and sustained. There are three main mechanisms.

Defining the right treatments and services

The National Institute for Clinical Excellence (NICE) is a special health authority with the remit of coordinating the production and dissemination of evidence-based clinical guidelines. Although many practitioners and managers in the field believe that the evidence base is poor, the real picture is more complicated. Although research on mental health is often weak, and much of it focuses on clinical not social outcomes, there is still a significant body of research within the UK and from the USA that needs to be disseminated and operationalized. NICE guidelines, at the time of writing, cover a range of mental health issues, most importantly the use of anti-depressants and anti-psychotics, the overall care of people with schizophrenia, and the use of anti-dementia medication.

Local implementation of high quality services

Clinical governance lies at the heart of local structures for improving quality, supported by moves to strengthen professional self-regulation and the development of values and structures that support lifelong learning. Clinical governance needs to be seen as a major opportunity for developing an effective quality framework. It has been suggested that an organization with a successful clinical governance framework will be characterized by:

- clinical staff with different attitudes and behaviour, including greater openness and willingness to address quality issues in a corporate way;

- managers who see themselves as responsible for quality of care, who are committed to a team approach to quality improvement, and who are willing to allow clinical leadership and responsibility to be developed. Changes in clinical governance will require similar changes in managerial governance.

One major problem with the concept of clinical governance is that the term itself implies a technical approach to improving quality focused on NHS services and does not describe the inclusive, often democratic nature of the quality process in the modern mental health environment. Partnerships with service users, carers and staff in local authority social services and other departments, and local community sector agencies, all have a part to play in delivering a quality mental health service and need to be involved in implementing the *NSF for Mental Health* effectively. It is clear, in particular, that the National Performance Assessment Framework for Social Services and the Best Value quality regime will serve the same purpose as clinical governance in social care. What is important here is that the underlying aim of delivering effective, quality services is seen as a partnership issue and that local quality systems are harmonized across and between the agencies to define local standards.

Lifelong learning

Lifelong learning is a concept which was originally used in industry, which recognizes the accelerating pace of change in technology, skills and society. As the nature of the work changes, so does the nature of employment. Skills quickly become obsolete at a time of great technological change. The UK government's strategy for lifelong learning has been set out in *Working Together, Learning Together, a framework for lifelong learning for the NHS* (DH 2001).

Continuing professional development

These developments have set the context for the NHS human resources strategy *Working Together: Securing a Quality Workforce for the NHS*

(DH 1998b). Continuing Professional Development (CPD) has a significant role to play in supporting this strategy. National policy sends a clear message that maintaining profession specific isolation within CPD is not consistent with lifelong learning approaches.

> Integrated care for patients will rely on models of training and education that give staff a clear understanding of how their own roles fit with those of others within both the health and social care professions. The government will work with the professions to reach a shared understanding of the principles that should underpin effective continuing professional development and the respective roles of the state, the professions and individual practitioners in supporting this activity.
>
> (DH 1998b: 8)

The government's intention was that by April 2000 all NHS employers should have training and development plans in place for all staff. While progress towards meaningful plans has been variable across the health professions, the assumption appears to be that the majority of health professionals already have personal development plans. It is clear that the government's intention is that, in time, personal development planning will be extended to all staff groups in the NHS and beyond.

A developing framework for practice

Modern mental health services now require staff who can cope with:

- rising demand for emergency psychiatric admissions;
- working across settings and agencies in both health and social care;
- formal integration of CPA and care management;
- new evidence-based psychological, social and pharmacological interventions;
- increasing severity of illness and disability;
- the new policy context;
- anticipated changes to the legal context;
- assertive outreach for people with severe mental illness who do not engage with other services;
- home treatment and crisis-intervention services providing emergency psychiatric care in the community;
- psycho-educational and behavioural approaches to family work;
- working in partnership with carers and users.

The capable practitioner

The current situation

From an older style institutional system of care has emerged a more open but complex community-based system of care delivery. The vision of the comprehensive, integrated community mental health service with specialized functional teams of multi-disciplinary practitioners providing an array of evidence-based medical, psychological and social interventions based on user and carer need, represents a quantum leap in organizational development (cf. Chapter 29).

Forces for change

Several key developments in the last few years have created the context for the more effective development of the workforce through education and training.

Workforce Development Confederations

The setting up of 27 new Workforce Development Confederations (WDCs) throughout England, to replace the old education and training consortia, will be a key factor in reshaping the landscape of higher education and professional training for mental health practitioners. This will facilitate a more strategic approach to education, training and workforce development with education providers as key partners in the enterprise.

The National Institute of Mental Health (England)

The creation of the National Institute of Mental Health (England) (NIMHE), along with its regional structures of regional development centres, with the workforce as one of the declared early programmes of work, represents an increasing recognition that the state of the workforce is a real 'Achilles heel' in the implementation of the *NSF for Mental Health*.

The Workforce Action Team

The Workforce Action Team (WAT), an advisory committee set up by the DH to advise on the workforce implications of the *NSF for Mental Health*, in its own analysis of the requirements to secure and retain a workforce needed to deliver a mental health service fit for the twenty-first century, set out some 'guiding principles' for positive change. These include the following:

- The education and training provided must ensure that the workforce is competent to understand the evidence base of their work (and its limits) and be able to take this into account appropriately in delivering services.

- Pre- and post-qualifying education and training must provide the competencies required to deliver the *NSF for Mental Health*.

- Lifelong learning and continuing professional development should be actively promoted, with staff given the necessary supervision and support to enable them to ensure their continuing fitness for practice.

- The workforce should be trained to deal with the emotional impact of their work and to actively seek lifelong support and supervision within the framework of an appropriate human resources policy.

- Staff involved in the delivery of training and supervision in the workplace should be trained and supported in these roles.

- Staff involved in the delivery of education and training should have an understanding and experience of contemporary practice.

- Service users and carers should be involved in planning, providing and evaluating education and training.

- Education and training provided must ensure that the workforce can operate collaboratively and effectively in multi-professional and multi-agency contexts.

The Mental Health Care Group Workforce Team (MHCGWT)

The MHCGWT will build on the earlier work of the WAT and is one of seven groups covering areas which include heart disease, children's services, services for older people, emergency care, and other long-term conditions (e.g. diabetes or renal services).

It will work closely with WDCs and the NIMHE to develop a national overview of workforce issues particularly with regard to numbers as well as the capabilities required to deliver on planned services. This will also involve making recommendations on innovative solutions to identified gaps in the skills and competencies of the multi-disciplinary workforce.

The Capability Framework

A key component of the WAT Report is the work completed by the Sainsbury Centre for Mental Health, *The Capable Practitioner* (Lindley *et al.* 2001). This document describes a framework of capabilities, which encompass the requisite skills, knowledge, values and attitudes of the multi-disciplinary mental health workforce to effectively deliver the type of services envisioned in the *NSF for Mental Health*.

Capability as a concept not only includes the element of competence or skill, but in addition captures the more fundamental requirements of effective practice, namely appropriate attitudes, values and relevant knowledge. Moreover, the concept of capability emphasizes the necessity of the transfer of acquired learning into the workplace.

To be capable in mental health care practitioners need:

- the ability effectively to implement evidence-based interventions within the service configurations specified in the *NSF for Mental Health*;

- judgement and decision-making capacity to apply appropriate effective interventions under complex, potentially stressful conditions, which adhere to agreed performance levels in the workplace;

- the ability to manage their own learning in the workplace, and to learn from experience, so as to build in the capacity for continuous improvement through lifelong learning;

- awareness of ethical considerations which integrate awareness of culture and values into professional practice; and

- the ability effectively to problem-solve and remove barriers to effective practice in the workplace, and to develop a working environment more conducive to the delivery of effective interventions.

Parameters

Development of the framework included an analysis of the requirements of both professional and professionally non-affiliated staff needed to deliver effective care to all working-age adults (not just those with severe long-term mental illness) within the new services outlined within the *NHS Plan* and *NSF for Mental Health*. This included all the key professional disciplines of psychiatry, nursing, occupational therapy, social work and clinical psychology along with those workers described as non-professionally aligned.

There was no attempt within the framework to differentiate levels of expertise between the disciplines. This is rightly a matter for the accrediting and professional bodies to determine. However, there is a clear message with the framework that while it is essential that the various multi-disciplinary groups have some common foundation of capability or core competencies, there is also a need for specialization and development of higher levels of capability among the multi-disciplinary groups.

Underlying principles and structure

This section provides a summary of the underlying principles and structure of the Capability Framework. For a full description please refer to *The Capable Practitioner* report (Lindley *et al.* 2001).

The purpose of the framework is to ensure that interventions are 'capable' across the comprehensive range of settings that, within the specifications of the *NSF for Mental Health*, constitute an integrated mental health service. This encompasses primary care, acute inpatient care, community-based crisis resolution teams, assertive outreach, residential and day care, and specialist secure and forensic settings.

The Capability Framework can perhaps be best seen as a broad inclusive 'map' of the knowledge, skills values and attitudes required of the mental health workforce that will enable it to deliver such effective interventions, in this complex array of different settings. These domains of the framework include:

- ethical practice;
- knowledge;
- process of care;
- interventions;

Table 4.4 summarizes the content outlines of the framework. The *NSF for Mental Health* was critically studied to ensure that all the standards were carefully and comprehensively covered. The second column in Table 4.4 indicates for each domain of the Capability Framework the NSF standards

Table 4.4 Summary of content outline of the capability domains

Domains of Capability Framework	NSF standards	Indicative content
Ethical practice	1–7	Attitudes, values and codes of practice
Knowledge	1–7	Policy and legislation; models of mental health, evidence-based practice and mental health services
Process of care	14–16: NSF (1–7) 17–18: NSF (6) 19: NSF (1–7) 20: NSF (4, 5, 7) 21: NSF (4, 5) 22: NSF (22–25)	Effective communication; partnerships with users and carers; teamwork and team liaison; comprehensive assessment; care planning, care coordination and review; supervision, professional development and lifelong learning; clinical and practice leadership
Interventions	26–30: NSF (1–7) 31–34: NSF (2–7) 35–36: NSF (1)	Medical and physical care Social and practical Psychosocial interventions: • Early intervention • Early signs monitoring and relapse prevention • Psycho-education • Crisis intervention • Cognitive behavioural individual and family interventions • Therapeutic strategies for alcohol or drug misuse • Psycho-education

it is designed to apply to. There is also a final component, which is the application of these domains to a variety of mental health settings or systems.

Ethical practice

The framework of capabilities for modern mental health work makes basic assumptions about the underlying *NSF for Mental Health* values and principles of care (Table 4.1). Such standards are at the core of mental health practice and are seen as cross-cutting themes throughout all the domains of the Capability Framework. For the purpose of this model it is assumed that as a starting point, all mental health workers will base their practice on these values.

Knowledge

Knowledge is the foundation of effective practice. The capability of a single practitioner involves constant interplay between knowledge and the practical application of mental health skills. The framework suggests the need for four kinds of specialized knowledge: policy and legislation, current understandings of mental health and mental illness, research evidence on effective care and treatment to optimize recovery, and models of mental health service delivery.

This includes knowledge of the policy outlined in this chapter and knowledge of any new legislation once enacted. A good understanding of the CPA and its operation would also be required. Other important components of knowledge include the various explanatory models of mental health and the evidence, which underpin them, and knowledge of mental health and mental illness in terms of causation, incidence, prevalence, description of disorders and the impact on individuals, families and communities. Understanding of the evidence base for effective interventions, including medical, psychological, social and environmental interventions along with service delivery models is also essential.

The statements in the framework for this domain denote the knowledge required by *most* of the mental health workforce.

Process of care

The process of delivering mental health care involves working within a social system (the NHS, Social Services, the community at large), a legal system (such as the Mental Health Act), within policy frameworks (the Care Programme Approach and clinical governance) and with the range of services available in the community and resources and expertise that exist within teams of multi-disciplinary practitioners.

Specific capabilities are required to optimize the relationship with carers and families and the network of care available to the service user. Finally, the relationship with the service user must encourage user participation and utilize the understanding of each individual's experience.

The capabilities for effective care coordination in the Capability model are divided as follows:

1 effective communication;
2 effective partnership with users and carers;
3 effective partnership in teams and with external agencies;
4 comprehensive assessment;
5 care planning, coordination and review;
6 supervision, professional development and lifelong learning;
7 clinical and practice leadership.

The statements in the framework for this domain denote the process of care capabilities required by *some* of the mental health workforce.

Interventions

The *NSF for Mental Health* undertakes its own 'evidence-based review' of psychosocial interventions, on the basis of which it recommends the implementation of those interventions, which it believes are empirically supported. The review for each particular intervention is brief and far from comprehensive. The interventions and services described by the *NSF for Mental Health* with respect to people with severe mental illness include:

• early intervention;
• early signs monitoring and relapse prevention;
• cognitive behavioural interventions;
• behavioural family intervention;
• assertive outreach;
• crisis resolution and home treatment;
• medication adherence;
• dual diagnosis.

The Capability Framework recognizes that part of effective care co-ordination is the capability to deliver these evidence-based interventions for facilitating recovery and meeting the needs of mental health service users, their carers and families.

Historically this has been the domain of professional specialists, where specific interventions were linked to professional groups. This model outlines a range of interventions that need to be delivered, but does not specify which group of practitioners should deliver them. The capabilities described in the framework offer a range of interventions beyond the standard psychological models:

1 medical and physical health care;
2 psychological interventions;

3   social and practical interventions;

4   mental health promotion.

The statements for this domain reflect the increasing specialization of the framework and denote interventions required by *only a few* of the mental health workforce.

Applications

The provision of mental health care in the UK has moved towards the development of comprehensive services. The mental health workforce will need to draw on values, knowledge, process skills and a range of interventions that will enable them to practice effectively. But in reality, this practice will relate to specific service settings.

While the model attempts to map a broad brush of capabilities not specific to any setting or professional level, the final section of the model addresses the specific applications required for each of these areas that are distinct from the essential capabilities described in the previous section. These are:

1   primary care;

2   Community-based care coordination (CMHTs);

3   crisis resolution and early intervention;

4   acute inpatient care;

5   assertive outreach;

6   continuing care;

7   services for complex needs (such as dual diagnosis clients).

The Capability Framework is best understood as a conceptual map with sufficient detail to define the skills development agenda established by the NSF. Ethical practice is seen as the underpinning domain that *all* mental health workers must possess. Most workers should have good knowledge of mental health issues, such as policy and legislation, and models of mental health. Capabilities to practise effective care coordination (i.e. process of care) should be applied by *some* workers, and interventions, perhaps the realm of the more specialist worker, should be practised by *only a few* workers. The final domain in the framework describes the specific service settings in which practice takes place (i.e. their application).

Future practice

By way of a conclusion to this chapter we summarize its content and examine its implications for mental health nurses. Mental health problems are common and affect all of us in one way or another. In the past the psychiatric hospital was the only place for specialist mental health care and all qualified nurses worked in these hospitals. Gradually hospital care has become less prominent. Mental health nurses have for many years been working in community settings and more recently in community mental health teams with other professionals. From 1998 onwards there has been a flood of policy initiatives that are beginning to influence care. Nurses need to know about the Safe, Sound and Supportive strategy, the National Service Frameworks and the Policy Implementation Guides as part of the knowledge base towards becoming capable practitioners. Equally, they will need to practise ethically and be skilled at delivering effective interventions within the framework of a sound process of care delivery. The presentation of mental health problems is also beginning to change, with a doubling of drug dependency problems in just seven years.

For mental health nurses there are massive implications, as our crystal ball shows:

- **User-centred practice**: nurses of tomorrow will be expected to work in partnership with people who use mental health services, their families and their communities.

- **Specialization**: there are already an array of different types of mental health care service based in many varied settings. Nurses will no longer be able to shift effortlessly from one service type to another. They will develop highly specialized skills in their chosen service area and they will identify more with this service area and the other professionals they work alongside than with the nursing profession.

- **Multi-disciplinary working**: working in integrated teams with a number of other professions will no longer be an aspiration, it will become the accepted norm.

- **New staff groups**: as mental health services expand they will have to recruit a more varied workforce who do not hold traditional qualifications. Nurses will more often become enablers, facilitators, educators, supervisors and consultants, rather than being expected to deliver most of the hands-on care.

- **Continuous development and change**: nurses can expect their roles and the world around them to keep changing. The expectation of life-long learning has emerged. Also, services need to keep improving and change management has become a core skill for nurses working at all levels. A good example is the way that dual diagnosis interventions for people with coexisting mental health and drug and alcohol problems have moved from a specialist service to a core skill for all mental health staff.

- **Information Management and Technology (IM&T)**: all nurses will be expected to use IM&T not just to maintain patient data, but also to manage patient care and access and use the knowledge base.

Acknowledgement

This chapter draws on my work whilst at the Sainsbury Centre for Mental Health, much of which was undertaken collaboratively with colleagues.

Questions for reflection and discussion

1 What are the three biggest challenges posed by policy to my personal practice or to my team?

2 How in my personal practice can I both empower users and improve public safety at the same time, or do occasions arise when this is impossible?

3 Is current UK government policy feasible and if not what elements of it need to go on hold?

4 How do my skills, knowledge and attitudes relate to the Capable Practitioner Framework?

Annotated bibliography

- Department of Health (1999b) *National Service Framework for Mental Health*. London: The Stationery Office. The basis for mental health services in England, the NSF for Mental Health contains not only the standards but a wealth of readable information as a rationale for each standard.
- www.nimhe.org.uk. The National Institute for Mental Health in England websites carry all the policy guidance. In particular the implementation guides are relevant to all people connected with the mental health field. The National Institute website also has a useful 'Ask NIMHE' feature.
- www.scmh.org.uk. The Sainsbury Centre for Mental Health (an independent charity) website has a number of topic guides relating to primary care, assertive outreach and crisis resolution.
- Bird, L. (1999) *The Fundamental Facts: All the Latest Facts and Figures on Mental Illness*. London: Mental Health Foundation. A favourite of both the authors. This short booklet is attractively presented and gives headline information on mental health problems and associated socio-economic factors. A new edition will be published shortly.
- Singleton, N., Bumpstead, R., O'Brien, M., Lee, A. and Meltzer, H. (2000) *Psychiatric morbidity among adults living in private households*: Summary Report. London: Office for National Statistics (available for

download from www.statistics.gov.uk). Straight facts and figures. At the time of writing further reports were due from this large scale survey.

References

Audit Commission (1999) *Children in Mind: Child and Adolescent Mental Health Services*. London: The Audit Commission.

Birchwood, M. and Tarrier, N. (1992) *Innovations in the Psychological Management of Schizophrenia*. Chichester: Wiley.

Bird, L. (1999) *The Fundamental Facts: All the Latest Facts and Figures on Mental Illness*. London: Mental Health Foundation.

Bracken, P. and Thomas, P. (2001) Postpsychiatry: a new direction for mental health. *British Medical Journal* **322**; 724–7.

Department of Health (1995) *Handbook on Child and Adolescent Mental Health*. London: HMSO.

Department of Health (1998a) *Modernising Mental Health Services: Safe, Sound and Supportive*. London: DH.

Department of Health (1998b) *Working Together: Securing a Quality Workforce for the NHS*. Wetherby: DH.

Department of Health (1999a) *Saving Lives: Our Healthier Nation*. London: The Stationery Office.

Department of Health (1999b) *A National Service Framework for Mental Health*. London: The Stationery Office.

Department of Health (2000) *The NHS Plan: A Plan for Investment, A Plan for Reform*. London: DH.

Department of Health (2001) *Working Together, Learning Together, A Framework for Lifelong Learning for the NHS*. London: DH.

Department of Health (2001a) *National Service Framework for Older People*. London: DH.

Department of Health (2002) *National Suicide Prevention Strategy*. London: DH.

Department of Health and Social Security (1975) *Better Services for the Mentally Ill*. London: HMSO.

Glover, G. and Barnes, D. (2002) *Mental Health Service Provision for Working Age Adults in England 2001*. Durham: Centre for Public Mental Health, University of Durham (www.dur.ac.uk/service.mapping).

Goffman, I. (1961) *Asylums*. Harmondsworth: Penguin.

Laing, R.D. (1990) *The Divided Self*. Harmondsworth: Penguin.

Lindley, P., O'Halloran, P. and Juriansz, D. (2001) *The Capable Practitioner*. London: Sainsbury Centre for Mental Health.

Norman, R.M. and Malla, A.K. (1993) Stressful life events and schizophrenia I: A review of the research, *British Journal of Psychiatry* **162**: 161–6.

McCulloch, A., Muijen, M. and Harper, H. (2000) New developments in mental health policy in the United Kingdom, *International Journal of Law and Psychiatry*, **23**(3–4): 261–76.

Rose, D. (2001) *Users' Voices*. London: Sainsbury Centre for Mental Health.

Sainsbury Centre for Mental Health (1998) *Keys to Engagement: Review of Care for People with Severe Mental Illness who are Difficult to Engage*. London: Sainsbury Centre for Mental Health.

Sainsbury Centre for Mental Health (2002) *Breaking the Circles of Fear: Review of the Relationship Between Mental Health Services and African and Caribbean Communities.* London: Sainsbury Centre for Mental Health.

Singleton, N., Bumpstead, R., O'Brien, M., Lee, A. and Meltzer, H. (2001) *Psychiatric morbidity among adults living in private households.* London: The Stationery Office.

Soni Raleigh, V. (1995) *Mental Health in Black and Minority Ethnic People: The fundamental facts.* London: The Mental Health Foundation.

Szasz, T. (1961) *The Myth of Mental Illness.* New York: Harper Row.

5

Rehabilitation and recovery

Rachel Perkins and Julie Repper

▌Chapter overview

> Recovery refers to the lived or real life experience of people as they accept and overcome the challenge of the disability . . . they experience themselves as recovering a new sense of self and of purpose within and beyond the limits of the disability.
>
> (Deegan 1988)

> Rehabilitation is the process of helping the psychiatrically disabled person to make the best use of his or her . . . abilities in as normal a social context as possible.
>
> (Bennett 1978)

Recovery and rehabilitation are not the same thing. Having serious mental health problems is a devastating and life-changing experience. There is no way of going back to the way things were before these difficulties started, but they are not the end of life. Many people who have experienced mental health problems have shown us that there is a way forward: that it is possible to recover meaning and purpose in life. Recovery is:

> . . . a deeply personal, unique process of changing one's attitudes, values, feelings goals, skills, and/or roles. It is a way of living a satisfying, hopeful and contributing life even with the limitations caused by illness. Recovery involves the development of new meaning and purpose in one's life as one grows beyond the catastrophic effects of mental illness.
>
> (Anthony 1993)

While recovery is an individual journey of rebuilding a satisfying and valued life, rehabilitation is the process via which mental health practitioners and services might help people to do this. Practitioners cannot 'rehabilitate' people, but we can facilitate (or impede) the process of recovery.

Traditionally, the primary aim of mental health services and the practitioners who inhabit them, is 'cure': interventions designed to reduce, and where possible eliminate, 'symptoms'. We judge our success in terms of the extent to which we have been able to do this and so 'discharge' people from our services. However, symptom reduction is neither a necessary, nor a sufficient condition for recovery. 'One of the biggest lessons I have had to accept is that recovery is not the same thing as being cured. After 21 years of living with this thing it still hasn't gone away' (Deegan 1993).

Recovery does not mean that all symptoms have been removed, or that functioning has been fully restored. Instead, it is about reducing the extent to which any remaining symptoms or problems interfere with the person's efforts to pursue their interests and goals. Both rehabilitation and recovery mean moving beyond 'cure' to thinking about how people can make the most of their lives.

In this chapter we:

- compare the concepts of 'rehabilitation' and 'recovery' and outline their underpinning principles; and

- consider how rehabilitation services can promote recovery.

Beyond 'cure': what are people recovering?

Mental health practitioners are accustomed to thinking about the experience of people with mental health problems in terms of their need for different types of interventions and services: medication, inpatient care, outreach services, psychosocial interventions, sheltered accommodation, occupational therapy, art therapy. This is not the best place to start. Before it is possible to decide on appropriate interventions it is necessary to understand the nature of the challenge that the person faces and what they wish to achieve in their life. Only then is it possible to consider how we might help their individual journey or recovery.

People who have experienced serious mental health problems are recovering from the multi-faceted calamity of that experience (Repper and Perkins 2002). They not only have to contend with the difficulties themselves, but also with the way in which people with such problems are treated both within and outside mental health services. These include:

- the multiple traumas of the often recurring, fluctuating, and/or ever-present symptoms themselves;

- the treatment of the illness, including the side effects of medication and the stigma associated with contact with mental health services;

- the sometimes negative attitudes and prognoses of professionals: 'You have a chronic illness', 'You will not be able to work, have children, live independently . . .';

- professionals whose primary concern is the relief of symptoms and who lack the skills necessary to help people to rebuild their lives;
- devaluing and disempowering services which encourage passivity, where 'them and us' attitudes prevail, and where the physical environment is often depressing and inadequate;
- the multiple manifestations of the prejudice and discrimination in a society where people with mental health problems are seen as dangerous, unpredictable, incompetent, unable to take control of, or make decisions about, their own lives; and
- the discrimination and social exclusion – lack of opportunities to engage in valued roles and activities – that people with mental health problems face.

These often combine to leave people feeling disconnected from themselves, from friends and family, from the communities in which they live, and from meaning and purpose in life. The identity of 'mental patient' eclipses all other facets of personhood and it is all too easy to lose hope – abandon any belief in the possibility of a positive future – and give up. 'When I was diagnosed I felt this is the end of my life. It was a thing to isolate me from other human beings. I felt I was not viable unless they found a cure . . . I felt flawed. Defective' (cited in Sayce 2000).

Anyone who experiences a catastrophe in their life – whether it be mental health problems, the death of someone we love, unemployment or the end of relationship – experiences a range of emotions (Kubler-Ross 1969; O'Donoghue 1994). These may include:

- **Denial:** 'It must be a mistake', 'It's not happening to me', 'Everything will be back to normal soon';
- **Anger:** 'Why me?', 'It's not fair';
- **Grief:** 'My life is over', 'Everything is hopeless';
- **Shame:** 'Oh dear, I hope no one finds out';
- **Isolation:** 'Now no one will want to have anything to do with me'; and
- **Terror:** 'Now what will happen to me?'.

Too often, practitioners fail to appreciate the range of traumas experienced by people with mental health problems. To be diagnosed as having serious mental health problems is a bereavement: it involves loss of the privileges of sanity; loss of the life the person had or expected to lead; loss of the person we thought we were or might become. Too often, when practitioners focus solely on symptoms and cures, such ordinary bereavement responses are seen as pathological – symptoms of the illness itself. Denial may be seen as the 'lack of insight' inherent in the disorder. Hopelessness, apathy and withdrawal may be understood as the 'negative symptoms' and 'lack of motivation' that characterize the 'illness'. Anger is seen as a symptom to be treated or as 'acting out'. 'This has left many people with mental illness feeling devalued and ignored and has resulted in mistrust and alienation from the mental health system' (Spaniol *et al.* 1997).

Unless we can understand and address the complex range of barriers that people face, and the ordinary human responses to the bereavement that the experience entails, then we may inadvertently impede recovery by alienating people from those very services that are supposed to assist them.

Beyond 'cure': what is rehabilitation and who is it for?

Traditionally 'rehabilitation' has been seen as synonymous with the resettlement of old long-stay psychiatric patients: helping people who have lived for decades in the neglected back wards of large asylums to move out of hospital and live more independently in the community. As this process nears its end, there are some who believe that rehabilitation is no longer necessary. It has been argued that as community services develop to treat and support people outside hospital settings, the deleterious effects of long-term institutionalization in remote psychiatric hospitals can be avoided, and there is therefore no longer a need for specialist rehabilitation services. However, it is important to draw a distinction between rehabilitation as a specialist service and rehabilitation as a process of helping people who are disabled as a consequence of their ongoing mental health problems and the social exclusion, disadvantages and discrimination associated with them.

The training of mental health practitioners, and the focus of mental health services, remains primarily the treatment of illness and the management of acute crises. People's problems are largely understood in terms of collections of symptoms to be treated, reduced and hopefully eliminated. Yet, despite a popular focus on acute services, some 80 per cent of people admitted to acute inpatient units (or treated at home during crises by 'home treatment teams') have experienced such crises before and will experience them again. If services are to facilitate recovery, then the treatment of symptoms and resolution of acute crises are only a part of the help that people need. If people are to be assisted to rebuild their lives, then the treatment of symptoms offers too narrow a focus to be a useful organizing principle for support and intervention.

Rehabilitation requires a change of focus: a move away from the 'treatment of acute illness' to the 'management of disability'. Although symptoms can be problematic in and of themselves, it is the way in which people with such difficulties are viewed and treated within society that is disabling: the prejudice, discrimination and exclusion and the barriers that they face in doing the things they want to do. Rehabilitation is about enabling people to retain or regain hopeful, satisfying and contributing lives: enabling them to live the lives they want to lead, pursue their aspirations and achieve their goals. While the treatment of symptoms, and help during acute crises may be important, they are only a part of a rehabilitation process which involves helping people to make the most of their skills, abilities and lives. Rehabilitation requires that we move beyond a consideration of symptoms and dysfunctions to a focus on skills and abilities; understanding what gives a person's life meaning and purpose; enabling people to accommodate what has happened to them; and helping them to access the ordinary relationships and opportunities that are available to non-disabled citizens.

The success of rehabilitation cannot be measured in terms of symptom reduction and discharge but in terms of the extent to which we are able to help people to do the things they want to do. This may or may not involve a reduction of symptoms. It may or may not involve a person being discharged from the services which provide them with support. Symptoms do not necessarily prevent people from doing the things they want to do, and ongoing support from services is not a problem if it enables people to do the things they want to do.

Rehabilitation is as important for the new generation of people with serious mental health as it was for their old long-stay forebears. Whether the service which facilitates recovery is called a 'rehabilitation service', or an 'assertive outreach service', or an 'early intervention service', the process remains one of helping people to make the most of their abilities and live satisfying, purposeful and valued lives.

Principles of recovery and rehabilitation

If people with serious mental health problems are to make the most of their lives, then they need access to a range of services, including: crisis support; interventions to help reduce and manage symptoms; a range of housing options including supported accommodation and intensive outreach support at home; help to access a range of work and education opportunities; support to maintain and develop relationships; and support from family and friends. However, the simple presence of this range of components does not guarantee facilitation of recovery in those whom they serve. Critically important are the principles and values of these services.

Recovery is about people's whole lives – not just their symptoms

There are a variety of different ways in which people may gain relief from distressing symptoms: these include medication, psychological therapy, counselling and a range of complementary therapies. However, people's problems extend well beyond the expertise traditionally found within mental health services. Difficulties with housing, money, employment, education, relationships, social and leisure activities are typically more important in the recovery process than are the mental health problems themselves.

It should not be expected that a single practitioner or agency can provide the full range of interventions, supports and assistance that a person needs. First, it is highly unlikely that a single worker/provider can simultaneously be an expert in welfare benefits; vocational rehabilitation and liaising with employers; individual psychological therapy and family interventions; the impact of various drug treatments; and putting together MFI furniture or making a washing machine work. Second, everyone needs the opportunity to be different people in different relationships and situations. We may be competent at work, delinquent with our friends, inadequate and needy with our nearest and dearest. In a single relationship with a 'key worker' or 'care coordinator' it is not possible for someone to simultaneously address their fears and problems, use/extend their skills and abilities, and achieve the social relationships on which most people rely so heavily for mutual support in their day-to-day lives. However, if a person is receiving help and support from a range of different individuals and agencies then effective coordination is required in order to ensure that the person gets all the assistance they need.

Therefore, if they are to facilitate *recovery*, then *rehabilitation* services need to:

- **Adopt a team approach:** If responsibility for the provision of all support rests with a single individual then the provision of effective support/ intervention across diverse domains is jeopardized; and

- **Ensure continuity across providers:** If people receive input from multiple agencies and individuals then these must work effectively together.

Recovery is about growth

It is very easy for people with mental health problems to become nothing other than the array of symptoms that characterizes their illness: 'a schizo-phrenic', 'a manic depressive'. 'Schizophrenia is an "I am" illness, one which may take over and redefine the identity of a person' (Estroff 1989).

If practitioners' focus is limited to symptoms and deficits simply then this process is reinforced. People are always more than their 'illness'. Recovery involves redefining identity in a way which includes these difficulties, but enables the person to grow, develop and move beyond them.

However, growth is often limited not by characteristics of the person, but by the barriers imposed by discrimination and exclusion. 'My recovery was about how to gain other people's confidence in my abilities and potential . . . in my own experience the toughest part was changing other people's expectations of what I could do. Combating a disempowering sense of being undervalued . . .' (May 1999).

The traditional focus of services is helping the individual to change: reducing their symptoms, helping them to develop new skills, helping them to adjust to what has happened. These may all be important in facilitating recovery, but it is important that practitioners also attend to reducing the external barriers that they face. Growth is not possible if you are debarred from doing the things you want to do.

Therefore, if they are to facilitate recovery, rehabilitation services need to:

- **Be strengths-based:** It is not possible to help people to rebuild their lives without focusing on their skills, interests, abilities and assets and helping people to make the most of these; and

- **Focus on changing the environment, not simply changing individuals:** A person's ability to access the things they want to do depends on the dynamic interaction between the individual and their environment. Changing the environment – providing support and adaptations to increase access – is at least as important as changing individuals to 'fit in'.

Recovery does not refer to an end product or a result

> Recovery is a process, not an end point or destination. Recovery is an attitude, a way of approaching the day and the challenges I face . . . I know I have certain limitations and things I can't do. But rather than letting these limitations be occasions for despair and giving up, I have learned that in knowing what I can't do, I also open up the possibilities of all I can do.
>
> (Deegan 1993)

People cannot be 'fixed' or 'rehabilitated' as one might mend a television or refurbish a building. If recovery is a continuing journey, then rehabilitation must be seen as a continuing process of supporting people in that journey. And this must involve not only helping the person to move forward, but also helping them to maintain what has already been gained. The original work on 'assertive outreach' of Stein and Test (1980) demonstrated that people did not simply require 'training in community living' but needed ongoing support to sustain their community tenure and the lives they had built for themselves. Likewise, there is now a wealth of evidence which demonstrates that people with mental health problems can be successful in open employment if they are provided not only with help to get work, but also ongoing, time-unlimited support, to sustain their employment (Bond *et al.* 1997, 2001; Crowther *et al.* 2001).

The critical yardstick of success is not whether the person can be discharged and function unaided – this may or may not be possible or desirable – but what they are able to achieve in their life in the presence of support. In the context of other impairments the efficacy of, for example, a wheelchair would never be judged in terms of whether it could be removed, but in terms of what it enabled the person using it to do.

It is also important to accept that recovery will not be a linear process – there will be problems and setbacks along the way. 'The recovery process is . . . a series of small beginnings and very small steps. At times our course is erratic and we falter, slide back, re-group and start again . . .' (Deegan 1988). Relapse is not 'failure', but a part of the recovery process. However, if a person is not to become dispirited or give up, they need people around them who can 'hold on to hope': believe in them and their possibilities, during those times when they are not able to believe in their own worth and future.

Therefore, if they are to facilitate recovery, rehabilitation services need to:

- **Focus on maintaining, as well as optimizing functioning:** Throughput models are inappropriate in the context of ongoing problems. The efficacy of an intervention/support should be judged in terms of what it enables a person to achieve, not whether it enables the person to be discharged from the service.

- **Adopt a long-term perspective:** If recovery is an ongoing process then people may require continuity of help and support, and over long periods of time.

- **Offer continuity of support over time:** If support over longer periods of time is to be effective, then it cannot be subject to the presence of a single member of staff. It is inevitable that practitioners will go on holiday, take sick leave, and move on to other jobs. In order to reduce the disruption and discontinuities to which this can lead, it is preferable if people know and trust a number of different team members, so that when one person leaves some continuity can be preserved. A team approach does not mean that individual relationships are unimportant, merely that everyone needs several such relationships.

- **Accept setbacks and relapse as part of the recovery process:** Practitioners must be willing to help people to persevere. We must be able to continue to believe in people even when everything seems to be going wrong.

Recovery is not dependent on professional intervention

Unlike medication or therapy, recovery is not a professional intervention and mental health workers do not hold the key (Anthony 1993). A person's own resources and those available to them outside the mental health system are central to the recovery process. The sources of meaning and satisfaction in most people's lives do not lie within mental health services – they lie in our work, our homes, our relationships, our leisure pursuits, our religion or spiritual beliefs. If people are unable to access the range of ordinary opportunities that their non-disabled peers enjoy then it is unlikely that they will be able to rebuild lives that they find satisfying and meaningful.

However, the expertise of experience can also be important. Many people have described the enormous support they have received from others who have faced a similar challenge (Chamberlin 1995; May 1999). This may be achieved via self-help groups and user/survivor organizations or more informal friendships and networks within which people can share experiences.

Therefore, if they are to facilitate recovery, rehabilitation services need to:

- **Emphasize social integration and reintegration:** Enable people to access and maintain those ordinary relationships, roles, activities and social supports that they value and which provide meaning in their lives;

- **Maximize opportunities for people with mental health problems to support and learn from each other:** People who have 'been there themselves' can often provide enormous encouragement, support, role models to others who face similar challenges; and

- **Successfully involve service users and their relatives/friends:** Tapping the expertise of experience at all levels – individual care planning; the monitoring and operation of individual services; service planning and development – is essential to the development of effective, accessible and acceptable services.

A recovery vision is not limited to a particular theory about the nature and causes of mental health problems

Just as professionals have developed a range of different organic, psychological and interpersonal models for understanding mental distress, so people who have experienced these difficulties understand their difficulties in different ways. Based on the narratives of 30 people with serious mental health problems, Jacobson (1993) identified six frameworks that they used to understand their difficulties: biological; interaction of biology and environment; abuse or trauma; spiritual or philosophical; political; and the dehumanizing impact of long-term contact with mental health services.

As Anthony (1993) points out, a recovery vision does not commit one to a particular understanding of distress and disability. People need to find ways of understanding what has happened to them, but whichever explanatory framework they choose, recovery is an equally important process. In order to facilitate recovery, such explanations need to make sense to the person and offer them hope for the future. If services insist that people adopt a single understanding of their difficulties then they are likely to alienate those who prefer alternative explanations.

Therefore, if they are to facilitate recovery, rehabilitation services need to be user centred and needs led. If services are to be successful in engaging those who are often reluctant to receive help, then their views, perspectives and wishes must be heeded.

Everyone's recovery journey is different and deeply personal

There are no rules of recovery, no formula for success: 'Everyone's journey of recovery is unique. Each of us must find our own way and no-one can do it for us' (Deegan 1993). 'Once recovery becomes systematized, you've got it wrong. Once it is reduced to a set of principles it is wrong. It is a unique and individualized process' (Deegan 1999).

It is easy for the destructive rigid routines and block treatment of old psychiatric hospitals to spill over into community services (Barton 1959; Goffman 1963; Brown *et al.* 1966; King *et al.* 1971; Ryan 1979). There remain services where a set of rules guide the way that people must use them: you cannot have lunch at the day centre unless you attend a group; in order to live in the hostel you have to cook a meal for all residents once a week and attend the community group each day. Similarly, the 'ladder' models used by some services insist that people start at point A and then move in an orderly fashion to point Z: you must start in the rehabilitation ward, and then show that you can manage in a staffed hostel before you can have a flat of your own. Such rules inevitably mean that services cannot be tailored to the individual needs and aspirations of the people who use them. Not only is this likely to impede recovery, it is also likely either to de-skill people – prevent them from using their skills/abilities to the full – or alienate them by offering things that are unacceptable to them.

Therefore, if they are to facilitate recovery, rehabilitation services need to:

- **Adopt an individualized approach to assessment and intervention:** People with serious mental health problems are a diverse group. The block treatment provided in institutions was not only destructive, it was also ineffective in ensuring that individual needs were met; and

- **Ensure flexibility in the use of services:** Different people need different things from services. Rules for the use of services tend to exclude those who cannot, or do not wish to, comply and make responding to individual needs difficult.

Recovery is a possible for everyone

Recovery is not the same as cure. Some people may never be free of their symptoms. But everyone, no matter how severe their problems, has assets they can use to develop sources of value and meaning in their lives. Sayce *et al.* (1991) have shown how easy it is for services to 'drift up market': focus on those less disabled people, with whom they believe that the greatest progress can be made, at the expense of those who are most disabled. The challenge for practitioners is to help people to identify and make the most of their abilities – especially when these are overshadowed by their problems. Some may need a high level of support and help indefinitely if they are to be able to use their talents.

Therefore, if they are to facilitate recovery for all, rehabilitation services must retain a focus on the most disabled individuals. Without this, services tend to move 'up market' and the most disabled do not receive the support they need to maintain their community tenure, thereby creating the risk of a new generation of old long-stay patients.

How can rehabilitation services promote recovery?

Each individual with serious mental health problems must set about rebuilding their lives in their own way. A brief glance at the writings of people who have faced the challenge of recovery demonstrates the unique and individual nature of their journeys (see, for example, Deegan 1988, 1993, 1996; Leete 1988, 1989; Spaniol and Koehler 1994; May 1999; Vincent 1999; Young and Ensing 1999). However, these authors have identified a number of common features that are important in the recovery process: hope; relationships; coping with loss; spirituality, philosophy and understanding; taking back control; finding meaning, purpose and opportunity. These do not constitute a recipe, or a set of predetermined stages, in the recovery process. For the purpose of description different facets are listed separately here, but they are in fact intimately interrelated and do not follow any set sequence. For example, some people cannot regain hope, or address what has happened to them, until they have the opportunity to do things they value. Others need to regain a sense of possibility before they are able to think about embarking on the rebuilding process.

Restoring hope

Hope has been described as the 'anchor stabilising our lives in the present and giving life meaning, direction and optimism' (Lindsey 1976), and is a critical factor in recovery. Indeed it is central to the lives of most people (Stotland 1969; Brunner 1972; Lindsey 1976).

There is a considerable body of research into the importance of hope in coping with physical illness (e.g. Hickey 1986). In the mental health arena, hope has long been recognized as a key to successful psychotherapy (Menninger 1959; Frank 1968). That there is a link between hopelessness and suicide (Drake and Cotton 1986; Beck *et al.* 1990) and the importance of practitioners' hopefulness has been emphasized as central in rehabilitation (Anthony 1993; Woodside *et al.* 1994; Kanwal 1997). Hope relates to the achievement of goals that have a significance for the person concerned, but may not relate to specific outcomes (Dufault and Martocchio 1985). Hope may be a generalized sense of some future positive development or related to a specific, valued outcome (like getting a job or getting married).

For people with mental health problems, hope lies at the heart of a person's willingness to take on the challenge of recovery and rebuilding: without hope there is no point. In the face of the prejudice and exclusion that many people with mental health problems have experienced it is very easy to lose hope. And if a person can see no possibility of a positive future then it is all too easy for them to give up trying to do anything at all (Lovejoy 1982; Deegan 1988, 1993, 1996).

Hope cannot exist in a vacuum – relationships are central to fostering and maintaining a belief in the possibility of a positive future. If everyone around you believes that you have nothing to offer – that you will never amount to anything very much – then it is difficult (if not impossible) to retain a belief in your own worth. Having people around who believe in your possibilities and support you in pursuing these, is critical in fostering hope.

Relationships are important not only as a source of succour: it can be a devaluing experience always to be on the receiving end of support and help from others. Giving is as important as receiving and reciprocity in relationships is critical. Relationships in which people can contribute to the well-being of others are an important source of value. But the contribution of people with serious mental health problems often goes unrecognized. If hope is to be fostered, then we must move beyond ideas about the 'carers' and the 'cared for'. Greenberg *et al.* (1994) have shown that people with a diagnosis of schizophrenia can and do contribute a great deal of practical, social and emotional support to other members of their families. Reciprocal relationships with friends and family in which people give and receive support and help are critical to the restoration of hope.

However, it is also the case that mental health services often fail to inspire hope. Many people have described the ways in which contact with such services, and interactions with mental health practitioners, have left them feeling discouraged and dispirited (see Deegan 1990). Russinova (1999) has described a number of practitioner 'relationship skills' that are important in developing effective hope-inspiring relationships that can enable people to gain the confidence and self-belief that are critical if they are to rebuild their lives and access the opportunities that they value.

- believing in the person's potential and strength;

- valuing the person as a unique human being;

- accepting the person for who he or she is;

- listening non-judgementally to the person's experiences;

- tolerating the uncertainty about the future developments in the person's life;

- accepting the person's decompensations and failures as part of the recovery process;

- tolerating the person's challenges and defeats;

- trusting the authenticity of the person's experiences;

- expressing a genuine concern for the person's well-being; and

- using humour appropriately.

However, relationships between practitioners and clients can never be truly reciprocal. The practitioner does not elect to enter the relationship with a particular client – they are paid to be there – and the purpose of the relationship is to benefit the client rather than the practitioner (except indirectly via the salary paid and job satisfaction gained). Therefore, the quality of a relationship between client and practitioner must be judged by the extent to which it supports, or enables people to develop, those elective, reciprocal relationships with friends and family on which most of us rely so heavily and within which we gain a sense of our own value and worth.

The restoration of hope in the face of serious mental health problems also involves the accommodation of that experience with all the losses it entails. As with any bereavement, people face the task of accommodating what has happened so that they can move on (Perkins and Repper 1996; Repper and Perkins 2002). Helping people in this process can be time-consuming and it is important to remember that there is no set formula: people choose to grapple with different issues at different times and they may repeatedly return to the same issue before they can move beyond it. If mental health workers are to assist in this process we must be able to respond flexibly to the individual's wishes and preferences in a number of ways.

Grieving that which has been lost

People need space and time to grieve, to tell their life stories – and to tell them over and over again if necessary: new issues, meaning and under-standing can emerge with each telling. In reclaiming a sense of identity and value in the present, it is often necessary for a person to talk of identities and valued roles of the past; and express at least some of the anger, fear, despair, resentment or shame that they may feel over what has happened. Sometimes anger and resentment may be directed towards the practitioner and the advantages that they have: we may not feel privileged, but in com-parison with many of those with whom we work, we are very fortunate. The process of grieving may be slow. It is difficult to live with mental health problems and there may be little we can do to substantially change the material realities of the person's situation. But we can share the person's burden: understand and accept their distress, help them to feel less alone. An initial sense of profound isolation is described by most people who have received a diagnosis of serious mental health problems. And for some this sense of isolation can be ongoing. If people are to feel less alone, contact with others who have shared similar experiences can be extremely important.

Information: Challenging the myths

Many of the popular myths and misconceptions that surround mental health problems are inevitably shared by those who experience them, and are regularly reinforced in the popular media. These make the experience even more frightening. Many of those who deny that they have such difficulties do so in order to reject the images of themselves as dangerous and incompetent. It is important that practitioners make active efforts to dispel such myths and in doing this the personal accounts of people who have succeeded in rebuilding their lives can be powerful. There are a number of anthologies in which these can be found (see, for example, Spaniol and Koehler 1994; Read and Reynolds 1996) and papers in journals such as *Schizophrenia Bulletin* (see, for example, Leete 1989). Information about the many success-ful people – great painters like Van Gogh, scientists like Einstein, writers like James Joyce, politicians like Churchill – who have had mental health problems can also be useful (see, for example, Jamison 1993, 1995; Post 1994, 1996). It may be helpful to acknowledge that things can be more difficult for people who have serious mental health problems, not only because of the difficulties themselves, but also because of the prejudice and discrimination that exists ... but not impossible with the right kind of opportunities, help and support.

Understanding what has happened

As we have already discussed, people need to find a way of understanding what has happened that makes sense to them and allows them a way forward: hope for the future. People adopt a range of different explanatory frameworks for understanding their experiences (Jacobson 1993), but the experience of serious mental health problems often prompts people to explore broader spiritual and philosophical issues concerning the meaning of their lives: 'Why me?', 'What's the point?' Without prescribing particular religious and philosophical frameworks, it is important that practitioners enable people to think about these issues as well.

Taking back control

Mental health problems are often presented and perceived as uncontrollable – the province of experts. An essential element of rebuilding a meaningful and satisfying life involves taking back control.

> To me, recovery means I try to stay in the driver's seat of my life. I don't let my illness run me. Over the years I have worked hard to become an expert in my own self-care. For me, being in recovery means I don't just take medications. Just taking medications is a passive stance. Rather I use medications as part of my recovery process. In the same way, I don't just go into hospital. Just 'going into hospital' is a passive stance. Rather, I use the hospital when I need to.
>
> (Deegan 1989)

In relation to cognitive and emotional difficulties, research has repeatedly demonstrated that people want to have control over their symptoms – predict relapse and manage crises – and can develop ways of doing so. People can recognize the early signs of impending problems and take remedial action to avert or minimize a crisis (Breier and Strauss 1983; McCandless-Glincher *et al.* 1986; Kumar *et al.* 1989; Meuser *et al.* 1992; Birchwood *et al.* 1998; Repper 2000). A number of interventions have been developed to assist people in managing their own symptoms and crises (see, for example, Chadwick *et al.* 1996; Nelson 1997; Birchwood *et al.* 1998; Kingdon 1998).

Sometimes managing cognitive and emotional difficulties involves seeking treatment (pharmacological or psychological) but it will also include self-help, support from friends, and a range of strategies that the person has developed for dealing with particular problems.

Over the years I have learned different ways of helping myself. Sometimes I use medications, therapy, self-help and mutual support groups,
friends, my relationship with God, work, exercise, spending time in
nature – all of these measures help me remain whole and healthy, even
though I have a disability.

(Deegan 1993)

. . . stress does play an enormous part in my illness [schizophrenia].
There are enormous pressures that come with any new experience and
environment, and any change, positive or negative is extremely difficult.
Whatever I can do to decrease or avoid high stress environments is
helpful in controlling my symptoms. In general terms all of my coping
strategies consist of four steps: (1) recognizing when I am feeling
stressed, which is harder than it may sound; (2) identifying the stressor;
(3) remembering from past experience what action helped in the same
situation or a similar one; and (4) taking that action as quickly as
possible after I have identified the source of stress.

(Leete 1989)

People can benefit from the experiences of others who have faced similar
difficulties, within self-help groups and networks (like the 'Hearing Voices
Network', see www.hearing-voices.org.uk) or the self-management programmes (like those run by and for people with manic-depression, see
www.mdf.org.uk) or via self-help 'work books', like *Victim to Victor*
(Coleman and Smith 1997a, 1997b).

However, if people are to take back control over their own lives, then
practitioners must give up that control. It is easy to support people in
making choices for themselves when they agree with you: the real challenge
arises when the person makes choices that the practitioner considers to
be wrong (see Perkins and Repper 1998). There are, of course, occasions
when it would be unethical or illegal for the practitioner to accede to the
individual's wishes: we may not, for example, help people to kill themselves
or obtain illegal drugs. However, such instances are few and far between.
More generally, people make decisions that the practitioner considers are
unlikely to be successful. Often from the best of motives, practitioners
are eager to help people to avoid failure and its potentially destructive consequences. For example, we may discourage a person going to the job centre
because we think they are not yet ready for employment; or recommend that
they live in sheltered accommodation because we do not think they will be
able to look after themselves; or suggest that they do not go out clubbing
with their friends for fear that they will get drunk or use drugs and make
their problems worse.

Making the most of one's life necessarily involves the risk of failure.
Entering a relationship involves the risk of rejection; trying to get a job
involves the risk of being turned down; studying for qualifications involves
risking failure of examinations or assessment. Growth and development
necessarily involve the risk of failure. And we can learn as much about ourselves, and our possibilities, from our failures as we can from our successes.

It is also the case that people with serious mental health problems are often more expert in coping with failure – because of the numerous losses and disappointments they have experienced – than are the practitioners who are helping them.

If mental health practitioners are to facilitate recovery – help people to take the risks necessary if they are to do the things they want to do – then we must be prepared to assist people in doing things that we may think wrong or sub-optimal. Instead of attempting to dissuade people from their chosen course of action we need to:

- offer any support and help that we can to maximize their chances of success;

- endeavour to find ways of circumventing the difficulties that might prevent a person from achieving their chosen goal; and

- help them to learn from their experiences and try again if they are unsuccessful (and always avoid saying, 'I told you so').

There are a number of ways in which people may be assisted to access the opportunities that they seek. So, for example, even if we think someone is not ready to get a job, we can maximize their chances of doing so by helping them to get to the job centre; thinking through what they will say when they get there; assisting them to complete application forms or prepare for interviews; and providing ongoing support to retain their job if they are successful. Similarly, if a person wishes to live independently, it is always possible to arrange for support to obtain and maintain the 'home of their own' they desire (obtaining furniture; maximizing welfare benefits and enabling them to obtain any grants to which they may be entitled; arranging home helps, service washes at the launderette, take-away or ready-made meals; introducing the person to inexpensive cafés; helping them to manage money and pay rent . . .). If the person wants to go out clubbing, then we might help them to find someone to go along with them and develop strategies for avoiding the temptations of illegal drugs or limiting their alcohol intake.

Increasing opportunity

It is impossible for a person to rebuild a meaningful and satisfying life without the opportunity to do the things they value. But prejudice and discrimination frequently limit the access of people with mental health problems to the opportunities that are available to non-disabled citizens.

In order to facilitate recovery, people with serious mental health problems require access to a range of accommodation possibilities; work/education, leisure and social opportunities; and sources of support (see Health Advisory Service 2000). However, Bates (2002) and Repper and Perkins (2002) have outlined things that individual practitioners can do to facilitate a person's access to valued roles and activities. At a general level, these may include:

- **Information:** providing people with information about the facilities, opportunities and services available in the local area;
- **Bridge building:** actively creating links with local facilities to facilitate access. This may involve getting to know key people at the local college, leisure centre, church or job centre; understanding the demands and expectations of these facilities; and the sort of people who use them; and
- **Capacity building:** increasing the capacity of community facilities to accommodate people who have experienced mental health problems. This typically involves two elements: breaking down myths and misconceptions about people with mental health problems and providing them with the support they feel they need to accommodate people with such difficulties.

At an individual level, practitioners might use the following strategies to assist a person to access the opportunities and activities that they seek:

- **Planning and target setting:** helping people to think about their goals and ambitions, break these down into manageable steps and plan the necessary interim goals and targets on the way;
- **Practice:** helping the person to rehearse what they are going to do and to practise it until they feel comfortable doing it;
- **Skills development:** using a variety of techniques – instruction, prompting, modelling, guided practice, feedback – helping a person to develop the skills they need to engage in their chosen activities;
- **Graded exposure/return:** helping people to overcome fears and anxieties that stop them doing what they want to do or resuming valued activities in which they have previously been involved;
- **Just visiting:** a place or activity beforehand as a way of becoming familiar with how to get there and what to expect;
- **Time-limited experience** (like work experience or college 'taster sessions'): in order to try something out before deciding whether it is what they want to do;
- **Providing transport:** to help the person to get to the activity, or actually going with them to help reduce their anxiety;
- **'Doing with':** helping someone to do something by doing it alongside them. This may involve a mental health practitioner, but having your nurse with you in a college class can be stigmatizing. There may be others who are better placed to join the person in the activity and who are less likely to attract negative attention: friends, relatives, volunteers, someone already engaged in the activity, others who experience mental health difficulties;
- **Subsidy:** helping to meet the costs of the activity by providing money for things like transport, refreshments, course registration fees and/or exploring other sources of subsidy like bus passes, or reduced rates of entry for unemployed or disabled people;

- **Special groups within ordinary settings:** for example, special groups or classes to introduce people with mental health problems to the local sports centre, college or library;

- **Staff from different facilities coming into mental health facilities:** to introduce them and to familiarize people with the activities involved before going to the community facility;

- **Mentoring:** arranging for someone who is already involved in the setting/ activity to provide information about what will be expected before they go, introduce them to the activity and provide advice and encouragement when they are there;

- **Helping people to make new friends:** often people lack the friendships and relationships on which most of us rely so heavily. Practitioners can help people to increase their social networks and contacts by, for example, enabling them to access activities where they are likely to meet people who share their interests; accessing internet chat-lines and e-groups (some of which are designed specifically for people with mental health problems like the Yahoo 'uksurvivors' e-group); placing or replying to advertisements in 'lonely hearts'/'contact' columns of local papers and listings magazines; befriending; or facilitating contact between service users who share interests/aspirations;

- **Help and support when difficulties arise:** the fluctuating nature of mental health problems often means that it is important to ensure that assistance is readily available when difficulties arise;

- **Working out ways of coping with symptoms/difficulties in the setting:** Leete (1989), for example, offers numerous examples of strategies that she has found useful in coping with the symptoms of her schizophrenia in a work setting;

- **Self-help and support groups:** where people with mental health problems who are engaged in similar activities (for example, working, going to college) can get together and gain encouragement and support from each other;

- **Negotiating adaptations and adjustments on the part of the provider:** these involve changing the physical or social environment, and/or the expectations on the person, so that they are able to engage in the activity. The UK Disability Discrimination Act (1995) not only outlaws discrimination against people with mental health problems but also requires that employers and providers of education, goods and services make 'reasonable adjustments' to ensure that people with such difficulties can access the opportunities they offer; and

- **Helping people to obtain their rights under the law:** as indicated above, the Disability Discrimination Act (1995) covers people with mental health problems and has been used by people with such difficulties to good effect (see Sayce 2001). Sayce (2001, 2002) has suggested that mental health practitioners should:

- Be aware of the rights and protection that the Disability Discrimination Act provides for people with mental health problems and inform people with whom they work of these. Such information can be obtained from the Disability Rights Commission Help Line or website.[1]
- Provide information about the assistance available from the Disability Rights Commission Help Line and casework team and help people with mental health problems to access this.
- Help employers, colleges and the providers of goods and services to decide what 'reasonable adjustments' people with mental health problems might need to facilitate access (either on an individual basis or as part of a more general 'capacity building' initiative – see above).
- Provide advocacy in relation to employment, education, leisure and other services.

There are many ways in which practitioners can enable people to access opportunities that they seek, but it is important that any such assistance is tailored to the needs/preferences of the person concerned. In choosing an appropriate approach practitioners might consider (Repper and Perkins 2002):

- **Individual acceptability:** What sort of help does the person want?

- **Social acceptability:** What sort of help would draw least negative attention to the person?

- **Amount and availability:** How much help does the person need and what support might be available?

- **Existing abilities and resources:** How can the person's abilities, social contacts and other resources be used to best effect?

- **Issues of control:** How far can the person themselves control the amount, timing and nature of the help they receive?

- **Evidence of past effectiveness:** What sort of help has been effective/ ineffective in the past?

- **The research evidence**: For example, skills development and practice are more effective when conducted in the setting in which the skills will be used because things learned in one setting do not always generalize to other situations (Shepherd 1977, 1978; Appelo *et al.* 1992; Ekdawi and Conning 1994). Similarly, Bond *et al.* (1997, 2001) have identified a number of factors important in the success of programmes to facilitate access to employment including rapid job-search and minimal pre-vocational training; the availability of time-unlimited workplace support and the integration of clinical treatment with vocational rehabilitation.

Images of possibility

Perhaps the most important factor in both recovery and rehabilitation is a belief in possibility. If a person is to embark on the task of rebuilding a valued and satisfying life with mental health problems then they must believe in the possibility of a positive future. If a practitioner is to be able to assist the person in this process then they too must believe in the person's possibilities.

The traditional focus of mental health practitioners on the remediation of symptoms, dysfunctions and shortcomings is not helpful in generating a framework that engenders such images of possibility in either practitioners or the people whom we serve. As Peter Chadwick, a lecturer in psychology who himself has a diagnosis of schizophrenia, has described:

> Deficit-obsessed research can only produce theories and attitudes which are disrespectful of clients and are also likely to induce behaviour in clinicians such that service users are not properly listened to, not believed, not fairly assessed, are likely treated as inadequate and are also not expected to be able to become independent and competent individuals in managing life's tasks.
>
> (Chadwick:1997)

If rehabilitation is to be effective in facilitating recovery, practitioners must extend their role beyond that of 'therapists who alleviate symptoms' to one of 'facilitators who assist people to rebuild lives'. We may hold a variety of theories about the nature and origins of mental health problems, but our primary role is to identify people's assets and possibilities and help them to recognize and exploit these themselves. If we are to be successful in these endeavours we must respect both the worth of people who experience serious mental health problems and the expertise of their experience.

A commitment, and ability, to learn from people with mental health problems, as well as their friends and relatives, is essential, as is an openness and willingness to be corrected by experience. Expertise does not mean never making mistakes but the ability to learn from those mistakes. Those whom we serve are our most important teachers.

Conclusion

To conclude, we summarize the main points of this chapter below:

- Recovery and rehabilitation are not the same thing. While recovery is an individual journey of rebuilding a satisfying and valued life, rehabilitation is the process via which mental health practitioners might help people to do this.

- Too often, practitioners fail to appreciate the range of traumas experienced by people with mental health problems. Unless we can understand and address the complex range of barriers that they face we may inadvertently impede recovery by alienating people from the very services that are supposed to assist them.

- If they are to facilitate recovery, then rehabilitation services need to:
  - adopt a team approach;
  - ensure continuity across providers;
  - be strengths based;
  - focus on changing the environment, not simply changing individuals;
  - focus on maintaining, as well as optimizing functioning;
  - adopt a long-term perspective;
  - offer continuity of support over time;
  - accept setbacks and relapse as part of the recovery process;
  - emphasize social integration and reintegration;
  - maximize opportunities for people with mental health problems to support and learn from each other;
  - successfully involve service users and their relatives/friends;
  - be user centred and needs led;
  - adopt an individualized approach to assessment and intervention;
  - ensure flexibility in the use of services;
  - focus on the most disabled individuals.

- Common features in the recovery process include:

  1 restoration of hope, which may involve:

  - grieving that which has been lost,
  - challenging the myths and misconceptions that surround mental health problems,
  - finding a way of understanding what has happened;

  2 taking back control;
  3 increasing the opportunities for people to do the things they value.

- Many things that mental health practitioners can do to facilitate a person's access to valued roles and activities are listed in this chapter. Crucial, however, is for the practitioner to believe in the person's possibilities for a positive future.

- If rehabilitation is to be effective in facilitating recovery then practitioners must extend their role beyond that of 'therapists who alleviate symptoms' to one of 'facilitators who assist people to rebuild their lives'.

Note

1 Disability Rights Commission Help Line: Telephone: 08457-622633, Text phone: 08457-622644. Disability Rights Commission website: www.drc-gb.org

Questions for reflection and discussion

1 The concept of recovery is not confined to mental health problems. Consider an event that has had an impact on your life (such as losing a job, the death of a loved one, serious illness, moving house . . .) and think about the effect this had on you, ways in which you coped, what helped you and what did not help. If possible discuss this with another person and note the similarities and differences in your experiences of recovery. How has the experience changed you/your life in the long term?

2 This chapter has drawn a clear distinction between recovery and rehabilitation.

   (a) Consider the differences between the two processes.
   (b) What does the concept of recovery contribute to ideas about rehabilitation?
   (c) How can rehabilitation services promote recovery?

3 Access to roles and relationships that are valued, both by the individual and within their society, is an essential part of recovery; facilitating such access is a critical component of rehabilitation. All mental health teams need to consider ways in which this 'socially inclusive work' could become a more integral and effective part of the service they provide. As a team, it might be useful to consider 'general level' strategies that might be introduced or strengthened within the team. Each one of these will need to be considered in some depth, and an action plan developed.

   (a) How could information about facilities opportunities and services within the local area be collected, compiled, maintained and presented?
   (b) How could bridge building be organized and facilitated within the service?
   (c) How might your team increase the capacity of community facilities to accommodate people who have experienced mental health problems through education, information and support?

Annotated bibliography

- Repper, J. and Perkins, R. (2003) *Social Inclusion and Recovery. A Model for Mental Health Practice.* Oxford: Elsevier Science. This text provides a more detailed analysis of recovery and inclusion by the authors of this chapter. It draws on service users' experiences of living with mental health problems, and their accounts of recovery to construct a model for practitioners seeking to promote recovery and inclusion.

- Leete, E. (1989) How I perceive and manage my illness, *Schizophrenia Bulletin* **15**: 197–200. Although this paper is somewhat dated, it still provides an inspirational account of the ways the author has developed to cope with the effects of her cognitive and emotional difficulties. Diagnosed with schizophrenia, Ms Leete now maintains her employment and social relationships through carefully considered and implemented strategies to cope with, for example, her anxiety, tendency to misinterpret situations, difficulties in concentrating and inability to respond quickly. Over twenty different coping strategies are described along with descriptions of the types of situations that are likely to be distressing or difficult.
- Sayce, L. (2000) *From Psychiatric Patient to Citizen. Overcoming Discrimination and Social Exclusion*, London: Macmillan. An in-depth analysis of the discrimination and exclusion experienced by people who have mental health problems with reference to extensive US and UK literature, research and personal contact. Various ways of overcoming this exclusion are debated through practical examples and theoretical debate.
- Perkins, R.E. and Repper, J.M. (1996) *Working Alongside People with Long Term Mental Health Problems*. Cheltenham: Stanley Thornes. Again, somewhat dated, but this remains one of very few texts available for direct care workers about the process of rehabilitation – facilitating access to socially valued roles, relationships, opportunities and facilities. It examines a range of different approaches that might be useful, and draws attention to the challenges that (still) remain.

| References

Anthony, W.A. (1993) Recovery from mental illness: The guiding vision of the mental health system in the 1990s, *Innovations and Research* **2**(3): 17–24.

Appelo, M.T., Woonings, F.M.J. and Van Nieuwenhuizen, C.J. (1992) Specific skills and social competence in schizophrenia, *Acta Psychiatrica Scandanavica* **85**: 419–22.

Barton, R. (1959) *Institutional Neurosis*. Bristol: Wright.

Bates, B. (2002) *A-Z of Socially Inclusive Strategies*. Unpublished text. First presented at 'Piece of Mind' Conference, New College, Nottingham, January 1999.

Beck, A.T., Brown, G., Berchick, J., Stewart, L.B. and Steer, R.A. (1990) Relationship between hopelessness and suicide: A replication with psychiatric outpatients, *American Journal of Psychiatry* **147**(2): 11–23.

Bennett, D. (1978) Social forms of psychiatric treatment, in J.K. Wing (ed.) *Schizophrenia: Toward a New Synthesis*. London: Academic Press.

Birchwood, M., Smith, J., Macmillan, F. and McGovern, D. (1998) Early intervention in psychotic relapse, in C. Brooker and J. Repper (eds) *Serious Mental Health Problems in the Community: Policy, Practice and Research*. London: Bailliere Tindall.

Bond, G.R., Drake, R.E., Meuser, K.T. and Becker, D.R. (1997) An update on supported employment for people with severe mental illness, *Psychiatric Services* **48**: 335–46.

Bond, G.R., Becker, D.R., Drake, R.E. *et al.* (2001) Implementing supported employment as an evidence based practice, *Psychiatric Services* **52**(3): 313–22.

Breier, A. and Strauss, J. (1983) Self control in psychiatric disorders, *Archives of General Psychiatry* **40**: 1141–5.

Brown, G.W., Bone, M., Dalison, M. and Wing, J.K. (1966) *Schizophrenia and Social Care*. Oxford: Oxford University Press.

Brunner, E. (1972) *Eternal Hope*. Westport, CT: Greenwood Press.

Chadwick, P., Birchwood, M. and Trower, P. (1996) *Cognitive Therapy for Delusions, Voices and Paranoia*. Chichester: John Wiley and Sons.

Chadwick, P.K. (1997) *Schizophrenia: The Positive Perspective. In Search of Dignity for Schizophrenic People*. London: Routledge.

Chamberlin, J. (1995) Rehabilitating ourselves: the psychiatric survivor movement. *International Journal of Mental Health* **24**: 39–46.

Coleman, R. and Smith, M. (1997a) *Working with Voices*. Gloucester: Handsell Publishing.

Coleman, R. and Smith, M. (1997b) *Working with Self Harm*. Gloucester: Handsell Publishing.

Crowther, R.E., Marshall, M., Bond, G.R. and Huxley, P. (2001) Helping people with severe mental illness to obtain work: Systematic review, *British Medical Journal* **322**: 204–8.

Deegan, P. (1988) Recovery: The lived experience of rehabilitation, *Psychosocial Rehabilitation Journal* **11**(4): 11–19.

Deegan, P. (1989) *A letter to my Friend Who is Giving Up*. Paper presented at the Connecticut Conference on Supported Employment, Connecticut Association of Rehabilitation Facilities, Cromwell, CT.

Deegan, P. (1990) *How Recovery Begins*, paper presented at the eighth Annual Education Conference Alliance for the Mentally Ill of New York State, Binghampton, New York.

Deegan, P. (1993) Recovering our sense of value after being labeled, *Journal of Psychosocial Nursing* **31**(4): 7–11.

Deegan, P. (1996) Recovery as a journey of the heart, *Psychosocial Rehabilitation Journal* **19**(3): 91–7.

Deegan, P.E. (1999) *Recovery: An Alien Concept*, paper presented at Strangefish Conference 'Recovery: An alien concept' at Chamberlin Hotel, Birmingham.

Drake, R.E. and Cotton, P.G. (1986) Depression, hopelessness and suicide in chronic schizophrenia, *British Journal of Psychiatry* **148**: 554–9.

Dufault, K. and Martocchio, B. (1985) Hope: Its spheres and dimensions, *Nursing Clinics of North America* **20**(2): 379–91.

Ekdawi, M. and Conning, A. (1994) *Psychiatric Rehabilitation – A Practical Guide*. London: Chapman and Hall.

Estroff, S. (1989) Self, identity, and subjective experiences of schizophrenia: in search of a subject, *Schizophrenia Bulletin* **15**: 189–96.

Frank, J. (1968) The role of hope in psychotherapy, *International Journal of Psychiatry* **5**: 383–95.

Goffman, E. (1963) *Stigma: Notes on the Management of Spoiled Identity*. Harmondsworth: Penguin.

Greenberg, J.S., Greenley, J.R. and Benedict, P. (1994) Contributions of persons with serious mental illness to their families, *Hospital and Community Psychiatry* **45**: 475–80.

Health Advisory Service (2000) *Review of Adult Mental Health Rehabilitation Services in Wandsworth, Merton, Sutton, Kingston and Richmond*. London: HAS.

Hickey, S.S. (1986) Enabling hope, *Journal of Cancer Nursing* **9**(3): 133–7.

Jacobson, N. (1993) Experiencing recovery: A dimensional analysis of recovery narratives, *Psychiatric Rehabilitation Journal* **24**(3): 248–55.

Jamison, K.R. (1993) *Touched with Fire: Manic-depressive Illness and the Artistic Temperament*. New York: The Free Press.

Jamison, K.R. (1995) Manic depressive illness and creativity, *Scientific American*, February, 46–51.

Kanwal, G.S. (1997) Hope, respect and flexibility in the psychotherapy, *Contemporary Psychoanalysis* **33**(1): 133–50.

King, R., Raynes, N. and Tizard, J. (1971) *Patterns of Residential Care*. London: Routledge.

Kingdon, D. (1998) Cognitive behaviour therapy for severe mental illness: strategies and techniques, in C. Brooker and J. Repper (eds) *Serious Mental Health Problems in the Community: Policy, Practice and Research*. London: Bailliere Tindall.

Kubler-Ross, E. (1969) *Death and Dying*, London: Macmillan.

Kumar, S., Thara, R. and Rajkumar, S. (1989) Coping with symptoms of relapse in schizophrenia, *European Archives of Psychiatric Neurological Science* **239**: 213–15.

Leete, E. (1988) The treatment of schizophrenia: A patient's perspective, *Hospital and Community Psychiatry* **38**(5): 486–91.

Leete, E. (1989) How I perceive and manage my illness, *Schizophrenia Bulletin* **15**: 197–200.

Lindsey, H. (1976) *The Terminal Generation*, Old Tappan, NJ: Fleming-Revel.

Lovejoy, M. (1982) Expectations and the recovery process, *Schizophrenia Bulletin* **8**(4): 605–9.

May, R. (1999) *Routes to Recovery – The Roots of a Clinical Psychologist*, paper presented at Strangefish Conference 'Recovery: An alien concept' at Chamberlin Hotel, Birmingham.

McCandless-Glincher, L., McKnight, S., Hamera, E. *et al.* (1986) Use of symptoms by schizophrenics to monitor and regulate their illness, *Hospital and Community Psychiatry* **37**: 929–33.

Menninger, K. (1959) Hope, *American Journal of Psychiatry* **116**(12): 481–91.

Mueser, K.T., Bellack, A. and Blanchard, J. (1992) Comorbidity of schizophrenia and substance abuse: implications for treatment, *Journal of Clinical and Consulting Psychology* **60**: 845–55.

Nelson, H. (1997) *Cognitive Behavioural Therapy with Schizophrenia*. London: Nelson Thornes.

O'Donoghue, D. (1994) *Breaking Down the Barriers. The Stigma of Mental Illness: A User's Point of View*. Aberystwyth: US, the All Wales User Network.

Perkins, R.E. and Repper, J.M. (1996) *Working Alongside People with Long Term Mental Health Problems*. Cheltenham: Stanley Thornes.

Perkins, R.E. and Repper, J.M. (1998) *Dilemmas in Community Mental Health Practice. Choice or Control*. Oxford: Radcliffe Medical Press.

Post, F. (1994) Creativity and psychopathology: A study of 291 world-famous men, *British Journal of Psychiatry* **165**: 22–34.

Post, F. (1996) Verbal creativity, depression and alcoholism: an investigation of one hundred American and British writers, *British Journal of Psychiatry* **168**: 545–55.

Read, J. and Reynolds, J. (1996) *Speaking Our Minds*. London: Macmillan.

Repper, J. (2000) Adjusting the focus of mental health nursing: Incorporating service users' experiences of recovery, *Journal of Mental Health* **9**(6): 575–87.

Repper, J. and Perkins, R. (2002) *Social Inclusion and Recovery: A Model for Mental Health Practice*. London: Bailliere Tindall.

Russinova, Z. (1999) Providers' hope-inspiring competence as a factor optimizing psychiatric rehabilitation outcomes, *Journal of Rehabilitation* **16**(4): 50–7.

Ryan, P. (1979) Residential care for the mentally disabled, in J.K. Wing and R. Olsen (eds) *Community Care for the Mentally Disabled*. Oxford: Oxford University Press.

Sayce, L. (2000) *From Psychiatric Patient to Citizen. Overcoming Discrimination and Social Exclusion*. London: Macmillan.

Sayce, L. (2001) Not just users of services, but contributors to society: The opportunities of the Disability Rights Agenda, *The Mental Health Review* **6**(3): 25–8.

Sayce, L. (2002) *Beyond Good Intentions: Making Anti-discrimination Strategies Work*, London: Disability Rights Commission.

Sayce, L., Craig, T. and Boardman, A. (1991) The development of community mental health centres in the UK, *Social Psychiatry and Psychiatric Epidemiology* **26**: 14–20.

Shepherd, G. (1977) Social skills training: The generalisation problem, *Behaviour Therapy* **8**: 100–9.

Shepherd, G. (1978) Social skills training: The generalisation problem – some further data, *Behaviour Research and Therapy* **116**: 287–8.

Spaniol, L. and Koehler, M. (1994) (eds) *The Experience of Recovery*. Boston, MA: Center for Psychiatric Rehabilitation.

Spaniol, L., Gagne, C. and Koehler, M. (1997) Recovery from serious mental illness: What it is and how to assist people in their recovery, *Continuum* **4**(4): 3–15.

Stein, L.L. and Test, M.A. (1980) Alternative to mental hospital I. Conceptual model, treatment programme and clinical evaluation, *Archives of General Psychiatry* **37**: 392–7.

Stotland, E. (1969) *The Psychology of Hope*, San Francisco: Jossey-Bass.

Vincent, S.S. (1999) *Using Findings from Qualitative Research to Teach Mental Health Professionals about the Experience of Recovery from Psychiatric Disability*, Presentation at the Harvard University Graduate School of Education Fourth Annual Student Research Conference, Cambridge, MA.

Woodside, H., Landeen, J., Kirkpatrick, H. *et al.* (1994) Hope and schizophrenia: Exploring attitudes of clinicians, *Psychosocial Rehabilitation Journal* **8**: 140–4.

Young, S.L. and Ensing, D.S. (1999) Exploring recovery from the perspective of people with psychiatric disabilities, *Psychiatric Rehabilitation Journal* **22**(3): 219–31.

|6

Law and ethics of mental health nursing

Philip Fennell

▎Chapter overview

Mental ill health and learning disability nursing pose more acute legal
and ethical issues than any other branch of medicine. The vast majority of
mentally disordered people consent to their treatment, and their decisions
about their health care pose no threat to their own health or safety or to the
safety of other people. However, a minority of people with mental disorders
cannot or will not accept that they are ill and may need treatment in their
own interests or those of others. Some may even be so afflicted by mental
disorder that they lack the capacity to make basic decisions about their care,
to consent to treatment, or indeed to complain when they are the victims of
abuse. These effects of mental disorder set it apart from other illnesses and
result in difficult ethical and legal tensions. Overshadowing all is the stigma
attached to mental disorder.

There are three main sources of legal rules governing good clinical
practice in mental health nursing:

1 the common law developed by the decisions of the judges over the
   years;
2 Parliamentary legislation which confers statutory powers and duties;
   and
3 the European Convention on Human Rights.

In legal terms mental disorder is given special status. This is reflected in
the special arrangements which exist to detain and treat mentally disordered
patients without consent, both under Parliamentary legislation (the Mental
Health Act 1983) and under judge-made common law. The Mental Health
Act (1983) allows for the detention and forcible treatment of patients
suffering from mental disorder of a sufficiently serious nature or degree to
warrant treatment in the interests of their own health or safety or for the

protection of others. Nurses have various statutory powers and functions under the 1983 Act. They may detain patients who are seeking to leave hospital using the nurse's holding power; or they may use reasonable force to administer treatment which a detained patient is required to accept under Part IV of the Mental Health Act (1983). Treatment without consent under the Mental Health Act is only possible if a patient is detained and the treatment is for mental disorder. Compulsory treatment of a detained patient is lawful provided it is sanctioned by a second opinion doctor, regardless of the patient's capacity to consent (Mental Health Act 1983, s 58).

The judge-made common law also allows for mentally incapacitated adults to be given any treatment for their physical or mental illness which is necessary in their best interests (*Re F (Mental Patient: Sterilisation)* [1990] 2 AC 1). Under common law mentally incapacitated patients may be treated without their consent, and even detained and restrained where such treatment is considered by the clinician in charge of their care to be necessary in their best interests (*R v Bournewood Mental Health Trust ex parte L* (1999)). Issues of confidentiality also loom large in psychiatric nursing, and there is a considerable body of case law both of the English Courts and the European Court of Human Rights on the circumstances where patient confidentiality may be breached to protect health or the rights and freedoms of others.

Nurses have other common law powers and duties. They owe a duty of confidentiality to patients not to disclose personal information about patients unless there is some overriding public interest. This duty of confidence is reinforced by terms in nurses' contracts of employment, and in *Ashworth Hospital v Mirror Group Newspapers* (2002) it was held that hospitals may, in certain cases, obtain an order that a journalist disclose the identity of any member of their staff who breaches professional confidence.

Where nurses exercise statutory or common law powers of detention or restraint of patients they would be likely to be found to be public authorities for the purposes of the Human Rights Act (1998). A public authority is any person or body certain of whose functions are of a public nature. Section 6 of the Human Rights Act (1998) makes it unlawful for a public authority to act in a way which is incompatible with a Convention Right, unless the public authority was required to act in that way by legislation. It is therefore important for nurses to understand the basic requirements of the European Convention on Human Rights.

This chapter covers:

- the sources of ethical guidance and legal rules and their interrelationship;
- ethical guidance and the powers of the Nursing and Midwifery Council;
- the nurse's duty of care and the common law of negligence;
- the powers of nurses to restrain a patient from leaving hospital under the Mental Health Act 1983;

- use of the common law power to detain and restrain mentally incapacitated adults;
- treatment of mentally incapacitated adults under common law;
- treatment of detained patients for mental disorder without consent;
- treatment of children;
- confidentiality and the duty to disclose information;
- the influence of the Human Rights Act 1998.

Sources of ethical guidance and their interrelationship with legal rules

There are two principal sources of ethical and policy guidance for nurses:

1   the *Code of Professional Conduct* of the Nursing and Midwifery Council (NMC), which has replaced the United Kingdom Central Council for Nursing and Midwifery (UKCC) and the Guidance issued by the Council on issues specific to mental health nursing;

2   the *Code of Practice on the Mental Health Act 1983* published by the Department of Health and the Welsh Office.

The Nursing and Midwifery Council *Code of Professional Conduct* is organized around seven core values shared by all health care regulatory bodies in the United Kingdom. In caring for clients and patients nurses must (*Code of Professional Conduct* (2002: 2)):

1   respect the patient or client as an individual;
2   obtain consent before giving any treatment or care;
3   protect confidential information;
4   cooperate with others in the team;
5   maintain professional knowledge and competence;
6   be trustworthy; and;
7   act to identify and minimize risk to patients and clients.

Nurses are personally accountable for their practice (*Code of Conduct* (2002), para. 1.3). This means that they are answerable for their acts and omissions, regardless of the advice and directions of another professional. In other words, the fact that a nurse has been directed by a doctor to do something will not relieve them of personal responsibility if that act was unethical or unlawful. For this reason it is important that nurses are aware of their ethical and legal position in relation to the key elements of patient care. Very often nurses are called upon to balance several different ethical values against one another, for example respecting the client as an individual may involve listening to their wishes, but it may also involve setting those wishes against the need to minimize risk to the client. The aim in such circumstances is to ensure that a fair balance is achieved.

In addition to the *Code of Professional Conduct* (2002) the NMC has issued special *Guidelines for Mental Health and Disability Nursing* (1998), *Guidelines for the Administration of Medicine* (2002) and guidelines on *Practitioner–Client Relationships and the Prevention of Abuse* (2002). Moreover there is an NMC *position statement on the covert administration of medicines – Disguising Medicine in Food and Drink* (2001). Nurses are subject to the disciplinary powers of the NMC, the statutory regulatory authority of the nursing profession. The purpose of the NMC is the protection of the public, and it has jurisdiction to consider cases of professional misconduct and unfitness to practise through ill-health. Failure, without good reason, to follow guidance in the nurses' *Code of Professional Conduct* or the *Mental Health Act Code of Practice* could form the basis of disciplinary proceedings for professional misconduct. It could also be referred to in an action for negligence for breach of the nurse's duty of care to the patient. If it involved assault or sexual impropriety it might also form the basis of a criminal prosecution.

The nurses' duty of care and the common law of negligence

Common law is the law developed through case-by-case precedent by the judges. Nurses owe a common duty of care to their patients, to avoid causing them injury by wrongful acts or omissions. The standard of care expected of a nurse is that of responsible practitioners skilled in the specialty. In order for a nurse to be liable in negligence, the patient or other person suing them must establish three basic elements:

1   that the nurse owed them a duty of care;

2   that the nurse breached that duty; and

3   that the breach of duty caused them injury.

The first question is who is owed a duty of care. Nurses owe a duty of care to people who they should reasonably foresee as being likely to be injured by their acts or failure to act. This means that patients and clients are owed a duty of care, as are work colleagues. So the nurse in charge owes a duty of care to a vulnerable elderly mentally-ill client who lacks mental capacity and who is seeking to leave the ward late at night in freezing temperatures. Equally, a nurse who is told by a patient that he or she intends to assault another member of staff would owe a duty of care to that colleague, to take reasonable steps to avoid that risk coming to pass.

The second issue in a negligence action is whether the nurse broke the duty, that is, fell short of the standard of care to be expected of a nurse. A nurse will not be negligent if his or her conduct is supported by a responsible body of professional opinion (*Bolam v Friern Barnet Hospital Management*

Committee (1957)), and that body of professional opinion is considered by the judge to be 'supported by logic', or logically defensible (*Bolitho v City and Hackney Health Authority* (1998)). This means that expert witnesses are called to state what they would have considered to be acceptable nursing practice. Judges only rarely find that a body of opinion put forward by reasonable, well-qualified expert witnesses is unsupported by logic. However, in the hypothetical example of the frail elderly person with mental illness seeking to leave the ward in freezing temperatures, it would be hard to imagine any responsible body of nursing opinion coming forward to support allowing her to leave. Even if there were, it is unlikely that the courts would find that allowing a frail incapacitated patient to put herself at risk in this way is in any way supported by logic.

The nurses' *Code of Professional Conduct* states clearly that, 'When facing professional dilemmas your first consideration in all activities must be the interests and the safety of patients or clients' (2002: para. 8.4). *The Mental Health Act Code of Practice* says that 'Every patient should have an individual care plan which states explicitly why and when he or she will be prevented from leaving the ward' (1998: para. 19.27), and that patients who 'persistently and purposefully' attempt to leave a ward, whether or not they understand the risk, should be considered for formal detention under the Act. In such a circumstance the nurse needs to be aware that if he or she is a registered nurse 'of the prescribed class' (Parts 3, 4, 5, 6, 13, 14 of the register) the patient may be held up to six hours so that an assessment of the need to detain him or her may be made. A nurse who is not of the prescribed class should be aware that he or she has a common law power to use reasonable force to restrain and detain mentally incapacitated patients where it is necessary in the patients' best interests (*R v Bournewood Mental Health Trust ex parte L* (1999)). This case study shows the need for nurses in carrying out their duty under the NMC *Code of Professional Conduct* to keep knowledge and skills up to date, and to ensure that they possess the knowledge, skills and abilities required for lawful, safe and effective practice (NMC *Code of Professional Conduct* (2002): paras 6.1–6.2). Professional guidance by the NMC and in other Codes and protocols will be referred to in assessing whether a nurse's conduct falls short of the standard to be expected, and for this reason it is important for nurses to ensure that they are aware of relevant professional guidance, and of the scope of their legal powers and responsibilities. Basic knowledge of the relevant law and ethical guidance is therefore a requirement for lawful practice.

The third issue in a negligence claim is whether the claimant has suffered injury as a result of the breach of duty. This means that the claimant must establish that his or her injury resulted from the negligence of the nurse and was not attributable to some other cause. Moreover the injury must be of a kind recognized by the law, which allows claims for recognized psychiatric illness or injury resulting from negligence, as well as for physical injury. The injury suffered must also be of a reasonably foreseeable kind. A whole vista of dire consequences would be reasonably foreseeable in the case of the frail elderly lady allowed to leave the ward late on a freezing cold night. If the lady died as a result of hypothermia, or falling into a river, the nurse could be sued for negligence. The employing hospital would be liable to meet the damages claim under the doctrine of vicarious liability whereby an employer is liable for the acts or omissions of his employee in the course of employment duties. In addition to suing for negligence, the relatives could ask the Health Service Commissioner (the Health Ombudsman) to investigate and report, and they could complain to the Nursing and Midwifery Council that the nurse was guilty of professional misconduct.

Compulsory admission to hospital under the Mental Health Act (1983)

The main source of statutory powers and duties for mental health nurses is the Mental Health Act (1983), which governs the care and treatment of people suffering from mental disorder. Although the Act allows for detention and the imposition of compulsory powers in the community, on people with mental disorder, the guiding principle, like its predecessor, the Mental Health Act (1959), is that informal admission is preferred to the use of compulsion. Section 131 reflects this principle by providing that nothing in the Act shall prevent a patient requiring admission to hospital from being admitted to any hospital, in pursuance of arrangements made in that behalf, without any application, order or direction rendering him liable to be detained. Informal admission does not necessarily mean that the patient has admitted himself or herself voluntarily. It may be used where patients lack the capacity to consent to admission, for example because of Alzheimer's, but are not resisting admission.

The *Mental Health Act Code of Practice* states that,

> Where admission to hospital is considered necessary, this should in general be arranged. Compulsory admission powers should only be used as a last resort. Informal admission is usually appropriate when a mentally capable patient consents to admission, but not if detention is necessary because of the danger the patient presents to himself or to others.
>
> (Department of Health and Welsh Assembly Government 1998: para. 2.7)

This means that detention should effectively be reserved for those who need inpatient treatment and are unwilling to be admitted informally. About 90 per cent of hospital admissions are informal (Department of Health, *Health And Personal Social Services Statistics*, 2001–2), but the numbers of compulsory admissions have increased from 18,000 in 1990–1 to 26,300 in 2001–2 (Department of Health Statistical Bulletin 2002/26). Informal patients have the right to leave hospital, but they may be restrained from doing so if a doctor or a registered mental nurse considers that it may be necessary to subject them to detention (Mental Health Act 1983, s 5, discussed further below).

In order to be liable to detention under the 1983 Act, a person must be suffering from mental disorder within the meaning of the Act. Mental disorder is very broadly defined as including 'mental illness, psychopathic disorder, arrested or incomplete development of mind and any other disorder or disability of mind'. Mental illness is not defined in the 1983 Act, yet it is the broadest category. It includes depressive illness, psychotic illness including bipolar illness and schizophrenia, dementia and Alzheimer's, anorexia and bulimia. Psychopathic disorder is defined as a persistent disorder or disability of mind, which results in abnormally aggressive or seriously irresponsible conduct. Psychopathic disorder essentially includes the categories identified in international diagnostic manuals as personality disorder, but the disorder must result in abnormally aggressive or seriously irresponsible conduct. Arrested or incomplete development of mind includes learning disability. The final element in the definition is the wide-ranging 'any other disorder or disability of mind'.

A person suffering from mental disorder in the broad sense described above may be detained under the 1983 Act for assessment for up to 28 days on the application of the patient's nearest relative or an approved social worker, supported by two medical recommendations, one of which must be from a doctor approved under Section 12 of the 1983 Act as having special expertise in the diagnosis or treatment of mental disorder (Mental Health Act 1983, s 2). A diagnosis of mental disorder is not enough on its own to justify detention. The disorder must be 'of a nature or degree which warrants detention for assessment 'with or without medical treatment'. Moreover, detention must be necessary in the interests of the patient's health *or* safety *or* for the protection of others. Only one of these grounds needs to be met, and a mentally disordered person does not have to be behaving dangerously to self or others to be compulsorily admitted (Department of Health and Welsh Assembly Government 1998: para. 2.6).

There is an emergency procedure under section 4 of the Mental Health Act (1983) for admission for assessment where only one medical recommendation is necessary. The conditions for admission for assessment under Section 2 must be met, and detention may continue for a maximum of 72 hours unless a second medical recommendation is furnished within that time to convert the emergency admission into a full 28-day admission for assessment. Until the second medical recommendation is furnished, the patient may not be given treatment without consent under Part IV of the Mental Health Act unless he or she lacks capacity to consent and the treatment is immediately necessary in his or her best interests (Mental Health Act 1983, s 56).

Section 3 of the 1983 Act provides for compulsory admission for treatment for up to six months, renewable for a further six months and thereafter at 12-monthly intervals. The patient must be suffering from one of four forms of mental disorder: mental illness, severe mental impairment, psychopathic disorder or mental impairment. Severe mental impairment means a state of arrested or incomplete development of mind, which includes *severe* impairment of intelligence and social functioning and is associated with abnormally aggressive or seriously irresponsible conduct on the part of the person concerned. Mental impairment is a state of arrested or incomplete development of mind, which includes *significant* impairment of intelligence and social functioning and is associated with abnormally aggressive or seriously irresponsible conduct on the part of the person concerned.

All the forms of mental disorder which apply to detention for treatment (or guardianship), except for mental illness, have a requirement of abnormally aggressive or seriously irresponsible conduct. Furthermore, in order for a person to be detained for treatment with a classification of psychopathic disorder or mental impairment, the doctors signing the admission form must certify that medical treatment for mental disorder is likely to alleviate or prevent deterioration in the patient's condition (Mental Health Act 1983, s 3(2)(b). Medical treatment is defined extremely broadly as including 'nursing, care, habilitation and rehabilitation under medical supervision'. The fact is that any of these interventions might well, if not alleviate, at least prevent deterioration in a patient's condition. This means that treatability is very much in the eye of the beholding treating doctor, who has considerable discretion to decide whether or not to accept a patient with this classification. Of all patients compulsorily admitted to hospital, 97 per cent have a statutory classification of mental illness (Department of Health, Statistical Bulletin 2002/26), and mental illness is clearly the core business of the compulsory psychiatric services.

For admission under Section 3 the patient must suffer from one of the four forms of mental disorder of a nature or degree which warrants medical treatment in hospital, in the interests of the patient's health *or* safety *or* for the protection of other persons. Finally the doctors must certify that the treatment which the patient needs cannot be provided unless he or she is detained under the Act. In other words, in US terms detention must be 'the least restrictive alternative', and in European Human Rights terms it must be 'a proportionate response'.

26,000 patients were compulsorily admitted to hospital each year of the last three years. An additional 20,000 were initially admitted informally, but were subsequently made subject to detention in hospital (Department of Health, Statistical Bulletin 2002/26). The 1983 Act provides holding powers for doctors and nurses where it is considered that an informal patient should be detained, and the doctor in charge has the power to hold that person for up to 72 hours if he or she considers that an application for compulsory admission should be made. This power can be delegated to another doctor nominated for that purpose (Mental Health Act 1983, ss 5(1), 5(2)). The doctor's holding power may be exercised even if the patient is not receiving psychiatric treatment as an inpatient but has come in for treatment of a physical disorder.

If neither the doctor nor the nominated deputy is available, the hospital managers have a power to detain for up to six hours an inpatient who is receiving treatment for a mental disorder, if a nurse of the prescribed class furnishes a written report in the prescribed form (Mental Health Act 1983, s 5(4)). The report must state that it appears to the nurse, (a) that the patient is suffering from mental disorder to such a degree that it is necessary for their health or safety or for the protection of others that he or she be immediately restrained from leaving hospital, and (b) that it is not practicable to secure the immediate attendance of a doctor empowered to use the doctor's holding power. Only nurses of a class prescribed in regulations may exercise this power, which means nurses whose names appear in Parts 3, 4, 5, 6, 13 or 14 of the Register (Mental Health (Nurses) Order 1998 (S.I. 1998, No. 2625). The decision whether to hold a patient is the personal decision of the nurse, who cannot be instructed to exercise the power by anyone else (Department of Health and Welsh Assembly Government 1998: para. 9.1).

Completion of the form recording the exercise of the nurse's holding power renders the patient immediately liable to be detained for a period of up to six hours or until the earlier arrival of a doctor with the power to hold the patient, whichever is the sooner. In a study carried out by Pym *et al.* of 100 uses of s 5(4), all were followed by an exercise of the doctor's holding power, and in 95 per cent of cases the doctor attended within three hours (Pym *et al.* 1999: 38). The Code of Practice states that the nurse must enter the reasons for invoking the holding power in the patient's nursing and medical notes, and must send an incident report to the managers (Department of Health and Welsh Assembly Government 1998: para. 9.4) A nurse invoking the holding power is entitled to use the minimum force necessary to prevent the patient from leaving hospital (ibid. para. 9.6). The purpose of both holding powers is to enable a full assessment of the need for admission under Sections 2 or 3 to take place, and this should be arranged as soon as possible.

In 1998, the UK government announced a root and branch reform of the Mental Health Act to ensure that the legislative framework supports mental health care. Proposals from an independent expert group were published in 1999 and following a Green Paper, a White Paper was published at the end of 2000. At the time of writing a draft bill, published in 2002 is out for consultation. Some of its main proposals are outlined in Chapters 20 and 21, in relation to the care and treatment of mentally disordered offenders and mental disorder and public protection.

The common law power to restrain and detain a mentally incapacitated patient

The nurse's holding power is limited to nurses of the prescribed class. Other nurses have a power at common law to restrain and detain a mentally incapacitated individual from leaving hospital if it is necessary in that person's best interests (*R v Bournewood Community and Mental Health Trust ex parte L* [1999] 1 AC 458). The person must lack the mental capacity to make a decision to stay in hospital, and it must be necessary in his or her best interests to be restrained from leaving. Hence, the profoundly confused elderly informal patient who wishes to leave the hospital could be restrained from doing so under the nurses' holding power in s 5(4) if a nurse of the prescribed class is present, or by a nurse acting under common law if the patient lacks the mental capacity to make the decision (incapacity in relation to consent to treatment is further discussed below).

Self-determination and the right to be respected as an individual

Respecting the client as an individual is a core principle of the nursing *Code of Professional Conduct*. It reflects the underlying function of the European Convention on Human Rights, the maintenance and promotion of the dignity of the individual. It is also reflected in the long title of the Council of Europe Convention on Human Rights and Biomedicine (1996) the convention for the protection of human rights and the dignity of the human being with regard to the application of biology and medicine (Beyleveld and Brownsword 2002).

Recognizing the individuality of the client requires that the role of the patient or client as partner in their care must be respected. This in turn involves identifying their preferences regarding care 'and respecting those within the limits of professional practice, existing legislation, resources and the goals of the therapeutic relationship' (*Code of Professional Conduct* 2002: para. 2.1). In relation to people with mental disorders the relevant 'existing legislation' is the Mental Health Act (1983) which authorizes detention and compulsory treatment. The nursing *Code of Professional Conduct* requires respect for the interests and dignity of patients and clients, irrespective of gender, age, race, ability, sexuality, economic status, lifestyle, culture and religious or political beliefs. The guiding principles of the *Mental Health Act Code of Practice* require that people to whom the Act applies, including those who are being assessed for the use of compulsory powers be given respect for: 'their qualities, abilities and diverse backgrounds as individuals and be assured that account be taken of their age, gender, sexual orientation, social, ethnic, cultural and religious background' (Department of Health and Welsh Assembly Government (1998), *The Mental Health Act 1983 Code of Practice*, para. 1.1).

However the *Code of Practice* is equally emphatic about the importance of not making assumptions on the basis of any of these characteristics. This means that everything possible should be done to overcome barriers to communication whether these arise from the fact that the service user's first language is not English or from other reasons, such as deafness.

Other contributors to this book have emphasized the importance of treating the service user as whole person, not just treating their mental disorder. Good mental health nursing is distinguished by its ability to respect personhood, to achieve the delicate balance between three aspects of respect for persons: respect for the service user's choices; respect for the service user's welfare, and respect for the rights and freedoms of other persons. At the same time there is a need to balance the choices of the sufferer against the rights of others, since mental disorder may impel sufferers, for example, through command hallucinations or severe depression to commit criminal acts. Respect for choices reflects the value placed on personal autonomy or the right of self-determination. Respect for welfare has connotations of paternalism or what some have sought less pejoratively to describe as 'parentalism'. Here emphasis is placed on making the treatment decisions that will promote the welfare and best interests of the person. Finally, respect for the rights and freedoms of others essentially means protecting the public against risks to their safety. Increasingly, government policy lays emphasis on risk assessment and risk management, and the goal of mental health policy is the management of the risk of suicide, self-harm, and violence to others.

A fundamental principle of all health care law is that adult patients with mental capacity have the right of self-determination, to determine what shall be done with their own body. In the case of *Re T* (1993) Lord Donaldson MR in the English Court of Appeal held that:

> An adult patient who . . . suffers from no mental incapacity has an absolute right to choose whether to consent to medical treatment, to refuse it, or to choose one rather than another of the treatments being offered . . . This right of choice is not limited to decisions which others might regard as sensible. It exists notwithstanding that the reasons for making the choice are rational, irrational, unknown or even non-existent.

Lord Donaldson was stating the position under common law, handed down by the judges in their decisions on individual cases, and developed over centuries. Adults with mental capacity have the right to refuse medical treatment even if their reasons are irrational or non-existent, and even if the result will be their own death. This principle was reiterated by Butler Sloss LJ in *Re MB* (1997: 549) where she said 'A mentally competent patient has an absolute right to refuse to consent to medical treatment for any reason, rational or irrational, or for no reason at all, even where that decision may lead to his or her own death.'

The right of self-determination is also reflected in the European Convention on Human Rights. Article 8(1) provides that, 'Everyone has the right to respect for his home, his privacy, and his family life.' In the case of *Diane Pretty v United Kingdom* (2002) the European Court of Human Rights held that the concept of private life included the right of self-determination.

> Though no previous case has established as such any right to self-determination as being contained in Article 8 of the Convention, the court considers that the notion of personal autonomy is an important principle underlying the interpretation of its guarantees. . . . The imposition of medical treatment, without the consent of a mentally competent adult patient, would interfere with a person's physical integrity in a manner capable of engaging the rights protected under Article 8(1) of the Convention.

(paras 61 and 63)

But the right of self-determination is not absolute. Under the European Convention an interference with the right of respect for privacy may be justified if it is legally authorized and is necessary in a democratic society to meet one of a list of legitimate policy aims contained in Article 8(2). The relevant aims that may justify interference with personal autonomy are the protection of public safety, health and the protection of the rights and freedoms of others. Where we afford more respect to the patient's welfare than we do to their wishes and intervene for the protection of the individual's own health we are acting in a paternalist or parental fashion. Intervention for the public safety or for the protection of the rights for freedoms of others is based on what Cavadino (1989) has called police powers. Both types of intervention are justified under English Law.

Before proceeding to examine the legal possibilities to treat a person without consent it is important to emphasize the fact that consent seeking is afforded high value as an ethical and legal principle. It enables patients to weigh up for themselves in accordance with their own value system the risks and benefits of proposed treatment and make their own decisions about what is in their interests. When treating mentally disordered patients whether or not detained, it is important to remember that the fact that they are mentally disordered or are detained under the Mental Health Act does not necessarily mean that they are incapable of giving a valid consent to treatment. The NMC *Guidelines for Mental Health and Learning Disabilities Nursing: A Guide to Working With Vulnerable Clients* (1998) stresses that nurses 'should not assume that patients are incompetent merely because they belong to a particular care group' and that it is 'important to devote as much time as necessary to explaining issues to clients in order to explore fully the consequences for them'.

The NHS Plan contains a commitment to 'patient-centred consent practice', and this is spelt out in detail in Health Service Circular HSC2001/023 Good Practice in Consent (www.doh.gov.uk/consent). The circular contains guidance on consent and competent adults, consent and mental disorder, learning disability, and children. The circular sets out the following 12 principles in relation to consent.

1   Consent is necessary before examination or treatment of a competent patient.
2   Adults are presumed to be competent.
3   Patients may be competent to make some health care decisions but not others.
4   Giving and obtaining consent is a process, not a one-off event.
5   Children can give consent for themselves in certain circumstances.
6   It is always best for the person actually treating to seek consent.
7   Patients should be given sufficient information about benefits and risks.
8   Consent must be given voluntarily not under duress.
9   Consent can be written, oral or non-verbal.

10   Competent adult patients are entitled to refuse treatment even where it would clearly benefit their health.

11   No one can give consent on behalf of an incompetent adult – the decision is for the doctor acting in the patient's best interests.

12   Advance refusal by a competent patient is valid if sufficient in scope to cover the situation which has currently arisen.

Treatment for mental disorder is defined very widely in the Mental Health Act 1983, s 145(1) as including 'nursing, care, habilitation and rehabilitation under medical supervision'. This includes physical treatment such as electro-convulsive therapy (ECT) and the administration of drugs, but it also includes basic nursing and care, as well as anything geared towards equipping or re-equipping the client with basic social and living skills. The Code of Practice emphasizes that it is essential for both informal and detained patients to have a written treatment plan, which should form part of a coherent care plan under the Care Programme Approach, and should be formulated by the multi-disciplinary team in consultation where practicable with the client. The written care plan should be kept in the clinical notes. The plan should be discussed with appropriate relatives, but if the patient is capable of consenting, his or her consent should always be sought to such discussions (Department of Health and Welsh Assembly Government 1998: paras 15.5–15.7).

There are three circumstances where English law allows a person to be treated without their consent. They are:

1   Where an adult lacks capacity to make the treatment decision under common law they may be given any treatment for mental or physical disorder which is necessary in their best interests.

2   Where a person is liable to be detained under the Mental Health Act 1983 they may be given treatment without their consent, regardless of their capacity or lack of it, as long as the treatment is for mental disorder and is 'necessary to alleviate or prevent deterioration in their condition'.

3   A child who is incapable of consenting or is refusing treatment may be given any treatment which is necessary in their best interests provided there is consent from a person with parental responsibility for the child or from the Family Division of the High Court.

Treatment of mentally incapacitated adults under common law

The common law provides that all adult patients who suffer from no mental incapacity have the right of self-determination, to determine whether to accept or refuse medical treatment, even if the result of refusal may be the patient's own death. All adults are presumed to be capable. 'Every person is presumed to have the capacity to consent to or to refuse medical treatment unless and until that presumption is rebutted' (*Re MB*, 1997: 553). It is therefore for those alleging that a patient is incapable to establish on the balance of probabilities (that it is more likely than not) that the patient lacks capacity. The more serious (life-threatening) the decision, the greater the level of capacity required. As Lord Donaldson MR put it in *Re T* (1993: 115–16): 'What matters is that the doctors should consider whether at [the relevant time] he [the patient] had a capacity which was commensurate with the gravity of the decision which he purported to make. The more serious the decision, the greater the capacity required.'

People may be deprived of their capacity by a range of factors including long-term mental incapacity or retarded development or by temporary factors such as unconsciousness or confusion or the effects of fatigue, shock, pain or drugs. The test for mental incapacity are set out in two cases. In *Re C (adult: refusal of medical treatment)* (1994: 295), C was a detained patient in Broadmoor suffering from schizophrenia who was refusing amputation of his foot which had developed gangrene. Thorpe J held that in order to demonstrate incapacity, the doctors who wished to treat C in the face of his refusal had to show that because of some disturbance of mental functioning he lacked the capacity to:

1   understand and retain the relevant treatment information;
2   believe the relevant treatment information; *or*
3   weigh it in the balance to arrive at a decision.

The judge held that the presumption that C was capable had not been displaced and upheld his refusal of amputation, which in the event turned out not to have been necessary as his gangrene was successfully treated by debridement.

The test from *Re C* was adopted by the Court of Appeal in *Re MB* (1997: 553–4) where Butler Sloss LJ held that

> A person lacks capacity if some impairment or disturbance of mental functioning renders the person unable to make a decision whether to consent to or to refuse treatment. That inability to make a decision will occur when:
>
> 1   The person is unable to comprehend and retain the information which is material to the decision, especially as to the likely consequences of having or not having the treatment in question.
> 2   The patient is unable to use the information and weigh it in the balance as part of the process of arriving at a decision.

Although this test appears to omit the second criterion from *Re C* of asking whether some impairment or disturbance of mental functioning is stopping the patient from believing the relevant treatment information, this was included as part of (2) in *Re MB* since if the patient is precluded by a disturbance of mind from believing that treatment is treatment they cannot possibly weigh the information in the balance. The example given in

Re MB was of a person being incapable of believing relevant treatment information in relation to a blood transfusion if he or she believed that everything red was a poison.

Incapable of understanding and retaining the relevant treatment information

The test of being unable to comprehend and retain material treatment information, means that a person will lack mental capacity if they cannot understand a simple explanation of the fact that the doctors think they are ill and that the treatment proposed is intended to alleviate the symptoms or cure the illness. So people with a profound learning disability might be incapable of consenting to treatment for cancer if they are not suffering pain from the illness and are not aware of it, whereas if they are suffering pain and the doctor can explain in simple terms that they are suffering pain because they are ill and that the proposed treatment will alleviate that pain they may have the necessary capacity. Capacity should always be assessed in relation to the actual treatment being proposed, and the 'broad terms' explanation of the treatment and its likely effects should be tailored to the level of mental ability of the client.

A person may comprehend the treatment information, but if they are unable to retain the information in their mind long enough to arrive at a decision they will lack mental capacity. This element in assessing incapacity is particularly evident in the mental illnesses of old age, Alzheimer's and dementia. The person may understand the information at the time it is imparted, but be nevertheless unable to hold it in their head long enough to make a decision.

Incapable of believing the relevant treatment information

If the person has sufficient cognitive ability to be capable of understanding the relevant treatment information, and has the ability to retain it, they may still be incapable if they are incapable by reason of a disturbance of mental functioning of believing that information. This may occur with psychotic illness where the sufferer has a delusional belief about the treatment, for example not believing that an injection is medical treatment for their mental disorder, but instead thinking it is inserting listening devices on behalf of MI5. Or a person with an eating disorder may not believe that he or she is on the point of death from self-starvation but instead thinks that he or she is overweight. In each case the mental disturbance is stopping the person from believing the relevant treatment information.

Incapable of weighing the information in the balance to arrive at a decision

A person who is able to understand and retain the treatment information and who is not precluded from believing that information by some mental disturbance may still be incapable if they are incapable of using the information and weighing it in the balance as part of the process of arriving at a decision. In *Re MB* the woman had a needle phobia which, when the time came to have an injection, overwhelmed her ability to make any decisions. Another example would be a person suffering from depression or reacting to the shock of a relationship breakdown who takes an overdose. That person may be perfectly capable of understanding the need for treatment by stomach wash or neutralizing drug, perfectly capable of believing that information and perfectly capable of understanding and believing that they will die if they do not have the treatment. But, if they say that life is not worth living because they have lost their partner or their job, are they capable of weighing the information in the balance to arrive at a decision? The effects of the shock and trauma of the relationship breakdown or of the depressive illness may be so disturbing their mental processes that they are unable to weigh the information in the balance to arrive at a decision. If they were to have treatment for their condition their decision might be very different. In such a case the doctors in casualty would assess the person as lacking mental capacity, and would administer the life-saving treatment as being necessary in the patient's best interests, using reasonable force if necessary. It is important to note that both under English law and under the European Convention concept of proportionality, no more force must be used than is reasonably necessary to give the treatment which is necessary in the patient's best interests.

Best interests

If an adult patient lacks capacity to decide, it is the duty of the doctors to treat him or her in whatever way they consider, in the exercise of their clinical judgement, to be in his or her best interests. This means that they must consider the range of treatment options available and choose the one which is best for that patient. This in turn means that the treatment should involve the least invasion of the sanctity of person commensurate with clinical effectiveness. The power and the duty to treat mentally incapacitated adults in their best interests apply to treatment for physical disorders and treatment for mental disorders. It also extends to authorizing detention of an informal patient. This means that informal patients who lack capacity to consent may be given whatever treatment for mental or physical disorder is necessary in their best interests. They may also be restrained and detained if it is necessary to do so in their best interests *R v Bournewood Community and Mental Health Trust ex parte L* [1999] 1 AC 458).

Treatment under Part IV of the Mental Health Act 1983

Part IV of the 1983 Act has two basic purposes. First, to make clear that treatment for mental disorder may be given to detained patients without their consent, and second, to subject certain treatments to regulation by a system of statutory second opinions. The second opinions are binding, not advisory. There are two groups of treatment which are subject to second opinion procedures. Section 57 treatments, psychosurgery and the surgical implantation of hormones to reduce male sex drive, require the patient's valid consent, and a medical second opinion. Consent to Section 57 treatments must be certified as genuine by a three-person panel appointed by the Mental Health Act Commission. Before treatment can be carried out, the medical member of the panel must certify that the treatment should be given having regard to the likelihood that it will alleviate or prevent deterioration in the patient's condition. Before issuing a certificate, the doctor must consult with a nurse and another person who have been professionally concerned with the patient's treatment (Mental Health Act 1983, s 57). Section 57 procedures apply to all patients, whether detained or informal.

The Section 58 procedures apply only to patients who are liable to be detained. Section 58 provides that medicines or ECT for mental disorder may only be given to a detained patient if the patient is either capable of consenting and actually consenting, *or* if there is a second opinion from a second opinion appointed doctor (SOAD) nominated by the Mental Health Act Commission. If the patient is capable of consenting and consents, the Responsible Medical Officer (RMO) certifies this on statutory Form 38, and describes the treatment consented to. If the patient is either incapable of consenting or refusing consent, the RMO must contact the Mental Health Act Commission who call in a SOAD. If the treatment is ECT and the patient is incapable or refusing consent, the treatment may not be given at any time without a second opinion to the effect that the treatment is likely to alleviate or prevent deterioration in the patient's condition. The only exception to this is where there is an emergency covered by Section 62. If the treatment is medicines for mental disorder, there is a three-month stabiliing period from the first time during that period of detention when medicine was administered, during which the patient may be required to accept medicine for mental disorder without recourse to a second opinion. A second opinion will be necessary if treatment is to continue beyond three months. When the SOAD visits to give the second opinion he or she must consult a nurse and another person (not a doctor or a nurse) who have been professionally concerned with the patient's treatment.

Section 62 of the Act authorizes emergency treatment which may be needed before a second opinion visit can be arranged. Section 62 provides that the procedures in Sections 57 and 58 do not apply to any treatment which:

(a) is immediately necessary to save the patient's life; or

(b) (not being irreversible) is immediately necessary to prevent serious deterioration in his condition; or

(c) (not being irreversible or hazardous) is immediately necessary to alleviate serious suffering by the patient; or

(d) (not being irreversible or hazardous) is immediately necessary and represents the minimum interference necessary to prevent the patient behaving violently or being a danger to self or to others.

Section 63 of the Act provides that any medical treatment for mental disorder not specifically identified as requiring a second opinion may be given to a detained patient without consent, if it is given by or under the direction of the RMO. Since treatment is defined in Section 145(1) of the 1983 Act inclusively – it includes 'nursing, care, habilitation and rehabilitation under medical supervision' – it can also include other treatments. In *B v Croydon Health Authority* (1995) medical treatment for mental disorder was held to include force-feeding, and to include any treatment for the symptoms and sequelae of the mental disorder as well as treatment for the core disorder itself. So a stomach wash for a detained patient who had attempted suicide as a result of a depressive illness could be treated under Section 63 as treatment of the sequelae of mental disorder. In this context it should be remembered that patients detained under provisions which authorize detention for 72 hours or less (Mental Health Act 1983, ss 4, 5, 135 and 136) may not be treated without consent for their mental disorder under the Mental Health Act, although they may be treated under common law (Mental Health Act 1983, s 56).

The Mental Health Act Commission has issued a Guidance Note entitled *Nurses, the administration of medicines for mental disorder*, and the Mental Health Act 1983 GN 2/2001, which draws attention to the three-month rule and states that it is the responsibility of the nurse administering the prescribed medication to patients detained under the 1983 Act to ensure that he or she is legally entitled to administer the medication. A copy of Form 38 (on which the patient's consent is certified and a description of the treatment is given), or Form 39 (on which the SOAD certifies that the treatment outlined on the form should be given) should be kept with the medicine card. The nurse administering the treatment should:

Check the medicine card for date of entry of prescription for the medicine, its dose and route of administration

I. Ensure that the three-month period has not been exceeded by checking the date of the first administration;
II. Ensure that where the patient has consented to medication beyond the three month period, the form 38 is in place and correctly completed;
III. Ensure that where a second opinion has been obtained the Form 39 is in place and correctly completed;
IV. Ensure that the administration of medicine is consistent with NMC professional Guidance.

The Guidance Note also refers to PRN or 'as required' medication and states that this should be authorized on the Form 39 if a second opinion has been obtained.

Children and consent

The position of children in relation to consent to treatment is that a child under 16 may consent to treatment in their own right if they are *Gillick* competent. In essence, *Gillick* competence means that the child has the necessary understanding and maturity to be capable of understanding, retaining and believing the relevant treatment, and of using it to make a decision (*Gillick v West Norfolk and Wisbech Health Authority* [1986] AC 112). The consent of a competent child between 16 and 18 shall be as valid as if the child were of full age (Family Law Reform Act 1968, s 8). The refusal of treatment by a child under 18 may be overridden by the parents, by anyone with parental responsibilities or by the Family Division of the High Court, if the treatment is necessary in the patient's best interests. The refusal may be overridden even if the child is *Gillick* competent, although this is a step which would only be taken in extreme circumstances.

Covert administration of medication

The UKCC issued a position statement in 2001 covering the covert administration of medicines, disguising medicine in food and drink. Since this involves treatment without consent, this may be authorized under common law if the patient lacks mental capacity and the treatment is necessary in their best interests, or under Section 58 of the Mental Health Act (1983). Where medication is disguised in this way, the position statement says that the nurse will need to be sure that what they are doing is in the best interests of the patient, and be accountable for this decision.

The Guidance Note states that the covert administration of medicines is only likely to be necessary or appropriate in the case of patients who actively refuse medication but are judged not to have the necessary mental capacity to understand the consequences of refusal. The UKCC, therefore, recognizes that there may be exceptional circumstances where covert administration may be necessary to prevent a client from 'missing out on essential treatment'. In such cases the nurse must consider the best interests of the client at all times, and the medication must be considered essential for the client's well-being. Any decision to administer medication covertly must be client specific, following discussion with the care team and any concerned relatives or supporters of the client. Covert administration should not be considered routine. There should be a written local policy, and decisions should be minuted and entered in the care plan. It is very important that the method of administration be agreed with a pharmacist, since crushing tablets or dissolving them may alter the bio-availability of certain drugs (UKCC (2001) *Position Statement on the Covert Administration of Medicines, Disguising Medicine in Food and Drink*).

Confidentiality and the duty to disclose information

Doctors and nurses owe a duty of confidentiality to keep private information which they have obtained in the course of treating patients. This is a general duty which is reinforced by nursing contracts of employment, and by the Code of Professional Conduct. Article 8 of the European Convention on Human Rights guarantees the right of respect for home, correspondence, privacy and family life. The right of respect for privacy includes the right of medical confidentiality (*Z v Finland* (1998) 25 EHRR 371). Information which is the subject of medical confidentiality may be disclosed with the consent of the patient if competent. Otherwise it can only be disclosed if it is in accordance with the law, and necessary in a democratic society for (*inter alia*) the protection of public safety, health or morals, or the protection of the health and rights of others. So a breach of confidentiality might involve a breach of the nurse's common law duty, a breach of the contract of employment, breach of the Human Rights Act, and professional misconduct.

The duty of confidence is not absolute. Under the European Convention Article 8(2) it may be interfered with if the interference is in accordance with law and necessary in a democratic society. As a matter of English law, the duty of confidence may be overridden if disclosure is necessary in the public interest. In *W v Egdell* (1990) the court held that a psychiatrist engaged to provide an independent report for a mental health review tribunal not only owed a duty to the patient, but also owed a duty to the public. His duty to the public enabled him to put before the proper authorities the results of his examination, if in his opinion, the public interest demanded it. The public interest means more than something which the public might be interested in. In order to be justified under the European Convention Article 8(2), disclosure must be for one of a number of purposes. They are national security, public safety, economic well-being of the country, prevention of crime or disorder, the protection of health or morals, or the rights and freedoms of others. The disclosure must be authorized by law, and must be necessary in a democratic society. This means that it must be 'proportionate', that is, the disclosure must be only to the extent necessary and to the proper officials necessary to achieve the legitimate purpose.

Take the example of a responsible medical officer considering the discharge of a detained patient, and that patient has told the nurse that he intended to kill his mother if discharged to her care. The nurse owes a duty of confidence to the patient, to keep confidential information obtained in the course of the nurse–patient relationship. However, there is also a duty under the Code of Professional Conduct to cooperate with others in the team and to act to identify and minimize risk to patients and clients. Moreover, there is a duty of care owed to the mother who is an identifiable foreseeable victim of the patient if he is discharged. In such a case the nurse would be justified in passing this information to the RMO, and if the RMO did not take it seriously, to the hospital managers. The important aspect of decision making in these circumstances is to ensure that disclosure is justi-fied under one of the heads of public interest in Article 8(2), that the public interest cannot be served without disclosure, and that disclosure is only to those who need to know to avert the threat to the public interest.

The influence of the Human Rights Act (1998)

The coming into force of the Human Rights Act (1998) has prompted a considerable body of case law in which the English Mental Health Act (1983) has been tested in various ways for its '*Convention compliance*'. The 1998 Act requires '*public authorities*' to act compatibly with Convention rights. 'Public authority' includes any body or person certain of whose func-tions are of a public nature. It covers health authorities, trusts, primary-care groups, responsible medical officers and second opinion doctors. Where a person is a victim of a breach of a Convention right as a result of the decision of a public authority they may have the decision quashed, as breach of a Convention right is a ground of judicial review, and may obtain dam-ages in an appropriate case. If the public body had to act in the way it did because of a statute which cannot be interpreted compatibly with the Con-vention, the High Court or any court above may grant a declaration of incompatibility which means that the appropriate minister must consider bringing forward amending legislation.

The case law can be divided into two groups: first, cases concerning detention and its review which mostly involve the protections against arbitrary detention in Article 5 of the European Convention on Human Rights (ECHR); and second, cases concerning the general rights of detained inpatients, engaging *inter alia* the right to life under Article 2, the protection against inhuman and degrading treatment in Article 3, the right to respect for correspondence, privacy and family life under Article 8, and the right to an effective remedy for human rights infringements under Article 13. What follows is not a comprehensive analysis of the case law, but a selection of some of the key issues which have been raised since the 1998 Act came into force.

Under Section 6 of the Human Rights Act (1998) it is unlawful for a public authority to act in a way which is incompatible with a Convention right. A public authority is defined as any person certain of whose functions are of a public nature. NHS hospitals are public authorities, and in *R (on the application of A and others) v Partnerships in Care Ltd* [2002] 1 WLR 2610 it was held that the managers of a private mental hospital were a functional public authority for the purposes of the Human Rights Act (1998). It is clear that an RMO renewing detention would be acting as a public authority, and that a nurse exercising the holding power would be too. In Convention terms the use of the nurse's holding power is a detention on grounds of unsoundness of mind under Article 5(1)(e). For a psychiatric detention to be lawful, unless it is an emergency the *Winterwerp* criteria must be met. There must be (1) Objective medical evidence before a competent authority of a true mental disorder which is (2) of a kind or degree warranting confinement and (3) there must be opportunities for review to ensure that conditions justifying initial detention continue to be met (*Winterwerp v Netherlands* (1979)). Most detentions using the nurse's holding power will be emergency measures to prevent immediate threat to the patient or to others, and so it will be sufficient for the medical evidence to be obtained immediately after detention (*Varbanov v Bulgaria* (2000)). The nurse will need to ensure that detention is necessary in the circumstances. In *Withold Litwa v Poland* (2001) 33 EHRR 53 the European Court of Human Rights held that detention of an individual is such a serious measure that it is only justified where other, less severe, measures have been considered and found to be insufficient to safeguard the individual or public interest which might require the person concerned to be detained. The deprivation must be shown to be necessary in the circumstances.

Inpatient's rights

States have a duty under Article 2 not to kill people by the use of force. They also have positive duties under Article 2 to take steps to protect the right to life. Those detaining psychiatric patients owe a duty to take reasonable care to prevent them from committing suicide. This was held as a matter of English law by the House of Lords in the case of *Reeves v Commissioner of Police for the Metropolis* (2000) decided before the coming into force of the Human Rights Act where it was held that this duty arose from the complete control which those detaining a person have over them, and the vulnerability of detainees to suicide.

The European Court of Human Rights held in *Keenan v United Kingdom* (2001) that the UK government had not breached Article 2 when a prisoner who had been placed in solitary confinement for disciplinary reasons killed himself. However, there were breaches of Articles 3 and 13. The court held that in respect of a person deprived of his liberty, recourse to physical force, which has not been made strictly necessary by his own conduct, diminishes human dignity and is in principle an infringement of Article 3. Treatment of a mentally-ill person could be incompatible with the standards imposed by Article 3 in the protection of fundamental human dignity, even though that person might not be capable of pointing to any specific ill-effects in terms of physical injury or psychiatric illness. Mark Keenan had been punished in circumstances disclosing a breach of Article 3 of the Convention and he had the right, under Article 13 of the Convention, to a remedy, which would have quashed that punishment before it had either been executed or come to an end.

Article 2 was held to have been breached in the case of *Edwards v United Kingdom* (2002) where a mentally ill and vulnerable prisoner was placed in the same cell as L, a mentally ill and violent prisoner. The Strasbourg Court concluded that the failure of the agencies involved in this case (medical profession, police, prosecution and court) to pass on information about L to the prison authorities and the inadequate nature of the screening process on L's arrival in prison disclosed a breach of the State's obligation to protect the life of Christopher Edwards. These cases show that detaining hospitals owe a duty to patients to carry out a risk assessment and to take reasonable care to avoid placing patients in a situation where they are at risk of suicide or being killed by others.

Control and treatment

Once detained, the decision of the House of Lords in the case of *Pountney v Griffiths* [1976] establishes that patients may be subject to a regime of control and treatment, which may vary in strictness according to the assessed level of risk. This power to control and treat compulsorily was held to be implicit in the Mental Health Act (1959). The power to treat compulsorily is now explicit in Part IV of the 1983 Act, and the English courts have held that the implied power to exercise reasonable control over detained patients still exists but is subject to the Human Rights Act (1998). This means that there could be inhuman or degrading treatment contrary to Article 3 if medical treatment, control, restraint or seclusion (1) causes physical or mental injury or (2) infringes human dignity by being more than strictly necessary to control the patient's behaviour (*Herczegfalvy v Austria* (1993); *Keenan v United Kingdom* (2001)). However, medical treatment deemed necessary by responsible medical opinion will not in principle infringe Article 3 (*Herczegfalvy v Austria* (1993)).

Nevertheless, treatment which is not severe enough to be inhuman or degrading may still breach Article 8 which states that everyone has the right to respect for his home, his correspondence, his family life and private life. However, interferences with these rights may be justified if they pursue a legitimate aim, and are proportionate, that is, strictly necessary in a democratic society to achieve that aim. The legitimate grounds for states to interfere with Article 8 rights include the economic well-being of the country, protection of health or morals, and protection of rights or freedoms of others.

Policies

In a series of cases the English courts have been asked to review different hospital policies towards detained patients. Restrictions on children's visits to offender patients in special hospitals were held to be justified in a democratic society for the protection of the rights of children (*R on Appn of L v Secretary of State for Health* (2001) 1 FLR 406). Ashworth Hospital's policy on random monitoring of phone calls was held not to breach Article 8 as it was necessary to pursue a legitimate aim, and in *R on Appn of H v Ashworth* (2001) (64) 1 BMLR 124 the hospital's refusal to issue condoms to patients was held not to breach Articles 2 or 8.

The decision to treat forcibly can engage the right of respect for privacy under Article 8, with the consequence that decisions to treat without consent must be proportionate and must be of the minimum interference necessary in order to achieve a legitimate aim such as health (including the health of the individual), or for the protection of the rights of others (*R (Wilkinson) v Broadmoor RMO and others* (2001) (CA). Moreover, reasons must be given by RMOs and second-opinion doctors that explain which justification under Article 8(2) (health, the rights of others, etc.) applies to the treatment authorized.

Seclusion can engage Article 3 if the conditions or duration reach a minimum level of severity causing physical or recognized psychological injury. Article 8 can also be engaged. However, neither Article 3 nor Article 8 can be breached merely by the fact of general segregation from the hospital population. The *Mental Health Act Code of Practice* (1998) provides guidance on when seclusion may be permitted, and how it is to be reviewed by nurses and doctors. In *Munjaz* and *S v Airedale* NHS Trust (2002) the Court of Appeal held that the safeguards in the Code of Practice governing regular observation and the attendance of doctors at intervals were intended to give effect to the government's positive obligations to prevent breaches of Articles 3 and 8. Therefore, the Code of Practice could be departed from only if there were reasonable grounds for doing so in an individual case.

The Court of Appeal considered that it should afford a status and weight to the Code of Practice consistent with the state's obligation to avoid ill-treatment of patients detained by or on the authority of the state. Seclusion would infringe Article 8 unless it could be justified under Article 8(2) in the interests of health, for the prevention of crime, or for the protection of the rights and freedoms of others. The justifications in domestic law were very broad. The Code of Practice had an important role to play in securing that the justification for this interference had the necessary degree of predictability and transparency to comply with Article 8(2). The Court of Appeal held that the doctrine of necessity provided a general power to take such steps as are reasonable and proportionate to protect others from the immediate risk of serious harm. This applies whether or not the person lacks the capacity to make decisions for himself or herself. Where the patient does lack capacity, there is also a power to provide whatever care and treatment is necessary in his or her own best interests. However, in every case medical necessity must convincingly be shown.

Conclusion

To conclude, the main points made in this chapter are summarized below:

- Mental health and learning disability nursing pose more acute legal and ethical problems than any other branch of medicine.
- There are two principal sources of ethical and policy guidance for nurses:
  - the *Code of Professional Conduct* of the Nursing and Midwifery

Council, and the Guidance issued by the Council on issues specific to mental health nursing; and

- the *Mental Health Act 1983, Code of Practice* published by the Department of Health and the Welsh Office.

- There are three main sources of legal rules governing good clinical practice in mental health nursing:
  - the common law developed by the decisions of judges over the years;
  - Parliamentary legislation which confers statutory rights and duties; and
  - the European Convention on Human Rights.

- Nurses owe a duty of care to their patients, to avoid causing them injury by wrongful acts or omissions. Case law demonstrates the need for nurses in undertaking their duty of care to keep knowledge and skills up to date, and to ensure that they possess the knowledge, skills and abilities required for lawful, safe and effective practice.

- The main source of statutory powers and duties for mental health nurses is the Mental Health Act 1983, which governs the care and treatment of people suffering from mental disorder.

- Respecting the patient as an individual is a core principle of the Nursing Code of Professional Conduct; this is reflected in the underlying function of the European Convention on Human Rights, which is the maintenance and promotion of the dignity of the individual. Recognizing the individuality of a patient requires that their role as a partner in their care be respected.

- The important issue for mental health nurses and all those who exercise statutory functions under mental health legislation is that they are aware of the legal and ethical context in which they operate; that they are aware of the circumstances where the different Convention rights, common law rights, statutory rights and ethical principles may be engaged, and of how to ensure that their decision making achieves a fair balance between protecting those rights and the need to detain, control and treat mentally disordered people.

▌Questions for reflection and discussion

1 When considering the circumstances where you should use your common law or statutory powers to override a person's decision to reject treatment for mental disorder reflect on how you would feel in such a situation if you were that service user. What steps would you want those making decisions on your behalf to take to find out your values, views and preferences? What decision would you expect a competent professional carer to make in your best interests?

2 Reflect on the circumstances when you would be entitled to communicate confidential medical information about a service user to

a third party. Reflect on the balance required by Article 8 of the European Convention on Human Rights between the right of respect for privacy and the need to protect health or morals or the rights and freedoms of others. Reflect on the fact that if information should be divulged it should only be to the extent necessary to remove the risk, and to the proper authorities.

3   Reflect on the need for careful use of language when discussing decisions about care and treatment, on the fact that psychiatric diagnoses carry with them a degree of fear and stigma, and on the fact that insensitive remarks about diagnosis or prognosis may add greatly to the burden of carers and service users.

Annotated bibliography

- R.M. Jones (2003) *Mental Health Act Manual* (8th edn). London: Sweet and Maxwell. The Mental Health Act 1983 and the accompanying rules, regulations and Code of Practice. The materials are annotated and the explanations are comprehensive and informative on all the key practical issues.
- Peter Bartlett and Ralph Sandland (2004) *Mental Health Law, Policy and Practice* (second edition). Oxford: Blackstone Press. An excellent guide to mental health law, policy and practice with very good contextual material.

Cases

Ashworth Hospital v Mirror Group Newspapers [2002] 1 WLR 2033.
B v Croydon Health Authority [1995] Fam 133.
Bolam v Friern Barnet Hospital Management Committee [1957] 1 WLR 582.
Bolitho v City and Hackney Health Authority [1998] AC 232.
Diane Pretty v United Kingdom (App no 2346/02) [2002] 2 FLR 45 [2002] 2 FCR 97, 66 BMLR 147.
Edwards v United Kingdom (2002) 35 EHRR 19.
Gillick v West Norfolk and Wisbech Health Authority [1986] AC 112.
Herczegfalvy v Austria (1993) 15 EHRR 437.
Keenan v United Kingdom (2001) 33 EHRR 38.
Pountney v Griffiths (1976) AC 314.
R v Ashworth Special Hospital Trust ex parte Munjaz (No. 1) [2000] MHLR 183.
ex parte Munjaz (No. 2) (2002) [2003] EWCA Cio 1036 (CA).
R v Bournewood Community and Mental Health Trust ex parte L [1999] 1 AC 458.
R (on the application of A and others) v Partnerships in Care Ltd [2002] 1 WLR 2610.
R (on Appn of H) v Ashworth (2001) (64) 1 BMLR 124.
R (on Appn of L) v Secretary of State for Health (2001) 1 FLR 406.
R (Wilkinson) v Broadmoor RMO and others (2001) (CA).
Re C (adult: refusal of medical treatment) [1994] 1 WLR 290.
Re F (Mental Patient: Sterilisation) [1990] 2 AC 1.

Re MB (an adult: medical treatment) [1997] 2 FCR 541.
Re T (adult: refusal of medical treatment) [1993] Fam 95.
Reeves v Commissioner of Police for the Metropolis (2000) 1 AC 360.
S v Airedale NHS Trust [2002] EWHC 1780.
Varbanov v Bulgaria (2000) Judgment of 5 October 2000.
W v Egdell [1990] 1 All ER 835.
Winterwerp v Netherlands (1979) 2 EHRR 387.
Withold Litwa v Poland (2001) 33 EHRR 53.
Z v Finland (1998) 25 EHRR 371.

▌ Statutes

Family Law Reform Act 1968
Human Rights Act 1998
Mental Health Act 1959
Mental Health Act 1983
Mental Health (Nurses) Order 1998 (S.I. 1998, No. 2625)

▌ References

Beyleveld, D. and Brownsword, R. (2002) *Human Dignity in Bioethics and Biolaw.* Oxford: Oxford University Press.

Cavadino, M. (1989) *Mental Health Law in Context: Doctor's Orders.* Aldershot: Dartmouth Publishing (pp. 131 *et seq.*).

Department of Health (2001) *Health Service Circular HSC2001/023 Good Practice in Consent*, http://www.doh.gov.uk/consent.

Department of Health (2001–2) *Health And Personal Social Services Statistics*, http://www.doh.gov.uk/HPSSS.

Department of Health (2002) Statistical Bulletin 2002/26 *In-Patients Formally Detained in Hospital under the Mental Health Act 1983 and Other Legislation, England 1991–2 and 2001–2002*, http://www.doh.gov.uk/public/sb0226.htm (November 2002).

Department of Health and Welsh Assembly Government (1998) *Mental Health Act 1983 Code of Practice.*

Nursing and Midwifery Council (2002) *Code of Professional Conduct.*

Nursing and Midwifery Council (1998) *Guidelines for Mental Health and Disability Nursing.*

Nursing and Midwifery Council (2002) *Guidelines for the Administration of Medicine.*

Nursing and Midwifery Council (2002) *Practitioner–Client Relationships and the Prevention of Abuse.*

Nursing and Midwifery Council (2001) *Position statement on the covert administration of medicines – Disguising Medicine in Food and Drink.*

Pym, N., Bell, C. and Salib, S. (1999) A review of 100 applications of section 5(4) Mental Health Act, *Nursing Standard* **13**(20): 37–40.

UKCC (2001) *Position Statement on the Covert Administration of Medicines, Disguising Medicine in Food and Drink.*

PART 2
Interventions

7

Assessment and care planning

Iain Ryrie and Ian Norman

Chapter overview

> It is difficult to say anything concrete about psychiatric nursing assessment except to say that it is in its infancy and is often gravely misunderstood.
>
> (Barker 1997: 14)

This statement presents quite a challenge, though we do broadly concur with Barker. It can be difficult to comprehend the breadth of activity that represents assessment, and even harder to disentangle different approaches and their associated methods. We draw on Barker's work to provide a 'map' of assessment that allows all its 'bits and pieces' to be understood collectively. Each is accorded its legitimate place in the framework, allowing each to be judged for its utility in relation to the person being assessed. The chapter is divided into two sections. The first deals in general with the principles and practice of assessment, from which the framework is developed. The second provides specific examples of selected assessment strategies and examines also care planning. Further detail on the assessment of people with specific mental health problems can be found in relevant chapters of this book.

This chapter covers:

- defining assessment;
- the purpose of assessment;
- the scope of assessment;
- methods of assessment;
- assessing the whole person;
- care planning.

Defining assessment

In its broadest sense assessment permeates all aspects of nursing care. It is not just a discrete activity that initiates the 'nursing process' or 'problem-solving cycle', leading to a plan of care, which is implemented and evaluated. The preferences people have for different health care options (planning) necessitate assessment, as do their abilities to engage meaningfully with the intervention itself (implementation), and evaluation requires still further assessment activity. Even then, it would be incorrect to suggest that assessment occurs only at these key points in the nursing process. It is an ongoing cycle of activity that all nurses perform in all nursing situations.

Assessment may be implicit or explicit, informal or formal. It may involve simply noting a person's appearance and behaviour during a home visit or observing someone who is deemed to be at risk over extended periods. It can involve structured instruments that specify the type or severity of problem that someone experiences, or it may take the form of a seemingly casual conversation. Common to all types of assessment is the collection of information.

The information we collect as nurses must be meaningful and necessary. Assessment data traditionally describe a person's appearance and behaviour, or their presentation and performance, or again, the form and function of their thoughts and feelings. Barker (1997) emphasizes the importance of these two viewpoints and their use by nurses to better understand a person. However, Barker cautions also against simply collecting data on the form and function of a person's thoughts and feelings, which can contribute to the formation of a medical diagnosis but will tell us little else about the person in the broader context of their life. Diagnosis is therefore one 'bit' of assessment, which focuses typically on problems, deficits and abnormalities. More broadly, assessment information encompasses a person's overall sense of self and their position in life, including not only problems and diagnoses but also their assets and strengths (Barker 1997).

The collection of information is only one part of the assessment process. Savage (1991) and Barker (1997) point to the inferences nurses draw from the available data, and the decisions they make regarding a person's need for care. Assessment is therefore a two-stage process. It is not enough to simply gather information; we must be able to do something useful with it, and that use is nursing's purpose. Hence, assessment is central to all nursing activity.

Barker has defined mental health nursing assessment as 'the decision-making process, based upon the collection of relevant information, using a formal set of ethical criteria, which contributes to an overall evaluation of a person and his circumstances' (Barker 1997: 6). This definition is useful since it implies the ongoing nature of assessment by referring to 'the decision-making process', which we take to be continuous and ever present in the activities of a nurse. Barker highlights also the importance of a '. . . formal set of ethical criteria', referring to such issues as confidentiality, note keeping, our style of interaction, how we ask questions, what we ask and why.

We would add to Barker's definition by stating that evaluations can be made also of groups and communities. Group programmes may involve assessment of the group's cohesion, the balance of its members or their aggregate characteristics. Community assessments are increasingly important in contemporary care. For example, knowledge of a locality's geography, social structures, deprivation and resources is important for outreach teams that work with drug users or with those who experience severe symptoms of mental disorder.

The purpose of assessment

We have emphasized two assessment stages, the collection of information and the use of that information to infer the need for nursing or other health care interventions. Though medical diagnosis is an important part of assessment, and one we fully acknowledge, mental health nursing is interested not in medical diagnoses per se, but in the way a person functions as a result of their condition. We need to comprehend their life problems (and strengths), and to understand the context within which these problems arise. Nursing diagnoses have been advocated for this purpose, which describe the nature of a person's problem and the effect it has on their functioning (Ward 1992). For example, 'I feel under threat and am angry with everyone I encounter.' This nursing diagnosis could be present in several medical diagnoses including paranoid schizophrenia or generalized anxiety disorder. Better then to deal with the nature of the problem and its implications, than with overlapping categories.

We have to confess that neither of us have been strong advocates of the term 'nursing diagnosis', preferring to use other, non-medical, terms to describe nurses' activity. But we agree fully with Ward (1992) and Barker (1997) that the exploration of relationships between a person's thoughts, feelings and behaviour is a diagnostic process, and one that nurses perform. Whether this procedure is referred to as nursing diagnosis, problem identification or functional analysis may be less important to the person in care.

Barker (1997) identifies four assessment objectives (summarized in Table 7.1), the products of which provide the basis for nursing diagnoses. The information in Table 7.1 provides an assessment overview; it tells us something about the quality, content and context of a person's health concern, its relationship to contributing factors and its effect on the person's and others' functioning. These data allow us to make judgements about why a problem exists and the factors that seem to be associated with it. In turn we are able to identify areas of need and so plan interventions. As a simple example consider the following problem statement, 'Arguments with my parents mean I don't like to be at home, so I spend my time alone in public parks where I smoke cannabis to make the day more interesting.' We can make several judgements about this person's need for care. The relationship

Table 7.1 Assessment objectives and outcome

Objectives	Outcome
Measurement	Key questions such as how often a person experiences a problem or exhibits a behaviour provide information on the scale or size of the problem
Clarification	Key questions such as where, with whom and under what circumstances problems arise provide information on the context or conditions associated with the problem
Explanation	Key questions such as the effects of a person's behaviour, their own and others' interpretation of its meaning provide evidence for the possible purpose or function of the problem
Variation	Key questions such as how the person's problem varies over time and in different situations provide evidence for its seriousness and the degree to which it dominates their life

(After Barker 1997)

between family tensions and personal isolation represents one possible area of need, and the lack of meaningful daily activity another. We might consider an opportunity to reflect on the positive and negative consequences of cannabis smoking to be a further need.

The concept of 'needs led' assessment is an underlying principle of the NHS and Community Care Act (1990) and the *National Service Framework for Mental Health (NSF)* (DH 1999). What is accepted as a need will vary across and within professional groups and, more importantly, between professionals and the people in their care. Bradshaw's (1972) definitions of need are often cited to understand these differences:

- *Normative needs* are defined by an expert or professional. This may involve a standard below which a person is considered to be 'in need'. For example, a community nurse who deems an isolated person to be in need of social skills training is making a normative assessment of their need.

- *Comparative needs* are identified by comparing the service provision received by one community or population, with the levels of provision received elsewhere. This approach may provide objective evidence for unmet needs in specific areas or localities.

- *Felt needs* are identified by the users of services and their carers. They are subjective and specific to them, for example the felt needs of a family or user group.

- *Expressed needs* represent the translation of felt needs into action. For example, an individual who feels isolated may attend a drop-in service, or the close family of a person who experiences a psychotic breakdown may attend a carers' group.

These different needs can conflict, for example normative and felt need and there will be occasions where identified needs have to be balanced against available resources. Thus, as Pickin and St Leger (1993) point out, a need may only be considered to exist in health care terms if there are the necessary resources to meet it. The possible relationships between these types of need and between need and resource are therefore far from perfect. But this is not true only of health care, it seems a good metaphor for life in general if we consider our own felt needs against the resources we have at our disposal. As Barker states, 'There is no obvious solution to this conflict. This is just one nettle of the assessment process that we must grasp without too much trepidation' (1997: 95).

The scope of assessment

Increasing emphasis is placed on assessment of the 'whole person', by which different authors may mean different things. We have suggested that mental health nursing assessments are concerned with how people function in relation to health problems as well as in relation to the broader context of their lives. This focus on functioning provides one way of understanding the whole person and thereby the potential scope of assessment.

Barker (1997) draws out a number of different levels on which people function or live simultaneously including their physiological self, biological self, behavioural self, social self and spiritual self. Actions as well as thoughts and feelings are included in Barker's 'behavioural self'. These levels reflect the four-quadrant schema we introduced in Chapter 1 (Figure 1.1) to integrate models of mental disorder. By so doing we proposed that human experience is made up of a *subjective* and *objective* sense of *self* and a *subjective* and *objective* sense of *community*, and each of the models tapped into a different aspect of the human condition. We employ these dimensions again to represent the whole person, and reproduce the schema in Figure 7.1, but without the various models of mental disorder.

Figure 7.1 presents a comprehensive, albeit general account of the scope of assessment. Consideration of each of the quadrants is necessary to understand and assess the whole person. The upper left quadrant (*subjective–self*) reflects a person's inner thoughts and feelings. It is concerned with the subjective meaning a person attributes to their life and/or their problems. We would position Barker's (1997) spiritual self and the thought and feeling components of his behavioural self in this quadrant. The upper right quadrant (*objective–self*) reflects a person's quantifiable, observable, external attributes. We would include the action component of Barker's (1997) behavioural self in this quadrant, along with the physiological and biological self. Similarly, we would place psychiatric diagnoses in this quadrant for their attempt to categorize people according to external, normative criteria.

The lower left quadrant (*subjective–community*) captures a person's collective sense of self. Their relations with family members and significant

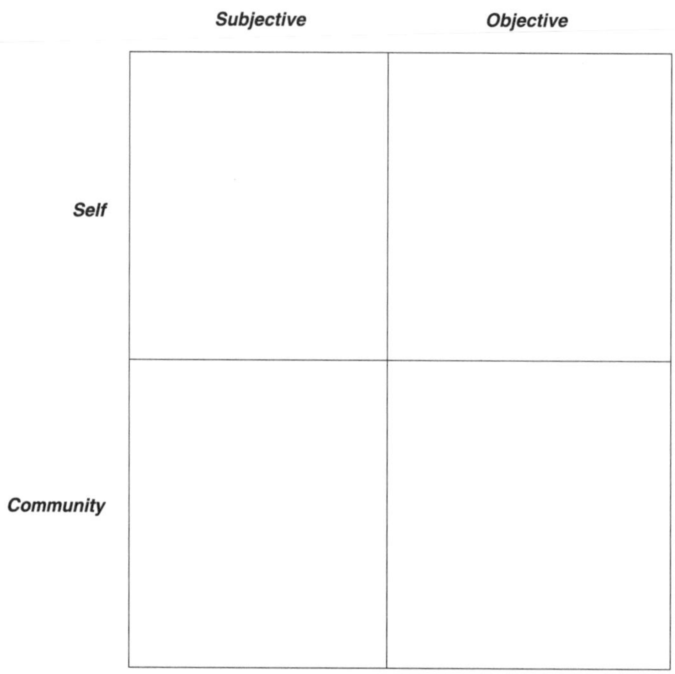

Figure 7.1 Schema for assessment of the whole person
(After Wilber 2000)

others are important here, as are their cultural roots and identity. But there is another side to our sense of self in community and this is reflected by the lower right quadrant (*objective–community*). As well as the inter-subjective experiences of culture and kinship there are interobjective social phenomenon in the form of health and social care systems (including the Care Programme Approach [CPA]), financial and other community resources that impact on our sense of self and thus on our sense of health or illness.

We would place nursing diagnoses or problem statements that deal with a person's thoughts, feelings or beliefs (written in the first person and using their words) in the upper left (*subjective–self*) quadrant. Those that deal with external, observable behaviour or actions are upper right (*objective–self*). In reality, problem statements can straddle both quadrants (or all quadrants) dealing with thoughts and behaviours in relation to self and community. This is to be expected since human experience is made up of all four quadrants. To repeat our earlier example, 'Arguments with my parents mean I don't like to be at home, so I spend my time alone in public parks where I smoke cannabis to make the day more interesting.'

Figure 7.1 therefore represents our framework for assessment of the whole person upon which all assessment approaches and methods can be mapped. We will continue to refer to it throughout this chapter. However, we must also consider in general terms the focus of any assessment in each of the quadrants. Following our discussion of the models of mental disorder in Chapter 1, problems can arise in any one of the quadrants. Equally though, particular personal or community strengths can reside in any one of the quadrants. Figure 7.1 depicts the experience of being human rather than the experience of human illness and thereby encourages us to think more broadly in terms of both health and illness.

Health and illness

In Chapter 1 we stated that mental health and mental illness are inseparable, they are relational terms, and the reality they describe is human experience. This is not to say that we only feel ill because *previously* we have felt healthy, but rather we feel ill against a background sense of health, we feel the two *simultaneously*. We can say we are ill because we experience limitations in our health, but it would be incorrect to say that we are ill because we have no health. Assessment therefore encompasses 'health' and 'illness', or 'mental health' and 'mental illness'. With some notable exceptions that we will come to, mental health nursing has focused largely on 'illness' in assessment practice. By this we mean deficits, problems, abnormalities, negative risks and so on. Their correlates (strengths, solutions, commonalities, positive risks) have received far less attention.

Health remains a poorly understood concept and is frequently used as a euphemism for illness (for example mental health problems). Tudor's work (Chapter 2) provides a valuable critique of this conflation and offers a number of models by which we can understand health without necessarily referring to illness. Pavis *et al.* (1998) have reviewed the psychology and health promotion literature to shed light on the factors that influence mental health in its positive sense, and have related these findings to the practice of mental health nursing. Common to these authors' work is the identification of such concepts as intersubjective relations, personal growth and development, self-esteem, autonomy and self-actualization. We draw on these concepts to provide examples of specific assessment strategies later in the chapter. For conceptual ease we also equate illness with diagnoses, dysfunctions, problems and abnormalities at both the individual and community level. Correspondingly we equate health with strengths, solutions, assets and skills at both the individual and community level. The following case study of Tom in Box 7.1 emphasizes the importance of health for an individual with a debilitating illness.

Although Tom's nurse was aware of his problems/illness (limited mobility and dementia) she was aware also of his strengths/health (outgoing and social). More importantly, in the second stage of assessment she used this information to promote Tom's independence, and sense of self, irrespective of his illness. Tom might have been discouraged from leaving the house alone and offered transport to attend a day hospital where he could mix with others. In this case the information gathered from the assessment would have been used with his limitations (illness) very much in mind.

> **Box 7.1** Case study: Tom
>
> Tom is an 80-year-old man with dementia whose mobility is limited, but who insists on a twice-daily walk. His insistence is borne of an inner belief that his ability to walk connects him with life as he has always known it, despite the fact that his mind seems to be deserting him quite literally. His morning walk connects him with the local newsagent where he buys a daily paper, which connects him with the wider world. Throughout his working years as a commuter he attempted to complete the crossword in this daily paper and he feels it is more important than ever to maintain that activity. His walks also expose him to society in general. He comes across people and does what he has always done, says hello, comments on the weather, strokes a dog or simply talks nonsense at the supermarket checkout. He has always been like this, outgoing and happy. He is also very proud of these abilities, these markers of himself, particularly as he knows something is terribly wrong.
>
> In fact, Tom is fast progressing in his dementia. His short-term memory has been virtually destroyed and he can no longer comprehend complex tasks. He has severe arterial restriction in his lower limbs and on two occasions Tom was found lying by the side of the road that leads from his home into town. Someone saw him fall once and commented that they thought he was drunk as he staggered up the road. At the time this hurt Tom deeply, he began to panic and refused any help.
>
> Now it is true that Tom is facing a progressively debilitating disease that will ultimately kill him (if he doesn't stagger into the path of traffic before then!). But what is far more apparent is his sense of health, those things that he can still do in spite of his illness. He may have lost his short-term memory to a ravaging, organic, pathological process, but Tom is still very much alive in his habits, his long-established routines and fundamental interactions with the world. Tom's community psychiatric nurse was an integral thinker who, while acknowledging the disease and its associated problems, set about assessing Tom's health with a view to preserving what was important to him.
>
> Tom now leaves the house with an urban version of a traditional shooting stick which allows him to rest when necessary. The nurse also asked one of Tom's children to write a message for him, which the nurse had laminated, and which now hangs on the back door next to his shooting stick. It simply asks Dad to remember to take his stick, and to enjoy his walks. Both his children's names are printed at the bottom of the message. On occasion Tom can now be found on the road leading back to his house, sitting on his stick and bothering anyone who passes with stories about his useless legs.

We can relate Tom's case study to Figure 7.1 to clarify the four quadrants. His 'inner belief that his ability to walk connects him with life as he has always known it' is an example of upper left, *subjective–self* information. His diagnosis of dementia and his limited mobility due to arterial restriction are upper right, *objective–self* data. The value Tom places on his social connections reflects the lower left quadrant, or *subjective–community*. Finally, the nurse's knowledge of Tom's family structure and the production of a laminated message by his family is evidence of lower right or *objective–community* awareness.

When considering what to assess we need then to take account of the context, the person's background sense of health, within which an experience of illness is felt. As well as gathering information on a person's problems and deficits we need to know something of their strengths and personal ideals. We need, in short, to develop an understanding of the whole person.

We can complete our framework for assessment by acknowledging that each of the quadrants has depth (Figure 7.1). Following Tudor (Chapter 2) this depth can be attributed to two continua, one that represents health and the other illness. Thus, we can experience both health and illness in terms of our subjective and objective sense of self, and in relation to our subjective and objective sense of community. This, we propose, represents the scope of assessment.

The scope of nursing assessment

We turn now to our vision for nursing assessment within this framework. We advocate the principle of holistic care and have presented a schema that we believe maps, in general terms, all that is the experience of being human. It follows that holistic nursing care, or assessment of the whole person, requires familiarity with, and assessment of, all quadrants in relation to both health and illness. Nurses are in an ideal position to champion this perspective given that they may have contact with service users over extended periods, which in turn provides opportunities to become involved in many areas of a person's life during different stages of health (Repper 2000). From this position nurses are well placed to provide holistic, integrated care which can be enhanced by enjoining with other workers who possess complimentary specialist knowledge and skills. Thus, the case for multi- and inter-disciplinary assessments in which nurses embrace the contributions of others to develop a holistic understanding of the person and their difficulties.

There is much talk of a holistic approach to nursing assessment but in practice there is a tendency for mental health nurses to focus on one side or other of the *subjective–objective* divide only. Thus, we have the 'qualitative camp' (all left-hand quadrants) and the 'quantitative' camp (all right-hand quadrants) as described by Burnard and Hannigan (2000) and Repper (2000) (see also Chapter 3). Neither is wrong, but each provides only a partial perspective, and both are incorrect for what they miss out and, at times, try to deny.

Methods of assessment

This section gives an overview of the main methods by which assessment information can be gathered. Selected assessment strategies for each of the quadrants are presented in the final section of the chapter. Information gathering for assessment can be more or less formal and explicit. Whether a formal or less formal approach is preferred depends on the circumstances. Take for example a person who is talkative and eager to communicate their experience. An informal approach that allows the person free expression would be recommended, particularly in the early stages of their contact with services. On the other hand, a withdrawn individual who finds it difficult to communicate may benefit from a more structured, formal approach. In both cases the information provided (or the information that is sought) is documented and arranged in a systematic way that tells us something about the person, the problems they encounter in relation to their condition and life in general, and the strengths or attributes they may possess.

Taking our cue from the person to be assessed, and the reason for assessment, methods are usually selected to increase specificity as the assessment procedure progresses. Thus, a broad overview of an individual leads to the collection of information regarding the nature and implications of a specific problem.

We outline three main data collection methods for mental health nursing assessments: interviews; questionnaires, rating scales and structured pro forma; and observations.

Interviews

The interview is a means of eliciting information by questioning people. Typically this will involve the person in care but may also include others who know the person well including their relatives, friends and other health care professionals. There is little benefit in asking questions if we are unable to listen properly to the answers that are provided. A good interviewer requires good listening skills.

Barker (1997) states that a good listener is someone who helps a person to elaborate and qualify what they have to say, and who is able to curb any desire to offer premature interjections or summaries. Active or reflective listening is an important skill in this respect. Reflective listening can involve repeating key words used by the interviewee, perhaps with an inflection in tone, which invites them to elaborate their point. It may be more appropriate to simply ask if someone could elaborate on a topic, or ask them to explain the meaning an issue has for them. Open questions that invite elaboration rather than closed questions, which need only a single categorical answer, are crucial for reflective listening. Summarizing at discrete points during an interview to check for understanding is another example of reflective listening.

Each of these techniques communicates accurate empathy in so far as they convey an interest in, and an understanding of, the person's experience. We emphasize this connection between reflective listening and accurate empathy since the two are often disassociated. When we ask groups of nurses how to convey accurate empathy, rarely do we get the response 'by listening reflectively'. And yet, research demonstrates that therapeutic change, and the necessary relationship between therapist and client for this to occur, is dependent on the manifestation of accurate empathy by the therapist (Miller and Rollnick 1991). This is a fundamental tenet of the therapeutic alliance.

Reflective listening is only beneficial if it is accompanied by appropriate non-verbal behaviour. It is no good asking someone to elaborate while we fumble to read our pager, or sit with our arms crossed admiring the view from a window, or position ourself in a room with constant interruptions. Interest can be conveyed as much through our non-verbal behaviour and the environment in which we choose to interview someone, as it can by what we say (or don't say). The verbal and non-verbal interpersonal skills that underpin effective listening and interviewing are thoroughly reviewed by Barker (1997) and have been described in dedicated texts such as Egan (1994) and Newell (1994). The latter having been written specifically for nurses.

Interviews may be more or less structured depending on their purpose and the type of information to be collected. Following Barker (1997), Table 7.2 represents a summary of the possible goals and aims of the interview, with the aims reflecting interpersonal functions between the nurse and the person receiving care.

Table 7.2 Interview goals and aims

Goal		Aim
Descriptive	Collecting information to form a broad overview or picture of the person and to develop a therapeutic, trusting relationship	Relationship building
		Trust building
Diagnostic	Investigation of a problem area in which relationships between a person's thoughts, feelings and behaviour are explored, and from which nursing or medical diagnoses can be formed	Professional collaboration
		Problem identification
Therapeutic	Ongoing face-to-face meetings to help the person through the process of care by clarifying problems, identifying solutions and reflecting with the person on their progress/response	Problem resolution

(After Barker 1997)

Questionnaires, rating scales and structured pro forma

Questionnaires and rating scales generate quantifiable measures of human experience. They stem from the objective right-hand quadrants in Figure 7.1 and therefore complement, but cannot replace, the subjective left-hand quadrants. Instruments of this type may invite simple categorical responses (for example, yes or no) to a question or statement. Many also invite the rating of a statement according to a series of possible responses that reflect different degrees of agreement with the statement.

These approaches can generate quantified summaries of the person in care. We may say that Tom's dementia is severe following administration of a questionnaire, on which he scored poorly. We could reduce this further by saying he scored 2 out of a possible 20, thereby indicating severe dementia. Such an approach can be advantageous. Questionnaires and rating scales are usually developed through extensive research during which the instruments are refined to enhance the accuracy (validity) and consistency (reliability) with which they measure a concept of interest. A well-researched instrument can assess comparative or normative needs, and provide a quantifiable basis to judge progress. However, to say that Tom's dementia questionnaire score was 2 tells us very little about the person behind this numeric.

We include various pro formas in this section, such as logbooks and diaries, which allow people to document specific experiences in a structured way (Barker 1997). A simple example is the 'antecedent', 'behaviour', 'consequence' framework, against which the context of a behavioural problem can be mapped. By substituting 'behaviour' for 'belief' in this framework we can map the context of a cognitive problem. Barker (1997) offers a further example using the headings 'action', 'emotion', 'thought', while Fox and Conroy (2000) advocate the acronym 'FIND' (frequency, intensity, number and duration of a problem).

Observations

Observation is a continuous form of data collection within the context of nursing care. It may be relatively informal, such as an overall assessment of a person's appearance and behaviour or the assessment of interactions within a ward environment. Structured observation methods include the prospective use of pro formas such as those described in the previous section. These can be completed by the person receiving care or by nursing staff. Observation schedules can yield important information but can also present a challenge to those who complete them. They require more or less continuous attention or good recollection in order to capture a representative set of data. This can be difficult for a person with a mental health problem and for their nurse who may not be available during periods when a problem is present.

Mental health care involves another type of observation that is concerned with documenting biochemical and physiological indices. Barker (1997) acknowledges this aspect of assessment but does not pursue it as a legitimate activity for the mental health nurse. We take a more integral view given that the *objective–self* is a part of human experience and would encourage nurses to familiarize themselves with the rationale and meaning of these observations (see, for example, McConnell 1998). To understand the implications and normal range of a human's white blood cell count is critical in today's health care environment (cf. Chapter 11). Furthermore, how would we know what to do and why would we be doing it if our assessment of a person's emotional and behavioural problems failed to incorporate an abnormal thyroid function test result? And if an overweight person presents with intermittent mental state changes, how can we provide a holistic assessment without comprehending the need to screen their blood glucose? Without these pieces of the jigsaw the how and why of nursing activity could be meaningless.

Assessing the whole person

In this section we provide specific assessment strategies for each of the quadrants in Figure 7.1. We begin with an exploration of the breadth of personal and social information that needs to be collected when people first enter a health care system. Those who are already known to services may have extensive past medical or nursing notes. Though the information contained within these notes may be useful they are not a substitute for the collection of contemporary data regarding a person's presenting problem, or for the opportunity to elicit someone's personal history in their own words.

Presenting problem and personal history

Gamble and Brennan (2000) have identified four core elements of the information gathering process that describe a person's presenting problem and history (Table 7.3). The core elements in Table 7.3 reflect predominantly the right-hand quadrants of Figure 5.1 (*objective–self and objective–community*). They are concerned with external, quantifiable attributes and phenomena, with the exception of 'personal insights'. This is not to

Table 7.3 Core elements of the information gathering process

Core element	Examples
History of psychiatric disorder and past physical history	• family and social background • past treatments, contacts with services and risk levels • current medication and any side effects
Current financial, social functioning and environmental factors	• personal relationships • employment
Psychiatric diagnosis and current symptoms	• to include effects of symptoms on behaviour
Personal insights	• evidence of the person's awareness and understanding of their difficulties

(After Gamble and Brennan 2000)

say that Gamble and Brennan (2000) are uninterested in a person's subjective feelings, as their work testifies. However, their main approach, in terms of identifying health-related need, tends towards objective assessment.

Barker (1997) provides a more integrated approach that begins with the generation of an admission profile and description of the presenting problem. By admission profile Barker refers to any point of entry into health or social care services, whether these be residential or community based. Tables 7.4 and 7.5 contain the key components of an admission profile and a presenting problem inventory.

It is evident that Barker's (1997) initial assessment draws on all four quadrants, incorporating both subjective and objective data of self and community. However, these data are firmly oriented toward problems, which Barker acknowledges. He believes it may be inappropriate to consider a person's strengths or assets at this stage, particularly as it may indicate a fear on behalf of the nurse to deal with a person's problems. We agree, but with one exception. And it is simply that: evidence of *exceptions* to the presenting problem. We have found it useful to ask people early in an assessment process whether there are ever any exceptions to the presenting problems they describe. If so, we would encourage exploration of those exceptions since this often uncovers potential solutions to the problem.

Having elicited an admission profile and inventory of the presenting problem Barker (1997) then recommends the development of this thumbnail

Table 7.4 Admission profile

Component	Examples
Name, age, sex, marital state	
Family	• whether any dependents and who they live with • siblings • whether part of an active extended family
Domestic	• living alone or with significant others
Occupation	• employment status • nature of employment
Socialization	• close friends and other acquaintances • membership of clubs or organizations including church
Financial status	• access to hard cash or other funds • record of outstanding bills or debt
Medical cover	• name and contact details of any physician/ social worker • current medication

(After Barker 1997)

Table 7.5 Inventory for presenting problem

Component	Examples
Functioning	• changes in bodily functions including limbs, speech and memory
Behaviour	• changes in behaviour including behaviours that might be upsetting the person or others
Affect	• specific feelings associated with problems
Cognition	• specific thoughts about the problems, including ruminations and recurring thoughts
Beliefs	• the meaning the problems have for the person
Physical	• physical problems associated with the difficulty for example pain, loss of appetite, listlessness
Relationships	• any changes in usual relations and whether associated with the problem
Expectations	• what the person thinks will happen to them now they are in touch with services

(After Barker 1997)

sketch. Specific topic headings are provided, which expand the available information to include past history, present circumstances and the way a problem interferes with the person's life experience (Table 7.6).

During this stage of the assessment process Barker (1997) places much greater emphasis on a person's strengths, assets and preferences while maintaining an interest in all four quadrants of human experience, as evidenced in Table 7.6. Barker (1997) also draws attention to exploring a person's hopes for the future having examined their past in some detail. Questions pertaining to their aspirations, their expectations and hopes, and their future plans are important in this respect. Through these enquiries a more holistic picture of the person begins to emerge, from which it is possible to identify areas where further investigation may be needed. This investigation may follow any one of the specific strategies we describe in the following sections.

Subjective–self

The upper left quadrant of Figure 7.1 represents a person's inner world, their thoughts feelings and beliefs. The psychodynamic model and its therapeutic approach (cf. Chapter 1) tap into this quadrant with their interest in assessing the ideas and feelings behind the words and actions that constitute human behaviour. Though some mental health nurses specialize in this tradition, the profession as a whole does not practise solely according to psychodynamic principles. Nevertheless, assessment of the *subjective–self* is a necessary component of holistic nursing practice.

Table 7.6 Developing the history

Topic	Example
Education	• description of schooling at basic and advanced level • attitudes towards schooling and adult learning
Occupation	• past and present occupations • feelings towards present job • any work aspirations • degree to which present problems interfere with work
Social network	• does the person enjoy going out? • do they have an extended social network? • what kind of social life would they prefer? • impact of problem on these social networks
Recreation	• way in which free time is used • hobbies and preferred activities • what changes might be desirable?
General health	• states of health throughout the person's lifetime • maintenance of health through diet, exercise, etc.
Drugs	• use of drugs whether prescribed, over the counter, or illicit • how does the person feel about drug taking • amount, route of administration, frequency and duration of any drug use • is present problem and use of any drugs connected?
Past treatment	• any past treatments for presenting problem? • effects of any treatments and preferences/feelings toward them
Coping	• coping strategies employed to deal with life's problems • successful strategies that have been employed previously
Outstanding problems	• problems that the person perceives to be beyond help • feelings towards them and likely reactions, including anger/attempting suicide

(After Barker 1997)

Barker (1997) refers to this as 'learning from the person', which necessitates listening to a person's life story or personal narrative. It is true that a personal narrative may allude to behaviours or social structures, which are external, observable attributes that belong elsewhere in Figure 7.1. But we can still ask for the meaning they hold for the person. This orientation lies at the heart of *subjective–self* assessments. It focuses on a person's thoughts, feelings, personal values and beliefs, which describe their sense of self and the meaning they attribute to their life experience.

Subjective–self assessments require the use of open-ended questions and reflective listening skills to elaborate a person's description of their experience. We might ask:

- What are your feelings about that experience?
- What thoughts did you have at the time?
- Could you say a little more about what that means for you?

It follows that the information we receive needs to be recorded in the person's own words, otherwise we are documenting our interpretations of what they say and are missing an opportunity to understand fully the person's *subjective–self*. Interpretations and judgements about their need for care will still be made, but in the case of the upper left quadrant these should be predicated on an individual's verbatim account of their inner world.

Barker's (2001) *Tidal Model* for person-centred recovery in mental health care places considerable emphasis on these verbatim accounts. A holistic nursing assessment format has been developed to document in a person's own words any significant and meaningful events in their life, and their personal perception of what needs to be done in response to any resulting problems. The philosophy underpinning this model, its practice implications and references for further reading are available at www.tidal-model.co.uk.

Frameworks

It is possible to bring order to the verbatim recording of a person's thoughts and feelings, though rarely are these separated from objective actions or behaviours. In Chapter 1 we introduced Ellis's (1962) ABC framework in which A stands for 'activating event', B stands for 'beliefs' about the event and C stands for the emotional (or behavioural) 'consequence' that follows. Barker (1997) offers a variation on this theme referring to 'actions', 'emotions' and 'thoughts'. Both frameworks provide a structure for eliciting and documenting aspects of a person's inner world, though each incorporates a behavioural component in its analysis.

Subjective–community

The lower left quadrant of Figure 7.1 represents the meaning, values and beliefs that a person holds regarding their sense of self in community. These include cultural identity, religious beliefs and world-views. Allied to these are negative correlates including racism, social exclusion and stigma. In Chapter 1 when describing the social model we demonstrated how these social forces have a bearing on people's mental health. For example, the experiences of African-Caribbean communities in the UK, which include poorer housing, higher levels of unemployment and lower average incomes than the indigenous population are sufficient to engender mental health problems (Modood *et al.* 1998). In this particular quadrant it is not the quantifiable attributes themselves but the meaning they have for people that contributes to the formation of mental health problems.

As with the *subjective–self* (upper left) we can only comprehend the personal meaning of these aspects of a person by asking them directly through open-ended questions and reflective listening. For example, someone may appear socially isolated or excluded but we cannot fully comprehend such observations without understanding the meaning they hold for the person himself/herself.

Of contemporary interest in this quadrant is the emergence of the UK user movement. A recent survey of its breadth, beliefs and ideals reveals a world-view that is very different from that which predominates among professional groups (Wallcraft *et al.* 2003). Mental health nurses need to understand these emergent cultures if they are to undertake holistic assessments in which a person's sense of self in community is accorded due regard.

Objective–self

The upper right quadrant of Figure 7.1 represents external, measurable, quantifiable attributes of the person. This includes their physiological and biological self, and associated indices, as well as measurements of their functioning or mental state through the use of questionnaires and rating scales. Functioning is a broad term that incorporates thoughts, feelings and behaviours associated with self as well as those associated with self in community. The latter is often referred to as social functioning, which is examined in the next section (*objective–community*). A number of instruments incorporate both self and community measures of functioning, particularly global assessments of need such as the *Health of the Nation Outcome Scale* (*HoNOS*) (Wing *et al.* 1995) and the *Camberwell Assessment of Need* (*CAN*) (Phelan *et al.* 1995). Each taps into personal attributes such as physical health and symptom severity as well as measures of social functioning such as interpersonal behaviours and social engagement.

Gamble and Brennan (2000) provide a detailed account of questionnaires and rating scales that are designed to capture in quantifiable terms the experience of illness. Less evident are instruments that tap into the experience of health, although some are cited in Barker's (1997) work. We draw on this literature to present a selected overview (in Table 7.7) of questionnaires and rating scales that are available for *objective–self* assessments. Readers may wish to review subsequent chapters for assessment instruments relevant to the specific problems/conditions that people experience.

Objective–community

The lower right quadrant of Figure 7.1 represents external, measurable, quantifiable attributes of the self in community. In the earlier section that described presenting problems and personal histories, the collection of information pertaining to these attributes was recommended. For example, in Table 7.6 Barker (1997) emphasizes the importance of enquiring about

Table 7.7 Instruments to assess illness and health in the individual

Instrument	Commentary
Brief Psychiatric Rating Scale (BPRS) (Overall and Gorham 1962)	One of the oldest and most commonly used instruments for assessing the presence of various forms of mental illness including anxiety, depression and thought disturbance. All items are rated on a 7-point scale from 'not present' to 'extremely severe'. Administered through direct questioning but relies also on observations made at the time of administration.
Beck Depression Inventory (BDI) (Beck *et al.* 1961)	Another much used instrument designed to measure the severity of depressive states. Containing 21 items, each is rated on a 4-point scale and can be completed by the person in care directly or through interview technique.
Positive and Negative Syndrome Scale (PANSS) (Kay *et al.* 1987)	Designed to assess key symptom types associated with schizophrenia. The instrument contains 30 items a proportion of which are completed through interview and the remainder through observation. Each is rated on a 7-point scale.
Beliefs About Voices Questionnaire (BAVQ) (Chadwick and Birchwood 1995)	Designed to elicit the feelings a person has about hallucinatory voices. The questionnaire contains 30 items, all of which are answered with simple yes or no responses.
Self-Esteem Scale (Rosenberg 1965)	This brief 10-item instrument taps into a key component of health or well-being. It is easy to administer with each item rated on a 4-point scale.
Self-Efficacy Scale (Sherer *et al.* 1982)	A further instrument to gauge aspects of a person's health. Of the 30 items the majority tap into general self-efficacy and the remainder examine social self-efficacy (lower right quadrant). Each is rated on a 5-point scale.

a person's occupation and social structures. These are examples of self in community data. In the *objective–community* quadrant these attributes are quantified according to questionnaires, rating scales and other objective data. However, we can also seek to understand a person's subjective experience of these phenomena (*subjective–community*).

For objective measurement, instruments that tap a person's social functioning and to a lesser extent their quality of life are important. We include the latter, which often straddle both the *objective–self* and *objective–community* quadrants of Figure 7.1, but which typically measure an individual's quality of life in its broadest sense, and are, therefore, grounded in the self in community. Measures of social functioning are often concerned with problem areas and deficits while quality of life measures are more broadly focused and accommodate measurement of a person's sense of health. We would include also in this quadrant the objective views of carers and significant others involved in a person's care. Table 7.8 presents a

Table 7.8 Instruments to assess illness and health of self in community

Instrument	Commentary
Social Functioning Scale (SFS) (Birchwood *et al.* 1990)	This instrument covers seven main areas of social functioning including independence in living skills and social engagement. All areas reflect aspects of day-to-day social functioning that can be adversely affected by mental health problems. The authors designed this instrument specifically for use in family intervention programmes.
Instrumental and Expressive Functions of Social Support (IEFSS) (Ensel and Woelfel 1986)	This instrument is designed to assess the function and emotional content of a person's social relationships. A 5-point scale is used to rate 28 problem areas, which cover demands, money, companionship, marital conflict and communication.
Quality of Life Scale (QLS) (Heinrichs *et al.* 1984)	This instrument has 21 items, each of which is rated on a 7-point scale. They cover three key areas deemed to be representative of a person's quality of life: interpersonal relations; occupational role; and richness of personal experience. The scale specifically taps into a person's capability to manage social roles and with this emphasis on capability is oriented towards health rather than illness.
Manchester Short Assessment of Quality of Life (MANSA) (Priebe *et al.* 2002)	In addition to gathering sociodemographic data this instrument asks 16 questions pertaining to employment, finance, friendships, leisure, accommodation, family, safety and health. Each is rated on a 7-point scale. As with the QLS the emphasis is upon health rather than illness.
Carers' Assessment of Managing Index (CAMI) (Nolan *et al.* 1995)	Designed to assess coping style and management of stress in the carers of people with mental health problems. Examples of coping strategies are given, which respondents report their use of and the degree to which they are effective.

selected overview of instruments that are available for *objective–community* assessments.

Care planning

The needs of an individual, which have been identified through the assessment process, and which can be realistically met by health and/or social services, form the basis of a care plan. The care plan in its simplest form is a documented account of how these needs are to be met. Typically it should include (Ward 1992):

- a statement of the goals to be achieved;
- a description of any actions to be taken;
- specified criteria against which an evaluation of progress can be made.

Goal statements should be SMART: **S**pecific; **M**easureable; **A**chievable; **R**ealistic; and **T**ime limited. They should also be formulated and agreed together with the service user, and as far as possible should reflect their preferences and priorities. This is an important point since several goals may emerge, not all of which can be tackled simultaneously, and priorities will have to be made. Of equal importance is the need for flexibility since priorities may change over time, or even from day to day depending upon the service user's overall health status. The care plan is then a living document, which is developed and refined throughout the care process.

Descriptions of any actions to be taken, or interventions offered, should reflect the preference of the service user. Ideally, nursing staff should be able to offer a menu of possible actions to tackle a particular problem. Their advantages and disadvantages for the service user can be explored and a preferred option identified. Actions may be carried out by the service user or by nursing and other health and social care staff. The care plan needs to specify who is responsible for which actions. Part 4 of this book provides examples of the types of action or interventions that may be useful for individuals who experience specific mental health problems.

A SMART goal statement provides detail on what should be achieved and when. Providing goal statements are SMART in their formulation they, therefore, contain the means by which a care plan can be evaluated and when. Once again this should be conducted in partnership with service users in a way that engages them in a collaborative problem-solving process. Even when goals are not achieved, much can be learned from the experience that will benefit both service user and staff in formulating alternative care plans.

The nursing profession has a well-documented history of care planning as part of the nursing process. Seminal texts for mental health nurses include Ward (1992) and McFarland *et al.* (1997), both of which we recommend. Gega discusses the practicalities of care planning with clients in Chapter 23.

Conclusion

We have presented assessment as an ongoing continuous process, which in its many forms underpins all nursing activity. Its purpose incorporates both the collection of information and the use of that information to make judgements about a person's need for health care. Traditionally these judgements are based on a person's problems, deficits and abnormalities though we encourage a broader perspective that accommodates strengths, assets and skills.

We advocate the principle of holistic assessment and have presented a schema for that purpose, which takes account of a person's *subjective* and *objective* sense of *self* and their *subjective* and *objective* sense of *community*. In each respect consideration needs to be given to a person's problems (illness) and their strengths (health).

This holistic framework does not require mental health nurses to be skilled in all areas of assessment, but does require acknowledgement of its scope and thus the need to collaborate with others who have complimentary assessment skills.

In summary, the main points of this chapter are:

- Assessment is an ongoing cycle of activity that all nurses perform in all nursing situations.
- Assessments can be more or less explicit and formal depending upon the person being assessed and their reason for assessment.
- The process of assessment involves decision making, which requires the collection and interpretation of information to make judgements about a person's need for care.
- Holistic assessment requires information on a person's *subjective* and *objective* sense of *self* and their *subjective* and *objective* sense of *community* and, in each area, indicators of both health and illness should be explored.
- Mental health nurses need to develop an integrated understanding of the scope of assessment to be demonstrated in collaborative partnerships with service users and professional colleagues.
- An individual's needs form the basis of a care plan, which should include a statement of the goals to be achieved, a description of any actions to be taken, and the specification of criteria against which an evaluation of progress can be made.

Questions for reflection and discussion

1   In relation to Figure 7.1 undertake an assessment of yourself, listing indicators for both health and illness in each of the four quadrants.

2   Reflect on the mental health care of someone you have nursed and consider whether their assessment and care incorporated an interest in their health. If not, what indicators of health are you able to recall and how might recognition of these have altered the care they received?

3   In a health care culture that deals primarily with the management of risk, deficits and problems, how feasible is it to redress this balance with health-oriented assessments? What factors might hinder such developments and how can these be overcome?

4   Reread Tom's case study in this chapter. How open you are to the possibility of health among people who experience mental illness, and, how willing are you to help people find a way to live in spite of their illness?

Annotated bibliography

- Barker, P. (1997) *Assessment in Psychiatric and Mental Health Nursing: In Search of the Whole Person.* Cheltenham: Stanley Thornes Ltd. This text provides a detailed contemporary account of theoretical principles, methodologies and instruments for conducting mental health nursing assessments. Practical examples of how to assess a range of disorders are provided, including anxiety states, psychotic experiences and human relations. The text includes an examination of the moral and ethical issues surrounding assessment, and provides a selected bibliography of assessment instruments.
- Gamble, C. and Brennan, G. (2000) Assessments: A rationale and glossary of tools, in C. Gamble and G. Brennan (eds) *Working with Serious Mental Illness: A Manual for Clinical Practice.* London: Bailliere Tindall. A valuable chapter in which the authors provide a rationale for systematic assessments, describe the core elements of information to be collected and provide an extensive glossary of standardized assessment tools. The chapter provides also some practical strategies to aid the interpretation and effective implementation of assessment data.
- Bowling, A. (1997) *Measuring Health: A Review of Quality of Life Measurement Scales*, 2nd edn. Milton Keynes: Open University Press. This text provides a comprehensive collection of quality of life measurement scales that have been selected for inclusion either because they have been well tested for reliability and validity or because considerable interest has been expressed in their content area. The author provides a useful discussion of the conceptualization of functioning, health and quality of life. The text includes instruments and methods to measure functional ability, health status, psychological well-being, social networks and support, and life satisfaction and morale.

- Bowling, A. (1995) *Measuring Disease*. Buckingham: Open University Press. Though not specific to mental health this book complements Bowling's 1997 text. The strengths, weaknesses and coverage of a range of instruments designed to measure aspects of disease are reviewed.

References

Barker, P. (1997) *Assessment in Psychiatric and Mental Health Nursing: In Search of the Whole Person*. Cheltenham: Stanley Thornes Ltd.

Barker, P. (2001) The Tidal Model: developing an empowering, person-centred approach to recovery within psychiatric and mental health nursing. *Journal of Psychiatric and Mental Health Nursing* **8**: 233–40.

Beck, A., Ward, C., Mendelson, M. *et al.* (1961) An inventory for measuring depression. *Archives of General Psychiatry* **4**: 561–71.

Birchwood, M., Smith, J. and Cochrane, R. (1990) The Social Functioning Scale: the development and validation of a new scale of social adjustment in use in family interventions programmes with schizophrenic patients. *British Journal of Psychiatry* **157**: 853–9.

Bradshaw, J. (1972) The concept of social need. *New Society* **21**: 640–3.

Burnard, P. and Hannigan, B. (2000) Qualitative and quantitative approaches in mental health nursing: moving the debate forward. *Journal of Psychiatric and Mental Health Nursing* **7**: 1–6.

Chadwick, P. and Birchwood, M. (1995) The omnipotence of voices II: The beliefs about voices questionnaire. *British Journal of Psychiatry* **166**: 11–19.

Department of Health (1999) *A National Service Framework for Mental Health*. London: The Stationery Office.

Egan, G. (1994) *The Skilled Helper* (4th edn). Monterey, CA: Brooks/Cole.

Ellis, A. (1962) *Reason and Emotion in Psychotherapy*. New York: Stuart.

Ensel, W. and Woelfel, J. (1986) Measuring the instrumental and expressive functions of social support, in N. Lin, A. Dean and W. Ensel (eds) *Social Support, Life Events and Depression*. New York: Academic Press.

Fox, J. and Conroy, P. (2000) Assessing client's needs: the semistructured interview, in C. Gamble and G. Brennan (eds) *Working with Serious Mental Illness: A Manual for Clinical Practice*. London: Bailliere Tindall.

Gamble, C. and Brennan, G. (2000) Assessments: A rationale and glossary of tools, in C. Gamble and G. Brennan (eds) *Working with Serious Mental Illness: A Manual for Clinical Practice*. London: Bailliere Tindall.

Heinrichs, D., Hanlon, T. and Carpenter, W. (1984) The quality of life scale: an instrument for rating the schizophrenic deficit syndrome. *Schizophrenia Bulletin* **10**: 388–98.

Kay, S., Fiszebein, A. and Opler, L. (1987) Positive and negative syndrome scale. *Schizophrenia Bulletin* **13**: 261–76.

McConnell, H. (1998) Psychological and Behavioral Correlates of Blood and CSF Laboratory Tests, in P. Snyder and P. Nussbaum (eds) *Clinical Neuropsychology for House Staff*. Washington, DC: American Psychological Press.

McFarland, G., Wasli, E. and Gerety, E. (1997) *Nursing Diagnoses and Process in Psychiatric and Mental Health Nursing*. Philadelphia, PA: Lippincott.

Miller, W. and Rollnick, S. (1991) *Motivational Interviewing: Preparing People to Change Addictive Behaviour*. New York: Guilford Press.

Modood, T., Berthoud, R., Lakey, J. *et al.* (1998) *Ethnic Minorities in Britain: Diversity and Disadvantage. The Fourth National Survey of Ethnic Minorities.* London: Policy Studies Institute.

Newell, R. (1994) *Interviewing Skills for Nurses and Other Health Care Professionals.* London: Routledge.

Nolan, M., Keady, J. and Grant, G. (1995) CAMI: a basis for assessment and support with family carers. *British Journal of Nursing Quarterly* **4**: 822–6.

Overall, J. and Gorham, D. (1962) Brief Psychiatric Rating Scale. *Psychological Reports* **10**: 799–812.

Pavis, S., Secker, J., Cunningham-Burley, S. and Masters, H. (1998) Mental health: what do we know, how did we find out and what does it mean for nurses? *Journal of Psychiatric and Mental Health Nursing* **5**: 1–10.

Phelan, M., Slade, M., Thornicroft, G. *et al.* (1995) The Camberwell Assessment of Need: the validity and reliability of an instrument to assess the needs of people with severe mental illness. *British Journal of Psychiatry* **167**: 589–95.

Pickin, C. and St. Leger, S. (1993) *Assessing Health Need Using the Life Cycle Framework*. Milton Keynes: Open University Press.

Priebe, S., Huxley, P., Knight, S. and Evans, S. (2002) *Manchester Short Assessment of Quality of Life*. Manchester: The University of Manchester.

Repper, J. (2000) Adjusting the focus of mental health nursing: Incorporating service users' experiences of recovery. *Journal of Mental Health* **9**: 575–87.

Rosenberg, M. (1965) *The Measurement of Self-esteem*. Princeton, NJ: Princeton University Press.

Savage, P. (1991) Patient assessment in psychiatric nursing. *Journal of Advanced Nursing* **16**: 311–16.

Sherer, M., Maddux, J., Mercandante, B. *et al.* (1982) The self-efficacy scale: construction and validation. *Psychological Reports* **51**: 663–71.

Wallcraft, J., Read, J. and Sweeney, A. (2003) *On Our Own Terms: Users and Survivors of Mental Health Services Working Together for Support and Change*. London: The Sainsbury Centre for Mental Health.

Ward, M. (1992) *The Nursing Process in Psychiatry* (2nd edn). Edinburgh: Churchill Livingstone.

Wilber, K. (2000) *Sex, Ecology and Spirituality: The Spirit of Evolution*. Boston, MA: Shambhala.

Wing, J., Curtis, R. and Beevor, A. (1995) *Measurement of Mental Health: Health of the Nation Outcome Scales*. London: Royal College of Psychiatrists Research Unit.

8

Assessing and managing risk

Steve Morgan and Andrew Wetherell

Chapter overview

In recent years the concept of risk has increasingly permeated the policy and practice agenda in mental health care. Legislative guidance and administrative documentation have introduced more bureaucracy, which can undermine confidence in practice and also promote a 'blame culture' where opportunities for positive risk-taking may be overlooked. This chapter unpacks the concept of risk and encourages the reader to look beyond its negative connotations to include the positive risks we must all take in the course of our lives. Types of risk and their associated factors are detailed and processes for assessing and managing risk are examined. The chapter places particular emphasis on the 'service-user perspective' and encourages the promotion of genuine involvement and collaboration with service users in the assessment and management of risk.

This chapter covers:

- an introduction to risk;
- policy guidance and legislative context;
- the service-user experience;
- positive risk-taking;
- risk assessment and risk management;
- risk categories;
- paper institution or practical tools?
- confidentiality.

An introduction to risk

Risk is enmeshed in all aspects of our daily functioning; it is essentially the art of living with uncertainty. For some, the emphasis is on the positive – a chance for gain; while for others, it takes on a more negative focus – the experience of pain. For many people, at least for some of the time, risk simply 'is', with little conscious acknowledgement of its influences. Whatever your personal standpoint, the passions for living or dying are sustained by the very existence and temptations of risk. A life devoid of risk is likely to have no challenge and very little real meaning.

In mental health, the term schizophrenia is broadly used as a diagnosis for conditions that are often represented by disjointed thinking and distorted perceptions. It may equally apply as a diagnosis of the diverse reactions observed in relation to the concept of risk in mental health. It becomes an emotive subject, generating conflicting priorities and agendas: a linked public safety and political policy agenda; an organizational bureaucratic and administrative agenda; and a clinical preventative and restrictive agenda. What these appear to have in common, when examined in some detail, is a 'cover-your-back' agenda. Seldom do we find a serious attempt to engage the service user's personal agenda!

The public safety agenda

For many people working in the field of mental health this is a relatively recent concept, perhaps only dating back ten years to the onset of a series of homicide inquiries. One of the repeated inaccurate messages is the implication of danger in pursuing a policy of community care, which may be serving to release dangerously deranged individuals into the community. In its more extreme implications, the suggestion is made that innocent members of the public are unknowingly being placed at risk by liberal minded policy makers and clinicians, who generally do not inhabit the same communities into which they have discharged the seriously mentally ill.

In defence of this position, there are detailed reports of inquiries which highlight the failure of treatment and care for individuals who did go on to commit horrendous and fatal acts of violence against family members or other members of the public (Ritchie *et al*. 1994; Sheppard 1996). The political policy reaction has carried implications of blame for those who provide mental health services, with the accompanying panoply of government guidance and legislation focused specifically on those who present a high risk (NHS Executive 1994; Department of Health 1995). The more general framework of managing care for the broader constituency of those diagnosed with mental health problems, the Care Programme Approach, is also taking on a stronger risk management focus (Department of Health 1999a) and the intention is very much directed towards the need to ensure public safety. The underlining premise appears to be that people experiencing mental health problems are primarily a threat to others.

To counterbalance this prevailing argument, less well publicized but researched evidence suggests that we do live in a more violent society than a generation ago. However, the progressive policy of community care has contributed nothing to the increase in homicide statistics during the second half of the twentieth century (Taylor and Gunn 1999). Either by a consistently high dose of luck, or the unnoticed application of some good practice, many risks are being effectively identified and managed, with the immeasurable outcome of potential incidents being prevented.

Undoubtedly, some horrendous tragedies have occurred that could otherwise have been avoided with attention to important principles of practice and a major dose of hindsight. However, we seem to have fallen into the trap of losing sight of realistic expectations in the face of sensationalist media headlines and political sound bites. The implications that risk can be accurately assessed and managed appear to be linked to measures of success based on the notion of 'risk elimination'. The unpredictability of human behaviour dictates that 'risk minimization' or reduction is a more realistic outcome to expect.

An organizational agenda

This is where senior management frequently find themselves caught between the ideals of guiding and supporting frontline staff to provide high quality services for those who need them, and the need to be seen to respond to the powerful external pressures and demands of the imagination-capturing, vote-winning, paper-selling public safety ticket. In its simplest form, it suggests that the staff are the organization's most valuable resource, that good service-user-involving practice is paramount, and that a flexible and creative response to individually assessed need is the way to deliver a first-class service. On the other hand, completion of the Care Programme Approach (CPA), risk assessment, carers' assessment, audit tools, daily notes and monitoring forms should be done on everyone seen by the service, primarily to meet externally determined performance targets. An inevitable consequence is the pressure put on to staff to manage the higher caseloads and workloads that accompany increasing expectations.

When, in this conflicting scenario, something goes wrong, the initial organizational response, at least as perceived by the majority of practitioners, is a 'guilty until proven innocent' stance. There often appears to be a management assumption that people with serious mental health problems can be comprehensively assessed with rigorous research tools. On this basis they can either be given the necessary support to live in the community without posing threats or fears to those around them, or they can be provided with varying degrees of restriction to ensure that no harm comes to unsuspecting members of the public. The unrealistic external expectations of those who know no better appear to be assimilated by people higher up within the organization, who should know better.

The challenge to this way of thinking is not a call to condone poor or negligent practice. Staff work daily with difficult challenges, and need to feel supported rather than blamed the instant things go wrong. Instead, their more usual experience leaves them with little doubt that in the quality versus quantity debate the organization stands on the side of high standards of service corresponding to high numbers being crunched! An 'us and them' divide within the organization leads to a belief in the stance that asks: What have you done today to ensure that your organization is beyond reproach? Can we count on you to have made a mistake that lets the rest of us off the hook when the real scrutiny begins?

The practitioner agenda

As the providers of direct treatment, support and care, most practitioners are fully aware of the place of risk and safety in their working lives. With few exceptions, their intentions are to provide a good quality of service that meets the needs of the people referred to them. They also expect reasonable resources, guidance and support in order to provide the necessary quality of care. Fears are that the role is gradually changing from primarily one of good nursing practice to a more generic notion of multi-disciplinary/multi-agency workers; to the administrator of care coordination; to the specific role of social policing; and where to next?

Mental health practitioners fear that their work has recently become dominated by risk, and maybe they are not doing the caring and supporting functions they came into the job to do, and from which they derive so much of their job satisfaction. They fear that external forces have conspired to make the mental health business into a risk business (Rose 1998). The news is that we are in the risk business simply because living is a constant risk. Risk has always been there – in the asylums, the mini-institutions, the development of community mental health initiatives, every time people come into direct contact; and the times when they do not. Perhaps the problem is not so much that we have become the risk business, but rather that we have become the 'bureaucratic and adminis-trative business of restriction' – a face of authority that it is easy to 'risk against'.

Many different and conflicting agendas have become established in relation to the conceptualization of risk in mental health. However, one significant question generally seems to be overlooked: Whatever happened to the notion that it could be the people experiencing the mental health problems who are the ones most at risk?

Definition of risk

> The likelihood of an event happening with potentially harmful or beneficial outcomes for self and/or others ... possible behaviours include suicide, self-harm, aggression and violence, and neglect; with an additional range of other positive or negative service user experiences.
>
> (Morgan 2000a: 1)

This is a helpful definition in that it does acknowledge risk as not totally negative by stating there can be beneficial outcomes for self and/or others. In addition, it registers that there are a whole range of additional service-user experiences, which need to be taken into account.

Policy guidance and legislative context

National Service Framework (NSF) for Mental Health (DH 1999b) and *NHS Plan* (DH 2000)

Most recently, these documents have set the scene as statements of intent and injections of resources, which imply that criticisms presented by repeated reports of inquiry are being dealt with. One positive development is the placing of a stronger emphasis on the category of suicide risk (*NSF for Mental Health*, Standard 7), thus recognizing the negative impact of circumstances on the service user, as opposed to the more usual inclination of media reporting and government policy towards service users as perpetrators of risk. The downside of this emphasis is a continued reliance on setting targets, in this instance the reduction of suicide rates by 20 per cent by 2010 (Department of Health 1999c). Any appreciation of the complexities that underpin the individuality of the suicidal act is only reflected in the statements of how Standards 1–6 will contribute towards the achievement of this ambitious target. Once again, expectations are set up, with the inevitable sense that they will become benchmarks of future service failures.

Overall, the *NSF for Mental Health* represents a more balanced view of risk than some of the earlier examples of guidance and legislation in the 1990s. Only in Standards 4 and 5 (covering 'Effective Services for People with Severe Mental Illness') does a more specific emphasis on assessing and managing risk appear, with reference to 'risk to others'; but, this is also counterbalanced by an acknowledgement of service users' potential risks of vulnerability. By implication, the emphasis of the whole framework will impact on the assessment and management of risk in the mental health population, through an integrated and partially evidence-based approach to service delivery.

Review of the Mental Health Act (1983)

This is awaited, but the detail of its reincarnation remains a cause for general concern on both sides of the mental health field – service users fearing further restrictions being placed on their liberties, and practitioners fearing more erosion of good practice for the pursuit of achieving a primary goal of public safety. It has potentially become delayed by the complication in interpreting Dangerous and Severe Personality Disorder (DSPD) legislation.

Human Rights Act (1998)

This legislation requires that all public authorities should act in a manner compatible with the European Convention of Human Rights (ECHR) (cf. Chapter 6). It will now be unlawful for them to act in a way that is incompatible with the ECHR, unless the specific requirements of other legislation appear to contradict the ECHR. How can the legislators marry together a promotion of human rights with a need for greater 'surveillance and supervision' of certain individuals, assumed to be required of mental health services charged with upholding public safety?

Briefing Paper 12 (Sainsbury Centre for Mental Health 2000) examines some of the potential impact of this legislation, highlighting:

Article 2: the right to life.
Article 3: prohibition of torture and inhuman and degrading treatment.
Article 5: the right to liberty and security.
Article 8: the right to respect for private and family life, home and correspondence.

It concludes that in this early stage, it is not possible to predict the type of mental health cases, which will be successfully pursued under the Human Rights Act (1998). Practitioners need to be aware of the likely wide-ranging impact of their work on the rights of service users and carers. They need to ensure that any perceived interference with individual rights needs to be clearly justified, reasoned and recorded. 'Risk' will be a significant area, as the issues of restriction and detention are generally closely aligned with the potential for risk.

Reviews of restriction at tribunal hearings may also pose a human rights' minefield; both in terms of scrutinizing the validity of the act of restriction in some individual cases, but also through unreasonable delays in arranging review dates. However, there may also be future potential for this legislation to be considered in support of reasoned positive risk-taking in mental health services.

Modernizing the Care Programme Approach (DH 1999a)

The Care Programme Approach (CPA) continues to represent the overall mechanism for coordinating care in UK services, including the management of risk. It has arguably taken more of an administrative function, in contrast to the more usual expectations of providing a 'clinical' service. The assumption across clinical services is that a risk assessment will be revised in line with at least the frequency of CPA reviews; and that risk management plans will be formulated either as an integral part of the CPA care plan, or separately but attached with the overall care plan. The risk-focused Supervision Register (NHS Executive 1994) is gradually being discontinued as the enhanced level of the modernized CPA is fully implemented to the satisfaction of NHS regional offices.

However, Supervised Discharge (Department of Health 1995), also referred to as Section 25 (Mental Health Act 1983), remains in operation as a method of administrating the management of risk through conveying people to places of treatment, education or meaningful activity, or determining where they should reside. This legislation has received widespread anecdotal practitioner apathy regarding its usefulness, being seen as more focused on multi-disciplinary meetings and paperwork, than on meaningful engaged working relationships.

The emphasis of inquiry findings on poor communication and failures to adequately coordinate care offer important messages for services to address. However, the overall legislative response seems to have created a role for care coordination that requires more administrative management of risk than actual clinical management of risk. While it has undoubtedly raised the profile of the risk agenda in the minds of all practitioners, it is highly debatable that it has brought about any of the desired improvements in safety that such changes are intended to achieve. Fearful quasi-administrators do not make for more skilled clinical practitioners; and service provision becomes much more negatively restrictive than the great majority of service users need or deserve.

The service-user experience

Some areas of government policy have been extremely disappointing to many service users, not least of which is the *National Service Framework (NSF) for Mental Health* (Department of Health 1999b). While this document is generally to be welcomed, the overwhelming view of many service users, and indeed practitioners, is that the standards it outlines should be regarded as minimums – not optimums. Therefore, the aim should be to try to build more effective and supportive services from those stated within the NSF.

It is important to note that a number of service-user participants on the government's External Reference Group, which helped to shape the *NSF for Mental Health* actually resigned from the group as they were unhappy not only with the process but also the general direction which was being taken. To highlight just one of the potentially serious areas in this context, it is worth considering the current proposals in relation to Compulsory Treatment Orders in the community (CTOs). Most service users and practitioners which the authors of this chapter have spoken to around the UK feel that this type of approach to community mental health will be a retrograde step which will have real potential to increase risk. Service users may be driven away from services rather than being properly engaged in an effective and sensitive way as the vital therapeutic relationship between service user and practitioner is broken down by inappropriate and highly unhelpful policy.

While the government policy agenda of reducing stigma and promoting social inclusion is warmly welcomed by most service users, the public safety agenda creates something of a paradox in that it only helps to stigmatize mental health service users even further by adding to some highly inappropriate and inaccurate myths connected with mental distress.

Further, the whole 'protection of the public' approach fails to fully register the far higher risks of self-harm, serious self-neglect and suicide, as well as abuse, attack and exploitation from other members of the public, which face many service users each day. In other words, mental health service users are more often than not vulnerable human beings who are far more likely to be victims of violence rather than the perpetrators of it (Wetherell 2000).

Taylor and Gunn (1999) looked at the homicide figures for the period 1957–95 and, overall, they found there was a fivefold increase in homicides within the UK. However, they found a decline of 3 per cent per annum in contribution to these figures by people with mental illness. Therefore, it is important to note that while we are now living in a significantly more violent society, proportionally, homicides by people with mental health problems are reducing.

While 35–40 homicides by people with a mental health problem is 35–40 too many, it is wholly unrealistic to expect this figure to be reduced to zero. As stated at the beginning of this chapter, risk is enmeshed in all aspects of our daily functioning; it is essentially the art of living with uncertainty. Therefore, in reality there will always be tragedies whether we deliver mental health care in the community, within large institutions, on acute wards or from specialist units. Most service users accept the above and are willing to live with risk in their lives so long as they are provided with accessible, person-centred, effective services, which are sensitive to their needs.

Service users are sometimes put at risk because inflexible systems and services are unable to respond to individual clinical needs as they occur. As an example, although Care Programme Approach (CPA) can be of great assistance in managing risk, systems failures can cause people to fall through the safety net despite good service-user focused planning. Therefore, it is essential that services are able to respond to specific risk management and crisis plans in a swift and appropriate manner at all times and such an approach should include the following:

- monitoring for early warning signs/relapse signatures;
- agreed crisis and contingency plans;
- proactive follow-up for service users who don't attend appointments; and
- a named care coordinator whose telephone number is available to all those in the network of care.

All of the above need to be supported with a thorough, detailed and up-to-date care plan which names the individual professionals responsible for each element of care, timescales and recommended responses, etc.

The service user's experience of risk in relation to acute care is another important area to consider. A survey of the quality of care in acute psychiatric wards (Sainsbury Centre for Mental Health 1998) highlighted that most acute ward environments have limited therapeutic input and can be dangerous places for both patients and staff. Service users commonly said that they felt unsafe on acute wards, and women in particular expressed concerns about their personal safety. In many areas, there is constant demand for beds that leads to inappropriate early discharge thereby putting service users at increased risk. Therefore, a comprehensive risk assessment needs to take place both for service users who are being discharged as well as for those being considered for leave.

As stated within Standard 7 (Preventing Suicide) of the *NSF for Mental Health*, care plans for those with severe mental illness should include an urgent follow-up within one week of discharge from hospital as it is recognized that this period carries a significantly increased risk of suicide. Although the suicide rate has fallen by more than 12 per cent since 1982 (Kelly and Bunting 1998), some people remain at a relatively higher risk of death by suicide. The following statistics taken from the *NSF for Mental Health* (Department of Health 1999b) help to highlight some of the higher risk areas:

- Men are three times more likely than women to commit suicide. It is the leading cause of death among men aged 15–24 and the second most common cause of death among people aged under 35.
- Men in unskilled occupations are four times more likely to commit suicide than are those in professional work.
- Among women living in England, those born in India and East Africa have a 40 per cent higher suicide rate than those born in England and Wales.
- Certain occupational groups are at higher risk, for example, doctors, nurses, pharmacists, vets and farmers, due to access to means.
- More than 1 in 10 people with severe mental illness kill themselves.
- Risk is raised further for those with depression and/or suffering major loss.
- Previous histories of self-harm, or drug and alcohol misuse are at relatively higher risk of suicide.
- There are high rates of suicide in prisons.

Positive risk-taking

Broadly speaking, individuals can only grow through measured and justifiable risk-taking. It would also be a rather dull world if it were devoid of all risks and associated choices. Life consists of exercising one choice over another, and this liberty should apply to service users as much as it does to other members of society. It is also important to remember that we all engage in risky behaviour to some degree as a normal part of daily living. Mental health managers, service commissioners, practitioners and service users alike all take some risks every day. It would be virtually impossible to actually live a normal life without some form of risk-taking.

Some obvious, common examples would include: smoking, drinking alcohol, poor diet, taking recreational drugs, driving while tired, breaking the speed limit, and crossing a busy road. Risk is often an important and positive element within our lives – people learn and grow through taking measured and justifiable risks, and so it is not all about danger and negativity, by any means.

While some would argue that positive risk-taking is a relatively new concept in risk management, it is true to say that many nurses and other practitioners have been working collaboratively with service users in this way for many years in their everyday working practice. The idea of positive risk-taking is usually most popular with service users and practitioners alike, as it takes a different approach by focusing on service users' strengths and positive attributes. This will be a different way of working to many practitioners as it is not problems oriented. However, it can be a useful, refreshing and empowering way to work collaboratively with service users (Morgan 2000b).

Any positive risks taken, together with the reasoning behind them, need to be clearly documented, and supported by a collaborative approach. To be 'defensible' in the face of opposition and scrutiny they need to be:

- justifiable;
- measured;
- intelligent;
- negotiated with the service user and carer(s) (Wetherell 2001b).

Some basic examples of what could be positive risk-taking are shown below and include some things which general members of the community would do as a matter of course in their daily lives:

- having a bank account;
- shopping;
- visiting family or friends;
- independent living;
- voluntary or paid work;
- going on holiday;
- 'controlled' self-harm;
- medication reduction or withdrawal.

Probably one of the most radical issues listed above is the 'controlled self-harm'. As a concept, self-harm needs to be more fully understood and accepted as a coping strategy that some people need to engage in order to prevent something even worse from happening. It should not simply be seen as behaviour associated with a suicide attempt. Therefore, if service users are going to engage in self-harm, from a risk perspective is it not better they do so with appropriate knowledge of harm minimization, which will help to reduce risk?

As an example, the National Self-Harm Network has produced some helpful literature in *The Hurt Yourself Less Workbook* (Dace *et al.* 1998) which is focused on harm reduction or minimization and includes information on informing service users of 'safer self-harm' approaches, effective first aid and wound dressing, etc.

When approaching the management of self-harm behaviours from a risk viewpoint, it is helpful to be aware of the following common inaccurate myths in this connection. Some people incorrectly believe that self-harm is:

- attention seeking;
- attempted suicide (although in some cases it has accidentally led to death);
- masochism;
- a form of manipulation; and
- unworthy for treatment within hospital settings, particularly accident and emergency departments.

Understanding why people engage in self-harm behaviours may also be helpful in assessing and managing risk. Some possible reasons include:

- to feel alive;
- preventing something worse from happening (for example, a suicide attempt);
- to reduce or stop intrusive thoughts;
- self-hatred;
- self-punishment;
- to achieve relief/release of emotions; and
- a distraction from 'intolerable reality'.

With a focus on effective management of self-harm behaviours, the following approaches may be of assistance within clinical practice:

- Encourage the individual to talk about how they are feeling.
- Show care and respect for the person behind the self-harm behaviour.
- Recognize that trying to extinguish self-harm behaviour can be unrealistic and can deprive the service user of a coping strategy. Working towards harm minimization or reduction may be a more realistic goal.
- Acknowledge the emotional distress and trauma that the person is experiencing.
- Even if self-harm is considered to be part of a 'Personality Disorder' try to remember that behind every 'personality disorder' there is a *personality* and; behind every personality there is a *person*.

Clearly, contingency plans need to be formulated just in case any positive risk-taking begins to go wrong or if the service user reaches a crisis at any time. Additionally, there can be value in making contracts with service users so that everyone is clear of the boundaries and any appropriate action to be taken should risk increase to an unacceptable level. At all times of any positive risk-taking process, practitioners, carers and service users themselves need to be monitoring for any early warning signs of relapse or increased risk, and an agreed course of action can then be taken in line with the contingency plan and/or the contract with the service user.

While we need to work towards a culture which accepts and positively encourages positive risk-taking, we need at all times to remember that there may be team conflict in this connection. This, of course, needs to be managed and constructive, objective dialogue needs to take place between all practitioners concerned, wherever possible leading to a negotiated consensus within the team.

Case study: Kate – a study in positive risk-taking

Personal history

Kate is 35 years old, born in Dublin, but moved to Manchester with her family (parents, older sister, younger brother) when she was 14. She was married at 26 and divorced at 33. Her ex-husband was awarded custody of their two sons owing to her mental health problems. Her working life was mainly spent in accountancy, before her marriage and parenthood. During the last 18 months, Kate held a part-time job (usually two days per week) in a local shop, using her accountancy skills. The shop owner has taken a flexible and supportive approach to employing Kate, even through numerous spells of time spent in hospital.

Psychiatric history

Kate was sexually abused by an uncle, between the ages of 6 and 14. Any attempts by Kate to discuss the abuse with her parents were quickly dismissed or denied. First contact with child and adolescent psychiatric services was at the age of 8, experiencing depressive episodes and low levels of self-worth and confidence. At the age of 10 the family GP prescribed Ativan, which Kate became addicted to, and was not properly supported to come off it until her late teenage years. Further developments in her teenage years included drug and alcohol misuse, and self-harm (cutting and burning).

A serious suicide attempt, through paracetamol overdose combined with vodka, followed her divorce. She was found by emergency services who were alerted by concerns of a close friend. Kate has had 11 hospital admissions during the last five years, most being short-term crisis admissions of up to three weeks' duration, with a couple of admissions extending up to six weeks. The longer-term diagnoses of depression and anxiety remain, but approximately four years ago Kate was diagnosed with borderline personality disorder, due to her chaotic lifestyle, self-harming behaviour and substance misuse becoming more pronounced features of her presentation.

Relationships

While the relationship with her parents is not very good, they are on speaking terms, and Kate usually sees them at least monthly. She maintains occasional contact and reasonably good relationships with her brother and sister. Weekly contact is maintained with two close friends from the local badminton club, and very good relationships are sustained with her two sons – they normally stay with her most Saturdays. Good relationships with mental health professionals are rare, and only established where she feels a strong sense of trust and safety; but on occasions she has become very attached to individual members of nursing staff, leading to unhealthy levels of dependency.

Current situation

Kate's ex-husband is due to remarry in the next few weeks. Concerns over her future contacts with her sons precipitated a series of arguments with him. She was admitted to the local psychiatric unit a few days ago following several days' drinking and drug use, leading to a serious incident of deep cutting, which damaged her arm. During the admission, a member of staff discovered Kate pushing paper tissue down her throat, in an attempt to asphyxiate herself. She was placed on one-to-one close observations. She has also attracted unwanted attention from young male patients on the unit, and feels a strong need for staff to ensure her safety over this issue.

Interests and aspirations

Maintaining the contact with her two sons is her main priority; and sustaining her part-time job in the local shop is something she feels respects her skills and abilities. Kate particularly values her few close friendships, and she has read some information on the psychiatric unit about the National Self-Harm Network. After discussions with another patient on the unit she is expressing a desire to contact the network, with the aim of meeting like-minded people and possibly taking some personal control and management of her self-harming behaviours.

Consideration of risk-taking

After a full multi-disciplinary discussion, with Kate proactively involved, a plan for early discharge was formulated based on:

- a counselling and coordination role provided by the community psychiatric nurse based in the GP practice (no referral to the community mental health team);

- establishing Kate's links with local people in the National Self-Harm Network;
- Kate's self-monitoring of an early warning signs and relapse signature plan, developed with an inpatient nurse with whom she has a trusting relationship;
- opportunities for Kate to occasionally initiate contact with the inpatient nurse to discuss her progress or concerns (the nurse will establish regular contact with the primary care CPN to coordinate such contacts);
- discharge on no medication, but with progress reviews established with the GP, and 6-monthly outpatient appointments; and
- clear documentation of the reasoned decision making: discussions, plans and contingencies for potential difficulties.

Risk assessment and risk management

For the purposes of a textbook, or training event, the concepts of risk assessment and risk management can be analysed separately. However, in reality they are closely inter-linked – risk cannot be effectively managed until it has been clearly identified and defined; and when a risk is identified we instantly respond with considerations of how it is best managed. In recent years, there has been a shift of conceptual thinking, from a singular and static determination of dangerousness, to a more dynamic and changeable concept of risk (Rose 1998). Risk assessment and management have become continuous elements of good clinical practice.

This development has coincided with some of the consistent requirements emerging from the homicide inquiry reports, namely that:

- high quality and up-to-date risk information is essential;
- information needs to be shared as widely as possible between agencies and individuals, as appropriate; and
- collaborative working between all individuals and organizations is crucial.

Risk assessment

A gathering of information and analysis of the potential outcomes of identified behaviours. Identifying specific risk factors of relevance to an individual and the context in which they may occur. This process requires linking historical information to current circumstances to anticipate possible future change.

(Morgan 2000a: 2)

Specific categories and risk factors will be discussed in detail in the next section; here we will focus consideration more on the skills and general areas of assessment. There is no mystique about risk assessment, as with all other types of assessment it depends on the accessibility and quality of information gathered. To this end, it requires persistence in pursuit of the relevant information held at multiple sources. The skill lies more in the delicate manner and approach to enquiring after appropriate information from the service user, and all others with relevant knowledge to contribute. The basic skills include active listening, empathic understanding and reflective communication, supplemented by alert observation of the non-verbal cues or signs of change.

Once information has been collected, the next skill required of the practitioner is that of reasoned analysis, towards the formulation of a plan of action. At this stage, accurate historical information needs to be evaluated against current patterns of behaviour. One previous incident, 20 years ago, does not necessarily indicate a high risk of reoccurrence; though such an eventuality should not be entirely ruled out. A repeated pattern of risk behaviours over time begins to present a stronger basis for predicting a reoccurrence. Never lose sight of the human potential to change behaviour patterns, even those that appear to be well established. The keys to a good assessment of risk are as follows.

Context

It is vitally important to look at any changing personal circumstances when assessing risk in relation to a particular individual. If someone is experiencing significant change within their life such as moving, the bereavement of someone close to them, or the allocation of a new care coordinator, there could well be increased risk present. An individual who may be at risk in one particular situation, or specific relationships, could actually be at little or no risk in another setting. For instance, the likelihood of self-injury or suicide may increase significantly in an individual faced with an inpatient admission, or in a specific relationship. On the other hand, inpatient admission could reduce risk for other individuals who feel safer within an acute hospital setting (Wetherell 2001a).

Environment

As well as assessing the individual, how well they are functioning, and their general behaviour, we need to look at the current environment, and the community in which the person lives (Morgan 1998). Whether the person may be at risk from local people needs to be considered – some service users are highly vulnerable and are open to abuse and/or exploitation in many ways. Local hazards have to be appreciated and taken into account, for example, a drug culture or robberies on the street. It is crucial to remember that these potential risks are faced not only by the service user, but also by the practitioner who might go to particular known areas to carry out home visits (Wetherell 2001a).

Another area of consideration is the degree of emotional arousal dependent upon the setting. For instance, one person may become emotionally aroused within a formal setting, whereas another person may find such a setting to be calming and safe. There is also the issue of potential weapons to be considered in the rare circumstances where a service user may pose the threat of violence to others. Anything can be a weapon, and practitioners need to give due consideration to this, in relation to the potential emotional arousal, as well as to the physical layout of the environment in any given circumstance.

Research information

Research information is a key part of risk assessment, and it can assist in identifying potentially risky circumstances or individuals (Department of Health 2001). For instance, men under 35 years of age are more likely to pose a risk of violence. If you then add the taking of drugs and/or alcohol, the risk increases further. Certain psychotic phenomenon, for example, persecutory delusions specifying an individual(s), or auditory command hallucinations then increase the risks even higher (Buchanan 1997). Risk factors are discussed in more detail in the next section.

Predictive ability

One expectation of risk assessment is that it enables predictive judgements on the probability of certain behavioural outcomes. Prediction is a very uncertain element, though its accuracy can be partly improved by shortening timescales. In this instance, risk has some parallels with trying to predict the weather (Monahan and Steadman 1996). A glance out of the window will tell you if you need to take an umbrella with you in ten minutes' time. Predicting whether you will need an umbrella at the same time a week later becomes a totally different, more complex and difficult to gauge scenario. Similarly with risk – events are generally easier to predict over the next few hours and days than the next few weeks and months.

Practitioner confidence in assessing risks grows with experience. However, the key to a good risk assessment process has to be a collaborative multi-disciplinary and multi-agency approach, where good quality information is shared as appropriate between all relevant parties, leading to shared decision making for good risk management.

Risk management

> A statement of plans and an allocation of individual responsibilities for translating collective decisions into actions. This process should name all relevant people involved in the treatment and support including the service user and appropriate informal carers. It should also identify a review date for the assessment & management plan.
>
> (Morgan 2000a: 2)

Risk management receives far less attention in the literature than risk assessment. The last decade has seen an overall change of emphasis, not just for the concept of risk generally, but also risk management specifically. The latter has shifted from a means of trying to control the volume of medical negligence, to a clinical initiative for addressing potentially harmful outcomes for service users (Vincent 1997). Morgan (1998) suggests that clinical risk management is now focused on the interpretation and implementation of individualized care plans, through targeting treatment, care and support options to the issues identified in a comprehensive assessment (including risk assessment). In reality risk management is about actions, and the responsibilities for ensuring they are carried out and monitored as effectively as possible.

Morgan and Hemming (1999) outline a structure for procedural risk management that stresses three levels of intervention:

- preventative risk management (including attention to the working relationship, education and early warning signs of relapse);
- management of escalating situations (including de-escalation techniques, rapid responses and crisis intervention); and
- post-incident supportive management (including positive support for victims and a culture of learning rather than instant retribution through blaming).

The effectiveness of risk management will be determined by the local team operational policies and daily procedures of clinical practice. The context that holds the most influence in this respect is that of team resources, space for imagination, reflection through individual and peer supervision, and attending to the tensions between the need for safety and least restriction of all people engaged in the process, not least the service user (Morgan and Hemming 1999).

One of the key messages for all nursing staff and other mental health workers is the need to move away from an approach relying on the sole responsibility of individual practitioners. The need for collaborative approaches and collective responsibility cannot be over-emphasized. It is recommended that this method of working is supported by organizational management, policies and procedures emphasizing the concept of collective responsibility. It is therefore vital that collaborative working takes place, where high quality information is shared and where colleagues use each other as sounding boards in order to check out thoughts, intuitive feelings, or concerns. In terms of good risk management practice, regular review at appropriate intervals is therefore required (Department of Health 1999a).

'A *collective approach* should lead to *collective responsibility* in the event of "*x*" ' (Wetherell 2001b: 15). We need to learn the valuable lessons from what has gone wrong in the past, and the 'near miss' situations, in order that similar risks can be minimized in the future. The current patterns of investigation immediately set up anxieties in practitioners, even before the full facts have been established. A sense of 'guilty until proven innocent' is established. It is highly unlikely that this approach generates the necessary confidence of practitioners, either in their own abilities or in the support of the organizations. This approach may also seriously contribute to a more fearful, and consequently closed attitude towards reporting events that nearly became incidents.

Therefore, we should welcome a culture that strives to encourage and support a 'blame-free, near-miss reporting' mechanism, in order to develop the confidence to learn. This may require a more confidential set of arrangements to be established within or across organizations, enabling people to pass on important messages to the people who can ensure they are heard without any attachment of blame to those doing the reporting (unless serious negligence has arisen). Similar arrangements currently exist in the aviation industry to learn about near misses without targeting blame to individuals.

Risk categories

Risk categories together with the various factors under each should assist nursing staff and other practitioners in their assessment and management of risk within their daily clinical practice. However, they should be used as a helpful aide-mémoire or as a tool to support professional judgement based on practical experience. This section is designed to help the reader examine the risk categories we are suggesting as well as the individual factors under each of the headings set out later on in this section.

Seven broad categories are considered:

- suicide;
- neglect;
- aggression/violence;
- risk associated with disability;
- physical/medical risks;
- self-harm;
- other risks.

Risk categories and their constituent factors can be used to develop tools that systematically gather these data in relation to individual service users. However, a few broad considerations will arise in practice:

- Provision for 'past' and 'current' (and possibly 'potential' in relation to the 'current' category). A frequent question raised by practitioners is, 'What constitutes "past" and what constitutes "present"?' One approach is to provide a cut-off date in the operational policy and on the risk documentation, for example, three months. However, this approach can lead to various problems including occurrences that are just a few days away from the cut-off point. Under which category should they be entered?

- Documenting 'potential' risks under the 'current' section. Arguably anything could be described as 'potential'. Therefore, the preferred option is to rely upon good clinical judgement, based upon sound professional approaches and experience. As far as possible where areas of potential confusion occur, it is preferable for practitioners to check out thinking, ideas and concerns with colleagues with a view to arriving at some sort of consensus on the issue in question.

- Inclusion of tick boxes for 'yes', 'no' and 'don't know' against each of the category factors (creating the opportunity for practitioners to highlight areas where more information or clarification is required by ticking the 'don't know' box). However, some documentation in use around the country only has provision for 'yes' or 'no', which can lead to people being forced to tick one of these when, in reality, it would be far more appropriate to be recording some items as 'don't know'.

Risk categories and associated factors

Tables 8.1–8.7 list the seven risk categories we are suggesting together with some of the associated risk factors for each. We pose a question to the reader regarding which categories they could come up with personally, and how they might re-arrange the individual factors, which are listed under each section.

Table 8.1 Suicide risk factors

	Examples (where appropriate)
• Helplessness or hopelessness	Severe depression
• Misuse of drugs and/or alcohol	
• Family history of suicide	
• Major psychiatric diagnoses	Manic depression, schizophrenia, clinical depression
• Separated/widowed/divorced	
• Expressing suicidal ideas	
• Unemployed/retired	
• Considered/planned intent	
• Attempts on their life	Taking of overdoses/hanging
• Expressing high levels of distress	Highly emotional, agitated
• Use of violent methods	Cutting of wrists
• Significant life events	Bereavement of close relative or friend
• Believe no control over their life	
• Other (to be specified)	

Table 8.2 Risk factors for neglect

	Examples (where appropriate)
• Periods of neglect	Neglect when abusing drugs
• Lack of positive social contacts	Abusive peer contacts
• Failing to drink properly	
• Unable to shop for self	
• Failing to eat properly	
• Insufficient/inappropriate clothing	
• Difficulty managing physical health	Ignoring dental needs
• Difficulty maintaining hygiene	
• Living in inadequate accommodation	
• Experiencing financial difficulties	
• Lacking basic amenities (water/heat/light)	
• Difficulty in communicating needs	Client with psychosis
• Pressure of eviction/repossession	
• Denies problems perceived by others	Lack of insight/denial
• Other (to be specified)	

Table 8.3 Risk factors for aggression/violence

	Examples (where appropriate)
• Incidents of violence	
• Paranoid delusions about others	'They are poisoning me'
• Use of weapons	
• Violent command hallucinations	Voices say 'Hit that nurse'
• Misuse of drugs and/or alcohol	
• Signs of anger and/or frustration	Shouting/banging fists
• Sexually inappropriate behaviour	Touching/stroking others
• Known personal trigger factors	Visit from family
• Preoccupation with violent fantasy	Rape/hostage taking
• Expressing intent to harm others	
• Admissions to secure settings	High, medium or low security provisions or use of seclusion
• Dangerous impulsive acts	Deliberate fire setting
• Denial of previous dangerous acts	
• Other (to be specified)	

Table 8.4 Risk factors associated with disability

	Examples (where appropriate)
• Sensory impairments	
• Intellectual impairments	Poor social skills
• Physical suitability of home	
• Mobility inside the home	
• Mobility outside the home	
• Risk of falls	Frail/elderly person
• Risk of wandering	Client with dementia
• Risk of accidental injury	Learning disability client drinking a boiling hot drink
• Communication difficulties	
• Expressing sexuality	
• Consequences of impulsivity	Assault on client
• Challenges to services	Poor service resourcing
• Risks associated with driving	Partial sighted or epilepsy
• Other (to be specified)	

Table 8.5 Physical/medical risk factors

	Examples (where appropriate)
• Physical impairments	Loss of limb(s)
• Medical conditions	Asthma/epilepsy
• Self-managing medication	
• Monitoring medication side effects	
• Risks of withdrawal	Relapse/fit/seizures
• Risks from smoking	Health/fire
• Manual handling risks	
• Incontinence	
• Other (to be specified)	

Table 8.6 Risk factors for self-harm

	Examples (where appropriate)
• Cutting	Use of razor blades/glass
• Burning	
• Insertion of objects	Pushing items into veins
• Overdosing	
• Eating disorders	Bulimia/anorexia
• Taking of laxatives	
• Hair pulling	
• Head banging	Striking head against wall
• Striking self with objects	
• Breaking of bones	
• Other (to be specified)	

Table 8.7 Other risk factors

	Examples (where appropriate)
• Exploitation by others	Finance issues
• Exploitation of others	Manipulation
• Stated abuse by others	Physical/sexual
• Abuse of others	Verbal/physical/sexual
• Harassment by others	Racial
• Harassment of others	Verbal
• Risks to child(ren)	
• Living alone (with no support)	Isolation
• Culturally isolated situation	
• Religious or spiritual persecution	
• Arson (deliberate fire-setting only)	
• Staff conveying clients in own vehicles	Volatile behaviour of client
• Other (to be specified)	

The following case study challenges you to consider risk categories and associated factors. The case study itself is a composite, for illustration purposes only, as it would be rare to find a service user who would exhibit major factors in all of the category areas.

Case study: Martha – a study to illustrate risk categories and factors

Personal history

Martha is 71 years of age, white British, and was born in Scotland. She experienced physical, sexual and emotional abuse from the age of 4 by her aunt who brought her up as her mother and father were unfit to look after her due to chronic alcoholism.

Martha did reasonably well at school despite the severe problems at home and subsequently obtained a job in a local bakery. She worked in various bakers' shops between 16 and 35 years of age. At 25, Martha married someone she met during one of her inpatient spells in hospital but unfortunately he was physically and emotionally abusive towards her and they eventually divorced when she was 36.

Approximately a year before the divorce, Martha was pushed down the stairs by her husband, through which she acquired a head injury leading to a mild learning disability. This incident also left her with epilepsy and she tends to get an attack every couple of months although she manages to cope with this quite well.

Residing in the Leeds area since the age of 23, Martha now lives alone in a 24-hour warden-assisted ground-floor flat where she normally copes reasonably well, receiving weekly support through her community psychiatric nurse (CPN) from the elderly service.

Psychiatric history and associated factors

Martha experienced her first episode of what is now known as bipolar disorder at the age of 19 and she had numerous hospital admissions up to 30 years of age. Fortunately, she was able to gain an immense degree of insight and applied herself to managing her illness and this led to dramatically reduced hospital admissions.

Following the head injury she sustained at the age of 35, Martha was admitted to Rampton High Security Hospital as she was considered too difficult to manage within her local hospital and, at that time, there were no other appropriate services to deliver her care. She was discharged from Rampton Hospital at the age of 40 to her local hospital in Leeds where she spent two months before being resettled into the community.

Three years ago, Martha had a major stroke that has left her right side very weak. Although she has responded well to physiotherapy, she still needs the aid of a stick when walking and she can be quite unsteady on her feet. In addition, it is impossible for her to climb stairs or walk much more than three-quarters of a mile without having to have a long rest. The following are some of the main risk factors that have been present at various times during the past ten years:

- *Self-harming behaviour*: Martha has been known to insert objects in her arm, swallow batteries and also cut herself when she is distressed.
- *Alcohol misuse*: She often drinks excessive amounts of gin when feeling depressed/not coping.
- *Exploitation*: Martha usually becomes very free and loose with her money when high and/or when she feels lonely and wants company.
- *Self-neglect*: When depressed and/or drinking heavily she usually doesn't wash or take a shower and fails to eat properly.
- *Aggression/violence*: During periods of psychosis, Martha has been known to lash out with her hands at various people who come into contact with her.

Martha has a standing agreement (by way of a 'contract' with her clinical team) to notify them when her clinical management requires inpatient care. This arrangement usually works well and short admissions of three weeks or so are usually sufficient to get her stabilized. She has the support of an advocate from the local advocacy service in relation to this set-up as well as for other issues which arise from time to time.

Relationships

She enjoys an excellent relationship with her CPN who previously worked in a challenging behaviour unit and is, therefore, well experienced in dealing with how she presents sometimes.

As well as a good relationship with her advocate, Martha enjoys a close friendship with a fellow woman resident who lives upstairs – they usually have tea and biscuits with each other at least twice a week.

Current situation

Martha's cousin passed away three days ago and this has led to a difficult period for her. Since receiving the awful news, Martha has been drinking heavily in order to escape from the intolerable reality and this has led to the usual problems of self-neglect.

In addition, she has been cutting her arm again and inserting objects into it as part of her coping strategy. On today's visit of the CPN, there were signs of psychotic symptoms in that Martha was talking rapidly and not making much sense at times. In addition, she became quite distressed twice during the visit and shouted abusively at her CPN.

The environment of the flat appeared to be extremely untidy with cigarette ends, ash, empty bottles and other items scattered around. Martha was also dishevelled and has been ignoring personal hygiene. Finally, as the CPN left the flat, he thought he heard Martha mumbling something about 'bringing an end to it all'. However, when he asked her if she was suicidal she said 'no'.

Service user strengths/positive attributes

- some insight when she is becoming unwell;
- excellent relationship with CPN;
- most of the time she manages to live relatively independently;
- sociable and reasonable communicator when well;
- normally requests support/assistance via her CPN when she needs it;
- good relationships with her advocate and fellow woman resident;
- normally does most of her own shopping as there is a helpful shopkeeper 300 yards from the flat.

Box 8.1 summarizes the risk categories and risk factors illustrated by the case of Martha, and associated risk management interventions.

Paper institution or practical tools?

One of the greatest fears currently has to be that the tools of bureaucracy are turning skilled clinicians into deskilled 'risk administrators'. The mechanisms for this change are the volumes of paperwork required in contemporary mental health practice, particularly in relation to risk. The need for the paper mountain (Morgan 2001) is driven by the culture of blame – something goes wrong and we all need to find a scapegoat.

The brick walls of the Victorian institutions were held together by mortar, but they seem to have been replaced by the paper walls of the modern institution held together by red tape (Rose 1998). However, is the issue of paperwork all seen as negative? Human services are essentially about

Box 8.1 Martha: Risk categories and factors and risk management interventions

Risk categories	Risk factors	Risk management
• Suicide	Manic depression diagnosis. Recent bereavement. Possibly expressing suicidal intent.	Increase CPN input to daily and encourage client to talk about how she feels.
• Neglect	Failing to eat properly. Not shopping for self. Not maintaining personal hygiene.	As above, plus try to see if neighbour can assist by offering practical help. Also, consider meals-on-wheels.
• Aggression/ violence	Misuse of alcohol. Signs of distress/ frustration. Previous admission to High Security Hospital.	CPN to closely monitor for early warning signs/ relapse signature(s) and consider short-term hospitalization.
• Risk associated with disability	Poor mobility and risk of falls. Poor communicator when unwell.	OT Home assessment. Try to get warden and neighbour to monitor the flat between CPN visits.
• Physical/medical risks	Risk of fire from smoking. Epilepsy condition. Frail following stroke.	Ensure smoke alarms are working. Arrange regular GP home visits.
• Self-harm	Cutting arm and inserting objects.	CPN to monitor on a daily basis – check for new injuries/dress wounds.
• Other risks	Possible verbal/ physical abuse towards others. Exploitation by others.	CPN to monitor on a daily basis and to liaise with Martha's neighbour and warden.

the giving and receiving of information, and the paperwork and computer systems are the currency for these transactions. The dilemma is how to create the right balance of time for doing, and time for writing. At another level, whether communicating important information, sharing good practice, or facing the rigours of a serious incident inquiry, written documentation is vitally important. What you knew and what you thought is what you have written. Without such a system requirement, we would be open to many abuses, through bad practices easily defended by the 'but I thought . . .' whim.

The types of paperwork currently in use are voluminous – referral forms, care programme approach documentation, comprehensive needs assessments, full risk assessments, supervised discharge documentation, Mental Health Act assessment forms, carers' assessments, detailed daily notes, copies to all, notes of all telephone conversations, letters of confirmation of all agreements, registers, lists, workload statistics, compatibility with team-organization-profession requirements, written requests on the relevant forms for the relevant organizations, incident report forms, and so on.

What is the purpose of all this documentation? For whose benefit is it? How much is necessary? Who has access to it? When do we arrive at the summit of this paper mountain? Who is involved or consulted in its design and implementation? What about the issues of duplication ... accessibility ... confidentiality? So many significant issues, yet often so little discussion at the local service level between all the relevant parties. Morgan (2001) suggests that one of the major challenges is that of shifting perceptions of paperwork, away from the negative demands of a remote bureaucracy, to one of a practical tool supporting good practice. However, this should not cloud the need to scrutinize the relevance of all the requirements, determining baseline minimum standards, involving practitioners and service users more in the design of relevant formats, and ensuring that there is a shared understanding of how these mechanisms are to operate.

One apparent answer would be to develop the technology by transferring all records to computer systems. The ideal situation would be a unified system of electronic patient record keeping. All practitioners would have access to desktops, laptops or palmtops as needed; so that relevant information could be entered or downloaded at the time of need. Records and assessments could be recalled and edited while in the review meetings. Duplication could be avoided, and new information could be shared with all relevant individuals as soon as it was available. People could search for key words or specific information without having to sift through what are often very bulky files, and different agencies would be using compatible systems that communicated with each other. At-risk individuals would be identified, and appropriate protocols implemented to ensure the risk information was passed to all people who need to know it.

In these days of information technology, this should be an achievable goal. However, the general experience in practice is that within individual organizations, even within the NHS, there are numerous different operating systems in place, which are not compatible with one another. The above scenario appears to remain a long way off and is only partly the answer to the paperwork conundrum. While it may save 'some' time for some people, services may still be populated by technophobes who require training and technical support; sufficient capital investment has been made into the supply of accessible equipment; and it still does not address the validity of all that is required to be recorded, or sufficiently addresses the confidentiality and accessibility of information issue.

How to shift from 'disabling' to 'enabling' risk assessments and management plans

A number of important principles would need to be established:

- information efficiently communicated, through a more collaborative process;
- a transparent 'need-to-know basis' established;
- a sense of ownership of documentation, developed through practical processes of consultation and testing of ideas;
- eradication of duplication;
- an awareness of realistic expectations openly acknowledged by all parties, that risks can be minimized or reduced but not eliminated;
- a recognizable culture shift to a more open use of risk-assessment information for the purpose of meeting service-user needs rather than just as a way to find out what went wrong, and who made the mistakes.

This type of development could have significant benefits: for the service manager, the possibility of collaborative working towards recognized good practice, supported by relevant research and practical evidence; for the practitioner, an appreciation of the place and function of essential administrative needs, able to both support and reflect the reality of working relationships; for the service user, fears heard and listened to, through more open discussion of the needs for minimum standards of essential documentation. The gathering of information needs to respect individual circumstances – achievements, strengths and personal priorities, not just to detail problems and difficulties.

Whether we are aiming towards the more difficult task of national standards for documentation, or supporting local decisions, an agreed minimum standard of what is needed has to be achieved. Essentially, what most people will want is the maximum information with the minimum time and effort – the impossible tension between being brief and comprehensive at the same time. It has been said, by some practitioners, that the best format for documenting a risk assessment is a blank sheet. While this will allow for complete individuality of the assessment recording process, it does not guarantee good practice in recording information by all nurses, and other practitioners. Furthermore, it offers no guidance on what a risk assessment should cover, and may encourage some people to write in a style that becomes inaccessible or not read. For many people, the absence of a structure will result in their attempting to devise a structure to their method of recording. There are no great merits in a system where the structure of recording is completely ad hoc.

Getting down to the basics – it is not so much the form, more the quality of the information. But, designed properly, the form structures the thought processes and the resulting information in a meaningful way (Morgan 2000a). It must be used with clear explanations to service users, about why, how and with whom it will be shared. Forms involving assessments of need and risks must incorporate equal attention to positive strengths, resources and opportunities for positive risk-taking.

The vitally important point to stress in this connection is that good risk documentation should always be a supportive tool to good clinical practice and not a burdensome hindrance. In a blame culture, it is important to remember that 'paperwork protects practitioners and patients' (Wetherell 2001b: 15). Where vital information was not accessed, it is still important in these instances to document the need for additional information, and the attempts to gain it. At all times professional training, practical experience and multi-disciplinary approaches arriving at sound clinical judgement should be the focus, supported, of course, by effective processes of risk assessment and management.

What about scoring mechanisms and numerical scales?

Some of the existing risk assessments on the open market have devised their own numerical systems of quantifying the risks identified (Worthing Priority Care 1995; O'Rourke and Hammond 2000). In practice and in workshops, the responses to this format are mixed. They seem primarily to be meeting the audit and research agenda for numbers that can be more easily analysed and evaluated. For this reason, they have some merit in comparison of assessments across time.

However, in the particular instant where clinical decisions need to be made about how a risk assessment may inform a risk management plan, they can become more misrepresentative of circumstances, and more inclined to the quantitative rather than qualitative values. Numerical systems are generally poor at representing the thinking and communication that informed a risk decision (Stein 1998). They may also be cynically seen as a useful tool for rationing services at times of pressure, rather than focusing on the reality of risks being faced.

What about risk management plans?

Clinical practice is fraught with demands on the practitioner's time, and the emphasis of many clinical tools is on the assessment of need, with a commensurate neglect of the management of the risks identified. In many instances, the design of clinical tools stops short at simply offering a final box headed 'management plan', lacking the guidance previously afforded to the process of assessment. Morgan (2000a) presents one example of how more space and guidelines may be offered, to inform the discussions that direct a risk decision to be represented in a more formal plan. This plan may equally be located within the overall 'care plan', or stand as a specific risk management plan attachment to the care plan. Accessibility and utility of the plan are the important issues.

The subsequent management of a risk, including the taking of risks, should be afforded at least equal importance and attention as the initial identification of risk through assessment. Ultimately, a thoroughly assessed risk that was haphazardly managed is still likely to result in negative consequences.

Confidentiality

One of the great paradoxes facing mental health professionals today is the need for greater disclosure and for confidentiality (Cordess 2001) (cf. Chapter 6). In conjunction with the inquiry reports calling for more sharing of information, we struggle to square the circle in mental health services. Guidance, legislation and local policy statements often exist, but serve to cloud the issues in the reality of day-to-day practice. Maybe it is one of the issues that simply defies clarity.

On the one hand, confidentiality is a crucial part of the risk assessment and management process, an essential cornerstone of the trusting working relationship. On the other, it has the potential for abuse, where playing the confidentiality card for all of the wrong reasons acts as a defence. In the latter circumstances, confidentiality may prevent the passing of information that should be communicated for important safety reasons.

Service users may not always be the people who use 'confidentiality' as a blocking mechanism. However, they are well within their rights to use it as a demand for more transparency in the use and communication of sensitive information about their personal lives. The person who is not told where information will be shared, and for what purposes, is understandably going to raise concerns about its widespread broadcasting. Where there is more transparency on behalf of the service providers there is likely to be more understanding and acceptance from most service users.

In its simplest form, transparency may be linked to the CPA network of care: indicating that these are the people who the information will be shared with, as they are all working together to offer care and support. As with ripples in a pond, this picture may spread further as we explain how some of these individuals will be part of working supervision relationships, and team-working, requiring some disclosure to aid ideas and care planning. Even where the information appears to be seeping through more widely, we may still be able to define reasoned boundaries to its sharing. We need to clarify the 'need-to-know' test.

Mental health services introduce many complications to this simple picture. Health and social services are often likely to operate different policies and procedures for information sharing and accessibility. The statutory sector services may express concerns about widely differing practices across a diverse voluntary sector. Some services, for example advocates, may actively refuse to accept information passed on, preferring to take a blank-slate approach to assessing individual needs (and taking their own precautions about the potential for risks as something you deal with if and when it arises).

A further complication arises when we are thinking about the mechanisms for recording information, their accessibility, and frequent incompatibility. Many practitioners experience that frequent heart-sinking feeling – so many different places to be recording so many types of data – that it becomes a challenge to determine where a specific piece of information should go; none of it is cross-referenced, and the thought of considering with whom it should be shared is a thought too far!

Some psychotherapeutic relationships are established on a strict basis of confidentiality. In this context, some disclosures may have been made on the premise that nothing is shared outside of the relationship. This approach is contra-indicated by the repeated reports of inquiries, which highlight a consistent factor of poor risk management, in the failure to pass on vitally important information to people who could have used it to possibly avoid a disaster. US and UK case law over the last 25 years has pointed towards the breaching of confidentiality, where information about a serious and imminent risk of harm to an identified individual is divulged (Monahan 1993).

There will be many 'what if' scenarios in relation to this issue, defying any attempts to secure an answer for all eventualities. What we do need, as a basic standard for practitioners, is guidance that indicates:

- service and team operational policy statements outlining the importance of confidentiality, and openly recognizing the dilemmas it throws up;
- development of leaflets/statements to present information about confidentiality and information-sharing to service users;
- the need for transparency with service users about how information is to be used;
- the setting of reasonable boundaries that recognize the rare circumstances where breaching confidentiality will be needed for personal safety of service user and/or others;
- clear documenting of the reasons for decisions to breach confidentiality;
- clear documenting of the reasons for decisions made not to share information with specific individuals; and
- inter-agency agreements about issues of confidentiality and information-sharing.

Conclusion

This chapter has examined the concept of risk and emphasized its importance in all our lives. Positive risk-taking can promote growth, while other types of risk can pose serious threats to the health and well-being of individuals and/or those around them. We summarize the main points of this chapter below:

- Risk cannot be eliminated. However, it can be reduced or minimized through good working practice and sound clinical approaches which, as far as possible are multi-disciplinary/multi-agency.

- Risk is dynamic and each case needs to be treated separately with due regard to its own particular elements.
- Risk assessment and risk management more often feel like 'done to' rather than 'collaborated with' processes for many service users. This promotes more stigma and hinders real recovery.
- Carefully considered positive risk-taking initiatives offer the most tangible form of defensible decisions.
- All people directly involved in mental health services need to collaborate in demonstrating the reality of everyday circumstances, and challenge the unrealistic expectations perpetuated by media misrepresentation, public perceptions and legislative bureaucracy.

Questions for reflection and discussion

1   Review the case study 'Kate – a study in positive risk-taking'. What are the potential outcomes of the stated plan, and what needs to be in place in your local services to make these types of decisions a reality?

2   What tensions exist between the roles of service documentation/ paperwork tools and clinical judgement, in the routine assessment and management of risk?

3   Confidentiality of service-user information is of paramount importance, and good risk assessment and management plans require the sharing of accurate information. How do you square the circle?

4   What elements should be prioritized in 'training' and 'practice development' programmes, for supporting the implementation of good practice in assessing and managing risks in local mental health services?

Annotated bibliography

- Department of Health (2001) *Safety First: Five-Year Report of the National Confidential Inquiry into Suicide and Homicide by People with Mental Illness.* London: Department of Health. This provides the most comprehensive statistics on the suicides and homicides in England and Wales. It focuses specifically on the populations in contact with mental health services, but importantly places these within the context of the figures for the whole population. Significant recommendations are drawn out for the wide-ranging areas of the service, from inpatient care to community support, and the vital place of primary care.
- Morgan, S. (1998) The assessment and management of risk, in

C. Brooker and J. Repper (eds) *Serious Mental Health Problems in the Community: Policy, Practice and Research*. London: Bailliere Tindall, pp. 265–90. This sets out to review the evidence and offer detailed clinical examples of the three main risk categories: suicide, neglect, and aggression and violence. Intensive outreach support is identified as a key service response to the repeated messages from the inquiry reports.

- O'Rourke, M. and Bird, L. (2000) *Risk Management in Mental Health*. London: Mental Health Foundation. A short practical booklet setting out clear bullet-point lists of the key themes and messages about the context and practice of risk assessment and management. In RAMAS it outlines one specific example of a locally developed and nationally recognized systematic approach to documenting and auditing the identified research risk factors and management responses.
- Rose, N. (1998) Living dangerously: risk-thinking and risk management in mental health care, *Mental Health Care* **1**(8): 263–6. A thought-provoking challenge to the way risk assessment and management have come to dominate the thinking and working of mental health services. It argues that we have become the 'risk business', with a greater emphasis on the administration of risk, rather than on the care and support of people experiencing mental health problems.

References

Buchanan, A. (1997) The investigation of acting on delusions as a tool for risk assessment in the mentally disordered, *British Journal of Psychiatry* **170** (Supplement 32): 12–16.

Cordess, C. (ed.) (2001) *Confidentiality and Mental Health*. London: Jessica Kingsley.

Dace, E., Faulkner, A., Frost, M. *et al.* (1998) *The Hurt Yourself Less Workbook*. London: National Self-Harm Network.

Department of Health (1995) *Mental Health (Patients in the Community) Act*. London: The Stationery Office.

Department of Health (1999a) *Effective Care Co-ordination in Mental Health Services: Modernising the Care Programme Approach*. London: The Stationery Office.

Department of Health (1999b) *A National Service Framework for Mental Health*. London: The Stationery Office.

Department of Health (1999c) *Saving Lives: Our Healthier Nation*. London: The Stationery Office.

Department of Health (2000) *The NHS Plan*. London: The Stationery Office.

Department of Health (2001) *Safety First: Five-Year Report of the National Confidential Inquiry into Suicide and Homicide by People with Mental Illness*. London: Department of Health.

Kelly, S. and Bunting, J. (1998) *Trends in Suicide in England and Wales 1982–1996*. London: Population Trends.

Monahan, J. (1993) Limiting therapist exposure to Tarasoff liability: Guidelines for risk containment, *American Psychologist* **48**: 242–50.

Monahan, J. and Steadman, H.J. (1996) Violent storms and violent people, *American Psychologist* **51**(9): 931–8.

Morgan, S. (1998) *Assessing and Managing Risk: A Practitioner Handbook*. Brighton: Pavilion.

Morgan, S. (2000a) *Clinical Risk Management: a Clinical Tool and Practitioner Manual*. London: Sainsbury Centre for Mental Health.

Morgan, S. (2000b) Risk-making or risk-taking?, *Openmind* **101**: 16–17.

Morgan, S. (2001) Scaling Paper Mountains, *Openmind* **107**: 20–1.

Morgan, S. and Hemming, M. (1999) Balancing care and control: risk management and compulsory community treatment. *Mental Health & Learning Disabilities Care* **3**(1): 19–21.

NHS Executive (1994) *Introduction of Supervision Registers for Mentally Ill People*. HSG(94)5. Leeds: NHSE.

O'Rourke, M. and Hammond, S. (2000) *Risk Management: Towards Safe, Sound and Supportive Services*. Surrey Hampshire Borders NHS Trust and South Thames Research and Development Fund.

Ritchie, J.H., Dick, D. and Lingham, R. (1994) *The Report of the Inquiry into the Care and Treatment of Christopher Clunis*. London: The Stationery Office.

Rose, N. (1998) Living dangerously: risk-thinking and risk management in mental healthcare. *Mental Health Care* **1**(8): 263–6.

Sainsbury Centre for Mental Health (1998) *Acute Problems*. London: Sainsbury Centre for Mental Health.

Sainsbury Centre for Mental Health (2000) *An Executive Briefing on the Implications of the Human Rights Act 1998 for Mental Health Services* (Briefing Paper 12). London: Sainsbury Centre for Mental Health.

Sheppard, D. (1996) *Learning the Lessons* (2nd edn). London: the Zito Trust.

Stein, W. (1998) *The Use of Standardised Scales and Measures for Identification, Assessment and Control of Risk in Mental Health*. Unpublished thesis. Glasgow Caledonian University.

Taylor, P.J. and Gunn, J. (1999) Homicides by people with mental illness: myth and reality, *British Journal of Psychiatry* **174**: 9–14.

Vincent, C. (1997) Risk, safety and the dark side of quality, *British Medical Journal* **314**: 1775–6.

Wetherell, A. (2000) Risk in Mental Health – Part 1, *Breakthrough* **6**(4): 22–3.

Wetherell, A. (2001a) Risk in Mental Health – Part 2, *Breakthrough* **7**(1): 17–18.

Wetherell, A. (2001b) Risk in Mental Health – Part 3, *Breakthrough* **7**(4): 15–16.

Worthing Priority Care (1995) *The Worthing Weighted Risk Indicator*. Worthing, Sussex.

9

The therapeutic milieu

Kingsley Norton

Chapter overview

> An ideal psychiatric hospital is not merely a sanctuary, a cotton-padded milieu that emphasizes the fragility, the incompetence, the helplessness, the bizarreness of patients. It is a sane society when it permits the optimal use of the intact ego capacities through its social organisation, its social supports, and its community values.
>
> (Talbot and Miller 1966: 367)

> There is no patient 'untreated' by his environment – only patients treated, well or ill.
>
> (Stanton: Foreword to Cumming and Cumming 1964)

In the second half of the twentieth century, in the West, high quality in-patient wards tended to draw, more or less deliberately, on the knowledge and skills base of the therapeutic milieu. In this sense they might be seen as having represented 'diluted' forms of the same. Later, in the UK, with changes to the ways in which health care was delivered and, in particular, the rising interest in and enthusiasm for care in the community, it is as if the inpatient environment underwent a crisis of confidence (Beadsmore *et al.* 1998; Ford *et al.* 1998). Not only was morale low for many of those still working in such environments but many skilled staff left to work in the newer community-based services. Consequently, as the community-based services flourished, the inpatient aspect withered. Not only were there fewer inpatient beds but also there were individuals with greater psychological disturbance occupying them. Those inpatient staff remaining thus had a more difficult job to do and low morale to cope with.

The changes to service delivery and the development of community care were reflected in the public's changing perception of mental illness, as this again became visible on the streets of large towns and cities. High-profile violent incidents perpetrated by the mentally ill on innocent members of the public, though small in number, meant an increasing political pressure on mental health staff to identify and admit to hospital those who might be at risk of violence. At the same time there was an increased awareness by users of the services of their human rights and their entitlement to freedom, dignity and, in particular, safety once hospitalized. Tellingly, in a survey of inpatients (MIND 2000): 57 per cent felt they had insufficient contact with staff; over half found their environment untherapeutic; 45 per cent claimed a detrimental effect on their mental health; 30 per cent experienced it as unsafe and 16 per cent reported having suffered sexual harassment. These patients' views may not be wholly representative but one result for inpatient staff, especially for the nurses who make up the largest number of these, is an enormous pressure to safely contain disturbance while at the same time providing the necessary conditions for patients to encounter therapeutic influences within a safe environment. Inevitably, there is a tension between the competing demands for security and therapy that is felt keenly by nursing staff.

Pressure to discharge and to admit to a smaller number of hospital beds requires more of the inpatient resource, yet there have been no relevant major advances or developments with inpatient care and, until recently, little attention was paid to this area. Many inpatient units are functionally isolated from their community services. Scant attention is paid to the continuing professional development needs of nursing staff within hospitals, adding to the problem with low morale. The much-vaunted multi-disciplinary team is often conspicuous by its absence from the inpatient environment. The roles and responsibilities of nurses are not always clear. In the light of all this, it is timely to reconsider the therapeutic milieu to see if its knowledge and skills bases can help restore some clarity of purpose and definition of method to an area of mental health working that has become more difficult but arguably of greater importance, partly due to its relative scarcity.

The objective of this chapter is to describe a set of values, flowing from a consideration of therapeutic milieu principles and practices in terms of its functions and relationships, that might be relevant to the internal workings of modern acute psychiatric ward environments. To achieve this, the chapter considers:

- the concept of the therapeutic milieu;
- its origins and functions;
- key therapeutic functions and how these relate to inpatients both collectively and individually;
- destructive processes that can undermine such functions;
- the workings of a democratic therapeutic community to demonstrate therapeutic principles in practice; and
- the relevance of the therapeutic milieu to acute care wards today.

Therapeutic milieux

A milieu is any environment in which a patient or anyone else lives. A therapeutic milieu represents 'a specialized environment which is designed to fulfil the general purposes of preventing "bad" things from happening and allowing "good" things to occur' (Gunderson 1978: 328). It represents less a different form of treatment, which rivals or threatens to supplant others, but more 'a metatreatment' (Abroms 1969), i.e. a general method for providing specific treatment techniques in an effective manner. The means by which this is achieved vary but involve 'constructing a stable, coherent social organisation which provides an integrated, extensive treatment context' (Abroms 1969: 554).

The aims of the therapeutic milieu, not always clearly stated, are summarized by Abroms as controlling or setting limits on the main kinds of pathological behaviour (destructiveness, disorganization, deviancy, dysphoria and dependency) and promoting the development of basic psychosocial skills (orientation, assertion, occupation and recreation). According to him, the organizational structure of the therapeutic milieu should be viewed in relation to its therapeutic aims or function, hence 'the milieu requires the consensus-making machinery characteristic of democratic social arrangements: a set of forums or meetings that encourage participation in information-sharing, decision-making, decision-execution, and interpersonal conflict-resolution' (ibid.).

Abroms acknowledges the value of such democratic institutions in their own right but claims that their main justification is their role in facilitating the achievement of specified treatment aims. An extension of the concept of a therapeutic milieu is embodied in those forms of milieu treatment where the milieu itself is recognized as an active therapeutic agent to promote and facilitate 'positive' changes in specified directions – a 'therapeutic community' (Gunderson 1978). This will be discussed in some detail below since, from the 1920s onwards, a range of therapeutic developments (milieux and prototype therapeutic communities) began to appear in Europe and the USA.

Origins

The history of such developments, however, can be traced much further back in time. For example, a provision for 'mentally afflicted pilgrims' had flourished from 1250 onwards in Flanders (Bloor *et al.* 1988). Centuries later, an English Quaker, William Tuke, introduced what came to be called 'moral treatment' for the severely mentally ill. In 1796, he set up the York Retreat, which, requiring high levels of staffing, provided 'a place in which the unhappy might obtain a refuge – a quiet haven in which the shattered bark might find the means of reparation or of safety' (Busfield 1986: 123).

The success and spread of this treatment meant that the numbers of individuals receiving it gradually outstripped the human resource required to maintain its sufficient quality. More bureaucracy resulted in a significant deterioration in atmosphere within these institutions, which therefore became 'impersonal, controlling, neglectful and harsh' (Busfield 1986: 124). Throughout the nineteenth and first half of the twentieth centuries in the West, psychiatric patients on both sides of the Atlantic continued to be housed in large numbers within institutions which all provided 'containment' but which, in addition, supplied only varying degrees of 'support' (see below, Gunderson 1978).

'Support', the contribution of Tuke and other reformers (such as Pinel in France), formed the basis on which all later therapeutic milieux would be constructed. Following the influence of, among others, Menninger (1936) and Bettelheim (1950) in the USA, 'structure' was added. Its contribution was to give the institutional environment a predictability that helped to orient the patient. This triad of containment, support and structure formed a new basis for the next generation of therapeutic milieux. This development required an evolution of existing hospital structures to include 'more open communication, less rigid hierarchy of doctors, nurses, patients, daily structured discussions of the whole unit, and various sub-groups' (Jones 1968: 63). The so-called 'democratic' approach followed, where patients were encouraged to help one another and gradually took a more equal role with staff in some administrative and social activities. The catastrophically destructive events of the two world wars in the first half of the twentieth century, which had shaken many belief systems, had thus revealed individuals within the mental health field who were willing to look at the relationship between the individual and wider society and to translate this ideology into the treatment setting, which to them represented a microcosm of society (Bloom 1997).

In essence, these new therapeutic developments were attempts to apply the principles of social psychiatry (Carleton and Mahlendorf 1979) and systems theory (von Bertalannfy 1967). The therapeutic milieux, which began to flourish in the 1960s, were thus based on the idea of 'social learning', that change could be effected through interpersonal interaction wherein conflict or crisis is analysed. Therapeutic milieux, and especially the therapeutic community, could function as 'living-learning' situations (Jones 1952), which represented a significant move away from the familiar and traditional 'medical model'.

Therapeutic functions

One of the problems with the development of therapeutic milieux was that their underpinning value systems were often presented and discussed at the expense of actual details of the method, its objectives and the extent to which these were regularly achieved (Abroms 1969). According to Wilmer, for example, the term therapeutic community stood not only for a system of treatment but also 'a battle cry, a charm and a password'. He argued that the term meant different things to different people and had come to signify a wide range of variations of milieu therapy, most of which had little in common (Wilmer 1958). However, as articulated by Gunderson, guidelines for those who would like to structure or select a milieu to accommodate particular patient needs, treatment goals or institutional requirements could indeed be produced (Gunderson 1978). The following five paragraphs on therapeutic functions and processes represent a brief summary of Gunderson's highly pertinent ideas and definitions.

Containment

'Containment' functions to sustain the physical well-being of patients and removes from them the burdens of self-control or feelings of omnipotence. It is effected through the provision of food, shelter, seclusion, etc. The aim of containment is to prevent assaults and to minimize physical deterioration and dangerousness in those who lack judgement. Its effect is to reinforce, temporarily, the internal controls of patients and to reality-test the omnipotent beliefs concerning the patient's destructiveness. However, there is a risk that a given setting could over-emphasize containment, thereby suppressing initiative, reinforcing feelings of isolation and leading to hopelessness and despair.

Support

'Support' refers to deliberate efforts, effected through the social network, to make patients feel better and to enhance their self-esteem. There is an acceptance that patients have needs, which staff can fulfil and limitations to which staff need to make accommodation. Relevant activities include the provision of escorts and other behavioural provisions (such as advice and education) aimed at supporting ego functions. This may also include assisting patients to do things which they protest are impossible but under circumstances where success is almost certainly guaranteed. Those milieux that emphasize support are recognizable as retreats that provide nurturance and permit, encourage and direct patients to venture into other, more specific, therapies such as psychotherapy, rehabilitation or family therapy.

Structure

'Structure' represents all aspects of a milieu that provide a predictable organization of time, place and person, i.e. act to make the environment less amorphous and to support reality-testing. It facilitates the safe attachment of patients to their environment since, ideally, they feel neither invaded nor alone. The function of structure is to promote changes in patients' symptoms and action patterns considered to be socially maladaptive. It aids them in considering consequences, thereby delaying their acting upon dysphoric feelings or destructive impulses. This is effected, among others, through: hierarchical privilege systems, the use of treatment contracts, desensitization programmes, etc. In so far as any of these uses of structure are jointly planned with patients, according to shared ideas of what is maladaptive, the structure ceases to be only an adjunct to treatment but itself begins to become an identified therapeutic approach, namely a democratic therapeutic community (see Jones 1952).

Involvement

'Involvement' refers to those processes that cause patients to attend actively to their social environment and interact with it. The purpose of involvement is to utilize and strengthen a patient's ego and to modify aversive or destructive interpersonal patterns. It particularly confronts patients' passivity, i.e. their wish to have others do things to or for them. Means of facilitating involvement include 'open doors', patient-led groups, identification of shared goals, mandatory participation in milieu groups, community activities, etc. Placing a high emphasis on the interpersonal meaning of symptomatic behaviours conveys the belief that the latter are within the patients' control and thus their responsibility. Patients who talk about their unmet 'needs' may find them restated (by staff of fellow patients) as unrealistic 'wants' (Gunderson 1978). The treatment aims to reinforce ego strengths by encouraging social skills and developing feelings of competence. Along with this, patients are expected to relinquish or subordinate private, asocial or unrealistic wishes. Wards that emphasize involvement will have a distribution of power and decision-making, some blurring of traditional roles, and an emphasis on expression of anger and on the group processes of co-operation, compromise, confrontation and conformity.

Validation

'Validation' refers to the ward processes that affirm a patient's individuality. This is effected through attention to individualized treatment programming, respect for a patient's right to be alone and to have secrets, frequent explora-tory one-to-one talks, providing opportunities to fail, an emphasis on loss, and encouraging individuals to operate at the limits of their known capacities. This requires an acceptance of incompetence, regressions or symptoms as meaningful personal expressions that need not be terminated or ignored. Validation might encourage patients to talk about their halluci-nations and to consider them as expressive of some unclear but important aspect of themselves. The 'wrist-slasher' might be asked to reconstruct the experience and explain why it had made sense to act in that way (Gunderson 1978).

Therapeutic processes

According to Gunderson (1978), these five functional properties can also reflect the patient's changing needs during the course of a given period of hospitalization. Thus, the grossly psychotic patient who is dangerously impulsive may profit initially from a simplified milieu that keeps him/her safe (containment). As the psychosis recedes, this patient may feel depressed, so the encouragement of their environment becomes essential (support). Emergence from this period may reveal the need to learn social skills, both in terms of consequences of actions and the impersonal nature of reality (structure). This period will frequently include learning about the effects of one's behaviour on other people and about the advantages of more sensitively recognizing one's potential to hurt or assist others (involvement). As patients plan to leave the hospital, they must resume full responsibility for their lives and suffer the knowledge that a safer world is being left behind (validation). Other sequences of these functions may be required for the hospitalization of other kinds of patients.

For a given individual and a particular milieu, each of the five functions depends to an extent on the successful negotiation and incorporation of those prior to it. Collectively, at times of crisis, however, a given milieu will need to 'regress' towards the simpler and clearer security of the earlier functions. Different milieux are likely to vary in their patient population, as well as in their valuing of different functions. In general terms, an over-valuation of the higher, 'later' functions of involvement and validation can prove costly. Also, the functions of involvement and validation can conflict with or obscure the importance of the first function – containment. The two extremes – closing down to contain and opening up to permit understanding or to facilitate expressiveness – require flexibility in milieu structure and a high tolerance for uncertainty on the part of the staff.

Within a psychiatric milieu, it cannot be assumed that the relationship between patient and professional is automatically or necessarily therapeutic. There always remains the potential for a 'bad', as well as, a 'good' therapeutic outcome. This possibility is true also of all the relationships encountered within the therapeutic milieu, not just those with the professional or clinical staff. Establishing a sufficiently high quality of relationships within a given hospital-ward environment clearly requires much communication and effort from all parties involved. A range of aspects need to be included: ideological; organizational; practical implementation; and quality monitoring. To achieve a correct weighting and integration of such aspects is the hallmark of a successful, i.e. therapeutic, milieu. As a bare minimum, aims need to be clearly stated and methods developed to enable them to be achieved (Abroms 1969).

A question arises as to the definition of a 'therapeutic' relationship. This may be hard to define especially where the treatment course is long and arduous, as with much long-term work with psychotic or severely personality disordered patients (cf. Chapters 13 and 21). There may be a need for compulsory admission or treatment without consent, both of which situations can strain the limits of what is, and, as importantly, what feels like a therapeutic relationship. Maintaining staff morale can be problematic under such conditions, especially where the aims of treatment are unclear, or not agreed within the whole team treating a given individual, or where teamwork is fragmented and uncoordinated. For many patients, encountering an inconsistent approach is all too familiar and consequently it offers little cause to make them think differently about themselves, i.e. what motivates them or about the effect their behaviour has on others, i.e. how others are left feeling by them. Such a set of circumstances does not represent a 'therapeutic' challenge to deeply-ingrained and maladaptive patterns of thinking, perceiving and behaving. So-called 'sick role' behaviour can be inappropriately reinforced.

With individual psychotherapy, it has long been recognized that the quality of the professional relationship should not be taken for granted. Mainly based on work with non-psychotic patients, there is a concept of 'therapeutic alliance'. This has been variously defined but many authors appear to describe central features in common. It refers to: 'the relatively non-neurotic rational relationship between patient and analyst, which makes it possible for the patient to work purposefully in the analytic situation' (Greenson 1967: 46). Recognizing the importance of the quality of human relationships that are encountered within a ward environment is crucial to the therapeutic functioning of any milieu. However, there is not an adequate research base from which to derive this conclusion. Little systematic work has been reported about what actually goes on in the standard psychiatric ward, if indeed there is any ward that can be regarded as 'standard'. Even less exists to indicate the superiority of one approach or 'model' of inpatient care over another.

It might be expected that the existence of a model, rather than its absence, would confer therapeutic advantage but there is insufficient evidence to support or refute even this conclusion. Potentially, a model brings with it a clear statement of aims and a method via which to achieve the same. Optimism and enthusiasm accompanying the application of a model perhaps makes a therapeutic result the more likely. Potentially, however, there are still pitfalls to be avoided. These derive from the necessity for teamwork, since the business of running an inpatient ward is a 'round-the-clock' enterprise involving many individuals, not all of whom are professionals or work in the environment voluntarily. It is highly unlikely that all will wish to behave therapeutically or, if they do, share a vision of how best to proceed!

Destructive processes

Processes that are destructive of the therapeutic endeavour have been described (Roberts 1980). Reflecting the complexity of the inpatient environment, Roberts classifies the processes as: the destructiveness of the isolated individual; destructive group phenomena; staff contribution to destructive processes; and structural manifestations of destructive processes.

A destructive individual may carry out actual acts of destruction, aimed at the fabric of the building or the individual's own body, rarely towards another member of the inpatient ward. Often this behaviour reflects alienation experienced anew within the treatment setting. Certain patients may be at especial risk of isolation: the new patient, the scapegoat, the psychotic patient, those with schizoid personality features, the borderline patient, those who repeatedly act out early rejection experiences, and those dependent on alcohol and drugs (Roberts 1980).

Regarding group phenomena that exert a destructive effect, there are a number of different ways of construing these. Roberts mentions Bion's 'basic assumptions' (Bion 1963), which he sees as potentially operating for long periods without detection. Essentially, these assumptions represent periods of unconscious avoidance of the stated task of the group involved. In the ward situation the stated task is the set of overall therapeutic aims and the methods agreed and set up to achieve them. Another influence that impairs the work task is the phenomenon of 'splitting'. For an individual, this involves an inability of the immature self to adopt an ambivalent attitude, hence the self or 'other' is experienced as all good or all bad. For a group, such as the multi-disciplinary staff team, the phenomenon of splitting results in polarizations, often painful and marked by extreme animosity, which may collect allies to the different causes and lead to a paralysis of usual team functioning. Other manifestations may follow in the wake of splitting, such as 'sub-culturing', 'idealization' and 'splits in leadership'. The last can be particularly destructive in its effect. Thought and energy, which might be otherwise directed by the leaders at detecting the inevitable splitting effects within their team and within the whole ward environment, is expended in a futile battle between themselves, into which other staff may be drawn, or from which they retreat as excited or helpless onlookers.

Staff may collude with community defences, for example a denial of the significance of staff absences due to sickness or annual leave. Among others, this can have the effect of giving permission to patients to miss parts of the therapeutic programme. It is important to recognize the staff's contribution in such a situation, otherwise the responsibility or blame is seen to lie only with patients and action taken on this basis will be likely to both alienate the patients and fail to resolve the cause of the non-attendance. Frustrations may lead to staff burn-out. So can idealization, if staff try to live up to unrealistic expectations placed on them by patients, i.e. to accept idealizations as actually achievable. They can find themselves overworking, becoming stressed and eventually becoming mentally ill themselves. All of this can foster the development of further destructive splitting and contribute to the formation of disparate treatment aims leading to an inconsistent delivery of the overall treatment programme for a given patient.

Finally, Roberts refers to structural manifestations of destructive processes and identifies three main effects: 'autolysis', 'crystallization' and 'encapsulation'. Autolysis is the breaking down of internal structures, such as the dissolution of time boundaries for the treatment programme and a lack of clarity between the respective roles of staff and patients. Crystallization reflects an internal organization, which becomes so rigid and entangled that change is impossible and function suffers. Encapsulation is the situation where the institution has stopped interacting with its environment. All of these states can appear within a given environment and be so destructive that closure ensues, in the case of specialist or autonomous units, or serious untoward incidents occur within units where closure is not so readily conceivable.

Democratic therapeutic community

The therapeutic community has been referred to as a 'living-learning' situation (Jones 1952), which implies a different model of care from that of traditional psychiatry, with its focus on illness and the dependent position of the patient in relation to staff. With this model there is an emphasis on interaction and interpersonal learning from an examination and exploration of it. For Tom Main, who originated the term therapeutic community, it referred to 'a culture of enquiry into personal and interpersonal and inter-system problems as these are expressed and arranged socially' (Main 1946). The essence of this approach is therefore to facilitate learning in respect of self and others, i.e. to improve reality-testing, in terms of a more differentiated and accurate perception of self and others (Norton 1992). Couched in these terms it can be seen that the model could have wider application to those suffering from other forms of mental illness than personality disorder (for which Jones' community was set up).

In order for the setting to achieve its objective to raise reality-testing, it needs to have a predictable 'structure' (see pp. 245–6 for a summary of Gunderson's ideas). In this way patients can experience an environment which is understandable and, ideally, also responsive to their specific needs. Potentially, however, it is differences in the needs of those living in the ward setting that pose a challenge to the system itself. It tends to introduce complexity and this in turn can evoke anxiety in staff as the size of the work task increases. Raised anxiety is likely to impair performance. For all parties, staff and patients, it is optimal if, as far as is possible, the same rules, rights and responsibilities apply to all. Obviously this goal can only be achieved to an extent that will vary greatly over time. However, the ward environment and the implementation of its aims and methods should be understandable to all the staff that work there, including (at an appropriate level of detail) non-clinical staff. Otherwise it is possible, if not likely, for someone unwittingly to undermine or compete with goals of other staff to an unhelpful extent.

Ideally, the inpatient setting offers new and different models of relatedness to those who reside there (Gabbard 1988). To achieve this, staff frequently need to avoid automatic responses, either personal or professional.

This may be especially hard to do in the face of threatening or seductive behaviour. To facilitate a thoughtful response, the democratic therapeutic community model (following Maxwell Jones) has a number of inbuilt safeguards.

1 There is an emphasis, in the formal programme of treatment, on the deployment of group treatment as the sole approach. This minimizes, but can never eradicate (nor should it), the situation in which a given member of staff is repeatedly exposed to a particular patient, with the increased potential for inappropriate or unprofessional conduct to ensue.

2 Following from this, there is co-facilitation, i.e. there is always, in theory more than one member of staff involved with a particular group of patients. In practice, staff sickness and absence for other unavoidable reasons means that this ideal is not always achievable. Knowledge of the ideal, however, keeps alive the notion of what is optimal and highlights attempts, conscious or otherwise, of patients to draw staff out of their professional roles.

3 Following every group activity there is an 'after-group', during which the staff who took part will, in effect, offer one another peer support and supervision.

4 There is clinical supervision for all multi-disciplinary staff on a weekly basis, which allows staff from the various subgroups to pool their knowledge and present their ongoing clinical difficulties.

5 There is a weekly 'team awareness meeting' at which all staff (clinical and non-clinical) are invited to explore inter-staff difficulties in as much as they bear on the clinical task.

Timetable

The range of activities shown in Table 9.1 is organized to provide a predictable set of experiences, which enable both staff and patients to anticipate what is due to happen next. This predictability itself is important to those whose previous lives and experiences have lacked order. It represents an important aspect of 'structure' (Gunderson 1978). Beyond this, however, the shared nature of the knowledge about the treatment programme fosters a levelling of the traditional staff–patient hierarchy, where only the staff know what's going on and what to expect during a given day. It is important that the level of collaborative involvement of patients is consonant with their abilities to comprehend it, otherwise it will be counterproductive and replace one hierarchy with another. The aim is to facilitate a strengthening of the patients' ego functioning, therefore what is demanded of them needs to lie within their compass to achieve it.

A system that expects patients to be in certain places at certain times also needs to monitor attendance, to observe if what is intended actually obtains. There is, therefore, a mechanism, involving both the patients and staff, to record accurately whether patients attend as planned. There is

Table 9.1 Weekly programme

Monday	Tuesday	Wednesday	Thursday	Friday	Saturday	Sunday
9.15–10.30 a.m. '9.15' Community meeting						
10.30 a.m. Morning break						
Small groups	Cleaning & reviews or elections or community projects	Small groups	Visitors' group*	Small groups		
New residents' group		New residents' group	Women's group; Men's group	New residents' group		
		Leavers' group 10.30–11.30 a.m.				
11.00–12.00 noon	11.00–12.00 noon		11.00–12.00 noon	11.00–12.00 noon		
12.15–12.30 p.m.; 12.30 p.m.	Cleaning; Lunch break	Weekdays			Welfare phone slot 10.30–11.00 a.m. 12.30–1.00 p.m.	
Surgery 1.00–1.30 p.m.	Surgery 2.05–2.15 p.m.	Surgery 2.05–2.15 p.m.	Surgery 2.05–2.15 p.m.	Surgery 2.05–2.15 p.m.		
Floor reps' meeting 1.30–1.45 p.m. Sports and social 1.45–2.10 p.m.		GLO meeting 12.30–12.50 p.m.				
Psychodrama or art therapy	Selection/unit reception or welfare or sports and social	Psychodrama or art therapy	Work groups (art or gardening and maintenance)	Work groups (art, welfare or gardening and maintenance)		
2.30–4.15 p.m.	2.30–4.15 p.m.	2.30–4.15 p.m.	2.15–4.15 p.m.	2.15–4.15 p.m.		
				Tea 4.30–5.00 p.m.		
5.00 p.m.	Handover					
7.00–9.00 p.m.	Community meal					
9.45–10.30 p.m.	Summit meeting (Top 4 residents and staff)				9.45–10.30 p.m. Summit	
						10.05 p.m. Booking in
11.00 p.m.	Night round					

* Visitors' day (professional visitors) – Thursday 8.45 a.m.–5.00 p.m. Community Afternoon – last Thursday in month 2.15–4.15 p.m.

also a mechanism that allows patients to miss a scheduled activity if prior permission has been granted. In this way patients can be confronted with consequences of their behaviour resulting from the extent to which they do what they say they will do. This includes receiving feedback from staff, and particularly, from the patient peer group on any upset which may have resulted from non-attendance or breaking of trust through the patient's actions not marrying up with their words.

Community meeting

Confronting of patients with their failed attendance at any of the group meetings of the programme is mostly carried out in a meeting of the entire community, i.e. all patients and those staff on duty on a given day. This meeting has an agenda and is chaired by one of the senior patients, elected to one of three 'Top Three' positions for a month at a time. The meetings take place every day except Sundays at the same time – 9.15 a.m. Most days' agendas follow a similar format reflecting what is to follow that day, and what needs to be processed and assimilated from the previous day and night. This enables the community members to learn from experience – 'living-learning' – something which a personality disordered client group is said to have difficulties in doing (cf. Chapter 21).

A specimen agenda in Table 9.2 gives an impression of the amount of daily business that the community generates and offers a sense of the level of responsibility taken by the elected senior patients and the degree of authority that is delegated by staff to the meeting. This represents the giving up of a significant amount of traditionally held staff power. (In a more acute and general setting, relatively less power can be delegated but this is a matter of degree, based on judgement of the patient group at a given time, rather than an 'all-or-nothing' situation.)

Table 9.2 Specimen community meeting agenda

9.15am Welcome	Yesterday's feedback
Who's missing?	Summit discussion feedback
Wash-up rota for the day	Groups missed yesterday/why?
Cooks for the evening meal	Discharge votes to be taken
Staff feedback	Those asking for re-instatement
Emergency meeting feedback	Permission to be absent

Emergency meeting

Having elaborated some of the regular and predictable time structuring, it is now important to describe how this can be overridden by an emergency (referred) meeting, which can be called at any time of the day or night by the Top Three patients in collaboration with the two 'duty staff'. It is thus the latter with whom the Top Three liaise. Duty staff represent the whole staff team during the 9–5, Monday to Friday, but are the only staff present in the community at all other times – 76 per cent of the entire week.

It is this group of five who decide how to respond in the face of an unexpected or untoward event or issue. In essence their task is to establish the urgency of the situation. Having judged a given situation to be urgent, the next step is to call a 'referred meeting', usually within 15 minutes of having made the decision. This meeting provides a forum for reflective functioning and therefore represents an important modelling of responding thoughtfully, as opposed to automatically, i.e. according to past judgement of similar events or issues. Many patients will have an underdeveloped capacity to evaluate situations or self-states under conditions of stress and will, as a result, tend to rate everything as 'urgent' and act accordingly – with the expectation that others will necessarily concur and support. Failure in the past by others, including previous staff involved with them, to share their sense of priorities will have contributed to difficulties with treatment alliance and to breakdown of the professional relationship.

In these referred meetings, which are also chaired by one of the Top Three, the issue in question will be presented to the whole community for its thoughts and for any necessary decisions and action. These meetings often enact a risk assessment and risk management function. As stated, they can be called at any time and they take priority over all other activity, including any of the formal treatment ingredients. All patients on the unit are expected to attend and as many of the staff, but always the two 'duty staff', who were also party to the decision to call the meeting. It is in this forum that *all* important decisions are made, for example, the premature discharge of patients via the taking of a democratic vote. (NB Patients' numbers almost always outweigh those of staff, aiding an authentic empowerment of patients.)

Small psychotherapy groups

Three times per week there are small group psychotherapy groups, facilitated by three staff members (see above). These groups, which contain approximately seven or eight patients, allow an exploration of both remote and recent events. Insights gained from these groups can feed a cautious experimentation with new coping strategies (Whiteley 1986). This leads to new results that can be re-explored and interpreted in the forum of the small group. In this way a circle of interaction, exploration and experimentation can be repeatedly set up, with beneficial results. The idea of a 'living-learning' experience is not readily understood by patients. Their defensive actions tend to militate against any learning from experience and they continue to function in familiar ways. However, this is expected, since many in this client group lack a well-developed capacity to verbalize their distress and difficulties. Enactment of emotional and interpersonal conflict, in various ways, is thus desirable – provided this can be encountered safely enough.

Work groups

In order for the usual strategies, and more importantly interpersonal difficulties, to be re-encountered there is as much as possible of everyday reality within the therapeutic community. As part of this there are non-verbal groups, which serve a number of purposes, for example, giving those with non-verbal skills a chance to shine and those who 'talk the talk', but cannot quite 'walk the walk', opportunities to display their difficulties with everyday problems, such as being unable to work with others or to complete a concrete task. All of this, whether success or failure, is grist to the community's psycho- and socio-therapeutic mill. This is provided that the opportunities for exploration and experimentation are seized. In practice, most patients are reticent to expose their vulnerabilities. It takes senior patients, leading by example, to induce sufficient confidence or courage in newer patients, as in Jones's (1952) seminal observation that it was those patients senior in the psycho-educational programme he was running who were best at inducting new patients and explaining to them what was the intended message, i.e. he saw that patients were, in many respects, superior teachers to the trained staff.

Informal time

Many patients, especially those who are familiar with prison culture, appear to believe that it will be sufficient merely to abide by the rules of the thera-peutic community and attend all groups – 'to keep their noses clean' – for them to derive benefit. Such patients may be popular, at least initially, since they often become 'model' patients, eager to help others, especially with the more concrete and manual tasks. It may take some months before this coping strategy or defence is seen for what it is and, even then, it may be difficult to challenge it successfully. Individuals utilizing such a survival strategy seldom have many other resources on which to draw. However, since part of the unwritten contract of the therapeutic community is to actively participate, non-participation in the psychotherapy aspects of the pro-gramme, in which to reveal the more human side (revealing some vul-nerability) becomes a potential reason for discharge. Perhaps in recognition of the deep-seated nature of this defensive posture, there is the potential for such patients to have a week in which to prove that they are actually motivated to change in spite of the difficulty. At the end of the week there is a democratic vote to decide the issue.

The informal time is also part of therapy and what goes on during it, whether or not the activity is useful to the individual of the community, is legitimately open for discussion and challenge. Many find it difficult to structure their free time at the weekends, from mid-morning on Saturday till late Sunday evening. It is tempting then to resort to usual coping mechanisms, such as self-mutilation, getting drunk, taking drugs (illicit or previously prescribed) or indulging in violence to others. Clearly the capacity of the community to 'police' itself is limited and reliance is placed on honesty, which is hoped for rather than expected, at least initially. One of the 'jobs' within the community, therefore, is to monitor attendance at group meetings. This includes the referred meetings, to which failure of attendance means having to face a discharge vote. Patients are generally good at spotting in others what they themselves habitually do (or are tempted to do but are avoiding). Consequently, there is considerable vigilance, albeit 'grassing up' or 'snitching' a fellow patient is something which many are loath to do. Only slowly is it realized that being a true friend might include giving honest feedback and condemning certain anti-social or destructive behaviours.

Jobs

Ideally, all the patients in the therapeutic community will participate in its daily working. There are many tasks to undertake, which in a more traditional setting would be carried out by staff, particularly nursing and medical. Many of these are delegated to patients to do either alone or in collaboration with peers or staff themselves. These include important administrative aspects such as the chairing of: community meetings, referred meetings, selection interviews for acceptance into the community (see above), and the meeting which welcomes and orientates new members. The recording of content at certain meetings, namely 'referred' and 'selection' (see Table 9.1), is also delegated to the patients, although a record is kept independently by staff. It is the patient's record that is used as part of the business of the community, in the sense of being read out in the community meeting – another job to be done. The ordering of food, within an agreed budget, its storage and preparation for the meals are all led by the patients but with staff collaboration in some of the actual negotiation with the wider world outside. However, this does mean that, if insufficient food or inappropriate food is ordered, it is the whole community who suffers the consequences. Also, it will be the responsible patients (i.e. plural, since for most of the posts there is a substantive post-holder and assistant, requiring at least a degree of working together with another) who are called to account.

Some jobs are inevitably more important than others, and these are left to the more senior patients, i.e. those who have been in treatment for at least three months. They will have served an apprenticeship, working in an assistant capacity while more junior in the community. Patients can nominate themselves or be nominated to a particular post at the monthly 'elections'. This meeting, which is also chaired by one of the 'top three' patients, will attempt to fill all the posts since all fall vacant at the same time. This maximizes the chance for everybody to have an opportunity to perform each of the roles within the community during the year of their stay. It also makes it less likely that only certain personalities will dominate the principal roles, since this will be conspicuous and obvious to all concerned. While staff may comment on nominations, or indeed nominate, they do not have a vote in any post. This means that the patient subgroup is empowered and thereby in a stronger position to learn from the experience of their decisions and choices.

Leadership

The complexity of the programme (the prominence of two main subgroups, or subsystems, of staff and patients and the need to identify and integrate into the formal therapy time aspects from the unstructured time spent between 'groups') demands much of leadership. How best to achieve this is uncertain. Most seem to agree that there is a need for an overall 'leader', even though at first sight this may appear at odds with the 'flattened hierarchy' and even with the ideal of a 'democracy'. Thus most therapeutic communities do have an identified leader.

Leaders cannot lead everything, however, and in any case this would not be desirable. Delegation is therefore a skill to be acquired and exercised. As well as a need to delegate there is a need to design and operate a clear management structure, with distinct roles and responsibilities being identified in all staff, especially in terms of line management and in relation to the leader. It is important that all staff have an understanding of where they are placed in the organization. Only then are they in a position to safely and responsibly 'blur their roles, as required of a good therapeutic community worker' (see Burns 2000).

Before the hierarchy can be flattened there is first a need to construct it. The responsibility for the creation of such a clear and ordered set of structures resides with the leader. In keeping with the democratic and multi-disciplinary ideology, at Henderson, this function is shared within a management group – those who have management responsibility and two elected representatives of those who are managed. This group meets monthly to plan and oversee the implementation of strategy and to receive and respond to structures which are higher up in its own hierarchy, its host directorate within its host NHS Mental Health Trust. It also feeds back to the higher structures and this is particularly important when the unthinking application of an instruction might have deleterious effects on the therapeutic community treatment model, as illustrated by Example 9.1. This example shows that the organization, although hierarchical, is small enough and flexible enough to 'flatten', in order to involve its whole membership quite speedily and for this to translate into action, which received a favourable reaction higher up in the hierarchy. For this to happen there is a need to ensure and maintain open communication within and between the various systems. This does not always occur, as Example 9.2 testifies.

There are many aspects of the therapeutic community or ward life that require some level of management and leadership thus there are plenty of opportunities for staff who are not formally in positions of management or leadership to gain relevant experience. For example, all the small groups are co-facilitated, as mentioned earlier. As well as conferring advantages for continuity of staffing and for mutual feedback and supervision,

Example 9.1

There was a dictat to display a notice declaring 'Zero Tolerance' in all parts of the building. The message behind the headline, all could espouse, since it was aimed at eradicating various forms of stigmatizing and abusive behaviour, especially in relation to minority groups. However, its essentially negative tone was thought by the therapeutic community staff to be such as to be likely to stifle important and relevant discussion of these very issues – part of both permissiveness and reality confrontation, i.e. ideological cornerstones of the method. The patients also objected to the notice and together representation was made to the Trust, which was sensitive to the objection and agreed to the development of an alternative poster, jointly created by the staff and patients and designed to achieve similar ends.

Example 9.2

A senior nursing post had remained unfilled over several months, for a variety of reasons, necessitating others to 'act up', i.e. to take on aspects of that role in addition to their own. This was not an altogether satisfactory arrangement for anybody or indeed for the therapeutic community as a whole. At the time of a change between those standing in there was a discussion at the management meeting as to who was the most suitable replacement and there appeared to be agreement that X should take on the role. Not all the relevant managers had been present at the discussion in question and the 'minute' from the meeting was worded ambiguously. As a result, two things happened in parallel. First, X, the nurse in question, was approached by one manager and agreed to 'act up'. Second, another of the managers, who had not been at the meeting but who had merely received the minutes of that meeting, arranged for an interview to take place, but also formally reopened the field to all those potentially eligible – previously those eligible had been only informally and verbally canvassed. X was surprised to see the job that they had been offered and had accepted appearing as an advertised post!

co-facilitation allows for one staff member to assume the lead for that particular group. This may mean overseeing the writing of reports, which relate to the group's specific function. An example of this would be the 'welfare' group, which is led by a social worker. Other groups, which have a less clearly definable professional lead, nevertheless require a degree of leadership. This might simply relate to ensuring that holidays are taken so as to maintain cover for the group. The overall running of the whole is exquisitely affected by the running of its individual parts.

Relevance of therapeutic milieu to acute care wards

Therapeutic milieux vary, but how they are structured, i.e. organized socially, and how they function should depend on the overall treatment aims and objectives that apply. To be successful, the milieu needs to define its objectives but also demonstrate a capacity to be flexible in order to remain sufficiently patient-centred, as internal priorities change. If the environment is to optimize the patients' intact ego capacities, as advocated by proponents of the therapeutic milieu, there needs to be an accurate assessment of the patients' healthy capacities as well as the nature and amount of support required to effect this outcome. This may be difficult to achieve in practice since an individual patient's situation will fluctuate. One patient can require a disproportionately large amount of staff resource, usually in association with the perceived high risk of violence to self or others, thus depriving the remainder of the patients from the treatment to which they are entitled. The level of overall risk accepted by the management system needs to be clearly stated and communicated to ward-based staff.

The inpatient ward environment, as a therapeutic milieu, will vary to the extent that it can embody the range of functions required of it. Such functional properties are hierarchical, with later functions being dependent on the successful achievement of earlier functions. According to Gunderson (1978) the functional properties of 'containment', 'support' and 'structure' all need to be in place before the later functions of 'involvement' and 'validation' can be pursued meaningfully (see above). It will thus be important that a given inpatient ward system is clear about its objectives (and how these relate to the whole local mental health service of which it is but one part). To achieve this, each local system needs to identify a discrete role, or range of roles, for its inpatient resources and to identify suitable leadership. The functional properties required will depend on a large number of factors, including:

- the other local inpatient services, such as the presence of a psychiatric intensive care unit;
- the presence and role of any day facilities;
- the extent of development of community services; and
- the interface with other services within the wider community, for example, housing, employment, education, leisure and social services.

Local socio-economic, political and other factors may also exert an influence on the inpatient service which can ultimately be delivered. It is, therefore, not possible to argue simply for an uptake of therapeutic milieu ideas and practices as if the inpatient unit existed in a vacuum, when this clearly is not the case.

What could be advocated, assuming that the reader finds some value and sense in the above discussion of the therapeutic milieu and therapeutic community, is a cautious application of some of the principles underpinning these approaches to inpatient care, *in relation to the local and fluctuating circumstances that apply*. Those who have written critically about the application of such approaches have been keen to point out the need for clear objectives, and a reliable method of checking that what was intended has actually taken place (Abroms 1969). It is crucial that charismatic leadership does not put ideology before safe clinical practice or that it demands patient-centredness to the detriment of staff, i.e. when staff resources are used up or morale is too low. However, leadership is crucial and this function needs to be clear both in relation to the leader's role responsibilities and the authority invested in the leader, including its limits, i.e. where authority starts and finishes. An effective leader is likely to delegate much authority to the multi-disciplinary team membership but this needs to be explicit. Likewise, it needs to be clear when and why the leader is acting alone but within defined limits of responsibility and authority.

Many uncomfortable compromises need to be struck if the inpatient environment is to optimize its custodial and therapeutic balance. This means accepting some level of risk both by that unit and its management system. However, this level will necessarily vary over time, sometimes quickly and dramatically. If so, it is incumbent on each part of the system, managers or managed, to keep the other informed, i.e. for there to be an ongoing dialogue.

Conclusion

The ideology and practice of the therapeutic milieu, as reflected in key papers in the literature, have been presented. What has been emphasized is the need for the acute ward environment to function as 'a general method for providing specific treatment techniques in an effective manner' (Abroms 1969). The environment needs to embody an identifiable range of therapeutic functions and to be able to judge when to 'regress' towards containment in the face of an increased risk of violence. Knowledge of this range could help staff to avoid simply lurching between extremes of custodial and therapeutic care. However, trying to bear in mind the needs of all patients within the ward is problematic. Ultimately, therapeutic functioning relies on an adequate set of staff–patient and staff–staff relationships, the quality of which is readily eroded by staff shortage, the employment of temporary staff (unfamiliar with the ward rules and routines), a lack of clear objectives for the ward and no mechanism to audit activities. Staff, therefore, need to remain vigilant to the different ways in which destructive processes may operate. To this end they are likely to benefit from supervisory and support structures modelled on those of the democratic therapeutic community.

So, what is it practical for acute psychiatric care to import from therapeutic milieux?

- The objectives of the ward environment can be stated and even documented so that patients as well as staff can know what the enterprise is attempting to achieve.

- Related to this, a statement of methods used to achieve these objectives can be issued, for example, explaining the social organization of the ward and what treatment ingredients or sessions might be encountered by a patient in any given week in the ward.

- Staff need to describe the rules that apply and, equally important, the expectations placed by staff on patients (recognizing the latter's healthy functioning) in terms of responsibilities, for example, in relation to illicit drug use, and specifying also what supports are available to help patients flourish.

- It will help to indicate that ultimately the work of the inpatient ward is collaborative, not only between different staff disciplines but between staff and patients. It is all too easy for a 'them and us' situation to apply.

- In pursuing such collaboration it will be useful to state what aspects of the treatment programme support the empowerment of patients so that the latter can know where to voice concerns over particular aspects of their inpatient stay, for example, safety or sexual harassment.

- In following the above, many of the values espoused by the institution will have been communicated, but some of these may benefit from an explicit statement, for example, in relation to abhorrence of racism, sexism, etc.

How the above is communicated will convey much about the ethos of the ward. A balance needs to be struck, bearing in mind the patient's mental state on arrival, about how much is imparted, how soon and by whom. Ideally this should be only as much as can be readily assimilated by the individual patient, but this may be difficult to judge. The importance of imparting information about such aspects should be understood, and it is a task that should not be delegated to the most junior nurse. The early hours spent on the ward are likely to colour the patient's stay and getting off on the wrong footing can result in an unnecessarily onerous episode of treatment with adverse consequences for compliance and avoidable use of compulsion. The aim, in being patient-centred, is to maximize the likelihood that the patient will be able to fulfil their side of the staff–patient treatment alliance. However, to achieve this, patients need to know what is expected of them and what are appropriate expectations of the environment, especially the human environment of the inpatient setting: in reality mainly nurses. Ideally, they need to know both the 'what' and the 'how' of the ward's treatment ideology and therapeutic programme.

In summary the main points of this chapter are:

- Ward environment needs to be construed as a context in which specific treatments occur.

- This context can support or undermine treatment.

- The context should embody a range of functions and be capable of (re)organizing itself to do so.

- Therapeutic functioning ultimately relies on the quality of staff–patient and staff–staff relationships.
- Staff need to remain vigilant to destructive processes that may be deleterious to patients' care and corrosive of staff morale.
- Clear objectives for the inpatient environment can support staff, individually and as part of a multi-disciplinary team.
- Patients can be empowered by being made aware of the ward's ideology and therapeutic programme and expectations placed on them by staff.

Questions for reflection and discussion

1 Consider with colleagues the extent to which the ward in which you work, or are connected, embodies the principles and practice of a therapeutic milieu. The following checklist might be helpful:

   - Do staff and patients in the ward know what the enterprise is trying to achieve?
   - Do patients know how the ward is organized and what ingredients or treatment sessions they might encounter in any given week?
   - Are staff clear and explicit with patients about the rules that apply, what is expected of them and what supports are available to help them flourish?
   - To what extent do staff from the same and different disciplines work collaboratively with each other and with patients?
   - Does the ward regime empower patients and provide them with sufficient opportunities to voice their concerns?
   - Is there an explicit statement about the values of the inpatient setting, such as abhorrence of racism and sexism?

2 What practical steps might be taken to increase the therapeutic potential of the inpatient environment? In collaboration with others, draw up an action plan for implementation.

Annotated bibliography

- Abroms, G.M. (1969) Defining milieu therapy, *Archives of General Psychiatry* **21**: 553–60. This paper provides a clear framework for thinking about the concept of therapeutic milieu and its practical application.
- Gabbard, G.O. (1988) A contemporary perspective on psychoanalytically informed inpatient treatment, *Hospital, Community and Psychiatry* **39**: 1291–5. This paper describes a psychoanalytic approach to inpatient psychiatric treatment, introducing the reader to relevant terms and concepts that are more widely applicable to general psychiatry.

- Gunderson, J.G. (1978) Defining the therapeutic processes in psychiatric milieus, *Psychiatry* **41**: 327–35. Although discussed in detail in this chapter, the interested reader may wish to see the original to which complete justice has not been done by the present author (K.N.)
- Main, T.F. (1946) The Hospital as a Therapeutic Institution, *Bulletin of the Menninger Clinic* **10**(3): 66–70. This is a classic paper in which the term 'therapeutic community' is introduced. Much of the essence of later developments and understanding in the field are prefigured here.
- Norton, K.R.W. (1992) A culture of enquiry, its preservation or loss, *Therapeutic Communities* **1**(1): 3–26. This paper expands the notion of 'culture of enquiry' (first expressed by Main) in relation to a democratic therapeutic community, exploring the relationship between organizational aspects and quality of clinical functioning.

References

Beadsmore, A., Moore, C., Muijen, M. *et al.* (1998) *Acute Problems: A Survey of the Quality of Care in Acute Psychiatric Wards*. London: Sainsbury Centre Mental Health Publications.

Bettelheim, B. (1950) *Love is Not Enough*. New York: Free Press.

Bion, W.R. (1963) *Elements of Psychoanalysis*. London: Heinemann.

Bloom, S.L. (1997) *Creating Sanctuary: Toward the Evolution of Sane Societies*. New York and London: Routledge.

Bloor, M., McKeganey, N. and Fonkert, D. (1988) The historical development of therapeutic community approaches, *One Foot in Eden*. London: Routledge.

Burns, T. (2000) The legacy of the therapeutic community practice in modern community health services, *Therapeutic Communities* **21**(3): 165–74.

Busfield, J. (1986) *Managing Madness: Changing Ideas and Practice*. London: Unwin Hyman.

Carleton, J.L. and Mahlendorf, U.R. (1979) *Dimensions of Social Psychiatry*. Princeton, NJ: Science Press.

Cumming, J. and Cumming, E. (1964) *Ego and Milieu*. New York: Atherton Press.

Ford, R., Durcan, G., Warner, L., Hardy, P. and Muijen, M. (1998) One day survey by the Mental Health Act Commission of acute adult psychiatric inpatient wards in England and Wales, *British Medical Journal* **317**: 1279–83.

Greenson, R. (1967) *The Technique and Practice of Psychoanalysis*: Vol 1. New York: International Universities Press.

Jones, M. (1952) *Social Psychiatry*. London: Tavistock Publications.

Jones, M. (1968) *Beyond the Therapeutic Community: Social Learning and Social Psychiatry*. New Haven, CT and London: Yale University Press.

Menninger, W. (1936) Psychiatric Hospital Treatment Designed to Meet Unconscious Needs, *American Journal of Psychiatry* **93**: 347–60.

MIND (2000) *Environmentally Friendly: Patients' Views of Conditions on Psychiatric Wards*. The Mental Health Charity.

Roberts, J.P. (1980) Destructive Processes in a Therapeutic Community, *International Journal of Therapeutic Communities* **1**(3).

Stanton, A.H. (1964) Foreword to *Ego and Milieu*, by J. Cummings and E. Atherton. New York: Atherton Press.

Talbot, E. and Miller, S.C. (1966) The struggle to create a sane society in the psychiatric hospital, *Psychiatry* **29**: 365–75.

von Bertalannfy, L. (1967) General systems theory and psychiatry, in S. Arieti (ed.) *Volume One: The Foundations of Psychiatry; American Handbook of Psychiatry*. New York: Basic Books.

Whiteley, J.S. (1986) Sociotherapy and psychotherapy in the treatment of personality disorder, *Journal of the Royal Society of Medicine*, Vol. 79, December.

Wilmer, H.A. (1958) Towards a Definition of the Therapeutic Community, *American Journal of Psychiatry* **114**: 824–33.

10

Psychosocial interventions

Catherine Gamble with Jacqueline Curthoys

Chapter overview

The transition of mental health care from the hospital to the community has required the development of modern efficacious talking therapies, such as those to treat early symptoms, manage psychosis psychologically and family interventions. However, there is a lack of consensus regarding which 'new talking therapies' fit best with contemporary mental health practice and how they should be used to help clients and their carers to cope with the complexities of living with severe and enduring mental health problems. The challenge for mental health nurses and other professionals is to learn how to listen more carefully to clients and value and respect their views. This is essential if nurses are to harness the expertise of clients about their own problems and establish and sustain positive working alliances with them.

This chapter regards psychosocial interventions, or 'talking therapies' as therapeutic, non-judgemental, practically based windows of opportunity, which can be drawn on to develop working alliances with clients. It provides an introduction to these therapies, illustrates them through the use of case studies and considers their therapeutic usefulness through the eyes of one client with first-hand experiences of using such therapies in the context of contemporary mental health services. The chapter provides a foundation for Chapters 24 and 25 in which Gega considers the practical application of behavioural and cognitive techniques when working with clients. This chapter covers:

- developing working alliances;

- Rogerian principles;

- finding ways to promote positive attitudes;

- psychosocial interventions:

- engagement and outcome-oriented assessment,
- motivational interviewing,
- psychological management of psychosis,
- family interventions.

Developing working alliances

Developing working alliances between health professionals, clients and their carers is perceived to be an important step forward in promoting partnership in the new NHS (Stuart 1999). The challenge ahead is to develop and sustain these working relationships in clinical practice. Interpersonal skills and qualities are key to developing such alliances and therefore a necessary requirement for all mental health nurses. However, there is insufficient emphasis on developing these attributes during pre- and post-registration education for mental health professionals (McQueen 2000). Furthermore, as nurses deal with numerous situations and experience many different encounters with people from all walks of life, there is only limited consensus on what personal qualities and skills are required in every situation. Experience and intuition appear to be guiding principles and it is mainly left up to the individual practitioner to exercise self-awareness and reflect upon the effectiveness of their interpersonal skills. Nevertheless, there is a demonstrated positive correlation between therapeutic relationships and therapeutic outcomes for clients (Blaauw and Emmelkamp 1994). Thus it is important to examine these qualities in some depth.

Rogerian principles

Carl Rogers, the renowned psychotherapist promoted the client-centred hypotheses, which are now considered fundamental to the development and sustainability of therapeutic relationships. The guiding 'Rogerian' principles are:

- empathetic understanding, which shows sensitivity to others' feelings;
- genuineness, which is reflected in an open, honest approach;
- unconditional positive regard, which is achieved by accepting others as individuals who are entitled to respect and care.

Rogers (1983) believes that exposure to such attributes produces learning, or changes, in people. That is, they come to see themselves differently, accept their feelings more readily, become more accepting of others, and more self-confident and self-directing. Thus, they are more able to change behaviours and adopt realistic goals. The promotion of these attributes provides common ground regardless of which treatment philosophy or affiliated school of thought is adopted. Indeed, at the core of any contemporary practice is the recognition that people are unique, that irrespective of their diagnosis they are able to collaborate, and that no positive outcome will be achieved if these principles are not adhered to or utilized by practitioners.

However, in today's busy clinical settings nurses and other health care professionals can become easily harassed with the result that any negative feelings they hold can be expressed in their interactions with others. All too frequently this means that professionals do not apply Rogerian principles in their routine contacts with clients (McQueen 2000). In routine relationships with clients how far do we always:

- act in ways that are trustworthy, dependable and consistent?

- communicate unambiguously?

- promote positive attitudes, such as warmth, caring, liking, respect?

- ensure that our personal feelings do not negatively influence our interactions?

- encourage clients to be individuals, rather than expect them to do as we say and fit in?

- understand and acknowledge clients' feelings and experiences, and respect their cultural and spiritual beliefs?

- act with sufficient sensitivity when presented with behaviours that seem threatening?

These questions were deliberately set to challenge, raise consciousness and encourage reflection on current practice. Undoubtedly, it is hard to answer yes to all of them. If you have been able to, then the rest of us will be very envious. Utopia springs to mind! In addition to demanding workloads and professional responsibilities there are numerous other reasons why it is not always easy to portray these characteristics to all those with whom we come into contact. It is a fact of life that no one person gets on well with everyone all of the time, which is a good reason for working in teams! But either on a collective or an individual basis we need to strive to portray Rogerian principles in our practice. Where there's a will, there is always a way!

Finding ways to promote positive attitudes

Stereotypes and prejudices pervade society's perceptions of schizophrenia. Users with this diagnosis, in particular, are continually bombarded with old-fashioned attitudes and assumptions that do nothing to promote optimism for the future; indeed it can leave a person believing they are stuck in the murkiest cul-de-sac of certified insanity (James 2001). Turning pessimism into optimism is a challenge, especially when many 'off-duty' professionals continue to reinforce these negative viewpoints. Consider for a moment the following conversation overheard while waiting for a bus:

Psychiatric nursing … Yes, it's a real challenge [laughs!!!]! A really difficult job! Especially in today's NHS!! Thank you for acknowledging that – only yesterday, we were so short I ended up spending nearly the entire day, with one client who ended up being sectioned! Poor guy was a schizophrenic – he was **so** mad! The ward **is** full of them now and I can't remember a time when there wasn't a violent incident!

To a fellow professional this conversation would not necessarily seem detrimental to clients; after all, the narrator is recalling his experience and explaining the reality of working on one of today's busy acute psychiatric wards. But, what message is it giving to the layperson waiting in the queue? Might it be something like, 'Mental health nursing is a "them versus us" hard challenging job, which involves legally detaining mad violent people'?

To avoid such type-casting, practitioners need to consider carefully how to portray themselves and describe their jobs and roles. Rather than going for the tabloid headline approach by using the term 'schizophrenic' as a noun, it would have been preferable if the above narrative had described the person behind the 'label' and included an objective description of the 'talking' strategies the nurse had used before the 'section' had occurred. This would have instilled a more optimistic view of mental illness and the role nurses play in ameliorating clients' distress. Overall, there is need for us all to be willing to review our:

- attitudes and challenge our assumptions;
- listening skills, so we are more able to hear clients' and carers' views;
- speaking styles and thus avoid 'talking down' to clients;
- working relationships with other members of the multi-disciplinary team.

Challenging our assumptions and reviewing our attitudes and beliefs

Adverse views of mentally ill people stem from the following assumptions:

- People with mental illness are prone to violence.
- They 'choose' to behave as they do.
- They are unpredictable and don't behave 'normally', so interacting with them in social situations is very difficult.
- Their symptoms are difficult to treat and the prognosis is that their symptoms will become chronic (Haywood and Bright 1997).

Promoting and sustaining positive working alliances involves challenging these, unfavourable views, negative beliefs and assumptions about mental illness and clients' lack of ability to change. Mental health professionals are part of society that perpetuates these unconstructive suppositions and at one time or other, are likely to have shared all or some of them (Gamble 2000). Therefore, before entering into any relationship with a client, it is important to consider how to minimize these assumptions, so that a more optimistic outlook is endorsed. Haywood and Bright's (1997) adapted model, shown in Table 10.1, provides some guidance as to how this may be achieved.

Table 10.1 Methods to counterbalance maladaptive views

Assumption	Methods
Mentally ill are violent and dangerous	360 homicides are committed/year in the UK, 10 per cent of this population are 'mentally ill'. Use of such statistics help to challenge the view that all those with severe mental health problems are violent and dangerous (James 2001).
They 'choose' to behave as they do	Utilize your educational role as a nurse. Challenge this view whenever it is expressed, strive to portray clients as rounded individuals – severe mental illness is not self-inflicted.
Prognosis is chronic	Many people go on to lead meaningful and successful lives – quote examples such as Ron Coleman (James 2001) and the work of Romme and Escher (1993). Moreover, it is possible to challenge this view when contemporary PSI, such as family work can produce significant benefits for clients long beyond the term of intervention (Sellwood *et al.* 2001)
Mentally ill are unpredictable and don't behave 'normally'	Does everyone always behave predictably and 'normally'? If we did wouldn't the world be full of robots? Challenge yourself to consider what is 'normal'. Review potential or actual 'strange' behaviours or ideas you have, such as, déjà vu, a belief in the occult, ghosts, reincarnation, aliens, astrology and tarot, etc.
Symptoms are difficult to treat	Incorporate cultural, psychological and biological models of health care, in doing so you will have a greater sense that there are self-management steps that can be used with symptoms that are perceived to be hard to treat (Kingdon and Turkington 1994)
This client group is hard to work with	Promote discussions with service users – learning to listen in this way you will be more likely to realize that working with this client group is a privileged lifelong learning experience.

Learning to listen

Listening is a skill that requires practice. It does not merely involve repeating words – parrots do that. Listening takes intelligent concentration and necessitates paraphrasing what is said without changing the meaning of the words and paying attention to the context as well as content (Bostrom 1997). If you are prepared to practise the art of listening it is less likely that you will force-feed your ideas upon clients and their carers or contaminate what you hear with your own thoughts and opinions. To guide you through the art of listening try the strategies listed in Table 10.2.

Table 10.2 The art of listening

The art of listening involves four Cs:	Potential barriers include:	Methods to overcome involve:
Considering situations in which you may find it difficult to concentrate	Interruptions; noisy external exchanges; when there is more than one thing on the agenda, someone interrupting the session or going over the allocated time.	Planning for and reporting your unavailability. Put a 'do not disturb' sign up for the duration of the meeting; challenging interruptions if they are made. Setting an agenda, a realistic timeframe and adhering to it.
	Client's current symptoms may be too troublesome and distracting for them.	Assess how the client feels, is this the right time and place to be meeting? Negotiate where and when would be more appropriate and/or turn off the TV or radio.
	TV and radio on.	
Collating methods to facilitate being a 'better listener'	Not planning for the interaction and missing valuable cues.	Discuss your interaction with another experienced member of the team. Plan how to structure and evaluate the session.
	Others not agreeing to formalized approach.	Balancing note taking with personalized interaction.
	Tape recording and/or note taking perceived to be journalistic rather than therapeutic.	Adhering to trust and/or university guidelines, so it does not breach local confidentiality guidelines.
	Clients and/or carers will be suspicious, won't they?	Providing a rationale for note taking and or audio-taping. No harm in just asking and gaining consent to audio taping. Challenging own and others' assumptions.
Constructing a rationale for why you can't always listen	Being occupied by all the above and other clinical responsibilities.	Being honest.
		Acknowledging distractions and reporting other items on the agenda.
		Recognizing inability to time manage.

Table 10.2 (*continued*)

The art of listening involves four Cs:	Potential barriers include:	Methods to overcome involve:
Consolidating what you will do with the information	Information obtained challenges others' perceptions.	Listening attentively; Reflecting and summarizing. Encouraging others to listen to client's and/or carers' viewpoint.
	Unable to objectively document or report on what you had learnt.	Documenting what you have learnt in the case notes.
	Other members of the team don't want to acknowledge and there is no forum to feedback.	Disseminating to other 'listeners' such as, the client, their carers and others on the team.
		Attending the next possible clinical review meeting to feedback.

Promoting collaborative speaking styles

 Friendliness, confidence and attentiveness can encourage the development of a trusting relationship (McQueen 2000) but there is also a need to ascertain the extent to which clients want to participate in their care (Carhill 1998). Be aware that some clients may find initial approaches overwhelming especially if they have been used to being patronized by traditional methods of care. To promote collaborative speaking styles and thereby positive working alliances, it is essential to bear in mind the communication style used and the manner in which we portray ourselves. For example, consider your reaction when a hairdresser, using a singing inflection and a somewhat supercilious tone in their voice asks, 'Could you put your head on one side for **me**?' The phrase is said routinely and as matter of habit, which female clients seldom feel is worth challenging. Do nurses fall into the same well-meaning, but somewhat thoughtless practice when they change their tone of voice and ask things like 'Should **we** do this today?' The attitude behind this approach infantilizes the client and infers a weakness in their position, as supplicant. The client's weakness is reinforced by the depersonalizing change of voice. This inflection and style of approach is best avoided. The message that we all share a common humanity can be conveyed by the manner in which we treat and talk to people.

So the next time you interact with a client or carer – stop for a moment and take note of the tone you are using, and then ask yourself, 'Do I speak to colleagues whom I respect, in this way?'

Valuing contributions made by multi-disciplinary team members

Users and their carers often complain that despite every communication effort on their part they are at times confronted with an array of conflicting messages from different members of the team. This does not bode well when trying to enhance collaborative working alliances and promote service user empowerment. Unless professionals are willing to communicate effectively, share working practices and value each other's contribution, it is unlikely that sustained working partnerships and positive outcomes for service users will be achieved. A lack of nurse–doctor collaboration, in particular has been recognized to contribute to problems in quality and efficiency of client care (Zwarenstein and Bryant 2002). Furthermore, it has been postulated by a team who have facilitated a regional training initiative that one of the main barriers to implementing contemporary practice methods, such as family intervention, is the negative assumptions professionals hold about each other (Campbell 2000). All too frequently in clinical practice, clinicians can be heard to make sweeping generalizations and judgements about other team members. For example:

> Our manager never listens – he's not in the slightest bit interested in the valuable clinical work we are doing!

> Getting information from the psychologist is like getting water out of a stone – you need to be one of them to get recognition.

> The GP was given the date of the clinical review meeting months ago – and he still hasn't had the decency to turn up.

> I asked the psychiatrist about reviewing the medication – I won't do that again in a hurry – you think I'd asked her to rob the crown jewels – more than her job's worth or what?!

> It takes so long to get the social worker to come and see my client – and when he does he doesn't do anything about his benefits.

> You wouldn't believe she is a nurse she is so autocratic!

These examples are not the exception; unfortunately they are more likely to be the norm, in part, because any one professional has only limited opportunities to see things from another professional's perspective. It is generally taken for granted that everyone knows how to portray empathetic understanding and thus value and respect the knowledge and skills that each professional contributes. But, in fact, many professionals have inadequate access to regular team training or supervision opportunities to learn how to incorporate these principles into everyday team practice. Moreover, if clients and carers were aware that these sorts of derisive statements were being made then they would also begin to question the multi-disciplinary team's credibility and ability to act as a team to provide a non-critical, transparent and responsive service.

There is some evidence that collaboration between professionals can improve outcomes that are important to clients and to health care managers (Zwarenstein and Bryant 2002). Dennis (2000) suggests that this might be achieved if there was greater awareness and understanding of each other's roles and responsibilities and more negotiation between professionals. Thus team members would feel more valued, would identify and exhibit loyalty to the team rather than their own discipline alone and would be more likely to acknowledge and be more confident of each other's skills. Thereby the whole organization would begin to communicate more effectively and support a greater blurring and overlap between roles.

One device for promoting such awareness is the communications – interaction (disclosure and feedback) framework. Based on Luft's (1988) 'Johari Window' model of self-awareness, the framework divides the concept of disclosure and feedback into four compartments:

1   areas known to the organization and to others;

2   areas known only by the organization;

3   areas known only to others;

4   areas unknown to either.

As communication styles change and understanding increases the format shifts; the areas unknown to others and the organization reduce in size, and the areas known to others and the organization increases.

Such models can aid reflection upon our own and others' interactions, disclosures and feedback. Many complex dynamic inter-relationships pervade the organizations within which nurses work, but these are not an impenetrable barrier. Irrespective of whether you are communicating with a

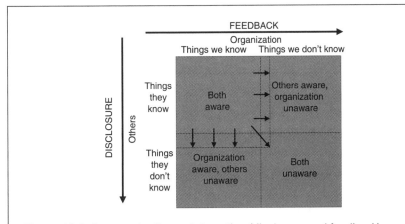

Figure 10.1 Communications – Interaction (disclosure and feedback)

(Adapted from Luft 1988)

fellow mental health professional or a client, the following cyclical aide mémoire, shown in Figure 10.2, may help you to reflect on the process of promoting working alliances.

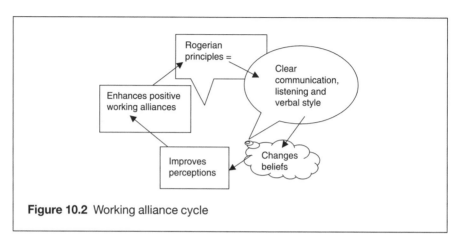

Figure 10.2 Working alliance cycle

This working alliance cycle combines Rogerian principles with the communication skills required to improve perceptions of people with severe and enduring mental health problems. These principles lie at the heart of contemporary interventions, such as psychosocial interventions.

Psychosocial interventions

Over the last decade it has been recognized that successful management of severe mental illness is rarely achieved by medication alone, but requires that this be combined with other treatment approaches, in particular psychosocial interventions (PSIs). These have been defined as formulation-driven interventions that ameliorate a client or their carer's problems associated with a psychosis, using an approach based on psychological principles or addressing a change in social circumstances. Psychosocial interventions include:

- engagement and outcome-orientated assessment;
- medication management, via motivational interviewing techniques;
- psychological management of psychosis, for example, formulation-driven interventions, such as coping-strategy enhancement, self-monitoring approaches and problem-solving training;
- family assessment of needs and intervention.

Engagement and outcome-orientated assessment

Outcome-orientated assessments encapsulate the extent to which interventions do what they are intended to do for a particular client or population. They are all about making sure that practitioners are doing the right thing, in the right way, at the right time and thus the best care possible is offered (NHS Executive 1998).

This chapter has emphasized the importance of developing therapeutic relationships, changing communication styles and has challenged clinicians to consider methods to address negative attitudes and beliefs that are sometimes held about this client group. Combining these attributes, with outcome-orientated assessment methods can engage clients, which in turn can help to ensure that objective reviews of need are undertaken to guide future interventions.

Undertaking a thorough assessment of a client may be perceived by some practitioners to be too complex, drawn out and time consuming. Furthermore, some may consider form filling to be a barrier to engagement especially if the assessment requires that clients are confronted with lengthy assessment tools. Obviously there is a limit. People do not want to be overwhelmed, therefore, it is very important to be pragmatic and considerate when selecting assessment tools. However, the assumption that all clients and their carers will feel bombarded has to be reviewed. Clinical experience suggests that many clients and carers perceive formal assessment approaches as a refreshing change. It can be very reassuring for them when sound, practical interviewing and rating procedures are therapeutically utilized, since this process demonstrates that assumptions are not being made, that accurate observations are sought and that systematic procedures are being followed. We may all expect these sorts of assessment procedures to be carried out in general medical settings, so why should this not happen routinely in psychiatric settings? Consider for example, visiting a close relative in a general hospital ward. The first thing many of us do is look at the charts at the end of the bed. Why? We are looking for formal reassurances that the person is getting better and the temperature chart, in particular provides visual evidence of this. It would be impractical and nonsensical to place charts at the end of our clients' beds, especially when the majority of them live at home, but sharing information obtained via systematic assessments at baseline, mid- and post-intervention provides overt evidence that change can occur.

Formulating a working hypothesis, through systematic assessment is an integral part of PSI implementation; the following case study of Claudette provides evidence of the therapeutic value of such an approach.

Case study: Claudette

Claudette is a 26-year-old African-Caribbean woman with a diagnosis of paranoid schizophrenia. She lives with her family and is currently unemployed. She was first admitted to hospital six years ago while she was studying hairdressing at the local college. She became concerned that another classmate was reading her thoughts and copying her ideas. Her coursework deteriorated and she became increasingly paranoid, irritable and secretive. She aggressively demanded screens to be erected in the classroom, lashed out at her tutors and despite every effort on their part her behaviour became so unmanageable she had to be asked to withdraw from the course. Her behaviour and symptoms worsened and she was eventually admitted to hospital. She made a satisfactory recovery and was in remission for nearly two years until she stopped taking her medication. She again became aggressive and paranoid, tried to strangle her mother and was readmitted. Despite being compliant with treatment, Claudette failed to respond fully to anti-psychotic medication with hallucinations remaining the most prominent and distressing symptom. At this point Claudette expressed feeling overwhelmed by her incapacity to socialize, concentrate or motivate herself and she expressed 'this is ruining my life'.

The initial phase of the assessment process included conveying to Claudette that her current concerns and problems would be addressed and taken seriously. In doing so it was possible to describe the process of therapy and introduce the idea that a formal review of symptoms and the problems she was experiencing via systematic assessment was required. She readily agreed to participate in this approach, because the supporting explanation conveyed to her that 'talking therapy' could be formalized and that there was hope for the future. Over the next six weeks she participated in the following assessments:

Krawiecka, Goldberg and Vaughn, Manchester Symptom Severity Scale

The KGV (M) is a standardized global semi-structured instrument which measures the severity of symptoms. It comprises 14 items, which are rated on a 0–4 scale: 0 = no symptoms, 1 = mild, 2 = moderate, 3 = marked and 4 = severe symptoms reported in the last month. The first 6 items are rated by the mental health professional on the basis of the client's verbal responses and next 8 are rated on observations made during the interview (Krawiecka *et al.* 1977). Claudette's main symptoms produced the following ratings:

Anxiety	3
Depression	3
Suicidal thoughts and behaviour	1
Hallucinations	4
Delusions	2

This assessment showed that anxiety, depression and hallucinations were Claudette's most prevalent reported symptoms but, through observation, it was clear also that others were evident, these included:

Flattened affect	2
Psychomotor retardation	2
Poverty of speech	2

By reviewing these ratings anxiety, depression and hallucinations appeared more prevalent than negative symptoms. At this stage it would have been easy to hypothesize about how to intervene, especially in relation to her reported anxiety. However, it is important not to rush in with a 'quick fix' anxiety-management programme; a fuller picture is always more preferable and further detail was recognized to be required. For instance, from this assessment it was not possible to measure the impact that some symptoms were having on Claudette's life and it was important to draw upon the initial concerns about her socializing, concentration and motivation capabilities.

Four further assessments were therefore carried out, as follows:

Hospital Anxiety and Depression Scale (HAD)

This validated self-report questionnaire assesses anxiety and depression. It comprises 14 items; half of these assess anxiety and the other half assess depression. Items are rated on a 0–3 scale. Thus, the highest possible score for each symptom is 21. The client is asked to report how they have felt during the past 1–2 days (Snaith 1993). The HAD was used in Claudette's case because it is more sensitive than the KGV (M) at measuring the current impact anxiety and depressive symptoms and it assesses depressive–negative symptoms. It thus complements the third assessment tool selected – the Schedule for the Assessment of Negative Symptoms (Hogg 1996).

Schedule for the Assessment of Negative Symptoms (SANS)

This scale assesses symptoms such as affective flattening (decreased range in emotional responses), alogia (poverty of thought), avolition (loss of motivation or drive), apathy, anhedonia (diminished capacity to experience pleasure), asociality and attention. All symptoms are rated on a 0–5 scale of increasing severity (Andreasen 1982).

In Claudette's case the HAD and SANS assessments produced the following scores:

Anxiety	9
Depression	4
Affective flattening or blunting	2
Alogia	2
Avolition–apathy	3
Anhendonia–asociality	4
Attention	1

The results from the HAD were illuminating. The score of 9 for anxiety was borderline, which contradicted the results of the KGV (M) which had rated her anxiety as 'marked'. Social anxiety and deficits in social functioning are viewed generally as core problems for individuals with psychotic disorders (Birchwood *et al.* 1990) and these results demonstrate why it had been essential to listen to Claudette's own appraisal of her problems, use more than one assessment tool and not to rush in with solutions.

Impaired social functioning is a recognized hallmark of schizophrenia either as an early sign or as residual symptoms. Therefore, before commencing any intervention a baseline of Claudette's abilities in this area was undertaken, using the Social Functioning Scale.

The Social Functioning Scale

Birchwood *et al.* (1990) designed this instrument to cover seven main areas of social functioning including: social engagement, relationships, independence in living skills (competence and performance) and employment. All seven categories are rated independently, high scores indicating higher social functioning. From Claudette's results (Table 10.3) it was possible to conclude that she seemed to be doing quite well in all aspects of social functioning since all scores exceeded 100 (the population mean), with the exception of social activities, which scored 98. The scores in this case, however, were not accurate or sensitive to her level of functioning with respect to 'relationships'. Claudette, since leaving college, had lost contact with many of her peers, had no 'real' friends and only socialized with her parents. In spite of this her 'relationships' score was 145, which is well above the population mean of 100.

Table 10.3 Social Functioning Scale data

Categories	Raw score	Transformed score
Social withdrawal	12	110.0
Relationships	17	145.0
Social activities	10	98.0
Recreational activities	21	113.0
Independence (c)	39	123.0
Independence (p)	37	124.0
Employment	4	103.0
TOTAL SCORE	140	816.0

Beliefs about voices questionnaire

By administering the beliefs about voices questionnaire time was spent reviewing Claudette's beliefs about her voice hearing experiences (Chadwick and Birchwood 1994). From this is was possible to conclude that in the past week, her voices had caused her to feel anxious, but she had been telling them to leave her alone and she felt confident in being able to control them.

As previously mentioned Claudette's assessment took six weeks. Throughout this period mental health professionals adopted a quizzical non-threatening approach and the rationale for going slowly trying to achieve a clear picture of Claudette was reiterated. Furthermore, as each assessment was completed Claudette was provided with feedback. It was imperative that this feedback was coherent and informative, because Claudette's previous experience of her 'case' being reviewed had not produced the results she had been promised and much of the information obtained had been filed and not used by the multi-disciplinary team. Claudette clearly appreciated the time that had been spent gathering this information; she described the experience as 'the detective period' and often questioned why she had never had the opportunity to do this following previous admissions.

The results of these assessments were drawn on to formulate a programme of care for Claudette, which could be monitored over time. Members of the mental health team discussed ideas for future interventions with her and with each other. These interventions included:

- activity scheduling and problem solving to increase Claudette's motivation, activity levels, social and independent living skills;
- cognitive therapy for voice hearing, utilizing, for example, coping-strategy enhancement techniques;
- reviewing Claudette's medication, the side effects she was experiencing and examining her motivation to continue to take what she had been prescribed (via motivational interviewing);
- monitoring progress by revisiting the previous assessments and continuing to gather further details from other reliable sources, such as her family;
- collaborating and working with her family.

Overall, the assessment process had proved valuable because:

- Assessment tools had been selected to meet the client's specific needs, rather than being part of a standardized assessment package.
- Being familiar with the tools enabled the mental health team to administer them sensitively and interpret their scores wisely.
- Assumptions about how to intervene were not made.
- The vital role that assessments can play in engaging clients and developing appropriate treatment strategies was demonstrated.
- It was responsive, flexible and tailor-made to suit Claudette's needs at the time she requested it.
- It provided a foundation from which successful collaborative intervention could be built.

Motivational interviewing

Motivational interviewing is not a new concept, and has long been utilized by those working with people with substance-use problems. It is not a panacea for activating change, but it does provide a way to challenge traditional treatment approaches and is a constructive method of exploring and resolving ambivalence; and reviewing lifestyles and treatment needs (Rollnick and Miller 1995). The aim of motivational interviewing is to increase a person's ability to recognize and do something about present or potential problems.

It is particularly useful when people feel hesitant or are ambivalent about change. People with schizophrenia have complex experiences and many find the idea of changing lifestyle patterns extremely difficult to understand. In many cases this is not because they do not have the motivation or inclination to understand the rationale for learning new methods of coping with their symptoms and experiences. The problem lies often in the limited treatment options that mental health professionals offer and the manner in which they present them to clients. Table 10.4 compares the characteristics of

Table 10.4 Characteristics of motivational interviewing

Motivational interviewing	*Tradition approach*
Individual responsibility	
Emphasis placed on personal choice regarding future lifestyle.	Emphasis placed on traditional disease model of schizophrenia which reduces personal choice.
Goal of treatment is negotiated and based on assessment, life experiences and personal preferences.	The treatment goal is prescribed and total adherence to medication is perceived as the panacea.
Self-medication use is a possible goal though not optimal for all.	Dismissed as impossible.
Internal attribution	
The individual is perceived as able to choose and make lifestyle modifications.	The individual is perceived as helpless and unable to work with or control his or her own symptoms.
Focus is placed upon eliciting client's own statement of concern regarding his or her experiences.	The evidence is presented and used to convince the client of his or her problem.
Denial	
Denial is seen as an interpersonal behaviour pattern.	Denial seen as a personal trait, requiring confrontation.
Denial is met with reflection.	Denial is met with argument and correction.
Labelling	
There is general de-emphasis on labelling. Stereotypical traits are seen as irrelevant.	Emphasis is placed upon acceptance of the person as 'schizophrenic' and therefore unable to make sensible choices without guidance.
Objective data of change in function and impairment are presented in a low-key fashion, not imposing any conclusion.	Objective date is presented in an confrontational fashion; as proof of a progressive disease.

Sources: Miller (1983); Bolton and Watt (1989)

motivational interviewing with traditional treatment approaches. Motivational interviewing dismisses the role of 'expert' versus 'recipient'. Instead it provides practitioners with an opportunity to adopt a partnership approach with clients which harness their ability to articulate and resolve their own ambivalence towards changing lifestyles or behaviours.

Kemp *et al.* (1996) found motivational interviewing to be an effective way to help clients with psychosis increase their insight into their treatment needs and their overall global functioning, and thereby significantly improve their willingness to adhere to treatment. Furthermore, the technique has been found to benefit those who have a dual diagnosis, those people who use substances as well as experiencing severe and enduring mental health problems. The approach appears to be successful, because it is non-confrontational and conveys a message of hope. It removes barriers and provides practitioners with an opportunity to address the client's situation as a whole (Sciacca 1997). The following case study of Paul demonstrates the potential benefits of motivational interviewing as a therapeutic approach.

Case study: Paul

Paul had been diagnosed with schizophrenia for four years. During this time he remained very ambivalent about his diagnosis, he took medication intermittently and rarely attended appointments, and was frequently absent when visited. He had never been admitted as an inpatient voluntarily and was always at loggerheads with either his psychiatrist or his parents who disapproved of his nomadic, drug-orientated lifestyle, and his inability to appreciate that he was unwell. One afternoon, he arrived dishevelled and 'stoned' at the mental health centre reporting that he was fed up and couldn't think of anywhere else better to go! He said he was tired of being hassled by everyone, having no friends, living in his squalid bedsit and, for the first time, openly reported hearing voices, which he included as part of the problem of being hassled. He clearly had weighed up the pros and cons of disclosing this information, and it was at this stage that the team recognized a potential window of opportunity to activate this motivation to change.

Over the next few months his key worker employed the five general principles of motivation interviewing, which are:

- expressing empathy;
- developing discrepancy;
- rolling with resistance;
- avoiding arguments; and
- supporting self efficacy to harness Paul's intrinsic motivation (Rollnick and Miller 1995).

'Motivation for change occurs when people perceive a discrepancy between where they are and where they want to be' (Miller *et al.*, 1992:8). Motivational interviewing involves working to develop this situation by examining the discrepancies between current behaviour and future goals. That is, clients are encouraged to recognize there is a 'discrepancy' between what they are doing or how they are behaving currently which prevents them from achieving goals. In so doing they become more motivated to make life changes.

In order to create a positive, empathetic atmosphere the authoritarian approach used previously by staff towards Paul was abandoned and a less intrusive role was adopted. Paul was very ambivalent about his diagnosis, so discussions surrounding schizophrenia and medical treatments were avoided. His feelings and perspectives were neither criticized nor judged and the Rogerian principles previously described were employed to develop a therapeutic alliance. His ambivalence towards change was anticipated and was recognized as a normal reaction, since reluctance to give up a particular lifestyle at the commencement of any intervention is perfectly understandable. Change can be daunting. Indeed, if it wasn't, Paul would have probably altered his lifestyle previously. Skilful listening was the key to helping Paul reflect upon his current lifestyle and provided him with an opportunity to review his present behaviour and his broader goals, i.e. where he was currently at, and where he wanted to be in the future. This triggered awareness of the discrepancy between his current behaviour and his longer-term goals, which included 'ditching the voices, wanting a decent flat and a girl-friend'. It was becoming clear to his key worker and the team that Paul wanted a change in his lifestyle and to be relieved of the symptoms he was experiencing.

However, at this stage it was important not to present this formulation to Paul. To override his attachment to his current lifestyle and behaviours, a motivational interviewing approach requires that the emerging discrepancy is owned and utilized by Paul himself. This is because hearing one-self explaining a perceived problem is more persuasive than hearing an explanation from others.

A further principle utilized was that of avoiding potential or actual arguments. While motivational interviewing is recognized to be confrontational in its purpose, it seeks to achieve this by increasing the client's awareness of his or her problems and the need to do something about them. Going 'head to head' with a client is unhelpful, because it may often lead to the client becoming entrenched and defending the opposing viewpoint. In Paul's case this was particularly pertinent, as he had been used to this style of intervention from both his parents and the mental health services. Resistance is strongly predictive of failure to change; therefore avoidance of confrontation was paramount. During the period when Paul was reflecting upon his lifestyle and discussing the pros and cons of changing it, he suddenly became very irritable. It was clear that he had experienced an insightful 'penny dropping experience' (Childs 1993), which had resulted in him feeling both vulnerable and resistive to the envisaged change.

Rolling with such resistance is another key principle of motivational interviewing. What to do about a problem is ultimately a client's responsibility, in this instance another view or goal was not imposed, but new perspectives were invited and Paul was asked to consider and generate other solutions. In this way it was possible to avoid a confrontation-denial trap and move on to consider Paul's belief in his own ability to carry out and succeed with his goal. Indeed it was important to ensure that the change he was contemplating was within his reach. If not, it would be unlikely that he would ever be motivated to make a real attempt to change and any efforts made would be in vain. This process was reinforced by asking open questions, which ranged from, 'What are your worst fears about what might happen if you don't change?' to 'five years ago did you think this is what you would be doing now – how is it different from what you envisaged?' The approach appeared to change Paul's perception of his current situation and thus it was possible to begin to generate some self-motivation statements (change talk). These encapsulated Paul's recognition of the problem, his concerns about it, his intention to change, and provided optimism for his ability to stick with his decision once it had been made. Some examples of Paul's self-motivational statements are given below.

Problem recognition

I like cannabis, but it doesn't like me any more, may be I should think about cutting down.

The voices hassle me, I never really realized how much I hate the way they tell me what to say and do.

Expressions of concern about perceived problem

I am really worried about what I look like to other people, I never thought I would end up like this!

Intention to change

Honestly, I don't want to be like this.

I didn't think I needed to change but now I think I am going to have to!

Expression of optimism

I think I could do this.

I am going to try, I am sure it can't be that hard!

Motivational interviewing is not a stand-alone therapy. It had helped Paul through a difficult period, but once these self-motivational statements had been expressed, the next key step was to connect Paul's new found enthusiasm with a cohesive, practical, collaborative plan of action. To sustain change, a variety of other resources had to be incorporated; it was imperative that Paul perceived the mental health team to be responsive, supportive and able to work alongside him. Hence, he was reintroduced to the team and a clear rationale was provided as to the role each member would play. Subsequently, a thorough assessment of his needs was undertaken and his accommodation and current financial situation were reviewed. Finally, he and his key worker started to examine alternative methods of coping with his voices and it was decided that they should also work with his family, so they could learn additional ways to value and positively reward Paul's efforts.

The lessons learned from this case study can be summarized as follows.

- Therapeutic alliances are paramount and reflective listening is a vital skill which provides clients with the opportunity to verbalize and reflect on experiences.

- Traditional treatment approaches can generate barriers in implementing motivational interviewing.

- Monitoring readiness to change ensures that windows of opportunities are utilized.

- Eliciting and selectively reinforcing self-motivation statements ensures that resistance is not generated by jumping ahead of the client (Miller 1998).

- Motivational interviewing is not a stand-alone therapy; it should work alongside the interventions described below.

Psychological management of psychosis: coping-strategy enhancement, self-monitoring and problem-solving approaches

These interventions draw their techniques from theories of education and methods used in cognitive behavioural therapy. All assume a complex interplay between biological, environmental and sociological factors which suggests that 'ambient stress' together with life events may trigger onset or relapse in some people (Zubin and Spring 1977; Neuchterlein and Dawson 1984).

Cognitive behavioural therapy (CBT) based on a structured form of psychotherapy incorporates problem-solving approaches, which teach clients and their carers ways to cope and alleviate their difficulties and/or symptoms. Thereby it is possible to change thinking errors or biases by appraising situations and stresses and thus clients and their carers are more able to modify assumptions they make about themselves, their experiences and the future (Blackburn and Davidson 1990).

The framework for CBT involves incorporating the ABC model. That is, by examining **A**ctivating events such as, what stresses exacerbate symptoms such as delusions or voice hearing and the **B**eliefs held about those ideas or thoughts, it is possible to understand the emotional or behavioural **C**onsequences that the **B**elief invokes. By understanding and utilizing these principles, it is possible to increase clients' self-esteem and ability to manage symptoms more effectively, thereby reducing levels of stress and anxiety associated with psychotic symptoms and the amount of medication they need (Haddock and Slade 1996).

Over the past decade, a number of studies have been undertaken to ascertain whether CBT-based treatment approaches have a part to play in ameliorating clients' psychotic experiences. In a randomized controlled trial Tarrier *et al.* (1993) compared the effectiveness of coping strategy enhancement (CSE) with problem solving in alleviating residual hallucinations and delusions. Improvements in functioning were noted in both groups and their delusions and levels of anxiety improved. Symptoms such as depression and wider areas of functioning and negative symptoms were not affected. However, the positive gains identified were maintained at six months follow-up and there was some evidence that CSE was superior. Kuipers *et al.*'s (1997) randomized controlled study allocated 60 outpatient clients with medication-resistant symptoms of psychosis to either CBT or standard care. CBT was individualized and lasted for nine months. Improvements were found only in the CBT group, in which there was a 25 per cent reduction in symptoms. Thus it was concluded that CBT could facilitate clients with long histories to talk about the meaning of their psychotic symptoms, which helped to improve their coping strategies and decrease their symptoms.

Other trials have subsequently been conducted with similar positive results (Garety *et al.* 2000), leading researchers to conclude that CBT is a promising new intervention for those who experience psychosis (Gould *et al.* 2001). However, Cormac *et al.*'s (2001) recent meta analysis highlighted that data supporting the wide use of CBT was far from conclusive. Thus, declarations of CBT-based treatment approaches as a universal remedy for psychosis are premature (Cormac *et al.* 2001; Paley and Shapiro 2002). However, research studies undertaken so far have challenged the widely-held view that people with severe and enduring mental health problems cannot learn strategies to cope with their symptoms or gain positive clinical outcomes and have to rely solely on pharmacological treatments.

Coping strategy enhancement

Coping strategy enhancement (CSE) involves undertaking a detailed assessment of a client's psychotic experiences, then constructing highly individualized coping methods to deal with each distressing symptom when they occur (Tarrier 1992). Many clients have developed and learned to use a labyrinth of strategies, such as dismissing, ignoring, selectively listening or distracting themselves from their symptoms and are very able to relay how they use these techniques to get on with their lives. Others may not be aware of doing this, or that it is possible to develop such methods.

CSE provides a pragmatic way of promoting awareness of such symptom maintenance techniques, as the approach involves incorporating cognitive restructuring and behavioural techniques which systematically train clients to think differently about their psychotic experiences, and develop a repertoire of idiosyncratic coping strategies such as thought stopping, focusing versus distraction, verbal challenging and belief modification (Romme and Escher 1993). Thus, clients learn to analyse the effectiveness of chosen techniques, review their limitations and make regular use of the ones they find effective (Yusopoff and Tarrier 1996).

Introducing CSE techniques involves a great deal of diplomacy and expertise and should not be rushed. It takes time for clients to talk about their experiences, especially if their symptoms are pervading and intrusive. Furthermore, it is important to review a client's overall motivation and be aware of the sort of terminology you are using when introducing the idea and rationale for using CSE. The importance of this was demonstrated by the reaction of a client who was being provided with a 'tried and tested' explanation of the learning element involved in the technique. This client, who was preoccupied with his voice-hearing experiences, suddenly responded, 'that sounds too much like school and I didn't learn anything there so I won't be any good at this!' Thereafter, and in spite of every reassurance, he was clearly put off the idea. On reflection it would have been preferable if further exploratory work had been undertaken, indeed perhaps this client's reaction may have been fuelled by his 'voice hearing experiences' which potentially could have been affecting his self-esteem by negatively commenting on his ability to achieve. To overcome such potential barriers Romme and Esher (2000) recommend adhering to the following principles:

- Be willing and able to focus on the client's experiences, remembering that it is they who are the experts, but some may find it difficult to talk about strange and intangible influences in an open way – it requires lots of practice.
- Take a journalistic approach to asking questions – use open questions until the picture is complete – try not to preempt what the client is trying to say and refrain from interpreting material too early. Practise introductions and interviewing – there are pitfalls which only experience can help you negotiate. A story may seem complete – but afterwards it may become clear that something is missing – this is not a disaster and can always be revisited. It will become less of a problem with time; you soon learn to get a sense of what is too vague and needs clarification.

Self-monitoring approaches: relapse prevention

The success of CBT in reducing positive symptoms led to a belief that self-monitoring could be used to help prevent relapse. The early work of Herz and Melville (1980) stimulated this interest as their study showed that by observing changes in thoughts, feelings or behaviours 70 per cent of clients and 93 per cent of families could predict when they, or their relative, were becoming unwell. Symptoms which acted as warning signs included eating less, sleep disruption, concentration problems, depression, seeing friends less, hearing voices, talking in a nonsensical way, thinking someone was controlling them and an increase in religious thinking. Therefore, as self-monitoring involves identifying signs of psychosis, it seemed logical to develop a structured way to help clients identify and manage their individual relapse signatures and offer interventions to prevent florid psychosis

(Spencer *et al.* 2000). This work may be undertaken on a one-to-one basis but a valuable strategy is to incorporate as many key stakeholders as possible. The approach involves five steps:

1   engagement and education;
2   identification of the relapse signatures, such as the signs noted above;
3   development of a relapse drill and a clear framework within which clients and/or their carers can voice their concerns: that is who will do what, when and how if particular signs or symptoms occur;
4   rehearsal and monitoring;
5   clarification of the relapse signature and drill, which involves ensuring that all concerned are aware of and willing to act if the drill is required (Spencer *et al.* 2000).

The first step in relapse prevention is to provide education as this offers one way to engage service users in the development of a collaborative management plan. Furthermore, it provides an ideal way to share goals and establish common ground with staff and services. One approach is to inform the client and his or her carers about the stress vulnerability model by relating stressful events such as, siblings moving away from home, parents divorcing, losing a job, moving house, etc. to particular personal experiences of increased psychosis. Clinical experience shows that clients and carers can learn how to anticipate and manage potentially stressful experiences.

Teaching self-monitoring methods is very rewarding for mental health professionals, particularly when undertaking the work as members of a team working with families. The procedure provides family members and all members of the multi-disciplinary team with opportunities to contribute, so it is highly valued by everyone involved. Information from this process is placed on a chart which incorporates the progression of symptoms, from minor to extreme and outlines what actions can be taken, by whom, and when to prevent escalation. With the client's consent, this chart can be circulated to all the key stakeholders involved in the client's care, and can act as a valuable aide mémoire for them. Sharing information in this way generates an open approach by all those most closely involved in the client's care, and if further potential relapse behaviours emerge, such as the client becoming isolative or withdrawing from usual activities, they can be tackled using a predetermined problem-solving strategy. An example of a self-monitoring and relapse chart is shown in Table 10.5.

Problem solving

As mentioned previously, problem solving is an integral part of a cognitive behavioural approach and a common element in successful PSI programmes, such as family work (Mari *et al.* 1996). Based on structured and comprehensive assessment, problem solving aims to elicit detailed information concerning the nature of the client's and/or carer's difficulties and thus generate specific goals, which can be formulated and tested. By

Table 10.5 Example of a self-monitoring and relapse prevention chart

Stage	Signs noted by client (*C*)	Signs noted by family (*F*)	Signs noted by staff (*S*)	Actions to be taken
3 = Extreme	Become obsessed with my mum. Not wanting her to go out. Not sleeping at all.	Won't leave mum alone. More arguments in the house.	Very irritable, increasingly suspicious and paces.	**C** = try to listen to the advice I am given!!! Don't panic. **F** = arrange a meeting with doctor, encourage to take increase in medication. **S** = monitor, take to clinic if family not able, increase contact to at least daily; liaise with doctor to review medication.
2 = Moderate	Sleep is disturbed.	Slightly clinging to mum, suspicious of other family members.	Becoming unkempt – less likely to go out.	**C** = talk to sister about feelings, ignore voices. **F** = be available to listen. **S** = encourage to go out with me. Feedback observations – encourage doing the actions outlined below.
1 = Mild	Feeling stressed, get cross with my mum.	Has a slightly odd look about the eyes.	Slightly irritable, not as interested in appearance.	**C** = go to bed earlier, take a break, visit mates. **F** = give space, encourage to do slightly less. **S** = reinforce the above, reflect on this in sessions.

identifying the problem or issues that are causing dissatisfaction it is possible to learn systematic methods to solve them and thus instil a sense of control. Ultimately this helps to tackle problems if and when they occur in the future (Hawton *et al.* 1989).

Some problems are easier to solve than others. Before considering how to help others find solutions, it is useful to review our own attitudes towards this skill. We have all encountered problems that we would rather avoid tackling and this is nearly always because we have to confront an emotive aspect of the problem. In these instances we have either wished for a magic wand, tried to brush it under the carpet and/or put off solving the problem until it turns from a molehill into a mountain! Experience tells many of us that in order to sort out problems, you have to detach yourself, address past experiences when you have tried and failed, and overcome a number of fears such as change, confrontation, others' expectations and losing control. This involves motivation and a personal disposition to sort it out amicably. Thus, problem solving involves clear communication, open-mindedness, flexibility and the realization that problems occur as a normal part of life and that finding ways to solve them is a skill that can be learned and practised like any other. Nevertheless, when you are living and dealing with serious mental illness on a day-to-day basis these attributes are hard to sustain especially if everything you try seems not to work. So, in many cases, it is preferable to stay in a state of inertia. It is, therefore, essential before commencing with problem-solving strategies to assess the degree of distress associated with the problem and the client's or carer's motivation to resolve problems. This information is needed to determine the degree of risk associated with problems and to review the chances of achieving realistic solutions.

The first step in teaching clients and carers effective problem solving involves promoting effective communication styles. Falloon and Graham-Hole (1994) advocate teaching these skills through specific behavioural tasks, which incorporate learning how to listen, praise, be assertive and make positive requests. Once these have been put into practice effectively, the likelihood of arguments occurring reduces and it becomes possible to amicably discuss previous coping strategies in response to problems, review past experiences and then move on to formulating a brief description or statement of the current difficulty, as the target for future work. This statement can incorporate behaviours, thoughts, feelings, material circumstances or individuals that the problem is affecting, such as the client, family, nurse, psychiatrist or neighbours.

Overall, the problem statement should indicate clearly who is involved in the problem, and describe specific thoughts, feelings or behaviours that constitute the problem. Those problems judged as having a reasonable chance of achieving improvement in a short time (weeks or perhaps months) should be targeted first, and progress measured.

The second step in a problem-solving approach is to develop a brief description of an agreed goal which the client, carers or practitioners have to pursue. For example:

Problem: John lies in bed all day, he is missing the work scheme he is supposed to attend which causes him to argue with his mother.

Goal: For John to get up every weekday morning by 11.00 a.m., attend the work scheme twice a week for the next month, and avoid arguments with his mother.

Step three is to generate a list of possible solutions, to the afore-mentioned problem statement and goal. The skill, at this stage is to merely devise solutions; not to discuss their pros and cons. Step four involves identifying advantages and disadvantages of the possible solutions. It is not uncommon for some aspects of the different possible solutions to be incorporated together and it is important to be flexible enough to allow an eclectic solution to develop. Figure 10.3 provides some examples of potential solutions to John's problem, and Table 10.6 lists the pros and cons of each.

Through the above process it is possible to choose the best solution which should be valued by all involved, i.e. they should understand the anticipated benefits and agree to its implementation. Furthermore, everyone should be clear about what to do if the best solution generated does not work. Indeed, specific cognitive or behavioural steps should be described and clearly stipulated so the person or people involved know exactly what part they will play. For example:

- John's sister will wake him up with a cup of tea at 8.00 a.m.
- Mum will prompt John at 9.30 a.m., set the alarm and go to work.
- John will get up at 11.00 a.m. and make his own way to the work centre.
- The solution's effectiveness will be reviewed at the next session and in the meantime no one will blame each other if it does not appear to work immediately.

At their next meeting the mental health worker and client, together with

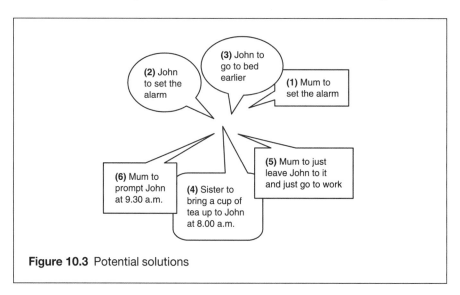

Figure 10.3 Potential solutions

Table 10.6 Advantages and disadvantages of potential solutions

Solutions	Advantages	Disadvantages
1 Mum to set the alarm	Mum would know it would have been set.	Places all the responsibility on Mum.
2 John to set the alarm	Places responsibility on John.	Might forget. Once it's switched off there will be nothing to wake him again.
3 John to go to bed earlier	Wouldn't be so tired in the morning. The house will be quieter.	Difficult to change routine. Miss late-night TV.
4 Sister to bring a cup of tea.	Nice thing to do. Good to see John before I leave for work.	
5 Mum to just leave.	Go to work and be there on time.	Would worry that nothing will change. More arguments.
6 Mum to prompt John at 9.30 a.m.	Would see him awake.	Might cause argument.

others involved, will review progress, identify potential barriers to further progress, and address how these may be overcome by, for example, either redefining the problem or reducing the goal into smaller, more easily accomplished components. When one target problem has been solved, the next is identified by mutual agreement.

In general there are numerous advantages to introducing clients and carers to problem-solving techniques, some of which are described above. However, easily avoided errors can commonly occur when implementing problem-solving strategies. It is important to remember, for instance, that many clients and carers will have tried repeatedly to overcome and cope with a maelstrom of problems, which they may never have had a chance to discuss or resolve, and which may lead them to display strong emotions. Furthermore, some clients and their carers may not consider that they have 'problems', therefore, introducing and using problem-solving terminology may cause irritation.

It is important for mental health care staff to recognize that it takes time for people to change and take on new principles. This highlights the importance of the worker developing therapeutic collaborative relationships with the client and his or her carers, and of utilizing the five general principles of motivation interviewing described earlier before embarking on a problem-solving approach. The preferred approach is to regard problem solving as 'team work' which involves identifying and working with the client's and their carer's personal strengths, resources and the supportive/confiding relationships they have and utilize. Problem solving should also include considering how other professionals might be involved to help clients reduce sources of external stresses, such as poor housing, inadequate finance and unemployment.

Family assessment of needs and intervention

Family work for psychosis is one of the most efficacious of all the PSIs. Over the past 20 years its effectiveness has been intensively evaluated in a number of different settings and cultures. Thus it has been possible to conclude that family work reduces relapse beyond the protection of medication, produces substantial long-term benefits for clients and provides families with the skills to cope more effectively with their relative's illness (Sellwood *et al.* 2001). In addition to incorporating many of the interventions described previously, family work may involve educating the family about the illness, teaching communication skills and problem-solving techniques to cope with symptomatic behaviour and reinforcing family strengths (Mari *et al.* 1996).

In spite of its strong evidence base, family work continues to be a difficult one to integrate into routine clinical practice. Faddon and Birchwood (2002) identify a number of reasons for this. The first appears to be directly related to service provision. Rigid service styles prevent integrating family work into existing caseload demands and practitioners are not routinely given time off in lieu for work undertaken in the evenings (which is when most family members are more likely to be able to participate). Second, there is a general lack of confidence and skill-experience in cognitive behavioural techniques, thus some practitioners feel ill-prepared to keep family sessions on track or tailor the approach to meet the family's needs. Third, professionals may feel themselves unable to deal with the maelstrom of problems professionals think they will encounter if they get involved with families, or they may fear breaching confidentiality or an escalating and unmanageable workload as further problems are unearthed (Leff and Gamble 1995; Furlong and Leggatt 1996; Faddon and Birchwood 2002).

What is clear, however, from clinical experience and the case studies presented in this chapter is that even if clients do not appear to be members of stereotypical families, it is rare to find them completely isolated. We know that family and friends are important in promoting recovery (cf. Chapter 5) and in helping clients find ways of coping (Baker and Strong 2001). Thus, it is essential that professionals overcome rigid working methods, revise their negative fears about undertaking family work, find practical solutions to overcome the risk of breaching confidentiality and embrace clients' families and friends as valued members of the care team.

The following case study of Sophie provides some ideas as to how the issues described may be addressed in order to work with carers more effectively.

Case study: Sophie and her son, Charlie

A referral for family intervention was received via a telephone call from a team who described themselves as 'desperate'. The mother of one of their clients was a 'terrifying, over-protective, management problem' and they needed help! It was agreed that the family workers should visit her to objectively assess her needs. On arriving outside the family home, thoughts of being lynched by an ogre were invoked by the image portrayed by the team. Then an ordinary woman (Sophie) in her late 60s walked up the road and went into the house. She was not 14 feet high and she definitely did not look like she could say boo to a goose. She was affable, welcoming and delighted when the idea of undertaking a comprehensive needs-led assessment was introduced.

The Knowledge about Schizophrenia Interview, which assesses a carer's knowledge about six broad aspects of schizophrenia was completed (Barrowclough and Tarrier 1992). From this it was possible to ascertain that she understood the diagnosis, recognized the positive symptoms and knew what her son was being treated for. She was also aware that its cause was stress related and knew his medication regime, the names of his drugs, the times they should be taken and was clearly worried that he would have problems again. She reported that 'services don't tell me anything and do nothing for him. I can't stop caring – I'm his mother and if I don't look out for him, who will?'

From her responses to the Relatives' Assessment Interview (Barrowclough and Tarrier 1992) it emerged that she was a lone carer who, after emigrating here 20 years ago, was left to bring up seven children on her own. One of her daughters, who still lived with her, had severe hearing problems and she had chronic arthritis. When her son Charlie became ill, she was the only one from whom he would accept medication, therefore the psychiatrist asked for her help. This was one of the main reasons why she now reported walking across town every day to ensure he took his medication. Following discharge, Charlie also experienced housing problems; the ceiling of his council flat fell in and he was without gas or electricity. Despite his mum asking – nothing was done about this for four months. Sophie had to start shouting at service personnel, and when she still wasn't heard she involved a solicitor.

The assessent process had elicited that Sophie was a great advocate, a deeply religious person who provided support not only for her immediate family – but also to her elderly neighbour. She endeavoured to maintain a life of her own; she was undertaking a creative writing course. Furthermore, it was clear that she had a clear set of realistic goals for Charlie – she stipulated that it was essential that he started to be more responsible, learn to take his own medication, take care of his flat and that she would like him to achieve this over the next year. But despite all this, the care team had 'pathologized' her behaviour and she had been labelled as demanding and over protective!

The sessions that followed involved reiterating that, from henceforth, rigid boundaries that had hitherto prevented Charlie's family from being fully involved in his care and care planning would be dismantled. Charlie welcomed this and described how he had previously felt like a 'pig in the middle!' The sessions also involved feeding back and reinforcing the family's strengths and providing all family members, including Charlie, with more information about Charlie's illness, especially with regard to negative symptoms (cf. Chapter 13), which family members reported never having heard of previously. It was clear that Charlie was experiencing some severe negative symptoms, which resulted in him being unable to motivate himself. Thus he had become increasingly socially withdrawn from his supportive family.

Charlie's family were keen to help him overcome these symptoms and were genuinely pleased when intervention ideas were proposed, as this provided them and Charlie with optimism for the future. Hogg (1996) suggests that activity scheduling is one of the simplest and most useful techniques to help clients overcome their negative symptoms. Initially Charlie and his family were encouraged to note down what he did throughout the day. By obtaining this baseline it was possible to monitor change in his activities and his progress. Engaging Charlie in activities that would give him the greatest sense of achievement is key to this work. Therefore, he and his family were asked to brainstorm all the activities he would like to undertake and Charlie was asked to rate on a 0–10 scale how pleasurable he would find them. Going to the gym, going back to college and visiting his mum emerged as Charlie's most pleasurable activities. It was clear that realizing some of these activities would be easier than others. In the short term, it was decided to focus on attending the local gym and visiting his mum. Ways to achieve these were problem solved, using the strategy outlined earlier in the chapter, and various members of his family volunteered to help Charlie to achieve these goals. Charlie's mum was clearly delighted, because increasing Charlie's ability to visit her meant that she would not need to travel across town as frequently as before to ensure that he took his medication.

Mum's dissatisfaction with mental health and other services was also addressed. The family's workers alleviated her concerns by liaising with Charlie's care team, which helped to defuse some of the myths that had been generated about this family previously. In turn, by observing the results that family interventions brought about, the whole multi-disciplinary team began to embrace the philosophy of family work and sought to implement Standard 6 of the *National Service Framework for Mental Health* (Department of Health 1999) (assessing the needs of carers – cf. Chapter 4) and thus integrate it into every client's treatment package.

A personal experience of 'talking therapies': Jacqueline's story

Hitherto this chapter has described the range of psychosocial interventions available, and their application by health professionals to the care of particular clients. The following section considers psychosocial interventions, not from the viewpoint of the professional, but as experienced by a client. There follows a personal account of the experiences of one client who has experienced 'talking therapies' within the context of mental health services:

My experiences as a user of mental health services have been somewhat unexpected. About five years ago, I was a happily-married successful professional planning to start a family. I was in good physical and mental health. Friends, if asked, would probably have described me as a lively outgoing individual who enjoyed socializing and liked to have a laugh and a drink in a variety of social circumstances. I enjoyed my job, and took an especial interest in the mental health list I was developing at the time, through which I was meeting a number of leading authors and practitioners.

The company I was working for was going through a sustained period of change involving major takeovers and changes in personnel. I was fortunate enough to be promoted to a job, which involved a great deal of travelling and considerable extra responsibilities. Within a matter of months, I started to feel the strain; suddenly it seemed as if I would arrive at my desk in the morning, turn on the PC and within an hour was sobbing uncontrollably behind the office door. I couldn't cope and the less I tried, the more insurmountable the workload became. Eventually, I went to my general practitioner (GP), desperate. I had no idea what could possibly be done, but had no idea what else to do. The GP signed me off with 'work-related stress', told me I was depressed (how could I be – I thought that meant staring at the walls?) and put me on Prozac. Bang, problem solved.

For a while, it was a miracle drug. I was back at my desk within a fortnight and felt like a new woman, completely back to my old self – in fact even better. I was the life and soul, confidence brimming, and could have become a passable stand-up comic.

If this sounds too good to be true, it indeed was. A few months later, I found my elation was getting to be a problem in itself. I started to wonder if Prozac might not be contributing to the over-excitement I experienced. I was not feeling depressed any more, so I weaned myself off it.

One of the 'problems' my over-confidence had caused was that I was now engaged in an affair, which my husband had discovered, and we were experiencing considerable marital difficulties as a result. Over the next 12 months, I went into another period of depression, deeper this time and my marriage began to break down irretrievably. During this period I went back on Prozac and was referred by my GP for six counselling sessions with the practice-based counsellor.

My initial reaction to this referral was one of suspicion. I had little belief that counselling would help. Frankly I felt my problems were of my own making and that my depression was my fault. Moreover, it would be 'cured' by Prozac not talking, although that seemed to be taking longer to work this time. My professional background made me quite curious about the approach that would be taken, but almost cynical about the efficacy. As it was, these suspicions appeared to be borne out by the experience.

The counselling itself took place in a room above the GP's, and the counsellor seemed young and inexperienced. My initial assessment of her was 'stereo-typical'. I believed her to be some kind of 'hello trees, hello flowers, hello sky' hippy chick in Laura Ashley, who clearly had no life experience to speak of. Unfortunately, she couldn't explain or justify the 'approach' she was taking although she described it as Rogerian and told me that this meant she would be positive about anything I said. We spent sessions mostly in uncomfortable silence as most of her questions seemed unworthy of response. Any response I gave would generally be repeated back to me parrot fashion in the form of a question. I could see little or no reason to trust her sufficiently to tell her personal or intimate details of my life as to me she lacked credibility, intelligence, or any ability to provide me with any of the 'answers' I so desperately sought. I now see that I was expecting advice, which she of course diligently withheld, and perversely I would never have taken from her anyway. It may seem immaterial, but I was never going to respect anyone who simply couldn't spell which was clear from the notes she showed me. She came across as pleasant, well-intentioned, but ultimately useless. We parted after the six free sessions came to an end.

Despite this experience, after a further year of coping with both the highs and lows, I became intensely depressed once more and had to take several weeks off work. The thought of returning filled me with fear and anxiety and in desperation I began to see another counsellor who I subsequently saw regularly for nearly a year.

From the beginning our relationship was helpful. The counsellor was considerably older than I was and her experience seemed to me to provide a secure environment of trust. She was open and explicit about the aims of counselling and the approach she was taking which she described as 'Rogerian with common sense'. The actual environment was very comforting; a large quiet slightly darkened room, where we both sat. She listened attentively and her questions always seemed pertinent and thought-provoking. She expressed herself well and helped me to do so, often prompting me to explain thoughts in ways I had not previously considered, to see them in new contexts. I was impressed by her apparent ability to recall details from previous sessions, which made the process seem very personal. She was non-judgemental and empathetic, yet did not avoid speaking herself or giving me advice, sometimes of a psychological nature, sometimes very practical. My only criticism, if I have one, is that as the agenda for each meeting was purely mine, the process lacked a certain structure and we would weave seemingly aimlessly across time periods and incidents. However, as I explained earlier, her skill lay in apparently extracting the themes which emerged and attempting to make me see a larger pattern to my thinking. Ultimately though, I was left feeling that we were looking for long-term solutions; for answers that were buried in some distant past that we might never find, while meanwhile my immediate problems in the form of deepening depression re-emerged. The counsellor did provide me with one hugely useful insight into my problems when she suggested that there was a bipolar element to my moods and in her opinion I ought to be seeking more expert psychiatric help than she was able to give.

Fortunately, shortly after this time I was referred to the local hospital and I began to attend a local clinic, seeing a psychiatrist there primarily for depression, which this time was crippling, and I was unable to work for three months.

As the depression began to lift, I was naturally keen to return to work, and anxious that although my employers had been supportive, this was not an open-ended arrangement. Work also meant to me self-esteem and returning to 'normality'. I cannot overstate at this time how important it was to me not to feel as if I had a long-term problem or was in any way 'mad'. One condition of my return was that I had to attend several private sessions with a consultant psychiatrist.

I find it difficult to discuss this experience. I was clearly quite ill and the anti-depressants I had been taking all winter were now swinging me into mania. I did not feel comfortable speaking honestly to someone I perceived to be in the pay of my employers. The formal setting which was intimidating compounded this and the manner of the psychiatrist was patronizing and distant. I was told I was fine and my company was being over-cautious as I was clearly no longer depressed. Just in case, the dose of anti-depressants I was taking was doubled. Striving to keep my job I tried to buy into the relationship. I was grateful to have access to some kind of support at this time, but I had no idea what purpose the sessions served. The relationship did not work, I was made to feel that I was a neurotic malingerer. In turn the psychiatrist often seemed distracted and bored and allowed long periods of silence to develop which I had no idea how to fill. I was galloping towards a major breakdown, he recommended inpatient treatment for what was described as 'treatment resistant alcoholism'. I was naturally terrified and summoned every remaining outward appearance of sanity I had in order to remain in control and to leave the premises.

One aspect I have not included in this account has been the often crucial role of family and friends. This is partly because of the selfish nature of depression which by its very nature turns you completely inwards and away from believing that help is available to you in any form. Compounding this is the fear that it often induces in those close to you who do not know as my mother succinctly put it 'where the old Jackie has gone', and fear the unknown country which mental illness often appears to be. I had some enormously supportive experiences of friendship during this period; people who were prepared to simply be there for me and tolerate having a miserable boring self-obsessed person in their homes through long winter evenings. Conversely, I also discovered that 'advice' from people perceived previously as friends, can be patronizing and destructive, simply confirming and compounding your own sense of worthlessness and inadequacy. Often these are the same people who enjoy the grandeur of your manic self-delusion as they confirm to you that all is well when in fact you are at your most unwell.

Ultimately, however, the important thing for health professionals to be aware of is that mental illness in any individual has a huge impact on their family and social networks, an impact which is often misunderstood or over-looked. There remains an almost Victorian sense that ultimately families provide the safety net for sufferers of mental illness, which in most cases is simply not practical in today's fractured society. How many of you reading this live within an hour's drive of your parents? How many of you come from nuclear families? Most of the time when I have been ill, I have spent alone, partly through choice but mainly through circumstance. Yet paradoxically there has been little or no attempt to involve family or friends in the treatment I have received or to acknowledge their role.

One illustrative example that is worth giving in brief concerns the manic breakdown I experienced. My account of this episode is by definition patchy. I have little recollection of much of the time that had elapsed – it is like a dream, leaving strong impressions which remain intensely vivid now at the time of writing almost exactly a year after the events.

As far as I know I spent a 48-hour period alone in a completely euphoric state experiencing intense delusions and hearing voices. During this period, I was convinced that my friends had planned a huge surprise party for me which was due to begin at any time. A CPN who was scheduled to visit me during this period arrived to assess me. I had been told I should not leave the house in case she arrived, so clearly she was simply a decoy, in fact some kind of minor celebrity brought in to launch the party. Hordes of friends were in hiding around my house, monitoring my every move via the use of Big Brother-type hidden cameras. When she finally arrived, three or four hours after the scheduled appointment time, I delighted in 'playing her game' and teasing her about the true nature of her visit. I was so excited about the party, and very pleased with myself that I had been clever enough to discover their plans. When she left, I felt as if I had been extremely cunning.

I had already spent the morning calling loads of friends, including my ex-husband, none of whom had any idea who to call or how they could help. Luckily a friend who is a senior mental health nurse had been contacted by one of my other friends and she came round to find me now intensely paranoid, cowering in my front room, terrified, knowing above all that I had gone completely mad. The counselling in crisis I received from her at that point was life-saving, literally and metaphorically. My friend spent several patient hours talking me back into something approaching normality and was able to liaise with the mental health services. It is unlikely that most people are as fortunate in their choice of friends as I was in this instance. She talked to me with patience, reassurance, and above all humour which promoted my sense of normality and trust in her and more importantly in myself. It still frightens me to realize now that under other circumstances I would have had to endure this alone.

I had been referred to the clinical psychology team via my psychiatrist at my local hospital in the previous January, but it took until December for this referral to come through. I was depressed following the mania of the summer recounted above (I had also lost my job), and I was as ever cynical about whether anyone could help me. Initially, a clinical psychologist and a student assessed me, and it was explained to me that a cognitive behavioural approach would be used. I knew something of CBT from my work and had heard that it had very positive results for depression in combination with anti-depressant drugs which I was taking once more.

The initial assessment was very reassuring. Both clinicians were open and explicit about the aims of the session and about the therapeutic approach. They explained themselves well and equally listened carefully to my answers to their questions. The session ended with a number of question-naires which I recognized as depression and hopelessness inventories, and I was then reassured that they would be able to help me. Their confidence astounded me at the time: they even put a limit on it – in 8–16 weeks I'd be better!

The therapy itself commenced after the Christmas break. From the out-set, I appreciated the structured nature of the sessions and the fact that the agenda was explicit and clear. Instead of feeling that I had to fill up the sessions, the therapist would provide a structure and guidance to which I contributed where I felt I could. I didn't feel at this stage able to contribute much at all, but I was pleased that we were going to focus on specific problems I was presently experiencing and how to alleviate them rather than dwelling on past problems, or far distant roots of psychological stress. The approach seemed refreshingly practical and grounded. A lot of time was spent in the initial sessions explaining the approach and encouraging me to 'buy into' each stage through understanding how it might work, even if results might take a little longer. The process was broken into manageable, and, above all, negotiated steps, addressing both mental and physical needs, and I was always given handouts to read as well as homework to complete, mostly diaries of my empty days. At each session the therapist was open and encouraging, and explicit in the aims and agenda of each session and what we wished to achieve in the following week. Terminology was explained and supported by reading matter and handouts. I felt supported while in some limited way able to take some charge of my own treatment in a way I hadn't been able to before. Even in a small way I was being encouraged to contrib-ute to and take control of my own well-being. From time to time, I com-pleted further mood inventories and these were used to show me how I was progressing. The benefits of monitoring my own mood changes and their triggers soon became clear and by working through these each week with the therapist, I was able to tackle some immediate negative thought barriers which I had thought not so much impassable as simply an intrinsic part of my life.

So is CBT the ultimate answer? I remain a partial convert. It is by far the most effective talking therapy I have encountered while in deep depression, but it has many downsides. It is intellectually demanding and jargon ridden. I am not a stupid person, but hypothesis testing as a concept is not a simple one, and one of the things you feel when you are depressed is stupid and unable to take on abstract ideas. The book from which my handouts were taken was a US text, no doubt seminal but the examples did not always seem really relevant to my experiences. Over-reliance on the agenda in a session can make the experience seem as if you are both simply working through a checklist and the sessions can seem limited and over prescribed. Most importantly, when you feel the therapy isn't working for you, it is easy to feel that you are simply too dumb to apply it properly and if you were less lazy and worked harder you'd be better. I felt guilty for leaving the homework to the last possible moment, yet that's hardly atypical of my character all my life! And thought records are really hard. Writing and thinking has been part of my professional life for almost 20 years and I found them and still find them a struggle.

My particular circumstances also taint my response to CBT. I was depressed and as ever the depression lifted. As I entered the inevitable following period of mania, the direction of the sessions became less focused. Two things have contributed to this: a lack of apparent understanding on the part of the therapist as to how CBT could be adapted from addressing the problems of depression to those of mania; and my own self-confidence, which in a manic state naturally leads me to assume that I don't need help anyway and that I am suddenly infinitely more intelligent than any therapist. I remain to an extent nervous of how CBT will be able to help me as I inevitably encounter depressive episodes in the future, as it requires self-confidence and analytical abilities that seem to desert me utterly when I'm depressed.

I'd also like to make the point that throughout this period I have also been seeing various psychiatrists to monitor the mood stabilizing medications I am on. Our sessions also involve communication though it is mainly restricted to discussion of the efficacy of medication. However, there is seemingly little or no cooperation or communication between the different personnel involved in my treatment, a situation which is not helped by the fact that both are on six-month rotations. It is left to me to try and keep the other informed of any significant goings on; they don't even share a single file for me. And of course each change in personnel involves a new period of attempting to establish a relationship, which each time feels like a potentially retrograde step.

I have reread what I have written above and would like to try and draw some conclusions. Although my experiences are as for any individual unique, I suspect they are not particularly unusual, and I have in fact been fortunate in the access to talking therapies I have had. However, the most important aspect is not the specific approach taken but the relationship of trust and security and mutual respect established. Acknowledging the reality and validity of the clients' experiences and life-situation, their key social and family relationships is crucial. What having a specific approach then contributes is that the therapist can provide an explicit framework of aims and outcomes, which the client can understand and hopefully buy into, thereby gaining joint ownership of the therapeutic relationship.

Conclusion

This chapter describes the requirements of therapeutic relationships with clients and the range of psychosocial interventions available to help people with severe and enduring mental health problems manage their lives. It includes also a personal account of the experiences of one client of receiving talking therapies within the context of health services.

The main points of the chapter are summarized below:

- A working alliance with a client is a prerequisite to the sensitive and effective application of evidence-based psychosocial interventions in clinical practice.

- The skills required by nurses to develop a working alliance with their patients can be learned and require practice.

- Rogerian principles are widely recognized as fundamental to the development of therapeutic relationships with clients. The challenge for nurses working in stressful health care settings is to demonstrate these principles in their everyday interactions with clients.

- Psychosocial interventions have been defined as formulation-driven interventions that ameliorate a user's or carer's problem associated with a psychosis, using an approach based on psychological principles or addressing a change in social circumstances.

- Formal assessment tools carefully selected and administered sensitively as part of assessment can be reassuring to clients because they demonstrate that mental health staff are seeking to identify and measure their problems accurately as a basis for care planning.

- Motivational interviewing aims to increase a client's ability to recognize and do something about present or potential problems. It is most helpful in cases where clients feel hesitant or are ambivalent to change.

- Coping-strategy enhancement, self-monitoring and problem solving are psychological management approaches for psychosis, which draw upon techniques from educational interventions and cognitive behaviour therapy. They all assume that ambient stress, together with life events may trigger onset or relapse in some people.

- Current research evidence suggests that cognitive behaviour therapy approaches are a very promising intervention for those who experience psychosis, however, their efficacy has not yet been conclusively demonstrated.

- Research findings show conclusively that family work for psychosis can reduce relapse beyond the protection of medication, produces substantial long-term benefits for clients and provides families with skills to cope more effectively with their relative's illness.

Acknowledgements

I am indebted to all the users, carers and those whose reported experiences have helped me shape this chapter, especially Martin Russell at the Department of Health for the disclosure feedback illustration, and Jacqueline Curthoys for her sincere, humbling contribution.

Questions for reflection and discussion

Read Jacqueline's personal account of her experiences of talking therapies, together with the case studies in this chapter and take time to self-reflect and consider the following questions.

(a) Am I willing to take time to listen, learn and communicate unambiguously with users, their significant others and my colleagues?

(b) Do I promote positive attitudes, such as trustworthiness, warmth, caring, liking and respect in my interactions with clients?

(c) Do I understand and encourage people to express their feelings and experiences?

(d) Am I able to utilize the skills and the interventions described in this chapter? If not what attributes, support and guidance do I require to be able to do this?

Annotated bibliography

- Romme, M. and Escher, S. (2000) *Making Sense of Voices: A Guide for Mental Health Professionals Working with Voice Hearers*. London: MIND Publications. This three-part easy to follow manual complements the discussion surrounding many of the interventions referred to in this chapter. The first coherently explains why it is necessary for mental health practitioners to develop new approaches to working with those who hear voices. The second provides step-by-step guidance as to how to interview clients and third, it describes the interventions that can help voice hearers learn how to deal with their experiences, in the short, medium and long term. Finally the appendices contain numerous user-friendly assessment tools.
- Birchwood, M., Fowler, D. and Jackson, C. (2000) *Early Intervention in Psychosis: A Guide to Concepts, Evidence and Interventions*. London: Wiley. This book helps to challenge the belief that early onset schizophrenia is hard to treat. It contains three parts, which cover the concept of early intervention, related strategies and their implementation.
- Lam, D., Jones, S., Haywood, P. and Bright, J. (1999) *Cognitive Therapy for Bipolar Disorder: A Therapist's Guide to Concepts, Methods and*

Practice. London: Wiley. Another excellent book to be published as part of the Wiley series! This has been chosen, as it is the first text to concentrate solely on working with manic depression. It consists of two parts – A and B. A provides readers with a basic knowledge of manic depression, and an overview of the interventions developed so far. B describes the treatment package and gives clear instructions as to how to introduce and use CBT with this client group.

References

Andreasen, N. (1982) Negative symptoms in schizophrenia: definition and reliability, *Archives of General Psychiatry* **39**: 784–8.

Baker, S. and Strong, S. (2001) *Roads to Recovery: How People with Mental Health Problems Recover and Find Ways of Coping*. London: MIND Publications.

Barrowclough, C. and Tarrier, N. (1992) *Families of Schizophrenic Patients: Cognitive Behavioural Intervention*. London: Chapman & Hall.

Birchwood, M., Smith, J. and Cochrane, R. (1990) The Social Functioning Scale: the development and validation of a new scale of social adjustment for use in family interventions programmes with schizophrenic patients, *British Journal of Psychiatry* **157**: 853–9.

Blaauw, E. and Emmelkamp, P.M.G. (1994) The therapeutic relationship: a study of the value of the therapist client rating scale, *Behavioural and Cognitive Psychotherapy* **22**: 25–35.

Blackburn, I. and Davidson, K. (1990) *Cognitive Therapy for Depression and Anxiety*. Oxford: Blackwell.

Bolton, K. and Watt, R. (1989) Motivating Change. *Drug Link*, July/August pp. 8–9.

Bostrom, R.N. (1997) The process of listening, in O. Hargie, *The Handbook of Communication Skills*, 2nd edn. London: Routledge.

Campbell, A. (2000) Evaluation of the West Midlands family intervention programme. Working with Families – Making it a Reality Conference. Stratford-upon-Avon, 20/21 March.

Carhill, J. (1998) Patient participation: a concept analysis, *Journal of Advanced Nursing* **24**(3): 119–28.

Chadwick, P. and Birchwood, M. (1994) The omnipotence of voices; a cognitive approach to auditory hallucinations, *British Journal of Psychiatry* **164**: 190–201.

Childs, D. (1993) *Psychology and the Teacher*, 4th edn. London: Cassell Education.

Cormac, I., Jones, C. and Campbell, C. (2001) Cognitive behaviour therapy for schizophrenia (Cochrane Review), in *The Cochrane Library*, Issue 2, 2002. Oxford: Update Software.

Dennis, S. (2000) Professional considerations, in C. Gamble and G. Brennan, *Working with Serious Mental Illness: A Manual for Clinical Practice*. London: Bailliere Tindall.

Department of Health (1999) *A National Service Framework for Mental Health*. London: The Stationery Office.

Faddon, G. and Birchwood, M. (2002) British Models for Expanding Family Psychosocial Education in Routine Practice, in H.P. Lefley and D.L. Johnson, *Family Interventions in Mental Illness – International Perspectives*. Connecticut: Praeger Publishers.

Falloon, I.R.H. and Graham-Hole, V. (1994) *Comprehensive Management of Mental Disorders*. Buckingham Mental Health Service.

Furlong, M. and Leggatt, M. (1996) Reconciling the patient's right to confidentially and the families need to know, *Australian and New Zealand Journal of Psychiatry* **30**: 614–22.

Gamble, C. (2000) Using a low expressed emotion approach to develop therapeutic alliances, in C. Gamble and G. Brennan, *Working with Serious Mental Illness: A Manual for Clinical Practice*. London: Bailliere Tindall.

Garety, P., Fowler, D. and Kuipers, E. (2000) Cognitive behavioural therapy for medication resistant symptoms, *Schizophrenia Bulletin* **26**(1): 73–86.

Gould, R.A., Mueser, K.T., Bolton, E., Mays, V. and Goff, D. (2001) Cognitive therapy for psychosis in schizophrenia: an effect size analysis, *Schizophrenia Research* **48**: 335–42.

Haddock, G. and Slade, P. (eds) (1996) *Cognitive Behavioural Interventions with Psychotic Disorders*. London: Routledge.

Hawton, K., Salkovskis, P.M., Kirk, L. and Clark, D. (1989) *Cognitive Behaviour Therapy for Psychiatric Problems*. Oxford: Oxford Medical Publications.

Haywood, P. and Bright, J.A. (1997) Stigma and mental illness: a review and critique, *Journal of Mental Health* **6**(4): 345–54.

Herz, M. and Melville, C. (1980) Relapse in schizophrenia, *American Journal of Psychiatry* **137**: 801–12.

Hogg, L. (1996) Psychological treatment for negative symptoms, in G. Haddock and P. Slade (eds) *Cognitive Behavioural Interventions with Psychotic Disorders*, London: Routledge.

James, A. (2001) *Raising our Voices: An Account of the Hearing Voices Movement*. Gloucester: Handsell Publishing.

Kemp, R., Hayward, P., Applewhaite, G., Everitt, B. and David, A. (1996) Compliance therapy in psychotic clients: randomized controlled trial, *British Medical Journal* **312**: 345–9.

Kingdon, D.G. and Turkington, D. (1994) *Cognitive Behavioural Therapy for Schizophrenia*. Hove: Lawrence Erlbaum Associates.

Krawiecka, M., Goldberg, D. and Vaughn, M. (1977) A standardised psychiatric assessment scale for rating chronic psychotic patients, *Acta Psychiatrica Scandinavica* **55**: 299–308.

Kuipers, E., Garety, P., Fowler, D. *et al.* (1997) London-East Anglia randomised controlled trial of cognitive behavioural therapy for psychosis. I: effects of the treatment phase, *British Journal of Psychiatry* **171**: 319–27.

Leff, J. and Gamble, C. (1995) Developing a training for schizophrenia family work: Implications for its implementation into clinical practice, *International Journal of Mental Health* **24**(3): 76–88.

Luft, A. (1988) Johari Window, in F. Quinn, *The Principles and Practice of Nurse Education*. London: Croom Helm.

Mari, J.J., Adams, C.E. and Streiner, D. (1996) Family intervention for those with schizophrenia, in C. Adams, J. De Jesus Mari and P. White (eds) *Schizophrenia Module of the Cochrane Database of Systematic Reviews*, Issue 3. Oxford: The Cochrane Collaboration.

McQueen, A. (2000) Nurse-patient relationships and partnership in hospital care, *Journal of Clinical Nursing* **9**: 732–1.

Miller, W.R. (1983) Motivational interviewing with problem drinkers, *Behavioural Psychotherapy* **2**: 147–2.

Miller, W.R. (1998) Enhancing motivation to change, in W.R. Miller and N. Heather (eds) *Treating Addictive Behaviours: Processes of Change* (2nd edn, pp. 121–32). New York: Plenum Press.

Miller, W.R., Zweben, A., Di Clemento, C.C. and Rychtarik, R.G. (1992) Motivational enhancement therapy manual: a clinical research guide for therapists treating individuals with alcohol abuse and dependence. Rockville, MD: National Institute on Alcohol Abuse and Alcoholism.

Neuchterlein, K.H. and Dawson, M.E. (1984) Information processing and attentional functioning in the developing course of schizophrenia, *Schizophrenia Bulletin* **10**: 160–203.

NHS Executive (1998) Achieving effective practice. A clinical effectiveness and research information pack for nurses, midwives and health visitors. London: DOH.

Paley, G. and Shapiro, D. (2002) Lessons from psychotherapy research for psychological interventions for people with schizophrenia, *Psychology and Psychotherapy: Theory, Research and Practice* **75**: 5–17.

Rogers, C. (1983) *Freedom to Learn for the 80s.* Columbus: Merrill.

Rollnick, S. and Miller, W.R. (1995) What is motivational interviewing? *Behavioural and Cognitive Psychotherapy* **23**: 325–34.

Romme, M. and Escher, S. (1993) *Accepting Voices.* London: MIND Publications.

Romme, M. and Escher, S. (2000) *Making Sense of Voices: A Guide for Mental Health Professionals Working with Voice Hearers.* London: MIND Publications.

Sciacca, K. (1997) Removing barriers: dual diagnosis treatment and motivational interviewing, *Professional Counsellor* **12**(1): 41–6.

Sellwood, W., Barrowclough, C., Tarrier, N. *et al.* (2001) Needs based cognitive-behavioural family intervention for carers for patients suffering from schizophrenia: 12 month follow up, *Acta Psychiatrica Scandinavica* **104**: 346–55.

Snaith, P. (1993) Measuring anxiety and depression, *The Practitioner* **237**: 554–9.

Spencer, E., Murray, E. and Plaistow, J. (2000) Relapse Prevention in Early Psychosis, in M. Birchwood, D. Fowler and C. Jackson, *Early Intervention in Psychosis: A Guide to Concepts, Evidence and Interventions.* London: Wiley.

Stuart, G. (1999) Government wants patient partnerships to be integral part of NHS, *British Medical Journal* **319**: 788.

Tarrier, N. (1992) Management and modification of residual positive symptoms, in M. Birchwood and N. Tarrier (eds) *Innovations in the Psychological Management of Schizophrenia.* Chichester: Wiley.

Tarrier, N., Harwood, S., Yosupoff, L. and Ugarteburu, I. (1993) A trial of two cognitive-behavioural methods of treating drug resistant residual psychotic symptoms in schizophrenic patients: I Outcome, *British Journal of Psychiatry* **162**: 524–32.

Yosupoff, L. and Tarrier, N. (1996) Coping Strategy Enhancement for Persistent Hallucinations and Delusions, in G. Haddock and P. Slade (eds) *Cognitive Behavioural Interventions with Psychotic Disorders.* London: Routledge.

Zwarenstein, M. and Bryant, W. (2002) Interventions to promote collaboration between nurses and doctors (Cochrane Review), in *The Cochrane Library*, Issue 2. Oxford: Update Software.

Zubin, J. and Spring, B (1977) Vulnerability: a new view of schizophrenia, *Journal of Abnormal Psychology* **86**: 260–6.

11

Pharmacological interventions and electro-convulsive therapy

Richard Gray and Daniel Bressington

Chapter overview

The introduction of psychopharmacological treatments since the late 1940s have undoubtedly revolutionized the treatment of psychosis, affective disorders and other mental health problems. As in many other areas of health care pharmacotherapy often requires long-term maintenance treatment to maintain health and prevent relapse. Mental health nurses have always had an important role to play in medication management; working with service users to help them manage their treatment so that it fits in with their lifestyle and maximizes their health. This chapter discusses pharmacological treatments for psychosis, affective disorder and other mental health problems and considers best practice in the light of current evidence. We include a brief section on rapid tranquillization, which is the use of drugs to control acutely disturbed behaviour; Sookoo discusses practical application of this procedure in Chapter 27. The chapter concludes with a section on electro-convulsive therapy, which is the main non-pharmacological physical treatment used to treat psychiatric problems.

This chapter covers the following:

- The brain;
- Pharmacology,
  - Antipsychotics:
    - acute extrapyramidal symptoms and other antipsychotic side effects,
    - clozapine,
    - atypical antipsychotics,
    - the economics of atypical antipsychotics,
    - NICE guidelines on the use of atypical antipsychotics,
  - Anti-depressants,

- Mood stabilizers,
- Anti-anxiety and sedative-hypnotic drugs;

- Rapid tranquillization;
- Electro-convulsive therapy.

The brain

The human brain is one of nature's greatest achievements. At a very simple level the brain is like a computer, it has an input (the sensory nervous system) and an output (the motor nervous system). Between these two systems the brain carries out mental processing such as thought, memory and interpretation of the world about us. However, as in a computer, things can and do go wrong causing neurological or psychiatric problems. The brain can be divided into a number of developmental and functional areas (Figure 11.1). The cerebral cortex at the top is the largest and most advanced region of the brain, responsible for our cognitive and conscious processes. Next is the limbic system, made up of the thalamus, hypothalamus, pituitary, amygdala and hippocampus. It is associated with preservation and emotions (such as fear) and behavioural patterns (such as eating). Below this are the basal ganglia and cerebellum involved in the control of movement at an autonomic level. The final part of the brain is the brain stem. The brain stem is made up of three parts, the pons, the reticular formation and the medulla, and is

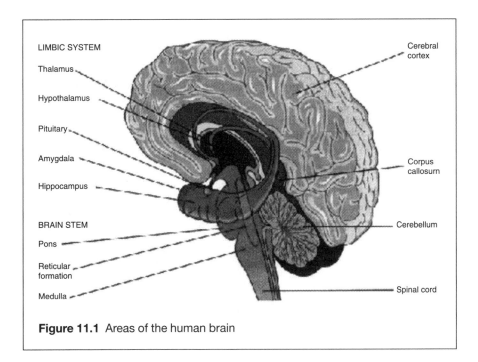

Figure 11.1 Areas of the human brain

continuous with the spinal cord. The brain stem is involved with keeping the person alive at a physiological level, controlling the heart, blood pressure and lungs and other essential functions.

The brain is made from either grey or white matter. Grey matter is made from the cell bodies of brain cells or neurones. White matter is made from the axons of neurones. The brain and the spinal cord are covered by three layers – pia mater, arachnoid mater and dura mater – of membrane called the meninges. The subarachnoid space between two of these layers, the arachnoid and pia mater, is the subarachnoid space containing cerebrospinal fluid (CSF), a watery fluid formed from blood plasma inside the brain that protects the central nervous system.

Blows (2003) has described the pathways between the different parts of the brain that are associated with mental health problems, psychotropic drug activity and medicine side effects. These are set out in Table 11.1.

Table 11.1 Key brain pathways involved in mental health

Pathway	From	To	Importance
Mesolimbic	Brain stem	Limbic system	Psychosis – positive symptoms (hallucinations and delusions)
Mesocorticol	Brain stem	Cerebral cortex	Psychosis – negative symptoms (isolation and withdrawal)
Nigostriatal	Substantia nigra	Corpus striatum	Extrapyramidal side effects
Diffuse modulatory systems	Brain stem	Limbic area and cerebral cortex	Depression and eating disorders
Median forebrain bundle	Brain stem	Frontal lobe of cerebrum	Reward pathways implicated in drugs of addiction
Dorsolateral prefrontal circuit	Frontal lobe	Basal ganglia	Deficits of frontal lobe executive functions
Lateral orbitofrontal circuit	Prefrontal cortex	Caudate nucleus	Involved in mood and personality changes

Neural communication

Neurones are the functional unit of the nervous system. They have a cell body bearing dendrites and an axon (Figure 11.2). All nerve impulses (or action potentials) originate in neurones. Nerve cells communicate with each other via these electrical impulses. An impulse travels along the nerve axon and stimulates the release of chemical messengers known as a neurotransmitter. They are released from storage vesicles in the presynaptic nerve and released into the synapse. The synapse is the gap between the presynaptic cell and the postsynaptic cell at a transmission site (Figure 11.3).

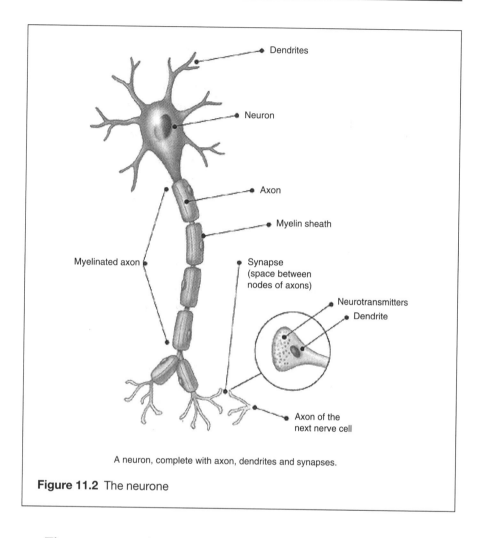

Dendrites

Neuron

Axon

Myelin sheath

Myelinated axon

Synapse
(space between
nodes of axons)

Neurotransmitters

Dendrite

Axon of the
next nerve cell

A neuron, complete with axon, dendrites and synapses.

Figure 11.2 The neurone

The neurotransmitter travels across the synapse and binds with the appropriate receptor on the postsynaptic cell membrane. Receptors are selective cellular recognition sites for neurotransmitters, hormones and many drugs. This usually sets up an electrical impulse (an excitatory effect) in the postsynaptic nerve cell and so the message is passed on. Sometimes neurotransmitters have an inhibitory effect and stop further transmission of the message. After transmission, the neurotransmitter usually leaves the receptor and is taken back up into the presynaptic cell (reuptake) or destroyed by enzymes such as monoamine oxidase (MAO) in the synapse. Some of the most important neurotransmitters in mental disorders are dopamine, serotonin (5-hydroxytryptamine or 5-HT), noradrenaline and gamma-aminobutyric acid (GABA).

It has been hypothesized that over- or under-response within neuro-transmission may be linked with some mental health problems. For example, psychosis may involve excessive dopamine neurotransmission (especially

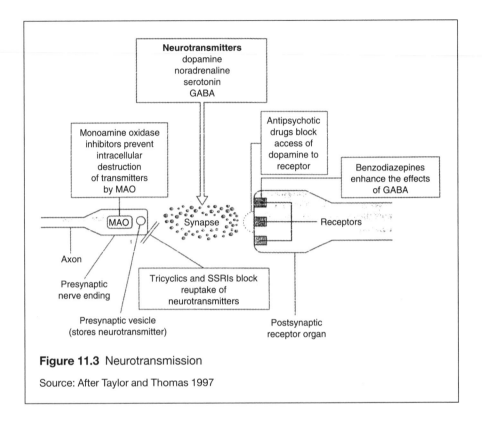

Figure 11.3 Neurotransmission

Source: After Taylor and Thomas 1997

in the mesolimbic pathway) while depression and mania may involve disruption in the normal patterns of neurotransmission of noradrenaline and serotonin. This thinking about neurotransmission has led to the development of a range of pharmacological strategies to try and treat mental health problems. For example, antipsychotic drugs stop the neurotransmitter from binding to the postsynaptic receptor site by blocking those receptors. This reduces the transmission of the message and activity of the nerves in that structure of the brain.

Anti-depressants stop the reuptake of noradrenaline and serotonin and regulate areas of the brain that make them. Monoamine oxidase inhibitors (MAOIs) prevent enzymatic metabolism of noradrenaline and serotonin. Both these actions result in increasing levels available at the synapse, thus increasing the activity between nerve cells. The clinical effects of medicines used in psychiatry do not, however, confine themselves to the specific areas of the brain associated with mental health problems. Medicines will often interact with many other receptors causing unwanted symptoms or side effects and potential drug interactions during concomitant drug therapy.

Pharmacology

It is important that practitioners have an understanding of the effect of the drug on the body (pharmacodynamics), the effects of the body on the drug over time (pharmacokinetics) and the cross ethnic, cross racial profiles (pharmacogenetics).

Antipsychotics

Antipsychotic medication has been the mainstay of treatment for schizophrenia since the 1950s when it was discovered that the dopamine antagonists – haloperidol and chlorpromazine – exert antipsychotic effects.

Dopamine is a neurotransmitter mainly associated with reward and control of movement. A deficit of dopamine (as a result of the degeneration of the substantia nigra in the mid-brain) results in Parkinsonism. This is characterized clinically by movement disorders including tremor, shuffling gait, stiffness and bradykinesia (slowed movement). Excessive dopamine results in symptoms of psychosis such as delusional beliefs and hallucinations. This can be demonstrated by administration of L-dopa (the precursor of dopamine) or amphetamines (dopamine agonists) in healthy subjects.

The dopamine hypothesis of schizophrenia proposes that excessive dopamine activity or hyperdopaminergia is associated with the pathophysiology of schizophrenia. Therefore reducing this activity should reduce symptoms. Drugs that are known to block these receptors, specifically of the mesolimbic dopamine pathway (Figure 11.4) are advocated as treatment for psychotic symptoms. This is supported by reports that the clinical potency of antipsychotics is proportional to the extent to which they block dopamine receptors.

Some reports suggest that a high affinity for D_2 receptors may not be the only basis for efficacy in antipsychotic agents. Although these drugs typically occupy these receptors within a few hours of administration, there is often a 1–3 week delay before therapeutic benefits are reported. This suggests that these drugs act via a series of secondary, and as yet unknown, processes that evolve over days to weeks. There are suggestions that a number of other neuroreceptors, peptides and amino acid systems may be involved. This is further supported by the fact that changes in systems other than the dopamine system have been implicated in the aetiology of schizophrenia (Gray 1999).

Chlorpromazine, the first effective pharmacological treatment for the symptoms of schizophrenia was introduced during the 1950s. Since then, a variety of antipsychotic agents have been developed (for example, haloperidol, trifluoperazine and sulpiride) some of which are available in a long-acting depot formulation (for example, flupenthixol and zuclopenthixol). Controlled clinical trials have repeatedly shown that these drugs are generally efficacious for the positive symptoms of schizophrenia. About

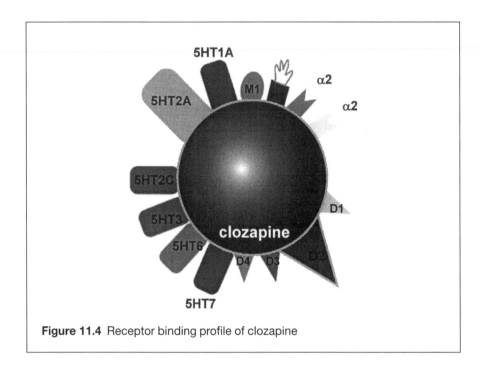

Figure 11.4 Receptor binding profile of clozapine

eight out of ten patients can expect to get some benefit from treatment, typically about a 50 per cent reduction in positive symptoms (hallucinations and delusions). However, blockade of D_2 receptors of the mesocortical dopamine pathway may make some negative symptoms (isolation and withdrawal) worse. Tolerability problems, especially acute extrapyramidal symptoms (EPS) (dystonia, akathisia and Parkinsonism) are common with these so-called conventional agents. Acute EPS has proved to be one of the most problematic side effects caused by these older medicines and to an extent defines them.

Acute EPS

Acute EPS refers to Parkinsonism, dystonia and akathisia, which develop soon after the initiation of antipsychotic treatment. Drug-induced Parkinsonism resembles idiopathic Parkinson's disease in many ways, manifesting itself as rigidity, tremor, postural abnormalities and bradykinesia. Although motor symptoms are the most prominent feature of Parkinsonism the mental effects, bradyphrenia (slow thinking) and cognitive impairment (mental clouding), are equally important as they impair patients' ability to undertake the activities of daily living. The most prominent feature of drug-induced Parkinsonism is rigidity of limbs, which are resistive to passive movement (cogwheel rigidity). Bradykinesia (or akinesia) is characterized by a reduction in spontaneous facial movement. This presents itself as decreased facial expression, a flat monotone voice, decreased arm swing during walking, and an inability to initiate movement.

Acute dystonic reactions are abnormal postures produced by sustained contorting and twisting muscle spasms. The muscles of the neck and head are most frequently affected. Symptoms include sustained contraction of the masticatory muscles (trismus), forceful sustained eye closure (blepharospasm), facial grimacing, oculogyric spasm (brief fixed stare, followed by upward and lateral rotation of the eyes so that only the sclera remain visible), dysarthia, dysphagia, glossopharyngeal constrictions and torticollis. Rarely abnormal movements of the limbs, with dystonic arm movements or gait are seen. Although dystonic reactions are generally fairly obvious, mild symptoms may go unnoticed.

Akathesia (literally can't sit still) is characterized by a subjective sense of inner restlessness, mental unease, unrest or dysphoria. This is commonly accompanied by a characteristic pattern of restless movements including rocking from foot to foot, walking on the spot, and shuffling and tramping of the legs. In severe cases, patients pace rapidly and are unable to sit or lie down for more than a few minutes.

Substantial variation in the course of each EPS has been reported. Acute dystonic reactions occur most commonly within 12 to 48 hours of initiating or substantially increasing antipsychotic treatment, akathesia typically occurs within a few hours or days of starting treatment, and Parkinsonism usually does not emerge for several days or weeks.

In a much-cited study, Ayd (1961) surveyed 3,775 patients treated with both high- and low-potency conventional antipsychotic drugs and reported that 38 per cent of the sample developed acute EPS. There appears to have been a steady increase in the prevalence of acute EPS in the past 30 years. This is almost certainly due to the increased use of higher doses of high-potency antipsychotics.

Although the presentation and incidence of acute EPS has been well described, the underlying pathophysiological mechanisms are far from clear. Antipsychotics' affinity for blocking dopamine receptors of the nigrostriatal pathway is generally cited as the underlying cause of acute EPS. Since all antipsychotics are potent dopamine D_2 antagonists it is often concluded that this characteristic is inexorably linked to acute EPS, although acetylcholine and, potentially, serotonin have an important, and as yet unclear, role to play.

The prevalence of acute EPS may be affected by a number of specific demographic and clinical variables. Dystonia appears to be affected by both age and gender. Young males have a significantly greater risk of developing dystonia. Akathesia and Parkinsonism are twice as common in women and almost all older patients develop Parkinsonism.

Treatment of acute EPS

The treatment of acute dystonia and Parkinsonism is broadly similar and is generally treated in two ways, dose titration, or more commonly, via the addition of other pharmacological therapies. The recognition that EPS, at least in part, results from dopamine/acetycholine imbalance secondary to dopamine blockade (Borrison 1985) has led to the widespread clinical use of anticholinergic drugs that reduce cholinergic activity. With anticholinergics, it is their antimuscarinic properties that explain their efficacy in EPS (Barnes and McPhillips 1996). A number of controlled studies have established the efficacy of anticholinergics in the treatment of acute Parkinsonism (Korsgaard and Friis 1986) and dystonia (Goff *et al.* 1991). Although anticholinergic drugs are commonly used prophylactically to prevent the onset of EPS the evidence for this strategy is weak, although in young patients such a strategy might be useful.

Anticholinergics are themselves associated with a range of side effects including dry mouth, blurred vision, constipation, tachycardia, urinary hesitancy or retention, and erectile dysfunction in men or failure of vaginal lubrication in women (Barnes and McPhillips 1996). Anticholinergics may also provoke or exacerbate tardive dyskinesia. Rebound phenomena including nausea, abdominal pain, restlessness and insomnia, and akinetic depression have been reported following the rapid cessation of anticholinergics. However, perhaps the most worrying effect of anticholinergics is their impact on cognitive functioning. Cholinergic blockade produces cognitive deficits similar to those observed in normal ageing. Anticholinergics may have specific effects on patients' short-term memory and their ability to sustain attention.

Acute Parkinsonism and dystonia respond relatively well to treatment with anticholinergics. Akathisia, however, responds in a less than satisfactory way. β-blockers (for example propranolol) have been shown to be effective in treating akathisia. Research has also shown that benzodiazepines are an effective treatment for akathisia, although their mode of action remains unclear.

The evidence for the efficacy of dose titration as a strategy for managing acute EPS is also uncertain. Data from studies using Positron Emission Tomography (PET) suggest that, *in vivo*, clinical response is achieved when 50–60 per cent of striatal D_2 receptors are blocked, but EPS only emerges when >80 per cent are blocked (Nordstrom *et al.* 1993). This suggests that a reduction in the dose of an antipsychotic to within this therapeutic window of D_2 blockade should minimize acute EPS. This hypothesis has not, however, been tested in large-scale clinical trials.

Given the specific efficacy and side-effect profile of anticholinergics and other drugs used to treat EPS their administration by mental health nurses on an as required (PRN) basis must be carefully considered. However, this does not appear to be the case. Gray *et al.* (1997) observed that 16 per cent of all administrations of PRN medication were for anticholinergic drugs. However, they were often administered in response to patients' request and without a formal assessment. There was also evidence of inappropriate administration. For example, anticholinergics were commonly given to treat dry mouth, blurred vision or restlessness.

Other antipsychotic side effects

Antipsychotics are also associated with a range of other common side effects that can be predicted by their receptor binding profile. The blockade of dopamine D_2 receptors in the Tuberoinfundibular dopamine pathway will cause an increase in prolactin levels and can cause sexual dysfunction, amenorrhoea in women, and gynocomastia.

The blockade of muscarinic (M1) receptors by many antipsychotic medicines causes characteristic anticholinergic symptoms that include dry mouth, blurred vision, sedation and constipation. The blockade of histamine (H1) receptors can cause sedation and weight gain. Antipsychotics can also cause a rare and potentially fatal idiosyncratic dose-independent drug reaction called neuroleptic malignant syndrome (NMS). The main symptoms are hyperthermia or fever and severe muscle rigidity. The incidence is unknown but may occur in up to 0.15 per cent of people treated with antipsychotics. There are many other side effects that are associated with antipsychotics that have not been discussed in this chapter.

Long-term effects

Many people who take antipsychotic medication are concerned about the long-term effects. For a long time it has been known that antipsychotics can cause tardive dyskinesia and, in a very few people, sudden death.

Tardive dyskinesia

Tardive (late onset) dyskinesia is characterized by abnormal oral and facial movements such as sucking or smacking, lateral jaw movements and flicking of the tongue. It is generally thought that 5 per cent of people treated with typical antipsychotics will develop these symptoms with each year of exposure to the medicine. Tardive dyskinesia is probably associated with dopamine blockade of the nigrostriatal pathway within the basal ganglia. Risk factors for tardive dyskinesia include:

- increasing age;
- increasing duration of illness and drug therapy;
- female gender;
- persistent negative symptoms;
- the presence of an affective disorder; and
- concurrent diabetes.

Tardive dyskinesia, especially when more severe, will make people stand out and contributes to the stigma of mental illness generally and schizophrenia specifically. It is important to remember that movement disorder similar to those seen in people with tardive dyskinesia have been observed in never treated individuals with schizophrenia.

Unexplained death

Unexplained sudden cardiac death in people taking antipsychotic drugs has long been a cause for concern. A search of the Medicines Control Agency (MCA) database for reports of unexpected sudden death with antipsychotic drugs from date of first marketing to 10 May 1996 found 31 reports of sudden death and 63 reports of fatal cardiac arrest arrhythmia (Gray 2001b). Antipsychotic drugs used in the treatment of schizo-phrenia are diverse and many affect cardiac function, causing relatively 'minor' adverse events such as postural hypotension, palpitations and tachycardia.

However, more serious arrhythmias, arising from prolonged QTc, and sudden death have also been associated with the use of some, but not all, antipsychotic drugs. These events have been reported to the Committee for Safety of Medicines (CSM) since the 1960s and have been a source of debate and concern among psychiatric health care professionals as the extent of the role of these drugs in cardiac events.

Prolonged QTc is a delay in ventricular repolarization, the key electrical event that prepares the ventricle for the next contraction. One of the ways in which this abnormality shows itself is by a lengthening of the QT interval on the ECG trace. The QT interval runs from the beginning of the QRS complex to the end of the T wave and represents the time between the onset of electrical depolarization of the ventricle and the end of repolarization. The QT interval varies according to the heart rate and correcting for this variation gives the QTc value or rate-corrected value.

At what point does QT interval become dangerous?

A study has shown that QTc prolongation (>420 milliseconds) is signifi-cantly more common (23 per cent) in a sample of chronic inpatients with schizophrenia receiving antipsychotic drugs than in age-matched drug-free controls (2 per cent). A QT interval that is longer than 500 milliseconds is considered dangerous and is associated with life-threatening arrhythmias and sudden death (Gray 2001a).

A particularly lethal cardiac arrhythmia known as *torsade de pointes* (Td P) has been implicated as a cause of sudden death in patients taking certain antipsychotic drugs.

The unacceptable side-effect profile of antipsychotic medicines and a lack of efficacy in treating negative symptoms has prompted further research into the development of improved novel and atypical agents such as clozapine, risperidone, olanzapine and quetiapine.

Clozapine

Clozapine is the original atypical antipsychotic. It was first marketed in the 1970s, to great excitement. It was said to avoid many of the drawbacks of conventional medicines; it reduced both positive and negative symptoms;

it was associated with few extrapyramidal symptoms (EPS), and it was effective for people who had not responded to other medicines. Unfortunately in 1975, 21 out of 6,100 people treated with clozapine in northern Europe developed agranulocytosis (a blood dyscrasia), and clozapine was voluntarily withdrawn from the market by the manufacturers.

Nonetheless, the advent of clozapine marked an important advance in the treatment of schizophrenia, and introduced to psychiatry the term 'atypical' to describe a new class of antipsychotic medicine. In 1988 a pivotal multi-centre trial demonstrated that clozapine was far more effective than conventional neuroleptics for people with so-called treatment-resistant schizophrenia (Kane *et al.* 1988). Subsequent studies have confirmed clozapine's efficacy in treating the positive and negative symptoms of schizophrenia with few EPS. In 1990 it was introduced to the UK, with strict guidelines for haematological monitoring because of the associated risk of agranulocytosis.

Clozapine has an effect on a complex and wide range of neurotransmitters including dopamine, serotonin, adrenergic, histaminic and muscarinic (Figure 11.5). As a result, clozapine is associated with a wide range of difficult-to-manage side effects of which the most clinically important are severe sedation (especially early on in treatment), hypersalivation, hypotension and seizures. However, for many patients the benefits of clozapine outweigh the problematic side effects.

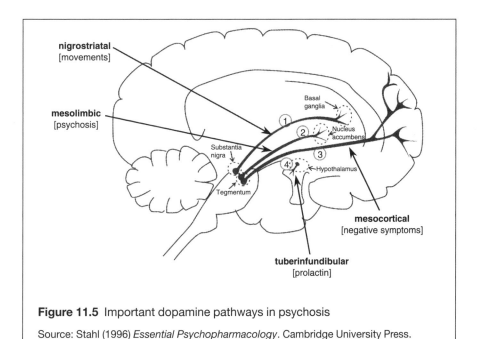

Figure 11.5 Important dopamine pathways in psychosis

Source: Stahl (1996) *Essential Psychopharmacology*. Cambridge University Press.

Additional benefits of clozapine

An improvement in quality of life is a frequently reported clinical observation in people with schizophrenia taking clozapine. Clinical observations suggest that perhaps more than any other drug clozapine enables people with schizophrenia to reintegrate back into society. Part of the reason why clozapine improves quality of life is because it improves cognitive functioning. Cognitive functioning has long been recognized as a feature of schizophrenia that may contribute to impaired social functioning. Treatment with conventional neuroleptics has been shown to produce only minimal improvement in – and may even impair – cognitive function. Several studies have examined the effects of clozapine on cognitive functioning and found improvements in, for example, attention and verbal fluency (Gray *et al.* 1997).

Atypical antipsychotics

Modern treatments that are safer and cause fewer side effects than typical antipsychotics or clozapine are clearly needed. Over the past decade a number of new atypical antipsychotics have been introduced to the UK. The first was risperidone in 1993, followed by sertindole in 1996, olanzapine in 1997 and most recently quetiapine in 1998. By definition, atypical antipsychotics cause fewer EPS; in fact they are no more likely to do so than a placebo drug (Gray and Gournay 2000). However, that is not to say that they are side-effect free. In fact, one of the atypical antipsychotics, sertindole, was voluntarily withdrawn by its manufacturers in 1998 because of fears over cardiac safety; nine patients treated with sertindole in the UK had died. Clinical experience with risperidone, olanzapine and quetiapine over a number of years has shown them to be exceptionally well tolerated (Gray 1999). Problems caused by raised prolactin, such as sexual dysfunction and period problems in women, are rare although these symptoms have been seen in some patients taking risperidone (Gray 1999). Risperidone can also cause postural hypotension, especially during the early part of treatment. Olanzapine and quetiapine are clearly sedative, and anticholinergic effects such as dry mouth and blurred vision are occasionally seen in patients taking olanzapine. Importantly, risperidone, olanzapine and quetiapine do not have the cardiac side effects reported with sertindole, thioridazine or droperidol (Gray 2001b). Finally, in the long term, atypical antipsychotics seem to cause much less tardive dyskinesia than traditional antipsychotics (Gray and Gournay 2000).

Additional benefits of atypicals

A dramatic reduction in side effects is not the only difference between conventional and atypical antipsychotics. When the data from a large number of clinical trials are pooled together it is clear that risperidone (Kennedy *et al.* 2000), olanzapine (Duggan *et al.* 2001) and quetiapine (Srisurapanont *et al.*

2004) are effective treatments for schizophrenia producing clinically meaningful improvements in symptoms. However, they are no more effective at doing this than conventional antipsychotics such as chlorpromazine or haloperidol. Emerging evidence suggests, however, that atypicals may be more effective than typicals (probably because of enhanced treatment adherence) at preventing relapse. There is also interesting emerging evidence that atypical antipsychotics may also be effective in treating negative symptoms such as social isolation and withdrawal (Tollefson *et al.* 1997) although further, long-term trials are needed to establish this effect. There is also interesting preliminary work suggesting that atypicals may also be useful in treating cognitive symptoms (Fujii *et al.* 1997), reducing violence and aggression (Rabinowitz *et al.* 1996), suicidality (Duggan *et al.* 2003) and perhaps most importantly, as with clozapine, improving patients' health-related quality of life (Franz *et al.* 1997). Based on this compelling evidence the most recent edition of the Maudsley prescribing guidelines (Taylor *et al.* 2001) recommends that atypical antipsychotics should be the treatment of choice for people with schizophrenia.

Issues in the prescribing of antipsychotics

Despite the obvious benefits to patients of atypical antipsychotics many psychiatrists and general practitioners continue to rely on older traditional drugs. In fact, probably only 25 per cent of UK patients are currently prescribed atypical drugs (Frangou and Lewis 2000). Alarmingly, those who are fortunate enough to get the new drugs are also likely to be getting the conventional drugs at the same time – so-called antipsychotic polypharmacy. For example, it is not uncommon to see patients prescribed risperidone, plus zuclopenthixol decanoate (depot Clopixol), plus as required (PRN) droperidol and procyclidine. Such prescribing practice makes little logical sense, is not grounded in any evidence and, most importantly, will not bring any additional health benefits to the patient.

Many clinicians report that they continue to use the conventional drugs because they have more experience with them and are concerned that there is not enough evidence about the safety of the atypicals. However, in the case of risperidone there is almost a decade of clinical experience and as Welch and Chue (2000) observe it is fallacious to say that the older drugs are safer when, primarily because of issues surrounding cardiac safety, it is highly unlikely that they would be approved for clinical use today.

The economics of atypical antipsychotics

Perhaps another reason why clinicians do not prescribe modern treatments is because of the cost of new drugs. Traditional drugs such as haloperidol or chlorpromazine only cost a few pounds for a month's supply of medication. Atypical antipsychotics are considerably more expensive. For example, at average clinical doses the price of atypical antipsychotics ranges from £117 per month for risperidone to £241 per month for clozapine (Taylor 2001). It is possible to curb these costs by using the lowest possible effective dose, for example 4mg/day of risperidone has been shown to work well in many patients and reduces the monthly cost of medication to £77. Primarily on economic grounds, the Maudsley prescribing guidelines (2001) suggests that risperidone should be the first choice antipsychotic for people with schizophrenia (Taylor 2001). Even if used carefully, if atypical antipsychotics are to be used first line there will be a substantial economic burden to the NHS and less money will be available to spend on other areas of mental health care.

Formulations

A final possible explanation of why atypical antipsychotics have not been more widely used is because of the formulations that are available. Many clinicians prefer to use medications that can be given as a long-acting injectable depot preparation (Walburn *et al.* 2001) primarily because they believe that compliance and therefore outcomes are better when the drug is given this way. Whether this belief is true and whether patients find this route of administration acceptable is unclear (Walburn *et al.* 2001). However, most atypicals are currently only available as tablets that are administered orally (some, such as risperidone, are also available as a syrup). Depot versions of atypical antipsychotics are being developed. A long-acting (two-weekly) version of risperidone was launched in 2002, and a depot version of olanzapine is expected soon.

The National Institute for Clinical Excellence (NICE) and antipsychotics

Based on the evidence that is available in the UK, much of which has been discussed in this chapter, NICE have recommended the following clinical practice guidelines for the treatment of schizophrenia and specifically about the use of atypical antipsychotics. The key points from NICE make excellent recommendations for practice:

- The choice of drug should be made jointly between the individual and the clinician involving the carer if appropriate.
- Atypical antipsychotics are the first line treatment for schizophrenia.
- Individuals on typical antipsychotics should be considered for atypical drugs if they experience unpleasant side effects.
- Clozapine is the treatment of choice for treatment-resistant schizophrenia.
- Clinicians should undertake a concordance assessment. If there is a risk of non-concordance a long-acting formulation may be indicated.
- The atypical antipsychotic with the lowest purchase price should be used if there is a choice.
- Antipsychotic medication is part of a comprehensive package of care.

• Atypical and typical antipsychotics should not be prescribed concurrently.

(NICE 2000a, 2000b)

Anti-depressants

It has been proposed that depression is caused by a reduction in either serotonin or noradrenaline and mania by an excess of noradrenaline. MAOIs (monoamine oxidase inhibitors) effectively inhibit the metabolism of these neurotransmitters (Figure 11.3) while tricyclic anti-depressants and SSRIs (selective serotonin reuptake inhibitors) prevent their reuptake at the pre-synaptic neurone (Figure 11.3). Both these mechanisms increase the amount of neurotransmitter at the synapse. Although this theory is widely taught to mental health nurses there are a number of substantial problems with it. Perhaps most importantly is the observation that 20–30 per cent of depressed service users do not derive any benefit from the medicines. Although mainly used in the treatment of depression and related mental health problems there is evidence that they may also be useful in the treatment of other illnesses such as obsessive compulsive disorder. It is important to remember that all anti-depressant medicines may take 4 to 6 weeks to begin to work and service users cannot expect to realize a quick response to treatment.

Tricyclic anti-depressants (TCAs) have been the mainstay for the treatment of depression for many years. Although clearly very effective in the treatment of depression it has long been known that they are poorly tolerated (common side effects include sedation, weight gain and anticholinergic symptoms) and, because of cardio-toxicity, are potentially fatal in overdose. Perhaps because of tolerability problems psychiatrists and general practitioners have tended to prescribe doses of TCAs that are known to be sub-therapeutic. Over the past decade their use in both primary and secondary care settings has reduced dramatically.

TCAs have now been largely replaced by SSRIs (such as citalopram, fluoxetine and sertraline) a group of drugs that inhibit the reuptake of serotonin at the presynaptic membrane promoting the neurotransmission of serotonin in the brain. Because they have specific affinity for serotonin receptors they have little effect at the transmission sites for other receptors and consequently are as effective as TCA but have fewer side effects. Venlafaxine is another newer anti-depressant and is a SNRI (selective noradrenaline reuptake inhibitor). It increases levels of both serotonin and noradrenaline, and although claims of increased efficacy have been made for this medicine in practice it appears to be equally as effective as SSRIs and TCAs. SSRIs do not cause many of the side effects associated with traditional TCAs and they are much safer in overdose. The main side effects associated with SSRIs are nausea and agitation; they have also been associated with sexual dysfunction in both men and women and, less commonly, dry mouth and sedation.

The final group of anti-depressant drugs to consider are monoamine oxidase inhibitors (MAOIs; for example, phenelzine and tranylcypromine).

Although they have been available for many years, and are generally well tolerated, they have not been widely prescribed because clinicians are worried about the hypertensive crisis when tyramine-containing foods and some other medicines are taken with these drugs. More recently moclobemide, a new MAOI, has been marketed. Unlike previous MAOIs it only temporarily inhibits monoamine oxidase and consequently the tyramine reaction is substantially reduced and there are no dietary restrictions.

Implications for clinical practice

Mental health nurses should note:

- Anti-depressants are effective in the treatment of depression.
- SSRIs are safer and better tolerated than TCAs.
- It takes several weeks for anti-depressant to begin to ameliorate depressive symptoms.

Mood stabilizers

Mood stabilizers are the most widely used drugs to treat bipolar affective disorder and other related conditions such as unipolar depression and schizoaffective disorder. There is also evidence that lithium is effective in treating some non-affective mental health problems such as borderline personality disorder. Lithium has been the front-line drug for bipolar disorder for many years although increasingly carbamazepine and sodium valproate are becoming more popular. There is also emerging evidence that some other drugs – most notably the atypical antipsychotics clozapine, olanzapine and risperidone – may also be effective in the treatment of bipolar disorder.

Lithium has been used as a mood stabilizer since the late 1940s when it was first recognized to have anti-manic properties. However, the exact mechanism of action is poorly understood. It has been proposed that lithium corrects ion exchange abnormality, alters sodium transport in nerves and muscle cells, normalizes synaptic neurotransmission of noradrenaline and changes receptor sensitivity. Lithium can be a complex drug to use. At high doses it can cause renal damage and reduce renal function. Hypothyroidism is also seen in service users taking lithium even at therapeutic doses. The maintenance dose for lithium must be individually tailored and carefully monitored and adjusted over time. Lithium is associated with a range of acute (such as tremor and fatigue), and long-term (such as thyroid dysfunction) side effects as well as the potential for toxicity (a clinical emergency).

Typically lithium is a first-line treatment. However, two anticonvulsants, carbamazepine and sodium valproate, have been shown to be effective mood stabilizers. Typically these drugs are only used if service users have not responded to lithium therapy or if it is contraindicated.

Implications for clinical practice

- Lithium is an effective mood stabilizer but requires close monitoring.
- Lithium toxicity is an emergency situation.
- Carbamazepine and sodium valproate are also well tolerated and effective mood stabilizers.

Anti-anxiety and sedative-hypnotic drugs

Benzodiazepines are the most widely prescribed group of drugs in the world although in recent years their popularity has waned because of their potential to cause tolerance and dependence. Benzodiazepines have a wide range of uses including anxiety, anxiety-related phobias, alcohol withdrawal and sleep disorders. They are also widely used in the treatment of acute agitation and aggression in services users with psychosis.

Benzodiazepines (for example, diazepam, lorazepam and temazepam) reduce anxiety by potentiating the inhibitory neurotransmitter GABA. There are few clinical differences between the different types of benzodiazepines except for different half lives (the time for the plasma level of the drug to reduce to half of peak level). Overdoses of benzodiazepines are almost never fatal (unless taken in conjunction with other central nervous system depressants such as alcohol and opiates) and the effect can be reversed by the specific antagonist, flumazenil. Side effects are rare and tend to be dose related. When used regularly tolerance increases therefore people need higher doses to obtain the same level of symptomatic relief. Prolonged use can result in physical dependency. Withdrawal symptoms range from insomnia and anxiety, to extreme agitation and convulsions. It may be fatal if not treated appropriately. However, if prescribed over a short term (around two weeks) dependence should not be an issue, especially if treatment is stopped gradually. It is also useful to advise service users to use benzodiazepines intermittently rather than regularly to reduce the risk of tolerance and dependence.

The use of barbiturates has largely been replaced by benzodiazepines as anti-anxiety and sedative-hypnotic drugs because of tolerability and safety issues (the range between therapeutic and toxic dose, leading to coma and respiratory arrest, is very narrow). Two drugs that are not structurally related to benzodiazepines and are licensed for the treatment of insomnia are zopiclone and zolpidem. Other drugs that may be useful anti-anxiety and sedative-hypnotic drugs include some antihistamines, propranolol and buspirone.

Rapid tranquillization

Rapid tranquillization (RT), the use of drugs to control acutely disturbed behaviour, is a high-risk and anxiety provoking procedure for both patients and professionals. It is a treatment of last resort when all other attempts to de-escalate disturbed behaviour have either been ineffective or are inappropriate. Each time RT is used, the risk of the patient harming themselves or others must be balanced against the potential side effects of drug interventions. Decisions may need to be taken rapidly as a situation evolves. Surveys of RT have consistently found practice to be idiosyncratic and suboptimal. A wide range of drugs and doses are used and polypharmacy is common, as is high dose prescribing (Mannion *et al.* 1997). There is also confusion regarding the desired outcome from RT and the timeframe over which it is expected that this will be achieved. Droperidol was widely used in RT (Pilowsky *et al.* 1992) and is the recommended antipsychotic in the current edition of the Maudsley prescribing guidelines (Taylor 2001). Although all antipsychotics have the potential to prolong the QTc interval in vulnerable patients, a renewed interest in the potential magnitude of this effect with droperidol led to its sudden withdrawal from use in early 2001 and widespread replacement by haloperidol. Although this action may seem to be in the best interests of the patient, it may have caused further confusion over drug choice in RT allowing more idiosyncratic practices to develop. Sookoo discusses the practical application of RT in Chapter 27.

Electro-convulsive therapy (ECT)

The main non-pharmacological physical treatment used to treat psychiatric problems is ECT which has been defined as: a medical procedure in which a brief electrical stimulus is used to induce a cerebral seizure under controlled conditions (Enns and Reiss 1992).

ECT was introduced in 1938 by Cerletti and Bini (Cerletti 1940) to treat severe psychosis and soon became the treatment of choice for the maintenance of chronic schizophrenia. After the development of antipsychotic medication, ECT was mainly used to alleviate severe affective disorders (Enns and Reiss 1992). Although there is a large body of literature from early studies many are seriously methodologically flawed. Early experiments using genuine ECT and 'sham' ECT as a control showed no benefit of using ECT in people with chronic psychosis. In people with depression there is robust evidence from systematic review and meta analysis that ECT is probably more effective that drug therapy (cf. LAN 361, 799–808). The main concerns with ECT are about its side effects.

The National Institute for Clinical Excellence (NICE) and ECT

NICE guidance (2003) recommends that ECT is used for treating only severe symptoms in people suffering with depression, catatonia or a prolonged and severe manic episode, and then only after an adequate trial of other treatments or because of life-threatening conditions. The decision to use ECT should adhere to strict recognized guidelines on informed consent, and the involvement of advanced directives, advocates and carers must be taken into account. The current evidence available does not support the use of ECT in the management of schizophrenia, the guidance recommends the development of national information leaflets and is to be reviewed in 2005.

Conclusion

In this chapter we have proposed that currently medication is the mainstay of mental health treatment. Modern medicines can offer safe and effective symptom reduction and relief for service users suffering from a range of mental health problems. Mental health nurses have a vital role to play in working in a collaborative partnership with service users in exploring and working through the multi-faceted concept and process of medication concordance.

In summary, the main points of this chapter are:

- Pharmacological treatments have revolutionized the treatment of mental health problems and are currently the mainstay of mental health care.

- Novel antipsychotics and anti-depressants are better tolerated and may offer efficacy advantages over older treatments.

- Many service users are concerned about psychiatric medicines and often stop taking them causing unnecessary morbidity; appropriate pre-scribing and a range of strategies can improve symptoms and quality of life.

- There is robust evidence that ECT is more effective than drug therapy for people suffering from depression, but it is not recommended for the treatment of schizophrenia. The main concerns with ECT are about its side effects. Any decision to use ECT should adhere to strict recognized guidelines on informed consent and the involvement of advanced directives, advocates and carers must be taken into account.

Questons for reflection and discussion

1   Reflect on each of the following and consider what elements of each may influence compliance with medication:

    (a) the person;
    (b) the illness/condition;
    (c) the medication/s.

2   Consider the rationale for the usage of medication. Could there be any negative effects from improving compliance?

3 Put yourself in the position of a person taking medication that gives you a feeling of inner restlessness, less energy and considerable weight gain. What changes would you like to make? How would you do this? What help might you need? How could you tell if things had improved?

4 Medications and ECT have side effects; there is a cost-benefit to usage. Think of a person you have known or nursed who has received one of these treatments. Make a list, one of the costs and the other of the benefits of the treatment that was used. What is your conclusion? Now give each element in the columns a weighting, from 1 (not important) to 8 (very important) then add the columns up. Are your findings the same? Has this highlighted any other issues?

Annotated bibliography

- Rollnick, S., Mason, P. and Butler, C. (2000) *Health Behaviour Change – A Guide for Practitioners*. China: Churchill Livingstone. This book offers a patient-centred framework for any behaviour change. The authors promote the idea of a generic change method and have looked for common ground across theories and models: motivational interviewing, problem-solving and brief solution-focused therapy. The result is a collection of strategies, rather than a discrete method. Some strategies have been evaluated while others have not.
- *Journal of Mental Health Practice*. Volume 6: 6. This volume focuses on the medication use in the treatment of schizophrenia. Two articles discuss the concept of psychopharmacology in relation to differing models of mental disorder in contemporary practice.
- Faulkner, A. and Layzell, S. (2000) *Strategies for Living: A Report of User-led Research into People's Strategies for Living with Mental Distress*. London. Mental Health Foundation. This report builds on the work of a large user-led survey and gives an understanding of how people live, cope and manage mental distress. Further reports and links can be found on the Mental Health Foundations website.

References

Ayd, F.J. (1961) A survey of drug induced extrapyramidal reactions, *JAMA* **175**: 1054–60.

Barnes, T.R.E. and McPhillips, M.A. (1996) Antipsychotic induced extrapyramidal symptoms. Role of anticholinergic drugs in treatment, *CNS Drugs* **6**(4): 315–30.

Blows, W.T. (2003) *The Biological Basis of Nursing: Mental Health*. London: Routledge.

Borrison, R.L. (1985) Amantadine in the management of extrapyramidal side effects, *Clinical Neuropharmacology* **6** (Supplement 1) 557–63.

Cerletti (1940) L'electroshock, *Rivista sperimentale di freniatria* **64**: 209–310.

Duggan, A., Warner, J., Knapp, M. and Kerwin, R. (2003) Modelling the impact of clozapine on suicide in patients with treatment-resistant schizophrenia in the UK, *British Journal of Psychiatry* **182**: 505–8.

Duggan, L., Fenton M., Dardennes, R.M. *et al.* (2001) Olanzapine for schizophrenia (Cochrane Review), in *The Cochrane Library*, Issue 2. Oxford: Update Software.

Enns, M.W. and Reiss, J.P. (1992) Electroconvulsive therapy, *Canadian Journal of Psychiatry* **37**(10): 671–8.

Frangou, S. and Lewis, M. (2000) Atypical antipsychotics in ordinary clinical practice: a pharmaco-epidemiologic survey in a South London survey, *European Psychiatry* **15**(3): 220–6.

Franz, M., Lis, S., Pluddeman, K. and Gallhofer, B. (1997) Conventional versus atypical neuroleptics: subjective quality of life in schizophrenic patients, *British Journal of Psychiatry* **170**: 422–5.

Fujii, D.E., Ahmed, I., Jokumsen, M. and Compton, J.M. (1997) The effects of clozapine on cognitive functioning in treatment-resistant schizophrenic patients, *Journal of Neuropsychiatry and Clinical Neuroscience* **9**(2): 240–5.

Goff, D.C., Arana, G.W. and Greenblatt, D.J. (1991) The effect of benzotropine on halperidol induced dystonia, clinical efficacy and pharmacokinetics: a prospective double blind trial, *Journal of Clinical Psychophamacology* **11**(2): 106–12.

Gray, R. (1999) Antipsychotics, side effects and effective management, *Mental Health Practice* **2**(7): 14–20.

Gray, R. (2001a) Medication for Schizophrenia, *Nursing Times* **97**(31): 38–9.

Gray, R. (2001b) Medication related cardiac risks and sudden deaths among people receiving antipsychotics for schizophrenia, *Mental Health Care* **4**(9): 302–4.

Gray, R. and Gournay, K. (2000) What can we do about extrapyramidal symptoms? *Journal of Psychiatric and Mental Health Nursing* **7**(3): 205–12.

Gray, R., Robinson, D. and Smedley, N. (1997) Nursing interventions with long term clients, in B. Thomas, S. Hardy and P. Cutting, *Stuart and Sundeen's Mental Health Nursing Principles and Practice*. London: Mosby.

Kane, J., Honigfeld, G., Singer, J. and Meltzer, H. (1988) Clozapine for the treatment-resistant schizophrenic. A double-blind comparison with clorpromazine, *Archives of General Psychiatry*, **45**: 789–96.

Kennedy, E., Song, F., Hunter, R., Clarke, A. and Gilbody, S. (2000) Risperidone versus atypical antipsychotic medication for schizophrenia (Cochrane Review), in *The Cochrane Library*, Issue 4. Oxford: Update Software.

Kosgaard, S. and Friis, T. (1986) Effects of manserin in neuroleptic-induced Parkinsonism, *Psychopharmacology*, **88**: 109–11.

Mannion, L., Sloan, D. and Connolly, L. (1997) Rapid tranquillisation: are we getting it right?, *Psychiatric Bulletin* **21**: 411–13.

NICE (2002a) Guidance for the use of newer (atypical) antipsychotic drugs for the treatment of schizophrenia, *NICE Technology Appraisal Guidance 43*. London: National Institute for Clinical Excellence. www.nice.org.uk

NICE (2000b) *Schizophrenia: Core interventions in the treatment and management of schizophrenia in primary and secondary care*. London: National Institute for Clinical Excellence. www.nice.org.uk.

NICE (2003) Guidelines on the use of electroconvulsive therapy, *NICE Technology Appraisal Guidance 59*. London: National Institute for Clinical Excellence. www.nice.org.uk

Nordstrom, A.L., Farde, I., Weisel, F.A. *et al.* (1993) Positron emission tomographic analysis of central D_1 and D_2 dopamine receptor occupancy in patients treated with classical neuroleptics and clozapine: Relations to extrapyramidal side-effects. *Archives of General Psychiatry* **49**: 538–44.

Pilowsky, L.S., Costa, D.C., Ell, P.J. *et al.* (1992) Clozapine, single photon emission tomography and the D2 dopamine receptor blockade hypothesis of schizophrenia, *Lancet* **340**: 199–202.

Rabinowitz, J., Avnon, M. and Rosenberg, V. (1996) Effects of clozapine on physical and verbal aggression, *Schizophrenia Research* **22**(3): 249–55.

Srisurapanont, M., Disayavanish, C. and Taimkaew, K. (2004) Quetiapine for schizophrenia (Cochrane Review), in *The Cochrane Library*, Issue 1. Chichester, UK: John Wiley & Sons.

Stahl, S.M. (1996) *Essential Psychopharmacology*. Cambridge: Cambridge University Press.

Taylor, D., McConnell, D., McConnell, H. *et al.* (2001) *The South London and Maudsley NHS Trust 2001 Prescribing Guidelines*. London: Martin Dunitz.

Taylor, D. and Thomas, B. (1997) Psychopharmacology, in B. Thomas, S. Hardy and P. Cutting (eds) *Stuart and Sundeen's Mental Health Nursing*. London: Mosby.

Tollefson, G.D., Beasley, C.M. Jr, Tran, P.V. *et al.* (1997) Olanzapine versus haloperidol in the treatment of schizophrenia, schizoaffective and schizophreniform disorders: results of an international collaborative trial, *American Journal of Psychiatry* **154**(4): 457–65.

Walburn, J., Gray, R., Gournay, K., Quaraishi, S. and David, A. (2001) Systematic review of patient and nurse attitudes to depot antipsychotic medication, *British Journal of Psychiatry* **179**: 300–7.

Welch, R. and Chue, P. (2000) Antipsychotic agents and QT changes, *Journal of Psychiatry and Neuroscience* **25**(2): 154–60.

12

Complementary and alternative therapies

Hagen Rampes

Chapter overview

This chapter describes the contribution of complementary and alternative therapies to the treatment and care of people suffering from mental health problems. It is written from the perspective of a psychiatrist in the National Health Service who is trained in a number of complementary and alternative therapies. The chapter covers the following:

- What are complementary and alternative therapies?
- Prevalence, and why patients use complementary and alternative therapies.
- Which complementary and alternative therapies benefit which conditions?
- Complementary and alternative therapies used among patients with psychiatric disorders:
    - acupuncture;
    - homeopathy;
    - herbal medicine;
    - aromatherapy.
- Research and complementary and alternative therapies.
    - qualitative studies;
    - systematic reviews.
- Placebo.
- Complementary and alternative therapies and the *National Service Framework for Mental Health*.

What is complementary and alternative therapy?

What is considered complementary and alternative therapy in one country may be considered conventional medicine in another. The Cochrane Collaboration (The Cochrane Library 2003) defines complementary and alternative therapy as a 'broad domain of healing resources that encompasses all health systems, modalities, and practices and their accompanying theories and beliefs, other than those intrinsic to the politically dominant health systems of a particular society or culture in a given historical period'. These practices: promote health, prevent and treat illness, complement conventional medicine by contributing to a common whole, satisfy a demand not met by conventional medicine, and diversify the conceptual framework of medicine. Examples of complementary and alternative therapies are listed in Box 12.1.

The National Center for Complementary and Alternative Medicine which is a department of the National Institutes of Health established by the Congress of the United States of America, classifies complementary and alternative therapies into five categories or domains:

Alternative medical systems

Alternative medical systems are built upon complete systems of theory and practice. Often, these systems have evolved apart from and earlier than conventional medicine in the West. Examples of alternative medical systems that have developed in Western cultures include homeopathic medicine and naturopathic medicine. Examples of systems that have developed in non-western cultures include Ayurveda and Traditional Chinese medicine.

Mind–body interventions

Mind–body medicine uses a variety of techniques designed to enhance the mind's capacity to affect bodily function and symptoms. These techniques include meditation, prayer, mental healing and therapies that use creative outlets such as art, music or dance.

Biologically based therapies

Biologically based therapies in complementary and alternative therapy use substances found in nature, such as herbs, foods and vitamins. Some examples include dietary supplements or herbal products.

Manipulative and body-based methods

Manipulative and body-based methods in complementary and alternative therapy are based on manipulation and/or movement of one or more parts of the body. Some examples include chiropractic or osteopathic manipulation and massage.

Box 12.1 Examples of complementary and alternative therapies

Treatments a person largely administers to himself or herself

Botanicals
Nutritional supplements
Health food
Meditation
Magnetic therapy
Treatments providers administer
Acupuncture
Massage therapy
Reflexology
Laser therapy
Balneotherapy
Chiropractic
Osteopathy
Psychological counselling certain types
Naturopathy

Treatments a person administers to himself or herself under the periodic observation of a provider

Yoga
Biofeedback
Tai Chi
Homeopathy
Hydrotherapy
Alexander therapy
Nutritional therapy
Ayurveda
Qi gong
Anthroposophical medicines
Unani medicine
Traditional African medicine
Bach flower remedies
Clinical ecology
Colon cleansing or irrigation
Music or sound therapy

Diagnostic techniques

Iridology
Kinesiology
Vega testing
Biofunctional diagnostic testing
Electroacupuncture by Voll
Hair analysis

Energy therapies

Energy therapies involve the use of energy fields. Biofield therapies are intended to affect the energy fields that surround and penetrate the human body. The existence of such fields has not been scientifically proven. Some forms of energy therapy manipulate biofields by placing the hands in or through these fields. Pressure or manipulation may be applied to the body. Examples include qi gong, reiki and therapeutic touch. Bioelectromagnetic-based therapies involve the unconventional use of electromagnetic fields, such as pulsed fields, magnetic fields, alternating current fields or direct current fields.

Prevalence of the use of complementary and alternative therapies

Survey data suggest that complementary and alternative therapy is used by a sizeable proportion of the population in a number of countries. Figures reported for some European countries in the early 1990s are between 20 per cent and 50 per cent. A study from Germany reported an overall prevalence rate for complementary and alternative therapy use of 65 per cent in 1996, which compared to a corresponding figure of 52 per cent in 1970 (Haussermann 1997). These figures are the highest reported anywhere. However, it is noteworthy that therapies such as herbal medicine, hydrotherapy and massage are firmly established in conventional medicine in many European countries.

An estimate of prevalence for the USA in 1997 was 42 per cent (Eisenberg *et al.* 1998). It is noteworthy that the US data demonstrate an increase in the use of complementary and alternative therapy during the last decade and it is reasonable to assume that this is reflected elsewhere.

It is estimated that in 1993, 8.5 per cent of the adult population in England had visited at least one complementary and alternative therapy provider of acupuncture, chiropractic, homeopathy, hypnotherapy, herbal medicine or osteopathy during the past 12 months (Thomas *et al.* 1993). This figure increased to 10.6 per cent in 1998 using similar methodology, suggesting a slower growth than that reported by Eizenberg in the USA over a similar time period. However, if data for reflexology, aromatherapy and remedies purchased over the counter were included in the analysis then the estimated one-year prevalence increased to 28.3 per cent. In this sample, the frequency of use was greatest for osteopathy (4.3 per cent) and chiropractic (3.6 per cent). Other popular therapies included aromatherapy (3.5 per cent), reflexology (2.4 per cent), acupuncture (1.6 per cent) and herbal medicine (0.9 per cent). Over 4 million adults made 18 million visits to practitioners of one of six therapies: acupuncture, chiropractic, homeopathy, hypnotherapy, herbal medicine or osteopathy in England in 1998. The National Health Service (NHS) provided about 10 per cent of these contacts. The majority of non-NHS visits represented direct out-of-pocket expenditures (Thomas *et al.* 2001).

Why patients use complementary and alternative therapies

Given the growing popularity of complementary and alternative therapy and the fact that the majority of complementary and alternative therapy use represents out-of-pocket expenditure, the issue of why people use complementary and alternative therapy is important. There are many different reasons. One important finding that has been reported consistently (Druss and Rosenheck 1999) is that the majority of complementary and alternative therapy use does not occur instead of conventional medicine care, but in addition to it. Patients report using conventional medicine for some complaints and complementary and alternative therapy for others. Patients may also choose to use complementary and alternative therapy alongside conventional medicine.

Explanations for complementary and alternative therapy use

Furnham (1996) has summarized the main hypotheses relating to why people use complementary and alternative therapies. Some he described as push factors. These include dissatisfaction with or outright rejection of conventional medicine through prior negative experiences or a general anti-establishment attitude. For these reasons, patients are pushed away from conventional treatment in search of alternatives. Other factors pull or attract patients towards complementary and alternative therapy. These include compatibility between the philosophy of certain therapies and patients' own beliefs and a greater sense of control over one's own treatment.

Kaptchuk and Eisenberg (1998) suggest that there are fundamental premises of most forms of complementary and alternative therapy, which contribute to its persuasive appeal. One of these is the perceived association of complementary and alternative therapy with nature. Complementary and alternative therapy is natural, pure and organic, whereas conventional medicine is artificial, synthetic and processed. Another fundamental component of complementary and alternative therapy is vitalism. The enhancement or balancing of 'life forces' known as qi, prana or psychic energy is central to many forms of complementary and alternative therapy. Another factor is spirituality. This bridges the gap between the domain of medical science with its search for causality and the domain of religion with its morals and values. Complementary and alternative therapy thus offers a satisfying unification of the physical and spiritual.

Another proposed explanation is that patients using complementary and alternative therapy are essentially neurotic and are drawn towards the touching or talking approach of many therapies. While levels of psychiatric disorder are reported to be high in patients visiting complementary and alternative therapists, and higher than those visiting a general practitioner (GP), this may simply be a reflection of the nature of the conditions being treated.

Several studies (Finnigan 1991; Resch *et al.* 1997) have compared patients' views of consultations with practitioners of conventional medicine and complementary and alternative therapy. Most studies have found complementary therapy practitioners to be perceived by patients as more friendly and personal, to have treated patients more like partners in care, and provided more time for the consultation. Patients were also more satisfied with the therapeutic encounter. The duration of consultation for complementary and alternative therapy is invariably longer than with conventional medicine; in Finnigan's (1991) study 68 per cent of patients reported a better relationship with the complementary and alternative practitioner than with their own GP. The hard-pressed GP can offer only a 10-minute consultation. Complementary and alternative therapy consultations involve more discussion and explanation than that offered by conventional medical practitioners in the NHS.

In general, complementary and alternative therapy does not replace conventional medicine. Rather it serves as a substitute in some situations and as an adjunct in others, while being disregarded when not considered appropriate for the condition in question. This has been described as 'shopping for health'. Patients simply perceive complementary and alternative therapy as one of a range of treatment options available to them and exercise their freedom of choice and discriminating power accordingly. The desire to try all available options may be for some an attempt to leave no stone unturned as they become increasingly desperate for an effective treatment.

Astin's (1998) survey of 1500 North Americans found a number of predictors of complementary and alternative therapy use. Complementary and alternative therapy users were more likely than non-users to be better educated, have a holistic orientation to health and report current poor health status. Their main complaints were anxiety, back problems, chronic pain and urinary tract infections. They had often had an experience that had changed their world-view. They were also more likely to be committed to environmentalism, feminism, spirituality and personal growth.

Astin found that dissatisfaction with conventional medicine was not predictive of use of complementary and alternative therapy. However, in addition to being more educated and reporting poorer health status, most complementary and alternative therapy users find these health care approaches more congruent with their own values, beliefs and philosophical orientations towards health and life than conventional medicine.

Which complementary and alternative therapies benefit which conditions?

Long *et al.* (2001) surveyed complementary and alternative therapy organizations to establish which therapies they recommend for particular medical conditions. The respondents were asked to list conditions they felt benefited most from their use of complementary and alternative therapy, the most important contra-indications, and the typical costs of initial and any subsequent treatments.

Aromatherapy, Bach flower remedies, hypnotherapy, massage, nutrition, reflexology, reiki and yoga were all recommended as suitable treatments for stress or anxiety. Long *et al.* (2001) report that there was supporting clinical evidence of varying methodological quality for all these therapies except reiki. They concluded that alternative therapy organizations were a reliable source of guidance to health care professionals wishing to advise or refer patients interested in using complementary and alternative therapy.

Complementary and alternative therapy use among patients with psychiatric disorders

Davidson *et al.* (1998) conducted a study to determine the frequency of psychiatric disorders in a random sample of patients receiving complementary medical care in the UK and the USA. Patients were randomly recruited from two sites. The UK study was conducted at the Royal London Homoeopathic Hospital. The North American component was conducted at a private complementary and alternative therapy practice in Durham, North Carolina. Patients were interviewed for demographic information and lifetime and current psychiatric disorders using a structured clinical interview.

Fifty patients (mean age 52.5, 79.6 per cent female) were interviewed in London and 33 (mean age 46.9, 78.8 per cent female) in North Carolina. Only 35.7 per cent of the patients in the British sample were married, whereas 66.7 per cent of the patients in the American sample were married. Of the British patients 78.3 per cent were white (13 per cent were Asian and 8.7 per cent were Black) whereas 100 per cent of American patients were white. Fifty-six per cent of the British patients had graduated from sixth form whereas 100 per cent of the American patients had graduated from high school.

Rates of lifetime psychiatric diagnoses revealed a total of 74 per cent of the British patients having a diagnosis and 60.6 per cent of the American patients. Major depression (52 per cent of UK and 33.3 per cent of USA) and any anxiety disorders (50 per cent of UK and 33.3 per cent of USA) were the commonest lifetime diagnoses. Only post-traumatic stress disorder was significantly different (UK was 10 per cent and the USA was 33.3 per cent). Rates of current psychiatric disorder revealed 46 per cent of the UK patients and 30.3 per cent of the US patients having a diagnosis. Six per cent of the total suffered from a major depression and 25.3 per cent of the total met the criteria for at least one anxiety disorder, with social phobia and generalized anxiety being the commonest. Social phobia was significantly more common in the US patients. While generalized anxiety disorder, simple phobia and major depression occurred more often in the UK patients, these were not significantly different from the US patients. The demographic differences of ethnic, marital and education status may have been due to the sources of recruitment. The authors found that psychiatric disorders were not rare among patients who sought complementary medical care and that anxiety disorders were particularly represented.

The Mental Health Foundation's *Knowing Our Own Minds* survey (1997) of mental health service users' views on complementary and alternative therapy found that of the 401 users who participated, 37 per cent had received osteopathy, acupuncture, massage, aromatherapy or reflexology. Of these, 85 per cent had found the therapies helpful. Thirty-one per cent had experienced exercise, yoga or movement therapy, of whom 85 per cent had found it helpful. Twenty-seven per cent had received nutritional therapy, homeopathy, naturopathy or herbal medicine; 63 per cent of whom found it helpful. In each of these groups 2–5 per cent found the therapies unhelpful and 1 per cent found them harmful.

What respondents valued most about complementary and alternative therapies was their relaxing and holistic nature. Some respondents found that the most helpful approach was to combine a number of different therapies and activities. In summary the survey found that mental health service users experienced complementary and alternative therapy as helpful in providing symptom relief and improving general health.

Some of the more popular alternative therapies are discussed below with particular reference to their contribution to the treatment of mental disorders.

Acupuncture

What is acupuncture?

Acupuncture encompasses differing philosophies and techniques. Acupuncture is the stimulation of special points on the body, usually by insertion of fine needles. How the points to be treated are selected depends on the teaching and background of the practitioner. At one end of the spectrum is the Traditional Chinese Medicine acupuncturist, who operates from a theoretical paradigm different to Western Conventional Medicine. Traditional Chinese Medicine includes the use of acupuncture, herbs, massage and dietary approaches. It has a belief in a vital force or 'Chi'. Disease results from imbalance of this 'energy'. The body has a number of 'energy' channels or meridians on which lie the acupuncture points. Traditional acupuncture theory sees illness in terms of excess or deficiencies in various exogenous and endogenous factors and treatment is aimed at restoring balance.

At the other end of the spectrum is the 'Scientific' or Western acupuncturist, who has divorced the Chinese theoretical basis of acupuncture and instead uses a set of acupuncture points to treat a variety of conditions empirically. Auriculo-acupuncture, i.e. acupuncture of the ears, although known to the Chinese, is a relatively new development advanced by Western doctors.

Following insertion of needles at acupuncture points, further stimulation of the points can be achieved by: manual stimulation of the needle by rotation, application of heat to the needle by burning the herb *artemisia vulgaris* over the needle (moxibustion) or by applying an electric current to a pair of needles (electro-acupuncture). Electro-acupuncture is a modern development, which the Chinese also use. Other developments include the use of lasers to stimulate acupuncture points.

Is acupuncture safe?

A review by Rampes and James (1995) revealed that serious adverse effects of acupuncture have been reported ranging from trauma to underlying organs (for example pneumothorax: puncture of the lung cavity) to infections (hepatitis B). Most serious adverse effects are preventable by appropriate practitioner training. In the past, practitioners used reusable needles, which required careful sterilization. Unfortunately, poor sterilization resulted in several outbreaks of hepatitis B worldwide. Overall, the conclusion of the review was that acupuncture is relatively safe.

Is there a role for acupuncture in mental illness?

There are Chinese studies on the treatment of mental illness with acupuncture. Unfortunately, the methodological quality of these studies is very poor. The majority are uncontrolled and do not meet the 'gold standard' of research for evaluating treatments, which is the randomized control trial. In the West, there have been a number of studies in the field of addiction: smoking, opiate and alcohol dependence and abuse. There appears to be a role for the use of acupuncture in the treatment of addiction. The use of acupuncture should be with a specific aim, for example to reduce craving for the addictive substance. Electro-acupuncture may have a useful role to play in the treatment of anxiety and depression and addiction. There is some evidence that electro-acupuncture (depending on the frequency of the current) modulates neurotransmitters such as dopamine and serotonin in the brain.

Acupuncture in smoking cessation

Acupuncture and related techniques are promoted as a treatment for smoking cessation in the belief that they may reduce nicotine withdrawal symptoms. White *et al.* (2003) conducted a review determining the effectiveness of acupuncture and the allied therapies of acupressure, laser therapy and electrostimulation, in smoking cessation in comparison with: (a) sham treatment, (b) other interventions, or (c) no intervention. A comprehensive literature search was conducted to identify all relevant clinical trials. Only randomized trials comparing a form of acupuncture, acupressure, laser therapy or electrostimulation with either sham treatment, another intervention or no intervention for smoking cessation were included in the review. Data were extracted and analysed in a standardized manner.

The authors assessed abstinence from smoking at the earliest time-point (before 6 weeks), at 6 months and at 1 year or more follow-ups in patients smoking at baseline. The authors used the most rigorous definition of abstinence for each trial, and biochemically validated rates if available. Those lost to follow-up were counted as continuing to smoke.

The authors identified 22 studies. Acupuncture was not superior to sham acupuncture in smoking cessation at any time point. The odds ratio (OR) for early outcomes was 1.22 (95 per cent confidence interval 0.99 to 1.49); the OR after 6 months was 1.50 (95 per cent confidence interval 0.99 to 2.27) and after 12 months 1.08 (95 per cent confidence interval 0.77 to 1.52).

Similarly, when acupuncture was compared with other anti-smoking interventions, there were no differences in outcome at any time-point. Acupuncture appeared to be superior to no intervention in the early results, but this difference was not sustained. The results with different acupuncture techniques did not show any one particular method (i.e. auricular acupuncture or non-auricular acupuncture) to be superior to control intervention. Based on the results of single studies, acupressure was found to be superior to advice; laser therapy and electrostimulation were not superior to sham forms of these therapies.

The authors concluded that there was no clear evidence that acupuncture, acupressure, laser therapy or electrostimulation are effective for smoking cessation. However, the fact that acupuncture is not more effective than placebo acupuncture for smoking cessation does not mean that it is entirely without effect. Acupuncture is associated with a sizeable placebo effect, which leads to immediate cessation in about 35 per cent of all patients. Thus, these placebo effects could be worth exploiting in clinical practice.

Does electro-acupuncture reduce craving for alcohol? A randomized control study

Rampes *et al.* (1997) conducted a randomized single-blind controlled study to determine whether auricular electro-acupuncture reduces craving for alcohol. Patients who met diagnostic criteria for alcohol dependence or alcohol abuse were randomized to specific electro-acupuncture plus treatment as usual (group 1, n = 23), non-specific electro-acupuncture plus treatment as usual (group 2, n = 20) or treatment as usual (group 3, n = 16).

Electro-acupuncture was carried out weekly for 6 weeks, each treatment lasting 30 minutes. The main outcome measure was craving for alcohol, measured by a visual analogue scale. Assessments were carried out by 'blind' investigators, at baseline, week 8 and week 24.

There was a significant change in the craving for alcohol scores in all three groups at week 8. A 59.8 per cent and 54 per cent reduction in mean craving scores was noted in electro-acupuncture groups 1 and 2 respectively. There was a 44.1 per cent increase in craving in the control group at week 8. Craving was low in all three groups by week 24 and not significantly different between them at week 8. The authors concluded that there was no advantage in treating auricular acupuncture points regarded as specific for addiction.

Who practises acupuncture?

The British Medical Acupuncture Society trains doctors and health care professionals. The British Academy of Western Acupuncture trains health care professionals. Physiotherapists and osteopaths have their own acupuncture training. The British Acupuncture Council represents non-medically qualified practitioners trained by several training colleges. Such practitioners are trained in traditional acupuncture.

Homeopathy

What is homeopathy?

Homeopathy is a school of medicine founded by Dr Samuel Hahnemann (1755–1843). The term homeopathy is derived from the Greek for 'like suffering'. It is based on the principle of 'let likes be treated with likes' or *similia similibus curentur*. This principle was known to Hippocrates but it was Hahnemann who coined the term 'homeopathy' and worked relentlessly in establishing it against much hostility from his contemporaries. Contemporary medical practice in Hahnemann's day consisted of techniques such as bloodletting, purging and prescribing toxic drugs. It was amid this background that Hahnemann developed his ideas on homeopathy. Homeopathy is used to treat a wide range of acute and chronic illness. Where a condition is beyond the scope of the body's normal self-repair mechanism, treatment is less likely to be curative, but may be palliative.

Homeopathic medicines

Homeopathic medicines are prepared from minerals, plant and animal substances. There are over 3000 medicines available. For example, a commonly prescribed medicine is lycopodium, which is derived from the plant club moss. The plant is macerated in 95 per cent alcohol and then this is filtered. This juice forms the basis of medicine preparation. A typical prescription would be lycopodium 30C. The number and letter refer to the degree of dilution of the original substance. One drop of the original substance is added to 99 drops of water and is then shaken vigorously. Then one drop of that is added to 99 drops of water and shaken vigorously. This is done 30 times! In fact by the laws of chemistry, lycopodium 30C is so dilute (ultramolecular) that not one atom of the original substance may be present in it. This is one of the most controversial aspects of homeopathy, which results in most people not being able to understand how homeopathic medicines may work.

Hahnemann hit upon the process of succussion or shaking by chance. This is said to potentize the medicine. It is important to understand that homeopathic medicines do not necessarily have to be very dilute. A substance can be prescribed homeopathically in its natural form. However, this would mean many toxic substances cannot be given for example, Arsenicum Album. Such toxic substances when used homeopathically are always prescribed very dilute to reduce or even abolish toxicity.

Is there a role for homeopathy in mental illness?

A systematic review by Kleijnen *et al.* (1991) of 107 controlled clinical trials of homeopathy concluded that the evidence of clinical trials is positive. Although there is now evidence that homeopathy in broad terms does appear to work, with regard to the homeopathic treatment of psychiatric disorder, the evidence base is poor. At the Royal London Homoeopathic Hospital, a significant proportion of the new referrals are for psychiatric disorders such as depression and anxiety. An evaluation of such treatment in conjunction with well-designed randomized controlled studies is required to evaluate homeopathy in the treatment of psychiatric disorder. In the meantime, it is important that patients do not have unrealistic expectations of homeopathy. They should avail themselves of all treatment options open to them.

Is homeopathy safe?

Dantas and Rampes (2000) conducted a systematic review to evaluate the safety of homeopathic medicines by critically appraising reports of adverse effects published in English from 1970 to 1995. A comprehensive literature search was conducted by using electronic databases, by hand searching, by searching reference lists, by reviewing the bibliography of trials and other relevant articles, by contacting homeopathic pharmaceutical companies and drug regulatory agencies in the UK and the USA, and by communicating with experts in homeopathy.

The authors found that the overall incidence of adverse effects of homeopathic medicines was superior to placebo in controlled clinical trials (9.4/6.1) but effects were minor, transient and comparable. There was a large incidence of pathogenetic effects in healthy volunteers taking homeopathic medicines but the methodological quality of these studies was generally low.

Anecdotal reports of adverse effects in homeopathic publications were not well documented and mainly reported aggravation of current symptoms. Case reports in conventional medical journals pointed more to adverse effects of mislabelled 'homeopathic products' than to pure homeopathic medicines. The authors concluded that pure homeopathic medicines in high dilutions, prescribed by trained professionals, are probably safe and unlikely to provoke severe adverse reactions.

Who practises homeopathy?

Homeopathy has spread from Germany to all over the world. At the start of the twentieth century it flourished in America, where there were homeopathic medical schools, hospitals and even asylums. The Faculty of Homeopathy trains medical doctors (and other health professionals). There are four main homeopathic hospitals in the UK: in London, Glasgow, Bristol and Liverpool. These have been part of the NHS from the beginning in 1949. The Royal London Homoeopathic Hospital has provided homeopathic treatment since 1840. The Society of Homeopaths, which represents non-medically trained practitioners, is the largest organization.

Herbal medicine

What is herbal medicine?

Herbal medicine utilizes the healing properties of plant substances to restore health. Since antiquity, mankind has used plants for healing. In fact, most of our modern drugs are originally derived from plant substances. In earlier times, plants were venerated because they were known to have valuable properties. During medieval times, the use of herbs was laden with superstition, incantation and ritual.

Modern science has analysed and studied the therapeutic effects of plants. This has led to the identification, comparison and classification of the various properties so that plants with similar effects may be grouped together, and the most effective selected for further investigation. Medicinal plants are defined as those, which produce one or more active constituents capable of preventing or curing an illness.

Is there a role for herbal medicine in mental illness?

There are many trade name products being sold with claims that they are effective in insomnia, stress, anxiety and even depression. Some of these have very seductive and inviting names such as 'Serenity'. People do find some of these preparations helpful. The risk and benefits of such preparations need to be compared with extant prescribed hypnotic medication. For example the propensity for benzodiazepines to cause addiction is well recognized.

Hypericum (St John's Wort)

Extracts of the plant *hypericum perforatum* have been used in folk medicine for a long time for a range of indications including depressive disorders. Extracts of hypericum are licensed in Germany for the treatment of depressive, anxiety and sleep disorders. In fact, Europe has a greater tradition of herbal medicine than the UK.

Hypericum has been the subject of a systematic review (Linde and Mulrow 2003). The aim of the review was to investigate whether extracts of hypericum are more effective than placebo and as effective as standard anti-depressants in the treatment of depressive disorders in adults. A comprehensive literature search was conducted. Clinical trials were included if they:

1   were randomized;

2   included patients with depressive disorders;

3   compared preparations of hypericum (alone or in combination with other plant extracts) with placebo or other anti-depressants; and

4   included clinical outcomes such as scales assessing depressive symptoms.

Data were collected and analysed in a standard manner. The main outcome measure for comparing the effectiveness of hypericum with placebo and standard anti-depressants was the responder rate ratio (responder rate in treatment group/responder rate in control group). There were 27 trials including a total of 2291 patients who met inclusion criteria. Seventeen trials with 1168 patients were placebo-controlled (16 addressed single preparations, one a combination with four other plant extracts). Ten trials (eight single preparations, two combinations of hypericum and valerian) with 1123 patients compared hypericum with other anti-depressant or sedative drugs. Most trials were 4 to 6 weeks long. Participants usually had neurotic depression or mild to moderate severe depressive disorders.

Hypericum preparations were significantly superior to placebo (rate ratio 2.47; 95 per cent confidence interval 1.69 to 3.61) and similarly effective as standard anti-depressants (single preparations 1.01; 0.87 to 1.16, combinations 1.52; 0.78 to 2.94). The proportions of patients reporting side effects were 26.3 per cent for hypericum single preparations vs. 44.7 per cent for standard anti-depressants (0.57; 0.47 to 0.69), and 14.6 per cent for combinations vs. 26.5 per cent with amitriptyline or desipramine (0.49; 0.23 to 1.04). The authors concluded that there is evidence that extracts of hypericum are more effective than placebo for the short-term treatment of mild to moderately severe depressive disorders. The current evidence is inadequate to establish whether hypericum is as effective as other anti-depressants.

Hypericum can be easily purchased over the counter. It would be preferable for patients wanting to take this anti-depressant to be supervised by their general practitioner or their psychiatrist. Many different preparations are available and this raises questions of quality assurance in the manufacture of these preparations. Hypericum extract LI 160 (0.24–0.32 per cent total hypericins), otherwise known as research grade hypericum, available in 300 mg coated tablet form and standardized to 900 µg of total hypericins per tablet is known as Jarsin 300®, and has been used in the majority of clinical studies. It is also the most commonly prescribed formulation in Germany. In the UK, it is available as Kira® tablets in two strengths standardized to 300 µg and 900 µg hypericins respectively.

How does it work? The method of action is uncertain. There is evidence for modulation of monoamine neurotransmitters. The leading constituent of the extract responsible for anti-depressant action via serotonin reuptake inhibition, appears to be hyperforin. Clearly hypericum will appeal to some patients simply because it is an herbal anti-depressant. Patient preference is important in terms of treatment adherence and therefore of importance for the effectiveness of anti-depressants.

Is herbal medicine safe?

Herbal medicines are different to the synthetic or non-synthetic drugs. Drugs can be measured with reliability and are tested out on animals and humans before they are allowed to be prescribed by doctors and in some instances nurses. Herbal medicines are not subject to similar scientific scrutiny. Many plants are toxic and can be fatal. The National Poisons Unit at Guy's Hospital collects information on overdoses and poisoning with plant materials.

Hypericum has an excellent safety profile that is superior to that of conventional anti-depressants. The available data suggest that hypericum is well tolerated and has an incidence of adverse effects similar to that of placebo. The most common adverse effects are gastrointestinal symptoms, dizziness and sedation. The only potentially serious adverse effects are photosensitization, which is extremely rare, and precipitation of manic symptoms in predisposed patients. However, problems may arise when patients take hypericum with other medications. Hypericum induces a hepatic enzyme through activation of the cytochrome P450 system. Thus hypericum can decrease the plasma level of a large range of prescribed drugs such as anticoagulants, oral contraceptives and antiviral agents with possible clinically serious consequences. Some evidence indicates that combination of hypericum with selective serotonin inhibitors can lead to the serotonin syndrome, particularly in elderly patients.

There is a growing market in the over-the-counter medicine field, with many pharmacists and supermarkets now selling herbal medicine products for self-use. This trend may not be in the best interests of patients, some of who may be misguided and desperately seeking help and self-medication inappropriately. Herbal medication should be supervised and general practitioners should be informed about any decision to take herbal medicines to ascertain whether the herbal medicine can interact with other conventional medication that one may be taking.

Who practises herbal medicine?

There are professional medical herbalists who belong to the National Institute of Medical Herbalists. They have good training in this discipline and often work in a private setting. However, the majority are not medically qualified.

Aromatherapy

What is aromatherapy?

Aromatherapy is based on the healing properties of essential plant oils. These natural oils are diluted in a carrier oil. Essential oils have been defined as 'non-oily, highly fragrant essences extracted from plants by distillation' which evaporate readily and have been used by doctors in France for their antibiotic and antiviral properties for many years. They are most commonly used in oil burners, in bath water, or massaged into the skin, thus the aroma of the essential oil evaporates and stimulates the olfactory sense. An aromatherapy massage is based on massage techniques, which aim to relieve tension in the body and improve circulation. This, practitioners believe, allows oil molecules absorbed into the blood stream during massage to pass efficiently through the body to the nervous system. Benefits of the aroma may also be obtained when oils are inhaled both directly and during the massage treatment bringing about a general feeling of well-being in an individual.

Is there a role for aromatherapy in mental illness?

Massage in general is mainly used to promote relaxation, and reduce anxiety. There is some evidence that aromatherapy massage reduces anxiety scores in the short term. The healing properties of aromatherapy are claimed to include promotion of relaxation and sleep, relief of pain, and reduction of depressive symptoms, the rationale being that the essential oils have a calming and relaxing effect. Aromatherapy might particularly be of use as an intervention with people who are confused, have little or no preserved language, and for whom verbal interaction is difficult and conventional medicine is seen as of only marginal benefit.

Aromatherapy may be useful in the management of disturbed behaviour in people with dementia. Behavioural and psychological symptoms in dementia are frequent and are a major management problem. Ballard *et al.* (2002) conducted a randomized controlled trial to determine the value of aromatherapy with essential oil of *melissa officinalis* (lemon balm) for agitation in people with severe dementia. Seventy-two people residing in NHS care facilities who had clinically significant agitation in the context of severe dementia were randomly assigned to aromatherapy with melissa essential oil (N = 36) or placebo (sunflower oil) (N = 36). The active treatment or placebo oil was combined with a base lotion and applied to patients' faces and arms twice a day by caregiving staff. Changes in clinically significant agitation and quality of life indices were compared between the two groups over a 4-week period of treatment. Seventy-one patients completed the trial. No significant side effects were observed. Sixty per cent (21/35) of the active treatment group and 14 per cent (5/36) of the placebo-treated group experienced an overall improvement in agitation. Quality of life indices also improved significantly more in people receiving essential balm oil. The finding that aromatherapy with essential balm oil is a safe and effective treatment for clinically significant agitation in people with severe dementia, with additional benefits for key quality of life parameters, indicates the need for further controlled trials.

A systematic review of aromatherapy by Cooke and Ernst (2000) identified 12 trials of which six concerned the relaxing effects of aromatherapy combined with massage. These studies suggest that aromatherapy massage has a mild, transient anxiolytic effect. However, Ernst concluded that the effects of aromatherapy are probably not strong enough for it to be considered for the treatment of anxiety. The authors state that national guidance on the use of aromatherapy and other complementary therapies within the health service is needed to inform purchasing decisions and to offer a rationale that can be passed on to patients.

Stevensen (1994) conducted a randomized controlled trial to assess the effects of aromatherapy and massage on post-cardiac surgery patients. Foot massage was given over 20 minutes with or without the essential oil of neroli. On day 5, post-operatively, there was a trend towards a greater and more lasting psychological benefit from the massage with the neroli oil compared to the plain vegetable oil.

Is aromatherapy safe?

Training in the safe use of essential oils is part of all reputable aromatherapy courses. Certain hazardous oils should be avoided, for example wormwood is known to have high toxicity. There are specific contra-indications for example certain oils induce menstruation and thus are contra-indicated in pregnancy. Other oils are thought to trigger epilepsy in susceptible people. Some oils are said to be phototoxic, or photocarcinogenic.

Who practises aromatherapy?

There are a large number of training organizations. The Aromatherapy Organisations Council has a national register of aromatherapists. The interest of nurses, midwives and health visitors in aromatherapy is considerable. There are many courses available, techniques can be learned relatively quickly and easily and it is possible to incorporate into practice. It might be argued that the use of this treatment brings many nurses back in touch with patients following technologically induced distancing. These nurses have rediscovered that caring touch can make a substantial contribution to patients' psychological well-being.

Research and complementary and alternative therapies

Qualitative studies

Nathan (2001) conducted a study of patients' perceptions and views on spiritual care in mental health practice in West London Mental Health NHS Trust. This study is an example of a qualitative study conducted by a nurse. This type of study is important since it raises interesting questions on how mental health professionals relate to patients.

The aim of the study was to establish patients' perceptions and views on spiritual care and to elicit whether or not mental health service users are of the opinion that spiritual care has any positive effects or benefits in mental health practice. A convenience sample of 13 patients from varied cultural and ethnic backgrounds were interviewed. Interviews were audio-taped, transcribed and the data were subjected to content analysis.

Four main themes that emerged were: religion, relationship, meaning making and work. Though all participants associated spiritual care with religion, none of them described spiritual care strictly as only religion. Patients described spiritual care as having to do with their relationship with others, daily activities that help them make meaning of life experiences and worship. Participants acknowledged that spiritual care is as important as all other aspects of care and its provision can contribute to their recovery and quality of life.

Patients were of the opinion that when spiritual care is appropriately provided it can enhance the effectiveness of other aspects of care (for example, social, physical and psychological). Elements of spiritual care were described as the quality that permeates all aspects of care and influences how each person provides or receives care.

One patient stated 'My religious belief is very important to me, without my faith in God I would not have been alive today.' Some patients described spiritual care as providing opportunities to participate in the following activities. 'Art or music acts as a door or window into an imaginary world, which provides meaning and understanding to things that one cannot explain in words. Spiritual world is very personal and each person's world is different and depends on one's needs.'

> Spiritual care is staff giving you time to talk through your problems . . .
> it is helping you to deal with your inner feelings . . . spiritual care is to do
> with your inner need, that which keeps you alive.

> Spiritual care is nothing more than the attitudes of staff to patients . . .
> it is when you are made to feel valued . . . it helps to bring dignity back
> to your life.

Nathan's and other qualitative research studies can make an important contribution to our understanding of the motivation and experience of users of complementary and alternative therapies. Practising nurses are well placed to contribute to this body of knowledge.

Systematic reviews

The Cochrane Collaboration is collating all randomized controlled trials and the Complementary Medicine Field within the collaboration is compiling those pertinent to complementary and alternative therapies. What constitutes good evidence that something works? The Cochrane database is an important resource for critically appraising the research evidence for treatments or interventions of complementary and alternative therapies. It is important to realize that non-randomized controlled studies also have a role in the assessment of complementary and alternative therapies. Current wisdom categorizes different types of evidence as a hierarchy of levels as follows:

1   Strong evidence from at least one systematic review of multiple, well-designed randomized controlled trial.

2   Strong evidence from at least one properly designed randomized controlled trial of appropriate size.

3   Evidence from well-designed trials without randomization, single group pre-post, cohort, time series or matched case-controlled studies.

4   Evidence from well-designed non-experimental studies from more than one centre or research group.

5. Opinions of respected authorities, based on clinical evidence, descriptive studies or reports of expert committees.

For each complementary and alternative therapy, there are differing levels of evidence. More research, particularly large well-designed studies need to be conducted in complementary and alternative therapy. The problem in the UK, as pointed out by Prince Charles's Integrated Healthcare Initiative (Foundation for Integrated Medicine 1997), is that there has been a lack of research infrastructure and lack of significant funding by the orthodox institutions. The hope is that this situation will change.

| Placebo

The term placebo effect is taken to mean not only the narrow effect of a dummy intervention but also the broad array of non-specific effects in the patient–clinician relationship. Such non-specific effects of treatment are taken for granted and have been under-researched. Clinicians can have potent placebo effects, which could be judiciously harnessed and exploited in clinical interactions. A clinician's bedside manner, his or her empathy, eye contact and smile in greeting patients have healing effects that are hard to quantify and measure.

In complementary and alternative therapy, the main question regarding placebo has been whether a given therapy has more than a placebo effect. Just as conventional medicine ignores the clinical significance of its own placebo effect, the placebo effect of complementary and alternative medicine is often ignored by its practitioners. The magic and ritual of medicine has ancient traditions. Perhaps complementary and alternative therapies have been better able to capture this magic for patients.

National Service Framework

Some of the guiding values and principles of the external reference group of the *National Service Framework for Mental Health* (DH 1999), states that people with mental health problems can expect that services will involve service users and their carers in planning and delivery of care. Users should have choices, which promote independence. Standard 1 of the *NSF for Mental Health* concerns mental health promotion. This standard is perhaps most relevant in terms of how complementary and alternative therapies could be involved in the *NSF for Mental Health*. In Standard 1 there is mention of individuals enhancing their psychological well-being. What better way is there of doing this than by the use of complementary and alternative therapies? 'Exercise, relaxation and stress management have a beneficial effect on mental health. Reducing access to illicit drugs, taking alcohol in moderation, maintaining social contacts, reducing smoking and talking things over are also helpful measures.' The *NSF for Mental Health* states also that not only physical but spiritual facets of mental health and mental heath problems should be looked at. The *NSF for Mental Health* provides an opportunity for greater use of complementary and alternative therapies in the NHS, which could result in significant improvements in the mental health of patients.

Conclusion

Complementary and alternative therapy is defined as a broad domain of healing resources that encompasses all health systems, modalities, and practices and their accompanying theories and beliefs, other than those intrinsic to the politically dominant health systems of a particular society or culture in a given historical period.

Complementary and alternative therapy use is common and increasing. Over 4 million adults made 18 million visits to practitioners of one of six therapies: acupuncture, chiropractic, homeopathy, hypnotherapy, herbal medicine or osteopathy in the UK in 1998. The NHS provided about 10 per cent of these contacts. The majority of non-NHS visits represent direct out-of-pocket expenditures.

Patients use complementary and alternative therapy for different reasons. In general, complementary and alternative therapy does not replace conventional medicine but complements it. Complementary and alternative therapy users tend to be better educated. They have a holistic orientation to health. Patients tend to be more satisfied with complementary and alternative therapy practitioners. Longer time for consultations is an important factor.

Currently there is some provision of complementary and alternative therapy in the NHS, but this is not readily available to mental health patients. These patients often lack knowledge and finances.

There is a growing database of research evidence for complementary and alternative therapies. It is no longer correct to state that there is no evidence for complementary and alternative therapies. Prince Charles's Integrated Health care Initiative has given complementary and alternative therapy a push in the right direction. There has been a lack of research infrastructure and funding. The question of combining therapies, i.e. what combinations of complementary and alternative therapy plus conventional might be most beneficial is one that deserves investigation. Compliance with medication is universally poor in medicine. The use of complementary and alternative therapy may improve compliance with medications. This is especially important now that there are newer generations of better tolerated antipsychotic and anti-depressant medications.

Many nurses are very interested in complementary and alternative therapies, and a number have been trained as practitioners in aromatherapy, in particular. Clinical experience suggests that there has been a move away from hands-on patient contact in nursing; complementary and alternative therapy has perhaps filled a lacuna in nurses' professional work. This raises questions about the role of nurses and their contact with patients. Mental health professionals need to be aware that their patients may be attending a complementary and alternative therapy provider and should enquire routinely about patients' use of complementary and alternative therapy.

The *NSF for Mental Health* and recent changes in the NHS such as formation of primary care trusts affords opportunities for the greater integration of complementary and alternative therapies within treatment and care delivered under the NHS.

In summary, the main points of this chapter are:

- Complementary and alternative therapies have been classified into five domains:

  1 alternative medical systems;
  2 mind–body interventions;
  3 biologically based therapies;
  4 manipulative and body-based methods;
  5 energy therapies.

- Survey data suggest that complementary and alternative therapy is used by a sizeable proportion of the population in a number of countries and that this proportion is increasing. One survey of a random sample of patients receiving complementary medical care in the UK and the USA found that almost three-quarters of the British patients, and just over three-fifths of the American patients had been diagnosed with a mental disorder; major depression and anxiety were most commonest.

- The majority of people who use complementary and alternative therapies do so in addition to conventional medicine, rather than as an alternative. Explanations for the increasing use of complementary or alternative therapy can be classified as 'push factors' – such as dissatisfaction with conventional medicine through previous negative experiences or anti-establishment attitudes – or 'pull factors' – such as compatibility between the philosophy of certain therapies and patients' beliefs, and a greater sense of control over one's own treatment.
- There is a growing database of research evidence for complementary therapies; it is no longer true to say that there is no evidence. For the therapies reviewed in this chapter the evidence base would suggest that:
  - Acupuncture has a role in the treatment of addictive disorders (smoking, opiate and alcohol dependence).
  - The evidence base for homeopathy is currently too poor to reach firm conclusions and well-designed trials are needed.
  - The evidence base for herbal medicines is variable. However, hypericum (St John's Wort) has been found to be more effective than placebo for the short-term treatment of mild to moderately severe depressive disorders.
  - There is some evidence that aromatherapy reduces anxiety in the short term. It might be particularly useful as an intervention with people who are confused, have little or no preserved language, for whom verbal interaction is difficult and conventional medicine is seen as of only marginal benefit; for example for dementia sufferers.
- There is an important potential role for nurses as providers of some complementary therapies.
- As researchers nurses are particularly well placed to conduct studies to contribute to our understanding of the motivation and experiences of users of complementary and alternative therapies.

▌ Questions for reflection and discussion

1 Enquire about complementary and alternative therapy use by the patients with whom you work.

(a) What are their perceived benefits?
(b) How much do they cost?
(c) Are there any safety concerns?

2 Assess the evidence base of the therapies you encounter in daily practice?

3 Examine the patient–clinician encounter for non-specific effects of treatment.

Annotated bibliography

- Ernst, E., Pittler, M.H., Stevinson, C. and White, A. (2001) *The Desktop Guide to Complementary and Alternative Medicine: An Evidence-based Approach*. London: Harcourt Publishers. Edzard Ernst has a chair in complementary medicine at the University of Exeter. With his team, he has made a significant scientific contribution to the critical appraisal of research into complementary and alternative medicine and has published many articles. This book is an excellent reference and has summarized the extant research in each field of complementary and alternative medicine.
- Boyd, H. (2000) *Banishing the Blues: Inspirational Ways to Improve Your Mood*. London: Mitchell Beazley. Hilary Boyd is a qualified nurse, journalist and author. This well-presented book has a section on depression and a section on use of complementary and alternative medicine in depression. It is aimed at patients but would be of interest to health care professionals in training as it gives pragmatic examples of how patients can help themselves. Dr Hagen Rampes was consultant editor for this book.
- Woodham, A. and Peters, D. (1997) *The Encyclopaedia of Complementary Medicine*. London: Dorling Kindersley. This is a comprehensive reference guide on the most important complementary and alternative medicine. The guide is aimed at patients but is a useful guide for health professionals.

References

Astin, J. (1998) Why patients use alternative medicine. Results of a national survey, *Journal of the American Medical Association* **279**: 1548–53.

Ballard, C.G., O'Brien, J.T., Reichelt, K. and Perry, E.K. (2002) Aromatherapy as a safe and effective treatment for the management of agitation in severe dementia: The results of a double-blind, placebo-controlled trial with Melissa, *Journal of Clinical Psychiatry* **63**(7): 553–8.

Cochrane Complementary Medicine Field. About the Cochrane Collaboration, *Cochrane Library*, Issue 1 (2003). Oxford: Update Software.

Cooke, B. and Ernst, E. (2000) Aromatherapy: a systematic review, *British Journal of General Practice* **50**: 493–6.

Dantas, F. and Rampes, H. (2000) Do homeopathic medicines provoke adverse effects? A systematic review, *British Homeopathic Journal* **89**: S35–S38.

Davidson, J., Rampes, H., Eizen, M. *et al.* (1998) Psychiatric disorders in primary care patients receiving complementary medicine, *Comprehensive Psychiatry* **39**: 16–20.

Department of Health (1999) *National Service Framework for Mental Health*. Modern standards and service models. London: Department of Health.

Druss, B.G. and Rosenheck, R.A. (1999) Association between use of unconventional therapies and conventional medical; services, *Journal of the American Medical Association* **282**: 651–6.

Eisenberg, D.M., Davis, R.B., Ettner, S.L. *et al.* (1998) Trends in alternative medicine use in the United States, 1990–1997: results of a follow-up national survey, *Journal of the American Medical Association* **280**: 1569–75.

Finnigan, M.D. (1991) The centre for the study of complementary medicine: an attempt to understand its popularity through psychological, demographic and operational criteria *Complementary Medicine Research* **5**: 83–8.

Foundation for Integrated Medicine (1997) *Integrated Healthcare. A Way Forward for the Next Five Years?* A discussion document.

Furnham, A. (1996) Why do people choose and use complementary therapies? in E. Ernst (ed.) *Complementary medicine: an objective appraisal.* Oxford: Butterworth Heinemann.

Haussermann, D. (1997) Wachsendes Vertrauen in Naturheilmittel, *Deutsches Arzteblatt* **94**: 1857–8.

Kaptchuk, T.J. and Eisenberg, D.M. (1998) The persuasive appeal of alternative medicine, *Annals of Internal Medicine* **129**: 1061–5.

Kleijnen, J., Knipschild, P. and ter Riet, G. (1991) Clinical trials of homeopathy, *British Medical Journal* **302**: 316–23.

Linde, K. and Mulrow, C.D. (2003) St John's Wort for depression, *The Cochrane Library* (1), Oxford: Update Software.

Long, L., Huntley, A. and Ernst, E. (2001) Which complementary and alternative therapies benefit which conditions? A survey of the opinions of 223 professional organizations, *Complementary Therapies in Medicine* **9**: 178–85.

Mental Health Foundation (1997) *Knowing Our Own Minds. A Survey of How People in Emotional Distress Take Control of Their Lives.* London.

Nathan, M.M. (2001) Overcoming barriers to spiritual care, *Sacred Space* **2**(4): 18–24.

Rampes, H., Pereira, S., Mortimer, A., Manoharan, S. and Knowles, M. (1997) Does electroacupuncture reduce craving for alcohol? A randomized control study, *Complementary Therapies in Medicine* **5**: 19–26.

Rampes, H. and James, R. (1995) Complications of acupuncture, *Acupuncture in Medicine* **13**(1): 26–33.

Resch, K.L., Hill, S. and Ernst, E. (1997) Use of complementary therapies by individuals with arthritis, *Journal of Clinical Rheumatology* **16**: 391–5.

Stevensen, C.J. (1994) The psychophysiological effects of aromatherapy massage following cardiac surgery, *Complementary Therapies Medicine* **2**: 27–35.

Thomas, K.J., Fall, M. and Williams, B. (1993) Methodological study to investigate the feasibility of conducting a population-based survey of the use of complementary healthcare. *Final Report to the Research Council for Complementary Medicine.* Unpublished.

Thomas, K., Nicholl, J. and Coleman, P. (2001) Use and expenditure on complementary medicine in England – a population based survey. *Complementary Therapies in Medicine* **9**: 2–11.

White, H., Rampes, H. and Ernst, E. (2003) Acupuncture for smoking cessation, *The Cochrane Library* (1), Oxford: Update Software.

PART 3
Applications

13

The person with a perceptual disorder

Geoff Brennan

Chapter overview

> At any one time one adult in six suffers from one or other forms of mental illness. In other words mental illnesses are as common as asthma. They vary from more common conditions such as deep depression to schizophrenia, which affects fewer than one person in a hundred. Mental illness is not well understood. It frightens people and all too often carries a stigma.
>
> (DH 1999: 1)

So begins Frank Dobson's introduction to the *National Service Framework (NSF) for Mental Health*. This chapter aims to explore the 'not well understood' condition that is schizophrenia from the viewpoint that such a disorder involves an extension or subtraction of normal functioning. In order to do this we need to consider how a normal person perceives the world. But there is a problem here given that there is no such thing as a 'normal person'. All we actually have is our own experience of the world. Accordingly, this chapter will ask you to consider your own experience with reference to its content. As you read, please ask yourself:

- How would this condition affect me?
- Have I ever had experiences approximating those described in the chapter?

Stigma arises when we cannot understand a person or group and judge them to be deviant. Therefore, it is important for nurses or anyone interested in mental illness to attempt to 'get inside the mind' of the individual they are trying to assist and understand what it is like for them in a manner which brings empathetic understanding of their experiences. You may be surprised, as you read, how you can relate in some small or large way to the mental experiences of people deemed 'mad'.

This chapter covers:

- What is a person?
- Perception;
- Schizophrenia;
- Symptom-focused treatments and interventions;
- Case studies.

What is a person?

It is often the simple questions that are the hardest to answer. Psychiatry is awash with seemingly simple questions that are, in reality, very complex. As a discipline which aims to promote health and well-being in society, it deals with *people*, either as an individual 'person' or grouped together into populations. But what makes a person a person? or What makes me '*me*'? Consider the following:

Imagine you are a judge in a legal system where only your opinion matters. You are hearing the trial of murder where the defendant freely admits to the crime, states they were of sound mind when they committed the crime and that the crime was premeditated with clear personal gain as a result of the victim's death. The defendant defiantly committed the murder. Their part in the crime was not discovered, however, until twenty years later. In that time, given the wonders of biology, every original cell in the defendant's body has been replicated in the natural process of cell regeneration. As a consequence their hotshot lawyer makes the defence that, although the person did, indeed, commit the murder, the present 'person' cannot be held responsible, as they are a completely different individual with different cells and therefore not responsible for the crime their earlier form committed. In his summing up the hotshot ends with the words 'How can we, in all seriousness, punish this person when it is true to say that not one cell was present when the murder was committed? How can we, when this hand was not there, when this brain was not there, when, by a process of clear logic, my client, in his present state, was not in that room, indeed, not even on the planet, when this crime was perpetrated.' The people await the verdict from you, the judge.

Obviously, you would find the defendant guilty, their hotshot lawyer would be chastened and you would be asked to join the House of Lords. But why?

In a nutshell, the hotshot lawyer's flaw is to argue that a person is a *body*. This does not take into account the mental, social, moral or spiritual aspects of an individual. While the body is *an aspect* of a person, it is only when this is combined with these other aspects, do we get the person, the individual, the 'me' that is a human being. The murderer committed the murder, and as the cells of the body changed, the person who committed the murder remained. If we accept the defence's argument, I did not pass (or fail) the exams I put on my curriculum vitae, my wife is not married to the man she exchanged vows with, I am not the father of my children, and my parents are impostors.

The aspects that are in addition to the physical aspect of the body are often called the 'mental' aspects. The hotshot lawyer has omitted the fact that the mental aspects stay in place while the physical cells change. They are the threads that connect the cells together into the whole. If we are to really get technical, the cells of the body have a memory of the previous cells, so that, although the cells 'change', they do not become new, autonomous cells but replicas of the old cells, including carrying the memory of the previous. Hence scars are carried on the skin as a memory of previous trauma, long after the original cells have been replaced and fingerprints are replicated as a unique marker of the individual. Therefore, even the physical body has a 'memory'. While it is true that the physical state changes, the mental is carried along.

Now all this is so obvious that the hotshot lawyer will be looking quite ridiculous. Despite this, they have been good enough to do us a favour. They have forced us into defining what makes up a person. If we agree that a person is a complex mixture of both the mental and the physical, we must acknowledge that there is some relation between them. The physical sense that we have, through our body's interaction with the world outside ourselves, feeds into the mental. This book exists in the real, physical world; the words exist as separate physical bits of ink on a physical bit of paper, which you are scanning with your eyes. The resulting images are carried through the optic nerve and are 'seen'. The meaning is then interpreted in the mental world of your thoughts as the words have mental meanings.

In turn our mental thoughts, ideas and drives influence our interaction with the world and can change this world as a result. For example, if your mental interpretation of what is written is that it is a load of rubbish, you can burn the book in the physical world, further deplete the ozone layer, increase the risk of skin cancer in yourself and others and have some responsibility for this.

As a consequence, our hotshot lawyer in disgrace has assisted us in getting nearer that very difficult question, 'What makes me "*me*?" They have helped us to see that the mental and the physical are two aspects of a person and that the complete person is the totality of both the mental and the physical. Moreover, the person also exists within the world and can interact with it. The physical body exists in the world and allows the mental aspects access to the world. It is this interactive pathway between the mental and the physical that we know as perception.

Perception

Perception, as described above, is a complex process of interpretation, which is described in its simplest form in Figure 13.1.

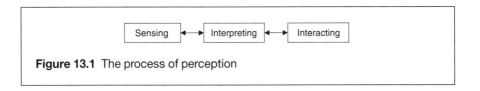

Figure 13.1 The process of perception

Sensing

We have five senses that operate on the edge of the mental physical interface. The mind without the senses would be like a computer without data. The potential to process would be there without anything to process. Provided you have no impairment to your senses, you can access all five of them easily. The sense you are using right now is sight. You are looking at the words on the page and literally seeing them. The other senses are there, but not so much in use. You are probably trying to not hear the world around you if you are concentrating on the words. If you wish to focus on hearing, you can do so effortlessly. Take a second to stop and listen. Likewise, your sense of smell and taste are there if you need them. What can you smell and taste? Finally, close your eyes, pick up the book and feel the weight of it in your hand. Rub your fingers over the cover. All these senses are there and you can generally focus on them or ignore them as you wish.

Interpreting

Whether you intended to or not, you probably entered into interpretation in the last section on the senses. For example, it is virtually impossible just to *see* words. It is much more likely that you *read* them. In other words you did not look at the sentence 'You are looking at the words on the page . . .' and *see* the words as individual words, but rather read them as a complete sentence and therefore interpreted their meaning. Hence, if the sentence had said, 'You are looking at the elephants on the page . . .' you would have reacted to the word 'elephant' because it was out of place. Thus you are interpreting the words that you are seeing. Also, when you were asked to listen, it is likely you would not have left it at just hearing, but thought: 'That was a police siren' or 'That was the television' or 'It's too quiet – the kids are up to no good/my partner has fallen asleep/I forgot to take my earplugs out.'

An important aspect of interpretation is that it is a purely mental activity. Once the eye has seen the words on this page and they pass the image into the brain, the process of sensing has finished, the interpretation of the image happens in the mind. Reading happens in the mind. Even if you read out loud, there is a point where the brain interprets the image and informs the mouth what to say. We know this because we can get a word wrong and read something that isn't there, but this isn't because we can't *read* but that we have *interpreted* wrongly.

There is an important aspect of interpretation that is summed up in the following:

> Instead of talking of seeing and knowing, we might do a little better to talk of seeing and noticing. We notice only when we look for something, and we look when our attention is aroused by some disequilibrium, a difference between our expectation and the incoming message. We cannot take in all we see in a room, but we notice if something has changed.
>
> (Gombrich 1960: 62)

This means that a vast majority of what we sense is ignored as it is deemed unimportant. The process of interpretation has a filtration system that allows for the focusing noted earlier. If you did have to stop reading for a minute to concentrate on hearing, this shows that the filtration system is working effectively. In other words, in order for you to focus on the words on the page, as you need to study and understand them, you need to lower your noticing of other senses. It would seem that the senses are wired into the brain like the control panel of a music studio, where certain inputs can be given higher or lower emphasis depending on the need. When you stopped and listened, you, in effect, turned up the hearing sense and lowered the seeing sense. While this was a conscious manipulation of the senses, the raising or lowering is an unconscious natural process necessary to function. As we shall see, the process of filtration and focusing can be both a problem when things go wrong and a possible benefit if we wish to change things.

We do have a complication here in that the 'interpretation' we are discussing could be seen to be an aspect of brain functioning, which would make it a physical activity. In other words, we could say that the processes are based purely within the brain and are really just a chemical reaction within the neurones in response to the stimulus of the senses. While it is probable that this is the case, the important thing within our discussion is that another person does not have access to this process. In other words, while you and I may 'see' the same thing, we could not agree that we 'interpret' it the same way. Imagine that we are both looking at a football match where we support opposite teams. Our interpretations of the event, while explicable by brain chemistry where our neurotransmitters will fluctuate depending on what is happening, will actually be at odds to each other. Similarly, we now know which chemicals are released in the brain if we see the person we love in a crowd of people, but why that person, and why doesn't everyone who sees them feel the same? Interpretation is in the eye of the beholder and brain function obeys it would seem.

Interacting

We live in and with the physical world. The purpose of sensing and interpreting is to keep us orientated within this world and to allow us to survive and thrive within it. In its simplest form, this interaction keeps us safe. An experience we all have in common is the reflex action of getting your hand off a hot object. There you are, the iron/cooker/bath water is too hot and will burn. Unaware, you place your hand on the hot object, sense how hot it is, interpret that this is dangerous (and if your mind was elsewhere, you certainly do now focus on your burning hand). What do you do next? You pull it away as quickly as possible.

This simple reflex action sums up the purpose of interacting with the world. Our sensing and interpreting the world allows us to move and function to the best of our ability. Sometimes this interaction is as simple as moving our hand from a burning object (reaction), and sometimes it is as complex as changing our attitudes and beliefs (learning) or storing sensory data or interpretations to assist with future interactions (memory).

Where does it all go wrong?

Are you just a complicated physical object? If not, are you a mind? If so, what are minds? What exactly is the relationship between the mind and the body? Are you a mind with a body, or a body with a mind? You are looking out of your body now. Does that mean you are your body or does it mean you are inside your body, or neither? Could we be immaterial souls, which survive our bodily death, or has that been ruled out by modern science? Are you your brain? How, if at all, is grey matter connected to our innermost thoughts and emotions? It is one of our peculiarities that we do not know what we are.

(Priest 1991: xi)

This quote is how Stephen Priest begins a 300-page examination of the interaction between the physical and mental from a philosophical viewpoint. Psychiatry has also pondered this question and also has not come to any firm conclusion. The difference between the two examinations is that philosophy deals with the issue in a theoretical manner. Psychiatry, however, is a practical discipline, and one that has been set up (and set itself up) to deal with those aspects of the interaction between mental and physical which can go wrong and cause distress to individuals, family and social systems. Philosophy aims to make the world more understandable through detailed examination of basic assumptions while psychiatry aims to change the individual who has been identified as having difficulties existing within the world.

Psychiatry, therefore, is necessary because things go wrong with people. Psychiatry exists to correct the things that go wrong, or to reorientate the people for whom things go wrong to cope with the things that go wrong. Psychiatry also has the function of identifying what can cause things to go wrong and attempting to change them to stop things from going wrong. There is a problem here. How do we know when things go wrong? Given that the mental, as defined above, is a private realm only observable to another within the physical world of interaction and observation of the individual, how can psychiatry definitively say that things are wrong?

Psychiatry is a younger sibling of medicine. What I mean by this is that medicine, as a science, came into existence to address the ailments of the body, or the physical. As medicine developed, so did the awareness of the need to address the mental. Hence psychiatry. As we shall examine later, there are problems with this inception and affiliation and the link between medicine and psychiatry can be to the detriment of a clear understanding of mental issues. For now, however, let us take it that psychiatry decides what is wrong in roughly the same way as medicine does.

So how do you know you have a cold? Well, in honesty, you don't. You wake up in the morning and notice that certain things are different about you. In other words, you have an understanding of how you normally wake up and (remembering what we said earlier) ignore the fact that everything is as it usually is. Lost you for a second there? OK, how many times have you woken up and consciously thought, 'Oh good. I'm not ill today.' My guess is (unless you have had a recent experience of illness) you do not have this thought as your automatic introduction to each day. Rather you wake up and . . . nothing. You just go about your business. The only time you would notice your state of health is when there is something wrong. Then you notice the things that are wrong. In the case of a cold you may notice a 'runny nose', 'blocked sinus', 'sore throat', 'raised temperature', 'lack of energy' and, possibly, a general feeling of 'being a bit low in mood'. Given your previous knowledge of this combination of things you say, 'I have a cold.' Percentage-wise, your guess would probably be accurate, but in reality you cannot know for sure. You may have influenza, or any number of conditions which can start with this combination of things, or you may notice another thing wrong which you have not come across before in the 'I have a cold' combination, such as vomiting, tremor or some other nasty physical ailment.

The point is, however, that you notice something is wrong. You wake up and notice. Then you notice the things that are wrong. These things, these signs are what we know as symptoms. Even if you visit the 'expert', the doctor or nurse, they will open with, 'Well, what is the matter with you then?' and you will not answer, 'My football team are rubbish, I hate my job and quite frankly, my partner better buck their ideas up or they are out!' Instead you know that they want a list of symptoms.

Psychiatry works in the same way with one massive difference. The similarity is that psychiatry also wants a list of the symptoms. The difference is that psychiatry will, however, take a note of symptoms identified through the observation of a third party. This does not mean to say that medicine will not, but it is often the case that a disorder of perception can also extend to a person's perception of themselves, particularly in reference to how they are relating to the world and other people. In addition, if you look at the list of

'I have a cold' symptoms, my bet is that the one you are least likely to notice is the 'bit of a low mood', which often accompanies physical illness. It would seem we are not as good at noticing changes in our mental state as much as our physical state.

As a consequence, the world-view of the person with the disorder of perception is often at odds with the world-view of others. This is particularly true when it comes to relatives or close friends who notice changes in a person's demeanour, behaviour and attitude as a cause of concern before the person themselves. Hence, psychiatry places a value on what is known as 'taking a history' from those who are in close contact with the person and who know them well. Usually the first part of this interview will begin with 'Have you noticed any change in X over the last few months?' Again, this is not without difficulty and we shall also come to this.

Another reason for calling on a secondary source of information in order to identify a mental health issue is that, where a physical illness can often call upon a secondary physical source to verify the presence or absence of symptoms, in psychiatry this is not possible. If you think you have a temperature you can use a thermometer to measure your temperature and know the measure it should be if you are to be considered of normal temperature. Higher than this mark would indicate you are correct. If you have a sore throat, a doctor can shine a light into your throat and see if there is the red swelling indicative of infection. If your nose is running, you will see evidence of the mucus secretions. In other words, another person can perceive the signs of physical disorder through various physical examinations. Despite the advances in various forms of brain scanning, disorders of perception are only truly elicited through the person relating their inner mental experiences to you – the private world of their mind. While there are various forms of behaviour that can be *associated* with mental disorders, *attributing* these to the presence of a mental disorder is guesswork until verified by the person exhibiting the disorder. What this means is that psychiatric examination should be an exceptionally cautious exercise and every effort must be made to verify the validity of disorders suspected and check with the person being examined. In my own experience psychiatric examination often feels like a detective story, piecing together the bits of evidence from as many different sources as possible, but always remembering that the eyewitness is the person themselves. In the absence of their individual testimony, everything else is second best, but sometimes all we have.

To get back to the symptoms and diagnosis of disorders of perception, we have one last dilemma before we can have a look at them. As with our example of waking up with symptoms that lead to a diagnosis of a cold, disorders of perception are categorized into diagnosis in the same way. In doing this, psychiatry attempts to emulate medicine's ability to clearly diagnose a problem in order to identify it and decide how best to manage it. In theory, once the psychiatric diagnosis has been identified, treatment can be prescribed according to what is known to work best for that particular diagnosis. The problem comes when we consider how much harder it is to categorize psychiatric symptoms because:

- They are harder to define given what we have already said about their reliance on a clear personal account of internal mental processes.
- There is, at present, huge crossover of symptoms between the diagnostic categories. This means that a specific symptom or even collection of symptoms can still meet several different diagnostic categories.
- There is an additional problem that many seemingly mental symptoms can be caused by physical problems. An example of this is confused thoughts caused by high or low blood sugar in diabetes or hallucinations caused by brain trauma or brain tumour.
- Some psychiatric diagnoses are not dependent on disorders of perception as much as identified issues with how the person relates to the world and other people. In this area it is less clear that the symptoms arise from disorders of perception so much as difficulties in interacting with others.

For the sake of clarity I am going to adopt the broad groupings of psychiatric diagnosis postulated by the psychiatrist philosopher Karl Jaspers (Table 13.1).

Table 13.1 Psychiatric diagnoses

Group	Defining features	Notes
I	Cerebral illnesses, e.g. • Trauma, • Tumour, • Infection of the brain and membranes, • Hereditary illnesses which cause gradual damage to the brain, • Mental deterioration due to age or age-related conditions.	The root causes of these conditions are in the physical realm of the body. These are essentially psychiatric symptoms resulting from brain damage.
II	The major psychoses: • Schizophrenia, • Bipolar disorder/manic-depressive illness, • Psychotic depression.	Jaspers originally included epilepsy in this category, which would now not be accepted. I have added psychotic depression, which would. Although the symptom presentation for these conditions is clear, there is huge sharing of symptom type between the three.
III	Personality disorders: • Isolated abnormal reactions that do not arise from the recognized conditions in Groups I and II, • Neuroses and neurotic syndromes, • Abnormal personalities and their developments.	There are problems in representing some of these conditions as abnormal, since to do so would indicate that there are personality traits that are 'normal'.

(Adapted from Jaspers 1963)

In order to proceed with our discussion I am ignoring Group I conditions on the grounds that the symptoms that indicate these conditions are the result of physical illness and deterioration. Group III is also ignored, but for more complicated reasons. In these conditions, it is not how the world is sensed, interpreted and interacted with as a consequence, but rather how a person's personality is perceived by the world. It should be remembered, however, that people do not fit neatly into the above groups, and it is possible for people to have experiences applicable to more than one group.

The major psychoses, symptoms and perception

Psychosis is 'a severe mental disorder in which the person's ability to recognize reality and his or her emotional responses, thinking processes, judgement and ability to communicate are so affected that his or her functioning is seriously impaired' (Warner 1994: 4). If you look closely at this thumbnail sketch of psychosis, we can see that we are back in the realms of the process of perception: sensing, interpreting, interacting, and that things are going badly wrong. It's that first sentence that particularly gives the game away, where the ability to recognize reality comes in. To recap on the first section of this chapter, we recognize 'reality', or the world as experienced by the vast majority, through perception. So what sort of things can go wrong?

The major psychoses are a mixture of disorders of perception and disorders of mood. The main disorder of perception is schizophrenia, and the main disorder of mood is manic depression. To confuse matters, as indicated above, the actual symptoms, which are diagnostic of these conditions, have major crossovers. In other words, many of the symptoms listed below will be present in all three listed major psychoses. Having said this, schizophrenia is also the most commonly diagnosed of the major psychoses.

The story so far

- A person is a complex amalgamation of a physical presence, which operates in the physical world and a private mind, which is unique to the person.

- The two interact together through a process of perception which includes sensing the world, interpreting this information and interacting with the world as a consequence.

- Individuals, while sharing vast commonalities in the physical world, still have unique experiences.

- The mental processes can go wrong in the same way as physical processes.

- The mental can result in people 'doing' wrong due to:
    - physical problems affecting the mental processes,
    - problems with the process of perception,
    - problems with the formulation of a basic personality.

- Schizophrenia is the most common example of problems with perception.

In the remainder of this chapter I will explore the major symptoms of schizophrenia to allow for a separate consideration of disorders of mood in Chapter 14.

Schizophrenia

Traditionally, symptoms of schizophrenia are categorized into two types: positive symptoms and negative symptoms.

If someone were to say to you that you had a symptom which was 'positive', what would you think? Would you think that there was perhaps, some benefit in having this particular symptom? Would you think that it meant that the symptom was the one that confirmed your diagnosis (like HIV positive), while a negative symptom meant the diagnosis was wrong? If you did, you would be incorrect in both instances. Many people who are given a diagnosis of schizophrenia and either read or are told that there are 'positive symptoms' respond with 'there is nothing positive about them!' They are correct. The positive here does not refer to some judgement of the symptom as a good one to have. The 'positive' in this case means that the symptom is a mental experience, which would be considered as an *additional* experience to the norm, or an *exaggeration* of the norm. Given our exploration of perception above, this means the symptoms where mental events are generated independent of the physical world.

It follows that, if positive symptoms are an additional experience, negative symptoms are a *reduction* in normal experience. This can be seen from the list given in Box 13.1. As a general rule, however, the more a person is affected by negative symptoms, the more disabled they will be by schizophrenia.

Box 13.1 The two symptom groups of schizophrenia

Positive symptoms	Negative symptoms
• Hallucinations	• Lack of volition
• Delusions	• Lack of excitement
• Thought disorder	• Poverty of thought
• Catatonia	• Poverty of speech

Positive symptoms

Hallucinations

The archetypal symptom of mental illness has to be hallucinations. Hallucinations are traditionally defined as a person experiencing false sensory perception. With hallucinations a person experiences a sense, which does not emanate from the world around them. As such, hallucinations are mental experiences that do not have the physical cause necessary from the experience to be a true sensory experience. Table 13.2 links the names of the hallucinatory types to the senses. Notice that hallucinations can come from physical trauma to the brain or other physical causes such as brain tumour, epilepsy, drugs and alcohol (the famous pink elephants!).

The fact that hallucinations are defined as 'false' in the real world does not mean to say that the mental experience is not 'true' in the person's mind, because it is. The person does, indeed, hear a voice, or see an object, but the voice or object is not real. Therefore, the experience is a true one, but there is no cause for it. The person would experience exactly the same as if the sense in question were activated by a true sensory experience. Therefore a noise or voice is 'heard' in the mind, despite their being no voice or noise in the physical world, an image is 'seen', despite their being no object to see in the physical world. To give some idea of how difficult this is to accept for the person experiencing a hallucination, imagine the following scenario happening to you. You are walking down the street and your mobile seems to vibrate in your pocket. You take it out and put it to your ear. After you say 'Hello', the person says, 'You won't get away with it you know.' The reception is a bit fuzzy, but the words are clear. When you ask who it is there is a silence on the other end. There is no more conversation. As you take the phone away from your ear, you notice that it is not switched on.

What would be your first reaction, do you think? I bet it would be some rational theory about malfunctioning mobile phones, or wrong numbers. Next you might think that you turned the phone off by accident after receiving a wrong number, or even consider the possibility of your

Table 13.2 Types of hallucination

Sense	Hallucination	Notes
Hearing	Auditory hallucination	Most commonly reported. Can be an individual voice, a combination of voices or simple noises.
Sight	Visual hallucination	Can be definite shapes, such as faces of people, or lights and flashes.
Smell	Olfactory hallucination	Often linked to other symptoms. Can be indicative of a physical problem such as brain tumour or epilepsy.
Taste	Gustatory hallucination	Often linked to other symptoms. Can be indicative of a physical problem such as brain tumour or epilepsy.
Touch	Tactile hallucination	Often linked to other symptoms. Can be indicative of a physical problem such as brain tumour or epilepsy.

phone receiving a rogue signal. Whatever the reason you came up with, you would not consider that the voice you had heard was anything but real.

Although all senses can be falsely experienced, auditory hallucinations (often called 'voices') and visual hallucinations are the most reported.

Auditory hallucinations

If you had the above experience with the mobile phone once, you would probably not even notice it as abnormal. You may ponder on it for a while, but as the experience does not happen again, you would gradually forget about it. If the experience happened again and again and again, you would begin, not only to notice it, but also perhaps to become anxious and upset by it. If you started to hear the voice without the mobile phone going off as if the person were in the same room as you, you would get a bit concerned. If the voice started commenting on your actions in a derogatory way, or talked about you with another voice or started to voice your worst fears, threatened and abused you, then you might become extremely anxious. You may even confront the voice and start shouting at it to go away. The psychotic experience of having auditory hallucinations is not truly captured in the phrase 'hearing voices'. In psychotic experience the voice can often become a dominant factor in someone's life experience and interfere grossly with their functioning. In schizophrenia, auditory hallucinations are experienced over a long period of time, are intrusive, often abusive and disruptive and generally cause the person anxiety and distress.

In the case of auditory hallucinations or voices a substantial amount of research has been conducted into both the experience of voice hearing and the means to assist voice hearers. This research has uncovered some very interesting facts, the most important of which is that auditory hallucinations are not confined to people who would be diagnosed as psychotic. The consequences of this are important, as it is evident that hearing voices alone will not indicate a 'full' psychosis. We need to explore this fact in more detail to get a clearer picture of the nature of auditory hallucinations.

Auditory hallucinations: a 'normal' mental experience?

Research indicates that the presence of auditory hallucinations is higher in people diagnosed with psychosis, but that they are independently present in the so-called normal population (see Table 13.3). As a consequence, auditory hallucinations have been explored as a separate mental experience as opposed to a symptom of schizophrenia.

Romme and Esher (1993) in the Netherlands have undertaken what is probably the most illuminating work on auditory hallucinations alone. Their research investigated auditory hallucinations with a view to seeing if people experienced them in different ways. In a nutshell, they found that not all hallucinations were disabling in the manner that is assumed in a diagnosis of schizophrenia. What was clear in their discussions with people who experienced auditory hallucinations was that some people felt that they had

Table 13.3 Prevalence of auditory hallucinations

Population	Percentage who experience auditory hallucination	Source
Diagnosed with schizophrenia	53	Landmark *et al.* 1990
Diagnosed with major affective disorder	28	Goodwin and Jamison 1990
The 'normal' population	2.3	Tien 1991

control, or could cope with the experience of hearing voices, and some could not. Those who could cope either experienced the voice in a pleasant way or had found methods to control the hallucinations and not allow it to disturb their lives. Those who were disabled by the hallucinations reported being persecuted by the voice and/or feeling that they had little or no control over the voice. As we shall see, people who are grossly affected by the voice, or experience it along with other positive and negative symptoms are those who will be diagnosed with a psychosis. The experiences and techniques of those people who learn to cope with the auditory hallucination has also been utilized to assist all voice hearers, and has become a standard approach in assisting people with psychosis (cf. Chapter 10).

Other hallucinatory experience

As mentioned before, although auditory hallucinations are the most commonly experienced, other senses can also be falsely perceived. Visual hallucinations are the next most common after auditory hallucinations. The other sensory hallucinations are much less common and would lead to some concern that there may be a physical problem such as brain trauma, or that the hallucination is linked with other symptom types. An example is someone who believes a part of their body is dead when it is not and who gets an accompanying smell to confirm their thought, although no one else can smell anything (see somatic delusions below). Sometimes a brain scan or other physical tests can be carried out to rule out any physical cause for the hallucinatory experience.

A spanner in the works: pseudo hallucinations

There are a number of experiences which can be defined as false sensory perception, but which are not hallucinations. An example of this is an illusion (where the 'eyes play tricks on you'). Imagine it is a dark windy night and you are walking home. You suddenly see a black dog sitting under a lamp-post moving its head. As you draw nearer you realize you were mistaken and the 'dog' is a black binliner left out for the dustmen. This is an example of an illusion where the interpretation part of the perception system has got it wrong. This is not a hallucination, however, because, regardless of whether it was a binliner or a dog, there was something there.

In ordinary experience we also know that it is common to hear the voice of a loved one who has recently died, and that people are particularly susceptible to hearing and seeing things in the process of falling asleep or waking up. It is fairly easy to see why these things should happen. A recently bereaved person is very susceptible, as they are both in a state of shock and adjustment. It is common to hear bereaved people say, 'I keep expecting them to walk in the door as if nothing has happened.' It seems it is a short step from this feeling to having a false perception that the person speaks to us, or gives us some form of message. Similarly, in the process of falling asleep and waking up, the mind is in a state of flux and again susceptible to abnormal perceptions.

These experiences are called pseudo hallucinations. With regard to auditory hallucinations, there is one very particular form of pseudo hallucination, which is worth knowing about. If a person says that they are hearing voices, but that the voice is inside their head as opposed to outside in the physical world, this is also thought to be a pseudo hallucination. This does not mean to say that there is not a problem, but rather that the problem is not considered to be an auditory hallucination. In this case an assessor would note the experience but look for some of the symptoms below to describe it, and would consider the voice inside the head to be part of the thought process, rather than the sensory experience process.

Delusions

A delusion is traditionally defined as a false belief based on an incorrect interpretation of an external reality, which is adhered to by a person despite evidence to the contrary. But what does this mean? Well, let us consider what a 'belief' is.

Beliefs

We come to believe something through a process. First, we perceive events as already discussed in perception. An example is that we see the sun in the sky every day and see it go down every night. We then draw an 'inference' from this sequence of events. We infer that the sun goes up every morning and goes down every night. We then firm this inference into a belief. 'I believe that the sun will rise every morning and set every night.' This belief is further strengthened by a number of facts, or new information:

- It always happens. The sun always rises and sets.
- We find factual information that confirms our belief. In school we are taught that the sun rises and sets, and the science behind it.
- We are able to flesh out the belief into a wider, more complex, belief system. We find out about the exception of eclipse, where the sun is

covered by the moon. We find parts of the world where the sun is not in the sky for a long period and, again, understand the factual science behind this. Our belief becomes, 'The sun always rises and sets in the sky outside my home, although the occasional eclipse covers it up and I know that people living elsewhere do not experience the sun in the same way.'

In this way many of our beliefs become complex and are open to change with new information. If we consider this process in a slightly different way and consider the historically held belief that the world is flat, we can see that people had this belief because they perceived the horizon or a limit to vision; that ships disappeared from sight, that the ships that went too far never came back and, besides, everyone else believed the world to be flat. In addition, some cultures had a model of the world which necessitated it being flat. The cultures that believed the world was carried on the back of a giant turtle, or the Norse belief that the world was contained as a flat disc inside the skull of a dead giant had whole factual systems which told the people not only that the world was flat, but why it was flat, in the same way as our scientific system tells us it is not. That this belief would be considered wrong today is just an indication that beliefs can be wrong, but held as true by entire communities. It is interesting to consider what beliefs we now hold as factual but will be proven to be incorrect.

There are obviously far more complex beliefs which, given the ability of human beings to absorb information, have complex sources. If we are to consider the extent of religious belief in the world and balance this with the fact that most of the individuals who founded the various religious institutions lived thousands of years ago, we can see that the power of belief systems are amazing. Often these belief systems are passed from generation to generation as part of orientating children to the world, but then these children adopt the belief as their own and, in turn pass them on to their children.

It is, in fact, very difficult to shift a commonly held belief in a population. For this reason, before a belief can be held as false and therefore delusional it has to be seen as divergent from the standard beliefs of the culture from which the individual comes. In some circumstances beliefs common to some groups, such as a belief in witchcraft, spirits or possession, can be misinterpreted as delusions. This is because in some cultures these beliefs are still held with conviction among a significant number in the same way that a significant number of people in western culture believe in faith healing, crystallography, tarot cards, or any number of esoteric healing systems. Our definition of delusion needs to expand, then, to a false belief held with conviction that would be recognized as false within the cultural context of the individual.

Care should also be taken in considering delusional thinking to be irrational. Often the delusion has a basis in a perceived reality, but the initial real thought has been exacerbated to the extent it becomes bizarre. An example from the author's experience is a man who saw his friend stabbed to death who later believed that people were trying to kill him. While this might seem to be a perfectly reasonable, although horrible assumption, the incident had happened several years before, he was not directly threatened when it happened, and he had moved several hundred miles away and yet believed that the people had moved with him and set up an observation flat next door to him to monitor his movements. In addition, he felt that the way the milk bottles were left outside various flats in his block were subtle signals among the group who were persecuting him. In a situation like this it is very important to acknowledge the previous real experience prior to discussing delusional thinking. In this situation the perception is based on a real and terrible incident, which would have left an indelible memory on any individual. In this person's situation, however, the development of a complex delusional system of beliefs was not a natural reaction to the trauma experienced. Hence, while this man suffered from delusions, they were triggered by a true-life trauma.

Types of delusion

The type of delusion a person experiences is extremely important (Table 13.4). Traditionally delusions have also been considered fixed in a person's mind. It is now known that a person can come to have doubts about the validity of their delusional belief (Garety and Hemsley 1994). This can be useful if a skilled therapist can help the person to test and challenge their thinking. Bridget's story at the end of this chapter (p. 380) gives a clinical example of challenging and modifying beliefs.

Thought disorders

Delusional thinking is really a very specific form of what is known as 'thought disorder'. In thought disorder a person experiences disruption or disturbance to normal thought patterns. These are usually named after the description given of the pattern observed. Hence, 'thought block' is a thought disorder described by the person as having thoughts that seem to get blocked in, as if they 'hit a wall in the mind' (client description). There are many other forms of thought disorder, and many individuals who experience thought disorder are aware of disruption to their thoughts.

Passivity phenomena

Passivity phenomena are a sub-type of thought disorder where a person feels their thoughts are being interfered with or accessed by the outside world. In our discussion of perception it would be a disorder of perception where the barrier between the mental and the world is felt to be breached. Specific examples of passivity phenomena are listed in Table 13.5.

Table 13.4 Types of delusion

Delusional type	Note
Persecutory delusion	'They're out to get me' type of thought. These delusions are part of the lay person's stereotype view of schizophrenia and many television or film portrayals use this stereotype.
	It is probable that we all have felt persecuted or harassed at some time in our lives, whether true or not. For the feeling to be delusional it must be a gross experience in that the conviction and feeling of danger and/or interference must be extreme. A personal example is a client who had moved house three times because neighbours were passing electric shocks through the walls and was asking for help with another housing transfer. My querying of this request and the simple fact that moving house three times had not stopped the experience was met with my being included as one of the persecutors. Therapeutic work could continue only when I agreed to write a letter to the housing department.
	It is sometimes very difficult to pin paranoia down as many people present with what I call 'plausible paranoia'. Examples are people who complain that they are being monitored by CCTV cameras, given that there has been a massive increased use of camera surveillance in England over the last 10 years. Another example is people who fear terrorist attacks on their homes. Given the recent world events, this fear could seem plausible. The important distinction with a delusion is the irrationality when referred to the individual, so that they would feel the terrorists were targeting them specifically, or that the cameras could read their thoughts. Interestingly, in western cultures, as the incidence of catatonia has gone down, the incidence of paranoid delusions has gone up, although no one knows why this is (Frangou and Murray 1996).
Ideas of reference	'They talk about me on the radio', 'David Bowie writes lyrics for me.' In this delusional type a person feels referred to, as in these examples. They can also feel that events or behaviours of others refer to themselves. A young client of mine who was a passionate supporter of a certain football club believed that certain goal celebrations related to whether he was accepted or rejected by the players.
Grandiose delusions	Where a client truly feels they have special powers, gifts or talents such as being able to heal the sick, change world events. The person can also believe that they influence powerful people or have powerful friends when they do not.
Religious delusions	Where the delusional type has a specific religious connotation. An example is a client who believed that God was communicating with him through various signs and asking him to do various things, which he would then do. A person can also believe that he or she is a religious figure, such as a profit or spiritual saviour.
Somatic delusions	Somatic means a physical manifestation or feeling. Hence a person can feel that they have cancer when they do not, or that a part of the body has died while they continue to live.

Table 13.5 Types of thought disorder

Thought disorder	*Explanatory note*
Thought broadcasting	As the name implies, the person feels as if the thoughts they have are broadcast and, therefore, become available to the outside world. In thought broadcast the person can often be suspicious of all social encounters and develop the belief that people react to them in such a way as to confirm the thought broadcast. An example is a client of mine who would interpret people smiling at them as people laughing at the thoughts being broadcast.
Thought insertion	Again, as it sounds, this is where a person feels that thoughts are being inserted into the mind by someone or something else, although clients can often be unsure who or what is inserting the thought. In my experience, thoughts inserted in this way are often at odds with the individual's related beliefs. An example is a black female client who had anti-black racist thoughts inserted by her neighbours.
Thought withdrawal	Thoughts being taken out of the mind wilfully by a third party. Different from thought broadcast in that a specific agent will withdraw the thought but others will not be able to hear it.
Thought echo	Thoughts continue to sound in the mind as an echo, or repeat, either in full or part. The person feels that they have no control over this process.
Made feelings	An emotion is experienced which a third party has generated.
Made actions	Can be both simple and complex actions. 'Look, see my leg twitching? It's not me doing that – it's the freak getting me to look a fool.'

Catatonic behaviour

There is one very unusual symptom linked with schizophrenia that deserves some separate consideration, and this is catatonic behaviour (also called catatonia). Catatonic behaviour is a very recognizable symptom in that the person exhibits bizarre behaviour and seems to be lacking in physical or psychomotor movement, but the symptom is not considered to be a negative symptom. With catatonic behaviour, individuals can alternate between extreme agitation and stupor. In its most dramatic form, the stupor can result in statuesque behaviour with one posture being maintained for a long period of time. The interesting aspect of catatonic behaviour is its gradual reduction in western societies, yet its continued presence in non-western societies. The theory given to explain this is that catatonia is a somatic form of a particular delusion called delusion of possession. In this delusional belief the person will believe someone or something has taken possession of the person's body and western societies have developed the means to articulate these delusions verbally (Craig 2000). Whatever the truth, catatonia and its variant presentation underlines the difficulty in being definitive with regards to schizophrenia.

Negative symptoms

The so-called negative symptoms are harder to define and separate as they tend to be grouped together in the person's experience. The presence of negative symptoms usually results in changes in behaviour and functioning, as will be seen. For this reason, it is often negative symptoms that lay people such as family and friends tend to notice first. Great care needs to be taken as the loss of functioning associated with negative symptoms can often be viewed as within the individual's control, whereas the positive symptoms, with their bizarre, but noticeable difference from ordinary experience, are not. This misconception can lead to the person being criticized for 'not trying' or 'being lazy'. In past nursing care, many interventions for clients with negative symptoms were questionable if not abusive, particularly in residential or inpatient units. Examples would include locking clients' bedrooms or pulling them out of bed against their wishes. Negative symptoms are not in the person's control but are a very real part of the disabling nature of the experience of schizophrenia.

The main types of negative symptom are summarized in Table 13.6. The strange words in the brackets are the complicated medical terms for the conditions.

We need to be aware that the symptoms and behaviours in Table 13.6 could be attributed to other conditions or causes. The following would therefore need to be ruled out for a clearer understanding of the symptoms presented.

- Behavioural consequences of positive symptoms

  People who have the mental experiences outlined in the above section on positive symptoms can respond in many ways. Sometimes their

Table 13.6 Types of negative symptom

Negative symptom	Possible observed behaviour
Poverty of thought or speech (alogia)	Monosyllabic conversation. Inability to follow conversation. Repetitious topics of conversation.
Impaired volition (avolition)	Reductions in social care skills. Passive acceptance of situations.
Blunt affect (anhedonia)	Reduction in emotion and ability to enjoy.
Social withdrawal	Social isolation, avoidance of social interaction.

behavioural response can look like negative symptoms. An example would be a person not leaving their room due to a voice telling them that they would be harmed if they were to do so or a person not talking because of a delusional belief that people were against them. A thorough assessment of the lived experience of the individual is obviously necessary in these circumstances to ensure we have a correct interpretation of the person's presentation.

- Clinical depression

  Sadly, having a major condition such as schizophrenia gives you no protection from any other of the nasty things that a person can be afflicted with. In fact, people with schizophrenia are prone to many other health disabling conditions. You are more likely to be clinically depressed if you have schizophrenia than if you do not. There can be many causes for this, including living with all the positive and negative symptoms listed above, or the fact that you are stigmatized by society, as indicated in Frank Dobson's words at the beginning of this chapter. Whatever the cause, if you are depressed, you will exhibit the behaviours above. A thorough assessment of functioning should attempt to assess mood as well as mental experience to explore the possibility of depression.

  If a person is thought to have both schizophrenia and depression, they are often given a diagnosis of schizoaffective disorder, which means they should be treated for both the psychotic symptoms and the depression. Care should be taken in their management to titrate the treatment so as not to control one set of symptoms to the detriment of the other.

- Side effects of medication

  As discussed in Chapter 11, medication given to counteract the symptoms of schizophrenia can also have side effects such as sedation and movement disorders. Again, a thorough assessment of medication is needed to rule out possible side effects. Having said this, recent advances in medication seem to cut down on those side effects, which can be mistaken for negative symptoms (Adams 1999).

The point was made earlier that a history could be taken from people who know the person well to elicit any changes in behaviour or functioning. It was also noted that there could be problems with this. It is clear from the above that care needs to be taken if assumptions are made on the basis of observed behaviour as there can be many causes for this behavioural change. If the behavioural change is due to negative symptoms the individual family and friends need to be informed that these symptoms are as much part of the condition as the more obvious positive symptoms. The negative symptoms can cause as much distress and disability as the positive symptoms if not acknowledged and taken into consideration when supporting the person.

It used to be thought that negative symptoms were also the result of people with a diagnosis of schizophrenia being treated in large institutions and loosing social skills as a consequence. The advent of community care has not eradicated the presence of negative symptoms, however, and their presence remains in people now living in group homes or independently (Hogg 1996).

So how do we diagnose schizophrenia?

Let us stop for a second and take stock. Schizophrenia, as we described, is diagnosed, in the same way as a cold is diagnosed, through the presence of a number of symptoms. These symptoms are split into two distinct groups, the positive and the negative. The positives are exceptional experiences which people who do not have a diagnosis would recognize as strange. The negative symptoms are the lack of skills, which lead people to seem flat and withdrawn, or who have limited social ability.

We have also seen that a large number of other factors have to be taken into consideration when considering any single symptom. Auditory hallucinations can be experienced by so-called 'normal' people. Brain damage can also account for some of the symptoms, along with other physical causes. Depression and even the medication given for schizophrenia can mirror some of the negative symptoms, and we are even unclear about whether or not catatonia is a positive or a negative symptom. So how do we put it all together and come up with a diagnosis? What are the things we need to consider when confronted with one individual with the mixture of mental experiences that are causing concern?

Let us examine the World Health Organization classification criteria for a diagnosis of schizophrenia, often referred to as ICD 10, to see if we can find some answers (Box 13.2).

We can see from Box 13.2 that diagnosis following the experience is dependent on two things:

- *Time*. It is important that we are not talking about fleeting experiences but ones that are experienced for at least four weeks.
- *Gross disturbance*. In order for schizophrenia to be diagnosed there must be some gross disturbance to an aspect of functioning. The disturbance can be to the mental experience of perception as described above or social functioning and social performance.

So there we have it. Significant disorders of perception experienced over a long period of time is what schizophrenia actually means. In addition, the course of schizophrenia can take many forms depending on the prominent symptoms and if they remain after the first episode. As a consequence, it is better to view the overall care of people with schizophrenia with reference to their symptoms because:

1   There can never be one generic approach to 'schizophrenia' because the condition, as the above criteria indicate, contains too many variables.

2   Research studies need to ensure that population samples have similar symptom presentation, and not just rely on diagnosis. In evaluating

---

Box 13.2 Diagnostic criteria for schizophrenia

At least one of the symptoms (a)–(d) or at least two of the symptoms (e)–(i) should have been present during a period of a month or more:

(a) thought echo, thought insertion or withdrawal, and thought broadcasting;
(b) delusions of control, influence or passivity, clearly referred to body or limb movements or specific thoughts, actions or sensations, delusional perception;
(c) hallucinatory voices giving running commentary on the patient's behaviour, or discussing the patient among themselves, or other types of hallucinatory voices coming from some part of the body;
(d) persistent delusions of other kinds that are culturally inappropriate and completely impossible, such as religious or political identity, or superhuman powers and abilities;
(e) persistent hallucinations in any modality, accompanied either by fleeting or half formed delusions without clear affective component, or persistent overvalued ideas, occurring every day for weeks or months on end;
(f) breaks in interpolations in the train of thought, resulting in incoherence or irrelevant speech or neologisms;
(g) catatonic behaviour, such as excitement, posturing, waxy flexibility, negativism, mutism and stupor;
(h) 'negative' symptoms such as marked apathy, paucity of speech and blunting or incongruity of emotional responses, usually resulting in social withdrawal and lowering of social performance; it must be clear that they are not due to depression or neuroleptic medication;
(i) a significant and consistent change in the overall quality of some aspects of the personal behaviour, manifest as loss of interest, aimlessness, idleness, a self-absorbed attitude and social withdrawal.

---

research into schizophrenia we need to ask if there has been an attempt to ensure comparability of sample selection in this regard.

3   Treatments and interventions should identify exactly which symptoms or group of symptoms they aim to influence.

4   The variation in prognosis between different ends of the spectrum of psychotic experience is vast. It is very likely that this is influenced by time of onset (i.e., at what age symptoms first become disabling, acceptance of treatment in early stages, time between first onset and treatment), symptom presentation, and ability to control symptoms.

5   We need to re-evaluate outcome measures in line with the above symptom variables. In this way services must move from pejorative terms such as 'revolving door clients' and 'treatment resistant clients' which seem to view the ineffectiveness of treatment as the clients fault, rather than the treatments.

(Brennan 2001)

Symptom-focused treatments and interventions

It is important to have some understanding of the advances in treatment that have been made over recent decades, as the policy of community care behind the NSF for Mental Health can only be realized if we can assist people to live with their symptoms in society. The best way to approach the treatment of psychosis is as a *process* rather than an *event*. This means that we take a long-term view of treatment. Our clients will often experience their symptoms for a considerable number of years (either as a residual symptom or florid episodes between periods of remission). Recent research into effective interventions has accepted this reality and evaluated benefits on a long-term basis (i.e., when follow-up assessments are carried out years after the intervention). Clinicians should also take this view. Any positive improvement on a person's ability to cope and manage the symptoms and consequences of schizophrenia can benefit the person long after the relationship with a particular clinician has ended.

Psychiatric medication

Treatments for schizophrenia need to focus on the symptom or symptom group they are intending to encounter. The most widely used treatment method remains the chemical treatments provided by medication (discussed in Chapters 11 and 26).

Psychiatric medication is used to address changes in the activity of various neurotransmitters in the brain. Schizophrenia has long been associated with neurotransmitter irregularities and it was once thought that it could be explained solely in terms of these abnormalities. We did not and do not, however, know enough about the action of neurotransmitters to justify this claim. For example, where schizophrenia was initially linked to the neurotransmitter dopamine, it is now recognized that:

- Serotonin also has a possible effect on symptoms;
- there is more than one type of dopamine.

It is very probable that mental health nurses will, in the future and after specific training, prescribe medication. In the meantime, they have a major role to play in monitoring medication and advocating medication review in multi-disciplinary teams. Monitoring medication is about ensuring the maximum benefit with the fewest possible side effects. To do this, we must ask ourselves:

1 What symptoms are being targeted by the medication?
2 What change in symptom has the medication achieved for the client?
3 What side effects does the client experience?
4 Does the benefit of the symptom change justify the side effect for the client?
5 Can we further reduce the side effect?

It should be obvious that we can only elicit this from constant discussion and negotiation with the client. To facilitate this, all clients should also be made aware of the specific side effects associated with any medication and encouraged to monitor these themselves.

Problem- and symptom-focused psychosocial interventions

One of the common complaints regarding psychiatric treatment of schizophrenia has been its over-reliance on psychiatric medication. Since the 1970s, however, various talking interventions have been used in conjunction with medication in an attempt to address symptoms. These interventions, which have come to be known as psychosocial interventions, are mentioned below and are discussed in detail in Chapter 10.

Cognitive behaviour therapy (CBT)

CBT was a treatment regime first used with good effect for the treatment of depression. As its title would suggest, the individual learns how to link feelings and emotions with thought processes and behaviours. CBT is most often targeted to positive symptoms. This is because, as we have seen, the diagnosis of schizophrenia is often given due to disruption to thought and perception. With CBT the individual is guided through a range of processes designed to either help the person to distract their mind away from their distressing thought or experience, to being able to challenge a positive symptom as they experience it. An example would be a client who believes that 'everyone is talking about me' being guided through a questioning process to test out the reality of this thought.

Social skills training

As will be appreciated, individuals with the above symptoms will find ordinary social interaction difficult. Social skills training is, as its name implies, a series of interventions geared to increasing the person's ability in social interactions. There have been a variety of methods used in social skills training, but the majority use role-play, practice and homework in a safe environment to allow the individual the opportunity to experiment, gain confidence and social skills. The desired result is increased ability to problem solve and socially interact (Smith *et al.* 1996; Midence 2000).

Family interventions

Family interventions are an advocated valid intervention for two reasons:

1   Families (and indeed any committed carer) can be a valuable resource for individuals who have symptoms. Unfortunately, if they respond to symptoms by being critical or doing too much for the person, this can have a negative effect on the prognosis (this fact is also true for professionals).

2   Families can be negatively affected if they are left to help the individual cope with symptoms and are not given support.

There is evidence to show that, if offered education about schizophrenia and assistance with problem solving regarding symptoms and relationships, both families and clients can benefit. Although these benefits were most pronounced in the early development of the interventions by dedicated research teams (Pharoah *et al.* 2000), the NSF for Mental Health has cited them as of benefit to clients and their carers (DH 1999)

Case studies

The following case studies illustrate the discussion above, and the human experience that is schizophrenia.

Case one: Bridget's story

History and experience

At the time of meeting and working with Bridget she was a middle-aged widow and mother who had lived with psychotic symptoms for nearly thirty years. Bridget was experiencing a relapse of her psychotic symptoms following the death of her husband, Cyril, the year before. Cyril died of cancer and was described by Bridget as a loving husband and father. Bridget's two adult children described their parents as loving and caring.

Bridget first experienced symptoms following the death of her mother and the birth of her second child. At the time her experiences took the form of a hallucinatory voice which called her a whore and a 'sex pig'. The voice accused her of being too sexual and yet suggested she perform various sex acts with various people. Bridget had a strong religious belief and found particularly distressing the voice's suggestion to seduce her priest. Gradually she gained control of her hallucinations through medication and what she termed 'the love of my family and my God'. Although Bridget gained control the voice stayed with her and her control fluctuated over the years. Accordingly, she needed admissions to hospital, which were always accompanied by a secondary guilt about not being a good mother. On analysis these admissions coincided with various stresses and life events. As a consequence Bridget, on assessment, felt that the voice had 'robbed her of years'.

In addition to the voice, Bridget also experienced various thought disorders, particularly passivity phenomena. At these times she experienced thought insertion and thought broadcast. The content of the insertion and broadcast would be predominantly anti-God. These experiences, in her account, were always the precursors to admission and, on two occasions had led to serious suicide attempts, one of which had left permanent organ damage.

Between highly florid episodes of positive symptoms, Bridget would also experience lowering of mood, energy and the ability to enjoy her children. It was unclear if these experiences were the result of depression or negative symptoms.

The death of her husband Cyril had, predictably, led to a crisis and an increase of all positive symptoms. What was particularly distressing her was the fact that she experienced the voice as Cyril abusing her 'from the grave' and saying he didn't love her, as she was a 'whore with a dirty mind'. At the time of referral there were serious concerns regarding Bridget's ability to keep herself safe. An increase in medication had not had the desired affect of reducing the positive symptoms.

Bridget, as can be seen from the above, was a remarkable woman who was very burdened by her symptoms, and was viewed as an amazing survivor in the face of extreme difficulties. Her schizophrenia was only one aspect of her life, an aspect which gained dominance over her abilities as a wife, mother and individual at times, but was not her defining feature.

Keeping Bridget safe

The first priority of work with Bridget was to keep her alive. This necessitated some clear and open discussions with Bridget as to whether she should receive care in her home or in an inpatient unit. She was adamant that she wanted to stay at home with her children. An open analysis of the risk that this posed had to be undertaken with the family. It was decided that Bridget could continue to receive care in her home, but under tight supervision and that admission (against her will) would not be ruled out should it become necessary.

Medication

A review was undertaken. Although the medication for positive symptoms was not changed, an anti-depressant was added. Bridget and her family were informed of the fact that the medication would take some weeks to start taking effect.

Dealing with the 'voice'

Two psychosocial techniques were used as indicated by the work of Romme and Esher. A system of distraction using a recording of the Pope saying the rosary (a sequence of prayers with relevance to the Catholic faith) was utilized where Bridget would listen to the recording when the voices became particularly bad. Distraction is a technique true to its name where the mind is 'distracted' from the voice experience by various alternative activities. If successful, distraction is really a short-term relief from the voice experience and teaches the individual that they can begin to control the voice experience themselves.

In addition to distraction, set sessions focused on the incongruity of Bridget's lived experience with her husband and the content of the hallucinatory voice. This technique is a direct challenge to the voice experience and is designed to show that the voice is not as powerful as it seems to the person. Bridget was encouraged to reread old letters from her husband and to consider the possibility that the voice was not, in fact, his. Bridget was encouraged to ask the voice why she should believe it, as her real husband would not say these things. In these sessions it soon became evident that Bridget was frightened that if the voices stopped, even though it was negative and cruel, she would truly lose Cyril. This was felt to be a reasonable concern and in keeping with the process of grief.

Eventually Bridget regained control of her experiences and the voice became less frequent and, sometimes, reverted to its old form. The distraction was extremely effective in enabling her to gain control and she found herself getting so involved in prayer that she was able to block out the voice completely.

Despite this, the thought insertion remained and Bridget came to the belief that 'God did not love me.' For Bridget this was a major concern, increasing the risk of suicide. As the belief was examined, Bridget stated that the only way she could prove to herself that God loved her was if a certain priest were to tell her. Bridget was encouraged to write to this priest explaining her situation. She did this and the priest duly responded with a letter and a set of rosary beads. The priest stated that the beads had been blessed and were to be used in 'times of hardship as an indication of God's love for you'. Bridget took great comfort in this letter and the beads and was able to use them to challenge her negative thoughts.

Although it took more than 12 months for Bridget to regain her normal level of mental experience, and even then she did have to continue in her grief, she was deemed as no longer presenting a suicide risk. More importantly, Bridget felt able to control her symptoms and experience pleasure in her family.

Bridget's story shows how a detailed knowledge of the lived experience can both help to understand and support a person with psychotic symptoms. Bridget's greatest asset in the process of care was her ability to use positive mental experiences (her memory of Cyril and the reality of their marriage), beliefs (her religious faith) and relationships (her children) to combat negative false perceptions (her psychotic symptoms).

Case two: Brian's story

History and experience

Brian is a young man who was diagnosed with learning disabilities at age 4. Brian and his family have lived for many years on a council housing estate in a close-knit inner-city community. Given Brian's learning disability, he was marked as different from his older brother and sister at an early age. The family had been used to being involved with services as Brian had attended special school and a work programme for people with learning disability. It was in the work programme, when Brian was 21 years of age, that his mental health problems were first noted. Having said this, he was initially thought to be having difficulties adjusting to the work placement following leaving school.

At the time Brian's problems were coming to light he moved into a shared home for people with learning disabilities. It was in this home he experienced his first episode of florid psychotic symptoms, believing that other people in the house were attempting to poison him as they knew he was the son of a famous gangster, which he was not. Brian's family became so concerned that they took him back home, but his mental experiences did not change and he eventually needed admission, as he would stay up into the early hours to 'protect his family from harm'.

Eventually Brian was admitted to a special unit for people with mental health and learning disabilities. This unit was sixty miles away from his family and this further heightened his paranoia. Following assessment, Brian was transferred to a local inpatient unit where he improved on an atypical antipsychotic.

Brian was discharged following a CPA (care programme approach) meeting to a local mental health hostel. When his family went to visit him they again found him frightened and saying his room-mate was stealing his benefits and physically and verbally abusing him. Another resident verified Brian's story and his family again took him back home, very angry at services. They refused to take Brian back to see his psychiatrist and insisted that all medication and treatment be coordinated through the local general practitioner (GP). Brian's GP referred him and his family to a primary care mental health service run by a voluntary organization. The care plan for Brian and his family focused on assisting the family to care for him in their own home in order to build a rapport with them.

On assessment, Brian was suspicious and had reverted to sitting up at night watching the house. It was decided, given the effect his behaviour was having on the family, to meet him and his parents in joint sessions to address the wider family implications. Accordingly, the first sessions were spent in answering any questions the collective family members had regarding Brian's diagnosis of schizophrenia. It soon became clear that neither Brian nor his parents were aware of the long-term effects of schizophrenia, and that a person with learning disabilities could experience psychotic symptoms. In these sessions the family also expressed confusion as to the increased number of professionals they now had to deal with.

Collaborative work

Brian's suspicion transferred into his relationship with his care team. He would not talk in sessions, in spite of the best efforts of his family. After sessions, Brian would say that he was frightened that members of his care team wanted to 'experiment on him' or that the community nurse was motivated by homosexual feelings towards him. The family would then phone the care team to relate these feelings and talk about the strain caused by Brian's suspicion. It was clear to the care team that the only way to maintain Brian in any form of collaborative work was through the family, and, in particular, his mother who was a dominant force within the family.

Working with a family system

In order to work with Brian, a series of family meetings aimed at assisting his family in their caring roles were conducted. While he remained a quiet, suspicious presence in these meetings, his family were encouraged to discuss their experience and concerns in front of him. Eventually, he was able to articulate his thought processes and related a series of both positive symptoms and realistic fears due to his experiences. The positive symptoms were mainly in the form of delusions of reference (various television programmes referred to Brian and his family), passivity phenomena, which led to Brian feeling that his body had been taken over by a 'bad person with bad ideas'. The realistic fears were that he would be taken away from his family if he told people what he experienced. At this stage in the work, Brian's mother related that she had a brother born with a severe learning disability who had been admitted into a learning disabilities hospital shortly after his birth and 'abandoned'. The fear of separation, given the family's life experiences and previous treatment decisions was viewed as realistic.

Medication

It was clear in the early stages of family meetings that Brian had stopped all forms of medication due to a mixture of suspicion that the medication was aimed at drugging him so that he could be 'taken away' (related to family members and not the care team) and side effects. The medication was reviewed and changed to an atypical drug under the supervision of his GP, whom he still trusted. The family was encouraged to administer and supervise the medication. After a few weeks, clear gains in Brian's communication were being seen in meetings, and the family related that they were pleased with his response as there were no reported side effects.

Problem solving

The main area of concern, once the situation had been stabilized, was Brian's lack of socialization outside of the family. A plan was made that Brian would leave the house for planned activities with his father and brother, with whom he felt safe. As this proved effective, Brain was encouraged to carry out small tasks in the locality to build his confidence. This proved very effective and, with the gains attributed to his taking regular effective medication, Brian began to leave the house by himself.

There followed a period of unforeseen problems as Brian began to spend his days drinking alcohol in his room. His drinking became an issue as he would get intoxicated and get into arguments with family members.

Brain related that he was now bored and it was clear that he needed more focused activities during the day when other family members were at work.

Service problems

Both family and care team were frustrated by an inability to find appropriate activities for Brian. A mental health day unit proved to be unsuccessful as he was frightened of again being exploited and learning disability work and day units were uneasy at accepting him due to his mental health problems. In the process of working through these issues, Brian began to deteriorate. He was now at home for long periods by himself, continued to drink and began to omit medication doses. Eventually, following an argument with his sister during which the police were called, he was admitted to the local inpatient unit.

Conclusion

Following a short admission, Brian stabilized. He continued to remain well at home, but the struggle to find appropriate activities continued. At the time I left Brian's care team it was clear that if a solution could not be found, he would continue to go through a sequence of improvement and relapse with his family bearing most of the caring role.

Conclusion

These case studies attempt to put a human face on the collection of symptoms that is schizophrenia. Take another look at the stories and you will note that these are two very different people in terms of age, gender and position within the family, but they have in common a set of mental experiences which many do not have – psychotic symptoms.

Brian and Bridget had one other thing in common, and that was they received treatment from a psychiatric team that included nurses. In doing this, the team worked together as best it could and used evidence-based interventions that were sometimes successful and sometimes not. Within this, however, a relationship was formed with both Bridget and Brian and their families. Relationship forming is, for me, the most basic, under-rated and essential aspect of the process of nursing and indeed psychiatry. However, for a number of reasons, it doesn't always happen that the connection can be made between client, team and nurse. Sometimes, as discussed above, it may be because the client's mental processes get in the way. It can also be that the person with schizophrenia perceives that the nurse is interested in their schizophrenia more than in them as the person they are. This is what I refer to as the 'professional disorder of perception', which is characterized by:

- *seeing* the schizophrenia and not the person;
- *interpreting* everything in terms of schizophrenia without reference to the person; and
- *interacting* exclusively with the disabled rather than the able part of that person.

This disorder may hinder the health care professional affected from functioning to the best of their ability and may lead them to be ostracized from their client group. In reality it is extremely hard not to be affected by the 'professional disorder of perception', particularly when in the acute stages of their illness the client is more or less hidden beneath their symptoms. Reflective practice and supervision can assist the professional to analyse their ability to stay in touch with their clients as people rather than relate to them as collections of symptoms.

It is right that people with schizophrenia live in the communities to which they belong and contribute. However, it is also right that these communities are assisted through quality mental health services run by professionals who are able to see the person through the disorders of perception that often mask their potential. Only then will we ever hope to overcome the fear and stigma still present in our society.

In summary, the main points of this chapter are:

- Mental processes can go wrong due to: physical processes affecting mental processes; problems with the formulation of personality; and problems with the process of perception.
- Schizophrenia is a mental disorder associated with serious problems with perception. The world-view of people suffering from schizophrenia may often be at odds with the world-view of others, in particular their relatives or close friends who notice changes in the person's demeanour, behaviour and attitude as a cause for concern.
- Traditionally, the symptoms of schizophrenia are classified as 'positive' symptoms – those that are an additional experience to the norm, or an exaggeration of normal experience – or 'negative symptoms', which represent a reduction in normal experience. As a general rule, the more a person is affected by negative symptoms, the more disabled they will be by schizophrenia.
- Treatment of people suffering from schizophrenia is best regarded as a long-term process, rather than a one-off event. Medication and psychosocial interventions in combination can help clients to manage their symptoms while living in the community. Nurses have a major role to play with regard to both these types of interventions.
- Crucial to high quality care is the nurse's ability to relate to people suffering from psychosis as people, rather than as a collection of symptoms.

Questions for reflection and discussion

1   Reflect on your own mental experiences. Can you relate to any of the mental experiences outlined above?

2   Reflect on your own belief systems. Are there aspects of your beliefs, such as religious beliefs, that others would not share? Why are your beliefs not delusional?

3   Consider what your own beliefs and attitudes were to people with schizophrenia prior to your training. Where did these come from? Have they changed? What has changed them?

4   What do you feel is the prevalent attitude to schizophrenia among the general population? If you wished to change this, how would you go about it?

5   Review Standards 4 and 5 of the NSF for Mental Health (listed in Chapter 4) with regard to the above case studies. Are these standards relevant to Bridget and Brian and their carers?

6   Review Standard 6. How is this standard relevant to Bridget and Brian? Who is this standard most relevant to and why?

7   How has Standard 7 been met in Bridget's case?

Annotated bibliography

- Chadwick, P. (2002) Understanding one man's schizophrenic experience, *Nursing Times* **98**(38): 32–3. In this short personal account, Peter Chadwick outlines his own experience of schizophrenia. The article gives a personal view of the issues presented here and is immensely worth the small effort that it takes to read. Peter Chadwick is an expert in many ways, being both a user of services and a teacher of professionals.
- Deveson, A. (1991) *Tell Me I'm Here*. London: Penguin. This is a personal account from the carer's perspective. The book is uncomfortable reading at times, particularly some of the family's encounters with professionals. The book again allows us to consider the perspective of non-professionals who are experts in their own right.
- Haddock, G. and Slade, P. (1996) *Cognitive Behavioural Interventions with Psychotic Disorders*. Routledge: London. A complex book, but a comprehensive exploration of talking interventions aimed at alleviating psychotic symptoms.

References

Adams, C. (1999) Drug treatments for schizophrenia, *Effective Health Care Bulletin: NHS Centre for Reviews and Dissemination*, Vol. 5, No. 6.

Brennan, G. (2001) Schizophrenia, diagnosis and introduction to interventions, *Mental Health Practice* **4**(7): 32–8.

Craig, T.K.J. (2000) Severe mental illness: symptoms signs and diagnosis, in C. Gamble and G. Brennan (eds) *Serious Mental Illness: A Manual for Clinical Practice*. London: Bailliere Tindall.

Department of Health (1999) *The National Service Framework for Mental Health, Modern Standards and Service Models*. London: Department of Health.

Frangou, S. and Murray, R. (1996) *Schizophrenia*. London: Martin Dunitz.

Garety, P. and Hemsley, D. (1994) *Delusions: Investigations into the Psychology of Delusional Reasoning*. Hove: Psychology Press.

Gombrich, E.H. (1960) *Art and Illusion: A Study of the Psychology of Pictorial Representation*. Princeton, NJ: Princeton University Press.

Goodwin, K. and Jamison, K.R. (1990) *Manic Depressive Illness*. New York: Oxford University Press.

Hogg, L. (1996) Treatment for negative symptoms, in G. Haddock and P. Slade (eds) *Cognitive Behavioural Interventions with Psychotic Disorders*. London: Routledge.

Jaspers, K. (1963) *General Psychopathology* (trans. J. Hoenig and M.W. Hamilton). Chicago, IL: University of Chicago Press.

Landmark, J., Merkskey, Z., Cernousky, Z. and Helmes, E. (1990) The positive trials of schizophrenic symptoms: its statistical properties and its relationship to thirteen traditional diagnostic systems, *British Journal of Psychiatry* **156**: 388–94.

Midence, K. (2000) An introduction to the rationale for psychosocial interventions, in C. Gamble and G. Brennan (eds) *Serious Mental Illness: A Manual for Clinical Practice*. Bailliere Tindall.

Pharoah, F., Mari, J. and Streiner, D. (2000) Family interventions for schizophrenia, *(Cochrane Review) The Cochrane Library*, Issue 3. Oxford: Update Software.

Priest, S. (1991) *Theories of the Mind*. London: Penguin Books.

Romme, M. and Esher, S. (1993) *Accepting Voices*. London: MIND.

Smith T.E., Bellack A.S. and Liberman, R.P. (1996) Social skills training for schizophrenia: review and future directions, *Clinical Psychology Review* **16**(7): 599–617.

Tien, A.Y. (1991) Distribution of hallucinations in the population, *Social Psychiatry and Psychiatric Epidemiology* **26**: 287–92.

Warner, R. (1994) *Recovery from Schizophrenia: Psychiatry and Political Economy*. London: Routledge.

14

The person with a mood disorder

Shaun Parsons

Chapter overview

This chapter discusses the care and treatment of people suffering from disorders of mood or what are referred to more commonly as affective disorders. It is in two parts: the first discusses depression and the second, bipolar disorder. Case studies are used to illuminate the conditions described and to highlight the experiences of service users. This chapter covers:

- Depression and dysthymic disorder;
- Treatments for depression;
- Principles of nursing a person experiencing depression;
- Bipolar disorder: manic episodes, mixed states, other symptoms;
- Treatment of bipolar disorder;
- Principles of nursing a person suffering from bipolar disorder.

Depression and dysthymic disorder

Depression is one of the most common of all psychiatric disorders. Even in its less severe forms, it is responsible for causing distress and disability to many people. An individual with depression described the experience in the following words 'it's not bad I don't feel like killing myself or anything but I can't be bothered, it takes all the joy out of my life'. This was someone who was experiencing what would be described clinically as mild depression and yet their life was blighted by the illness. Depression is also one of the primary causes of self-harm and suicide and Goodwin and Jamison (1990) have estimated that 15–20 per cent of depressed individuals go on to commit suicide. Depression, therefore, not only affects the sufferer but also has a profound effect upon their family and friends and is a major cause of work lost through sickness. It is estimated that 2 per cent of the population suffer from pure depression and a further 8 per cent suffer from mixed anxiety and depression (Hale 1997).

Depression is characterized by a variety of symptoms of which the most prominent is a pervasive low mood. The American Psychiatric Association's *Diagnostic and Statistical Manual* version IV (DSM IV) (APA 1994) defines depression as a condition where at least five of the symptoms summarized below are present:

- depressed mood most of the day, nearly every day;
- markedly diminished interest or pleasure in all, or almost all, activities most of the day, nearly every day;
- significant weight loss when not dieting or weight gain;
- insomnia or hypersomnia nearly every day;
- psychomotor agitation or retardation nearly every day;
- fatigue or loss of energy nearly every day;
- feelings of worthlessness or excessive or inappropriate guilt nearly every day;
- diminished ability to think or concentrate, or indecisiveness nearly every day; and
- recurrent thoughts of death, suicidal ideation.

The symptoms described above may be very severe, pervading all aspects of a person's life or they may be relatively mild. Mild depression or 'feeling blue' merges into the clinical condition of dysthymia (APA 1994), which is essentially a prolonged mild depression. However, as the APA point out in DSM IV periods of transitory sadness and even more intense feelings of grief are part of the human condition and we should not seek to pathologize them. Sometimes other symptoms of depression are present without the sufferer complaining of low mood; this is said to be masked depression. This kind of depression can be difficult to spot as sometimes symptoms are somatized, that is the depression is manifested as, for example, abdominal pain, headache or excessive tiredness.

For 80 per cent of individuals with depression the disorder is episodic and recurring, i.e. although the depression resolves it will reoccur at a later date. However, some 20 per cent of people with depression are said to have a chronic course, that is the symptoms do not remit but are continuous (Thornicroft and Sartorius 1993). A less severe form of chronic depression is dysthymic disorder which is discussed below.

Dysthymic disorder

Dysthymia is very similar to depression; however the symptoms are less severe and occur over at least a two-year time period.

DSM IV (APA 1994), states that for a diagnosis of dysthymia a person must have a range of symptoms, which must impair and impinge upon their daily functioning. These symptoms include a depressed mood for most of the day, which is present on most days for at least two years. While the individual is experiencing depressed mood they should also experience at least two of the following symptoms:

- poor appetite or overeating;
- insomnia (lack of sleep, inability to get to sleep and/or early morning wakening) or hypersomnia (excessive sleeping);
- low energy or fatigue;
- low self-esteem;
- poor concentration or difficulty making decisions; or
- feelings of hopelessness.

During the two years they have been feeling depressed the individual should not have been free from feeling depressed or from two of the six symptoms for more than two months at any one time and they should not meet the criteria for a 'major depressive episode' during the two-year period. Additionally there should never have been a 'manic episode', a 'mixed episode' or a 'hypomanic episode', and criteria for 'cyclothymic disorder' (these disorders are discussed later in this chapter). The symptoms should also: not occur during the course of a chronic psychotic disorder, such as schizophrenia or delusional disorder; not be due to the direct physiological effects of a substance, for example a street drug or a prescribed medication; and not be due to a general medical condition, for example hypothyroidism which can produce symptoms of depressed mood.

Treatments for depression

Over 90 per cent of people with depression are treated in primary health care with only a small number requiring a psychiatric admission (Scott *et al.* 1997). Therefore, practice nurses, primary care-based psychiatric nurses and community psychiatric nurses (CPNs) are the most likely nurse contact for depressed people. There are a number of treatment options for people with depression but broadly they fit into three groups:

- anti-depressant therapy;
- talking therapies; and
- combined talking and anti-depressant therapy.

In addition, electro-convulsive therapy is used for severe, life-threatening depression and for depression with psychotic features.

Anti-depressant therapy

As discussed in Chapter 11, there is a variety of anti-depressant therapies available. Some, such as the tricyclic group of drugs, have been available since the 1950s while others are more recent additions, for example, the selective serotonin reuptake inhibitors (SSRIs). In recent years these have become the dominant anti-depressant medication, especially in primary health care. Most anti-depressants are equally effective if given at therapeutic doses for sufficient periods (Hale 1997), the main differences between them being their side effects. It is important that anti-depressants are given in high enough doses to be therapeutic, in primary health care anti-depressants are too often given at sub-therapeutic doses and do not have an anti-depressant effect and additionally they may often be discontinued before they have their full effect (Hale 1997). This can lead to the mistaken belief that the depression is treatment resistant or that medication has failed.

There are three principal types of anti-depressants and also a combination therapy, and these are discussed below.

Tricyclic anti-depressants

This group has largely been replaced by the SSRIs due to the large number of anticholinergic side effects and, additionally, the drugs' lethality in overdose. Examples of tricyclic anti-depressants are clomipramine and amitriptyline. Tricyclic medications have a number of unpleasant side effects of which the most important from the user's point of view are anti-cholinergic side effects. Anticholinergic effects can include insomnia and tremor (which normally disappear after the first two weeks), dry mouth, blurred vision, constipation and difficulty in urination. There can also be more severe side effects including postural hypotension (drop in blood pressure when the individual stands up, which can cause fainting), tachy-cardia and sometimes cardiac arrhythmias even at a low dose. There are also side effects which are particularly distressing such as loss of sex drive, failure to maintain an erection in males, increased sensitivity to the sun, sedation (sleepiness) and increased sweating. Some of these side effects will disappear after a few weeks or if the dosage of the medication is decreased. A particularly distressing side effect is weight gain which can be as much as 450 grams a month with about 25 per cent of individuals taking the medication gaining 9 kilograms or more. Since tricyclic medication can cause cardiac arrhythmias even in normal doses, and especially in overdoses, they can cause sudden death. The lethality of a drug for depression is especially problematic since an individual who is depressed may attempt suicide and tricyclic medication is an effective method of suicide. Lofepramine is safer than other tricyclics in over dose and has relatively few anticholinergic side effects.

Serotonin reuptake inhibitors (SSRIs)

These are the most common anti-depressant medications in use at present and widely used examples include fluoxetine (Prozac) and citalopram hydro-bromide (Cipramil). SSRIs cause the amount of serotonin (5HT) available to neurones in the brain to increase. Serotonin is a chemical known as a neurotransmitter which is used to pass a signal across a gap in the neurone known as a synapse. By increasing the level of serotonin the way in which signals passing along neurones is changed and the effect of this change is, among other things, anti-depressant. SSRIs have the advantage over many other anti-depressants that they can be taken as a single daily dose and are free from sedative and anticholinergic side effects. In addition they appear to be safe in overdose making them a safer drug for those people at risk from self-harm. They do have side effects such as vomiting, nausea, lack of appetite, drowsiness, dry mouth, sleep disturbances, difficulty passing urine, and sweating, especially initially. However, compared with other anti-depressants these side effects are rare and resolve quickly for most people. The reduced side effects and the need to take only one dose per day helps to improve compliance in SSRIs and explains the rapid increase in their popularity. In a number of studies SSRIs have been shown to be as effective in treating depression as the tricyclics.

Monoamine oxidase inhibitors (MAOIs)

MAOIs are also an older anti-depressant drug and are rarely used today. Although effective, they place a number of dietary restrictions on people taking them. Any food containing tyramine, for example, yeast spread, can cause an extreme hypertensive episode, which is unpleasant and can be fatal, although this event is rare.

Combined drugs

A number of anti-depressants are available which combine two types of agent. An example of which is Venlafaxine, which is a mixed serotonin and noradrenaline reuptake inhibitor. It has a number of side effects including nausea and vomiting, headache and sweating but is relatively safe in overdose. Its main advantage is its speed of action compared to other anti-depressants, including SSRIs, with effects within seven days being reported (Porter and Ferrier 1999). It is, therefore, particularly suitable for severe depression with suicidal ideation.

Cognitive behavioural therapy

Cognitive behavioural therapy (CBT) is a behavioural modification technique which aims to challenge the negative thoughts and attributions associated with depression and replace them with positive, or at least neutral, attributions. It is based upon the theory that people with depression have different thought processes (cognitions) to people not experiencing depression and that by teaching the individual to change these thought processes the symptoms of depression can be reduced or even eliminated.

Attributions are the names and more importantly the causal explanations we give to the events that happen around us. The result of these events can be given a number of attributions. Firstly, the cause of events can be grouped into several categories. Some events are caused by us (i.e. they would not happen without an action from us), some of them would happen anyway, some events would have happened anyway but are affected by us. The effect of the event is also an attribution and this can be a negative, neutral or positive attribution. To make this clearer the event of dropping a glass of red wine is given.

Firstly, what are the attributions surrounding the cause of the event? The wine could have been dropped for a number of reasons. From the perspective of the person dropping the wine the causes attributed could be:

1   My hand was jarred and I dropped the glass.

2   The glass was slippery and I dropped it.

3   I was careless and I dropped the glass.

4   I'm so useless and worthless, everything I do is wrong, I'm pathetic.

As you can see from the example above it is possible to assign positive, neutral and negative attributions to causes. In attribution 1 the cause of the event is located entirely outside of the individual – their hand was jarred. In attribution 2 the cause is no longer outside of the individual but is mitigated by saying that the glass is slippery. In 3 the individual blames himself/herself for the event but perceives it as an act of carelessness, however, in attribution 4 the individual not only blames himself/herself for the event but uses it as evidence that he/she is a worthless and useless person. The type of attribution shown in 4 is known as a global attribution in that one small error is being applied to the rest of an individual's life and is used to reinforce a negative self-image.

A further important and related concept to be considered here is the individual's locus of control. The locus of control is the extent to which an individual feels in control of their day-to-day life. Crudely, this point of control varies between two poles either feeling that one is an active participant in events and has control of one's life, or that one is generally powerless and helpless and at the mercy of events. Most people will have a general view of their locus of control and a series of specific attributions of locus of control for different events. For example, imagine that you needed to travel to an important meeting and the train you are travelling in is late. As in the previous example, a number of attributions can be assigned which reflect the perceived locus of control:

1   The train is late, it's not my fault there is nothing I can do about it.

2   The train is late, there is nothing I can do about it now but I should have got an earlier train.

3 The train is late, I am so stupid and useless, I should have got an earlier train or gone down the night before.

4 The train is late I must be able to do something.

In the first three examples the locus of control is set externally. In example 1 the individual is exonerating themselves from the blame whereas in the second and third example the person, while acknowledging that there is nothing they can do about the train, blames himself or herself to a greater or lesser extent for being in that position in the first place. However, in example 4 the individual still feels that they are in control to some extent and feels, somewhat unrealistically, that they can do something about it.

It has been suggested that people with depression have a particular attributional style (see Rizley 1978). This style is one in which negative events such as failure are attributed to some internal factor, for example: 'My baby is always crying; I'm a bad mother.' Non-depressed individuals are more likely to try to attribute negative events to some external factor, for example: 'I failed that exam because my flatmates were so noisy; I could not concentrate to revise.' Generally, an attributional style which assigns internal, powerless attributions to daily events is a feature of thinking, or cognition, when depressed. In addition, it has been suggested that a locus of control in which the individual feels powerless most of the time, even when, in fact, they are not, is also associated with depression. Seligman (1975) suggested the theory of learned helplessness in which he proposed that when people no longer feel in control of their lives they become apathetic and depressed. It has been suggested that those people least likely to become depressed tend to feel in control of their lives while those most likely to become depressed do not feel in control of their lives for most of the time.

CBT aims to train the individual to stop thinking negatively about themselves, to adopt more neutral or positive attributional styles and, additionally, to begin to feel that they are in control of their lives to at least some extent. Readers are referred to specialist texts on CBT with bipolar disorder provided at the end of this chapter, and also Gamble and Curthoys's discussion of talking therapies in Chapter 10. However, two of the techniques used in CBT, which may also be useful in daily nursing care of depressed people are described below:

- *Thought catching or blocking*: Here the individual is taught to counter a negative thought with a more positive attribution. Therefore in the wine-glass example given earlier the individual who thinks that they are useless and always dropping things would counter the thought by thinking: 'That was clumsy but I did not do it on purpose and I don't do it very often.'

- *Reframing or re-authoring events*: Here events, which the individual sees as being negative or which are viewed as evidence of, for example, worthlessness are reviewed and an attempt is made to change the cognitions associated with them. This may be an event in the past such as a failed marriage or a current event such as a baby's repeated crying, which is being used to reinforce a mother's view that she is a bad parent. People are encouraged to see events in a wider context and to see that they are perhaps not entirely to blame for negative events such as a failed marriage or, in the example of a persistent crying that crying is not evidence of bad parenting but that the baby is simply hungry, or often has colic.

CBT has been shown to provide immediate benefits in terms of a reduction of depressive symptoms and reduces the relapse rate of major depression. The usual course of CBT is 15–18 treatments carried out by a mental health professional trained in CBT. However, Scott *et al.* (1997) has shown that even fairly brief CBT of four sessions delivered within a primary care setting can be effective in reducing depression symptoms.

CBT demands substantial investment of time by both the therapist and the client. Scott *et al.* (1997) point out that the therapist must be a skilled clinician trained in CBT techniques and that brief CBT in particular is a highly skilled intervention. Regrettably, there is currently a shortage of therapists trained in CBT. Therefore, although CBT is an effective intervention it is also an expensive treatment within primary and community health care settings.

Electro-convulsive therapy (ECT)

ECT is the passage of an electrical current through the brain with the intention of artificially inducing a seizure. For many years its mode of action was not understood, however recent research suggests that it works by stimulating dopanergic pathways in the brain causing an increase in levels of dopamine (a neurotransmitter) and its metabolites resulting a rapid anti-depressant effect (Porter and Ferrier 1999). It has been shown to be an effective treatment for all forms of depression but is particularly suitable for treatment of depression, which has not responded to anti-depressant therapy (Hale 1997), and depression with symptoms of psychosis or in individuals with learning disabilities who are experiencing depression (Porter and Ferrier 1999). In addition, it is a useful emergency treatment of severe, life-threatening depression due to the rapidity of the onset of its anti-depressant effect (Porter and Ferrier 1999).

ECT is not a stand-alone treatment of depression but should always be given in conjunction with anti-depressant therapy and/or cognitive therapy. It is also important to maintain anti-depressant therapy after a course of ECT (Hale 1997).

ECT has been, and remains, a controversial treatment for some mental health professionals and service users who fear that it causes permanent impairment of cognitive function and who, in the past, were able to point to lack of understanding of its mode of action. However, ECT is a safe procedure with a risk of death during treatment of two deaths per 100,000 treatments, which is the same rate as for other minor procedures carried out under general anaesthetic (Hale 1997). Although there is no evidence that ECT causes brain damage or intellectual impairment (Royal College of Psychiatrists 1995), it does cause short-term, transient cognitive side effects. These side effects include short-term memory loss, confusion and headache, the effects are particularly pronounced if the treatment is given three times a week, in the case of life-threatening depression, as opposed to twice a week. The symptoms normally resolve within a few hours of treatment. However, repeated studies have failed to find evidence for long-term cognitive impairment, for example, the American Psychiatric Association (1990) task force on ECT. In addition, the mode of action of ECT is now more clearly understood as described above. ECT, therefore, remains a useful treatment for depression, and when combined with anti-depressant therapy and CBT it can be a life-saving intervention.

Principles of nursing a person experiencing depression

The main role of the nurse is to build a collaborative relationship with the person experiencing depression. This relationship is the core of working with the depressed person. It is a relationship that must be built on genuine respect and openness in which the nurse is seen as a partner in the depressed person's recovery. When examining the principles of nursing an individual with depression, it is important to bear in mind the standards of the *National Service Framework (NSF) for Mental Health* (DH 1999), some of which are particularly relevant to the treatment of depression. Given the high prevalence of depression in primary health care, and the fact that 90 per cent of people with depression are treated in primary health care, Standard 2 is important. Standard 2 states:

> Any service user who contacts their primary health care team with a common mental health problem should:
>
> - have their mental health needs identified and assessed;
> - be offered effective treatments, including referral to specialist services for further assessment, treatment and care if they require it.

It is therefore important that nurses working in primary health care are familiar with the signs of depression and are able to detect them. It is also important that effective treatments are offered to people who have been detected as having depression. Again this is particularly relevant in primary care since research discussed earlier suggests that people with depression in primary care are often prescribed sub-therapeutic doses of anti-depressants, and there is a shortage of suitably trained professionals to offer cognitive behavioural therapy. It is also important that the provisions of Standard 3 of the *NSF for Mental Health* are met, that is:

Any individual with a common mental health problem should:

- be able to make contact round the clock with the local services necessary to meet their needs and receive adequate care.
- be able to use NHS Direct, as it develops, for first-level advice and referral on to specialist helplines or to local services.

Individuals with depression need to be able to seek help and feel able to discuss their feelings with primary health care staff. Many of the feelings and thoughts engendered by depression are intensely personal and difficult to discuss. Nursing staff need to be aware of this and should take time to build a relationship with depressed people and enable them to discuss their problems. Although this sounds simple, the demands of modern primary care mean that primary care practitioners are often busy and under considerable pressure, and it is difficult to spend time discussing an individual's feelings and problems. However, this is exactly what a person experiencing depression needs. It is important, therefore, that primary care staff recognize this need and ensure that adequate time is allowed for discussion when making appointments for people with depression.

The starting point for the nursing care of a person with depression is the preparation of a care plan. It is suggested that five areas are given particular attention, whether in the community or in hospital. These are outlined below and then illustrated through reference to a case study.

Monitoring of mood

Depression, as the title of this chapter suggests, is a disorder of mood, and perhaps the key role of the nurse is to continually monitor mood as part of an ongoing assessment. It is only through monitoring of mood and other symptoms of depression that the effectiveness of any treatment plan can be assessed. It is important to assess mood within three inter-related domains: physical, cognitive and behavioural.

With respect to physical signs, particular note should be made of a disturbed sleeping pattern especially difficulty in falling asleep or waking particularly early. A careful eye should be kept on any change in weight, as depressed people may not eat. Very depressed people may even not drink and therefore careful observation should be made of their fluid status and any signs of dehydration should be noted. A person who is depressed to the extent that they are not taking fluids should always be admitted to hospital.

Cognition can only be assessed indirectly through noting an individual's conversation and interactions with others. It is particularly important to note the attributions that people give the events around them and negative attributions should be noted and, if appropriate, challenged. As noted earlier, people with depression will often have very negative views of themselves and often attribute negative meanings to everyday events. Although CBT should be carried out only by those who are trained in the therapy it is appropriate for nurses to draw on CBT techniques, such as challenging negative attributions and cognitions and encouraging the depressed person to counter negative thoughts with more positive attributions.

Behavioural signs are assessed mainly through observation and are closely linked to the previous two domains, especially physical signs. However, what is being observed here is behavioural style rather than specific behaviours. Is the individual showing psychomotor retardation (i.e. are they carrying out actions more slowly)? Are they moving around less than usual? Are they neglecting their self-care, not washing or changing their clothes, or perhaps staying in bed?

Information about mood can be gathered from the depressed person himself/herself in response to the important open question, 'How do you feel?' This information together with information gathered within the three domains can be used by the competent nurse to make an accurate judgement of the person's mood.

Assessment of risk

Any assessment of depression requires that the risk of self-harm or suicide be assessed. This is highlighted by the *NSF for Mental Health* and is particularly relevant to depressed people since self-harm and suicide are prevalent. Standard 7 says local health and social care communities should prevent suicides by ensuring the other standards are enacted and additionally NHS services should:

• ensure that staff are competent to assess the risk of suicide among individuals at greatest risk; and

• develop local systems for suicide audit to learn lessons and take any necessary action.

It is particularly important that community health staff are competent at assessing suicide risk especially as people experiencing depression are at a greater risk of suicide and self-harm than the non-depressed population. When individuals talk about suicide and self-harm they should *never* be ignored. Anyone showing symptoms of severe depression, especially psychomotor retardation and/or psychotic symptoms, should be regarded as at high risk of suicide, as should anyone who has previously attempted suicide or self-harm. It should be noted also that a person determined to self-harm may not discuss their intentions for fear that they will then be prevented. Paradoxically, depressed people are at highest risk of suicide when they begin to recover. As their mood begins to lift, psychomotor retardation decreases and motivation increases, the individual may become more able and motivated to carry out a suicidal act, because they may still feel profoundly depressed. Therefore, as a depressed person begins to recover, assessment of suicide risk becomes increasingly important. Risk assessment is discussed in detail in Chapter 8.

Acting as an advocate

Nurses are uniquely placed to act as advocates to service users because they spend more time with them than most other mental health professionals, particularly with those users being cared for in hospital. People experiencing depression may be withdrawn and passive and may not be able to assert their rights or ask questions of those treating them. It is the nurse's role to facilitate these individuals to ask questions about their treatment plan and be active participants in their own care. Sometimes, despite the nurse's best efforts, the individual experiencing depression may still not engage in their care; in this situation it is the nurse's role and duty to ask questions on the individual's behalf, particularly when treatment is being enforced.

Respecting personal space and reserving time to talk

In the busy world of modern health care, and particularly in hospital, nurses may feel under pressure to 'get results', and they may also be extremely busy. It is easy to forget that the busy pace of the modern health professional may not be the pace of a person experiencing a mental health problem, particularly depression. A feature of depression is that people often feel the need to be alone with their sadness and to reflect on their thoughts. They may, therefore, spend a lot of time alone in their room or some other quiet place; if at home they may rarely go out, or answer the door or telephone. The nurse needs to strike a careful balance here. It would be wrong to drag the depressed person out into public situations, since this would deny their rights and does not respect their feelings. However, it would be equally wrong to ignore the person sitting alone and isolated. Instead the nurse should let the depressed person know where they can find them and when off duty who they can talk with instead. The nurse might go to the depressed person at regular intervals to let them know they are still around and try to engage them in conversation or perhaps to simply sit with them awhile in silence. If the depressed person is living at home, a brief visit or a telephone call by the nurse may be appreciated. At the same time reinforce the idea that recovery involves re-engagement of the depressed person with society and that, although their right to time to themselves will be respected, it is also part of the nurse's role to help them re-engage.

All these actions by the nurse will let the depressed person know that someone cares for them and that they are not alone. These two simple facts alone may provide the person with a foundation for recovery.

Valuing the individual

The concept of valuing the individual is an extension of the point made above. Often when the depressed person does engage in conversation they will be profoundly negative and self-blaming, and they may also apparently resist attempts to engage in treatment. It is important to try to respect and value what the person says even if it appears damaging or self-blaming.

This can be difficult for the nurse who is trying to maintain a one-sided conversation, when even the most apparently positive event is cast by the depressed person in a negative light. This does not mean that the nurse has to agree or reinforce the depressed person's negative or damaging beliefs about himself or herself, rather the nurse can explain that they respect their beliefs but, that from their perspective, events have different attributions and meanings and that perhaps, as their mood lifts they too will feel differently.

In summary, the role of the nurse in working with a depressed person is essentially that of support and monitoring and working with them towards recovery while keeping them safe. The importance of simply being with the depressed person and valuing their experience, while supporting medical treatment and interventions cannot be overemphasized.

Box 14.1 presents a case study of Jean who suffers from depression.

Bipolar disorder

Bipolar disorder or manic depression as it is sometimes known, is a disorder which, as its name suggests, consists of two categories of symptoms: depressive symptoms which are described in the first part of this chapter, and mania, that is periods of exaggerated mood, euphoria and psychotic episodes. The other key feature which needs to be present in order to diagnose bipolar disorder is cyclicity, which is a shift of mood between depression and normal mood and mania over periods which may vary between two to three days and several weeks or months; so there may be long spells of normality followed by reoccurrence of either a manic or depressive symptoms. Thus bipolar disorder can be said to be a mental illness characterized by the presence of one or more of the following:

- manic episodes,
- mixed episodes,
- hypomanic episodes.

Only one of these episodes needs to occur just once during the lifetime of an individual for that individual to be considered as suffering from bipolar disorder. The presence of a major depressive episode occurs in 90 per cent of those with bipolar disorder during their lifetime. However, a major depressive episode does not need to have occurred for a diagnosis of bipolar disorder to be made. Thus there are individuals suffering bipolar disorder who do not have a history of major depressive episodes.

The lifetime risk of bipolar disorder (i.e. the risk of developing bipolar disorder over the lifetime) is less than 1 per cent in Western countries with a range between 0.4 and 1.6 per cent (American Psychiatric Association 1994). The prevalence of bipolar disorder at any given time, that is the number of people who actually have the disorder, is estimated to be between 1 and 3 per

Box 14.1 Case study: Jean – a 34-year-old with dysthymia and depressive episodes

Jean is a 34-year-old woman who has experienced dysthymia, that is, persistent low mood, for most of her adult life. However, over the last five years this has become particularly distressing and her mood has often deepened to include long spells of disabling depression. These depressed spells began after the birth of her first daughter and were diagnosed initially as postnatal depression. Jean reports that she has always been a melancholy person but denies feeling depressed in the past. However, after the birth of her first child Jean became extremely depressed and after the midwife and health visitor became concerned about her low mood and lack of self-care, although she continued to care for her child, they arranged for her to see her general practitioner who prescribed an SSRI. After several weeks Jean's mood had not improved and her husband became concerned about her because on three occasions, she had talked about committing suicide. Jean was seen by the community psychiatric nurse (CPN) who arranged for her to see a consultant psychiatrist; the psychiatrist increased the dosage of her SSRI medication and referred her for cognitive behavioural therapy.

During this time Jean received regular visits from a CPN who monitored Jean's mood and spent time discussing how she felt. The CPN also ensured that Jean was taking her medication and, with Jean's permission, discussed Jean's problems with her husband with the aim of reducing his feelings of isolation and blame, and to help him support Jean. Jean did not notice any improvement in her mood at first. However, the waiting list for CBT was six months and while waiting for a place Jean noted that her mood had begun to lift. Over the following six months Jean's mood returned to what she described as normal and she told the CPN that she had not felt so well since before her first child was born. Jean did not want to continue to take the SSRIs but to take cognitive behavioural therapy alone to see if it could help her. In discussion with her psychiatrist it was agreed that Jean will attend for cognitive behavioural therapy and that she will be withdrawn slowly from her SSRIs while her mood is closely monitored. Jean agreed, in collaboration with the psychiatrist and the CPN, to recommence taking the SSRIs in addition to the CBT course if her mood deteriorates either from her perspective or, as importantly, from the perspective of her family.

Jean's case illustrates that early diagnosis of depression is important, as is evidence-based treatment, to a successful outcome. Although Jean has seen a psychiatrist, her care has been carried out in the community and her main point of contact and support has been her husband and the CPN. In working with Jean the CPN performs three key roles. She is: an advocate for Jean, a source of information for Jean and her family, and, as the key worker, she monitors the effect of Jean's treatment and changes in her mood. The case shows also that the resolution of depression takes place in the medium, rather than the short term and that individuals should not stop taking anti-depressant medication without support, continued monitoring and without having sought advice.

cent of the general population. The frequency of bipolar disorder, unlike major depression, is similar for men and women (APA 1994), and onset of bipolar disorder peaks between the ages of 15 and 25.

Manic episode

A manic episode is classically described as a period of persistently elevated, heightened mood, consisting of euphoria and expansive goodwill but also comprising negative emotions such as fear, irritability and anger. In DSM IV (APA 1994) this episode must last for one week, or less, if hospitalization is required. These moods are accompanied by other symptoms, such as an unrealistically increased level of self-esteem, which is sometimes even grandiose, a decreased need for sleep and sometimes an apparent ability to not need sleep. Some individuals with mania have reported that while in this state they perform some tasks better and are more creative. For example, the artist Edvard Munch maintained that he painted 'The Scream' while experiencing a manic episode. However, the evidence for these creative episodes is largely anecdotal (Rothenberg 2001).

Individuals experiencing mania are easily distracted and, in addition, individuals with mania often describe symptoms of racing thoughts. This is a particularly distressing symptom in which the individual's mind constantly flits from one thought to another and they are unable to hold an idea in their mind for any length of time as their train of thought jumps wildly, and often randomly, from one thought to the next across a range of topics. The nature of these thoughts can also be frightening as they may involve paranoid or persecutory ideas that the individual finds distressing. This rapid transition of thought is often evident through other symptoms of mania that include pressure of speech and flight of ideas. In their attempt to reflect and convey their rapidly changing thoughts the manic individual may speak almost constantly on a wide range of topics and there may appear to be almost a torrent of new ideas and concepts, which are rapidly forgotten, a phenomena known as flight of ideas. In less severe cases of mania and in hypomania the individual may simply talk quickly and appear easily distracted, but in more severe cases the individual may speak in a confused and/or nonsensical way. Such speech may also contain grandiose and impractical ideas or statements, which sound as though they could be true but, upon investigation are not, or are targets and goals that are unrealistic.

A hypomanic episode is essentially a less pronounced and extreme version of mania. In DSM IV (APA 1994) it is defined by a distinct period of persistently elevated, expansive or irritable mood lasting for at least four days. As in mania the elevated mood must be accompanied by additional symptoms, such as inflated self-esteem or grandiosity, a decreased need for sleep, pressure of speech and flight of ideas. Again the individual may be easily distracted and be agitated. In contrast to a manic episode, a hypomanic episode is not severe enough to cause marked impairment in social or occupational functioning or to require hospitalization.

Mixed states

Mixed states are a problematic and complicated feature of bipolar disorder. As the name suggests they are states in which the individual experiences features and symptoms associated with both depressive and manic phases. They are often described as transition states between mania and depression, but this is not always true and some individuals with bipolar disorder present with a mixed state only and not with either 'pure' mania or depression.

DSM IV (APA 1994) describes a mixed episode as characterized by a period of time lasting at least one week in which the criteria are met for both a manic episode and a major depressive episode nearly every day. Therefore the person experiencing the mixed state may experience rapidly alternating moods (sadness, irritability, euphoria) accompanied by symptoms of a manic episode and a major depressive episode.

In the late nineteenth and early twentieth century Emil Kraepelin (1896) described six main types of mixed states. These states are:

- depression or anxious mania, in which mood is depressed but the individual's activity can be described generally as manic and in which thought content is also what would be expected during a period of mania;

- excited or agitated depression in which mood and thought is depressed, but the individual's activity is, nevertheless, best described as manic;

- mania with poverty of thought in which mood and activity is manic, but in which thought appears to have a predominately depressive content;

- manic stupor in which mood is manic but activity and thought have more in common with an individual experiencing depression;

- depression with flight of ideas in which mood and activity are depressed, but in which thought has a predominately manic content and, as the name suggests, is exemplified by pressure of speech and rapid flow of ideas which may or may not have a basis in fact; and

- inhibited mania in which mood and thought are manic in content, but activity is mainly depressed.

Even though these descriptions appeared over 75 years ago, they remain highly relevant and accurate descriptions of the various forms of mixed states which present today. However, it should also be remembered that these are perhaps only six examples of what is in fact a wide range of differing presentation that can occur.

In modern psychiatric terminology bipolar disorder is also classified into a variety of subtypes which are outlined below:

- In Bipolar I Disorder an individual must have at least one manic or mixed episode (lasting for at least a week) within his or her lifetime. An episode of depression is not needed to warrant a diagnosis of Bipolar I, although, as discussed above, 90 per cent of people usually experience at least one depressive episode.

- In Bipolar II Disorder an individual must have had at least one hypo-manic episode and at least one depressive episode within their lifetime. However, they must never have experienced an episode of mania.
- In cyclothymic disorder the individual must have experienced many periods with hypomanic symptoms as well as periods of depressive symptoms over a two-year period that do not meet the criteria for major depressive episode. More than 50 per cent of days need to be either a hypomanic or depressive day. The individual will have been symptom free for less than two months in total, and should not have had an episode of mania.

Other symptoms

Sleep disturbances, which are a common feature of mania, may present in a number of ways. The individual may have difficulty falling asleep because rapid and changing thoughts constantly distract them and prevent them falling asleep. However, many people experiencing mania simply do not feel tired and therefore do not sleep. This is often reinforced by a belief that there is simply not enough time to sleep because there is so much to be done.

Depressive phase

During the depressive phase individuals with bipolar disorder will often describe their mood as bleak, black, despairing and futile. Many of their signs and symptoms are identical to those described earlier for major depression. The psychotic symptoms associated with depression are more common in bipolar disorder than with major depression.

Psychotic depression is characterized by the same low mood, psycho-motor retardation and slowing of thought that occurs in non-psychotic depression. However, the features of depression are often more severe in psychotic than in non-psychotic depression. Individuals with psychotic depression may present with irrational and improbable beliefs (delusions), which have no basis in reality. They may believe that they have a severe illness (hypochondriacal delusion), massive debts, or they may have para-noid ideas or ideas of reference (where they believe that they are the subject of conversations which, in fact, have nothing to do with them). It is impor-tant to be aware of psychotic features of depression as their presence may have implications for treatment.

Treatment of bipolar disorder

Treatments for bipolar disorder are aimed at either stopping the episode of depression or mania and preventing and lessening the severity of relapse. A variety of treatments can be used including medication and cognitive behaviour therapy. Treatments can be carried out in hospital, especially during acute manic episodes or severe life-threatening depression, and also in the community, especially during less severe depressive episodes and hypomania.

Medication

Three classes of medication are used and have been found to be helpful in the treatment of bipolar disorder, these are mood-stabilizing drugs, anti-depressant drugs and anti-psychotic medications.

Anti-depressants

The same anti-depressant medications used for major depression (described earlier) are also used for bipolar disorder. But in manic depression, anti-depressant medication should be prescribed in combination with mood stabilizers, otherwise there is a high risk of inducing a manic state. Anti-depressant medication may be reduced or discontinued once the depression has been relieved but some psychiatrists prefer their patients to continue taking anti-depressants to avoid having to continually change their medication regime.

Mood stabilizers

Mood-stabilizing drugs taken during bipolar disorder aim to reduce the number and severity of manic, hypomanic and depressive episodes. For nearly half a century the main mood stabilizer used in bipolar disorder has been lithium. Lithium has been shown in a large number of controlled trials to be more effective than a placebo in stabilizing mood and preventing relapses into either mania or depression (Baldessarini *et al.* 2002). However, it is a particularly toxic drug and it is important that blood lithium levels are monitored closely.

Recently other medications have become available for the treatment of mood stabilization, particularly carbamezapine and divalproex sodium. However, these are not as effective at long-term mood control as lithium which is therefore still a useful drug in the treatment of bipolar disorder (Baldessarini *et al.* 2002). However, carbamazepine, in particular, is noted as having few side effects other than initially a mild sedation which individuals get used to rapidly (McIntyre 2002). Unlike anti-depressants, mood stabilizers are taken continually by patients often for the rest their lives; the hope is that they will prevent relapses or reduce the severity and speed of onset of new episodes of bipolar disorder.

Some anti-psychotic medications such as risperidone and olanzapine have also been shown to be efficacious in stabilizing mood (Yatham 2002). A problem with the introduction of new mood stabilizing drugs is that clinical trials need to take place over many years in order to assess their effectiveness in reducing relapses. However, taking anti-psychotic medications as mood stabilizers also has the added benefit of reducing psychotic symptoms of bipolar disorder.

Psychotherapeutic techniques

Cognitive behavioural therapy (CBT) has been shown to be useful in improving the effectiveness of medications taken for bipolar disorder. For example, Fava *et al.* (2002) suggest that CBT reduces residual symptoms and enhances the effect of lithium in preventing relapse. During CBT individuals can be taught to recognize and monitor symptoms of mania or depression and can, therefore, report them to their mental health worker at an early stage. In addition, cognitive behavioural strategies can be taught which help the individual to reduce the distressing nature of some symptoms of mania, especially racing thoughts, and also of depression as described previously (Scott *et al.* 2001). A particular approach which is based upon the cognitive therapy aspect of CBT involves teaching people strategies so that that they learn to identify and modify the disordered and distressing patterns of thought associated with manic or depressive episodes. This approach can be effective for both depression and mania where individuals can be taught to focus upon the unrealistic and improbable nature of many thoughts which may occur while they are experiencing these episodes. However, as with treatment for depressive disorder Scott *et al.* (2001) warn that CBT for bipolar disorder requires skilled trained therapists and its use in bipolar disorder can be complex.

Principles of nursing a person suffering from bipolar disorder

Nursing people suffering from bipolar disorder requires a variety of nursing skills and behaviours. These are based on the same principles of nursing that apply to the care of people suffering from depression, which have been discussed previously. However, the nurse needs to be aware of the possibility of mood change and particularly the development of a mixed state.

Manic episode

The nursing care required by a person in a manic episode will depend to a large degree on the extent and severity of the episode. Some episodes of mania, which border on hypomania, may be manifested primarily by an exaggeration of an individual's usual personality. Other manic episodes may be characterized by marked lack of insight and irrational behaviour. One of the major challenges for hospital-based nurses is to care for an individual who is excited, euphoric and perhaps afraid. This person may be agitated and restless with marked pressure of speech and will often be unable to stop long enough to complete any task, including self-care tasks such as washing and dressing, watching television or reading.

Eating and drinking

It may be difficult to encourage a manic individual to eat and drink as they may feel that they have no time to eat and/or that they are not hungry. There is, therefore, considerable risk that they may become dehydrated and in the longer term, malnourished. Dehydration is a primary concern as it can cause the individual to become unwell and exacerbate their psychological symptoms. It is, therefore, important to check that the individual is taking adequate fluids and, if not, drinks should be offered and encouraged at regular intervals. Although nutrition is a less pressing problem than fluid intake, it is important that it is addressed. A manic person may engage in considerable psychomotor activity which increases their energy expenditure, and if they are not eating, they may lose weight quickly. Frequent snacks, such as sandwiches and biscuits, that can be eaten during activity is more likely to be accepted by a manic person than full meals. However, as mood stabilizes, providing a meal, which the individual must sit down to may be a way of making them stop and take time.

It is important to note that in mania the opposite effect may also occur with the result that an individual may drink large volumes of fluid or eat large amounts of food. Again, in the short term this may not be a pressing problem, but in the longer term, weight gain may be undesirable.

Restlessness

The manic individual in hospital will probably find the environment constraining and irritating, often wishing to leave the ward. This can be very difficult for nurses to deal with as it may not be in the individual's best interests to leave and, if restricted under the Mental Health Act (1983), it may not be possible.

It is important to engage the individual with mania in activities if they are restless. For some people it is appropriate to encourage them to carry out minor 'jobs' around the ward within the limits of health and safety regulations and therapeutic need; for example, allowing them to make a cup of tea for other residents or assisting with either setting up an activity or tidying up afterwards. It is important that such activities are the outcome of therapeutic decisions and not for staff convenience; inpatients should not act as unpaid help! Other activities may include residents organizing feedback forums and other similar administrative tasks. Such activities can provide a constructive outlet for individuals experiencing mania, which can make them feel useful and enhance their self esteem. It is important to supervise these activities carefully. Manic individuals may be overbearing, over-enthusiastic and over-zealous in their dealings with other residents. Nurses should be ready to step in if such activities become inappropriate or no longer therapeutic from the point of view of either the individual with mania or other residents.

Sleeping

An individual with mania may have difficulty sleeping. This may be due to disturbing racing thoughts, disinclination to go to bed or waking up after a short period feeling refreshed. There are a number of nursing interventions that the manic person may find helpful. Encouraging them to go to bed even if they are not feeling tired, ideally in a room of their own so that they do not disturb others, is good practice. Night-time sedation may be offered over a period, especially if the person has difficulty in going to sleep. However, in some cases the nurse may need to accept that while experiencing their current mood the individual may find sleep impossible and so it is less distressing for them to stay up. The main challenge for ward-based nurses is to help the manic person find activities that will enable them to pass the night without disturbing others.

Aggression and violence

An individual with mania may be irritable and even violent. A key role of the nurse in such cases is to maintain the individual's safety and that of others in the ward. Again, the key is to spend time with the individual, and to remove them from situations where they are being annoyed or are annoying others. Ensuring adequate personal space and outlets for their mood may often serve to defuse potentially violent situations.

It is important that prescribed medication is taken and this is another key part of the nurse's role. As discussed above, mood stabilizers will probably be prescribed and occasionally short-term anxiolytic sedation may be taken to promote sleep.

Racing thoughts and actions

An individual with mania in hospital is likely to have substantial problems with racing thoughts and actions. The individual may be constantly coming up with new and urgent ideas that they must act on. They may interfere with the actions of staff and of other patients. This can be distressing and exhausting.

Resolution of mania

As mania resolves the key challenge is to discuss the episode with the individual and to deal with their feelings about what has happened. They may have acted in a disinhibited way, perhaps through making sexual advances or making self-disclosures that they may not only regret but also find deeply embarrassing. They may also have to deal with the consequences of actions carried out while they were becoming manic. A particular modern problem encountered is debt via overdrafts and credit cards, accumulated while the person was manic but before the problem became clear. Individuals need opportunities to discuss these issues, and reassurance that their family and staff understand that such disinhibited acts were a feature of their illness.

A danger during the resolution phase is that the person's mood may continue to drop to the extent that they begin to show signs of a depressive or mixed episode. This may be exacerbated by problems that have arisen as a consequence of their manic episode, such as embarrassment or debt, which may serve to lower their self-esteem.

The individual with mania in the community

The individual with mania in the community should be approached in a similar way to the individual in an inpatient setting, and the same principles apply. However, two points should be considered. First, the family will be carrying out much of the care and will be experiencing strain. Secondly, it is far easier for individuals with mania in the community to make choices that may have negative financial, professional or legal consequences for them.

The family and friends of an individual experiencing mania, or even hypomania, in the community may be under a considerable strain. They may experience the physical strain of being with someone who is restless and perhaps sleeping little, and in addition they have to deal with the consequences of the individual's mood and actions. The family may experience hostility, anger and irritability or conversely may be bombarded with goodwill and the results of exuberant generosity. Both of these extremes can be difficult to deal with on a daily basis and may cause the family significant distress, of which the manic individual may be unaware. The role of the nurse here is primarily that of a listener and a provider of practical help and support. Giving the family information about the individual's mood and listening to family concerns is valuable as is reassuring the family that if the mania becomes more severe, inpatient treatment will be arranged, if it is deemed appropriate.

The person suffering from a manic state who is living in the community may make choices that they would not even consider when their mood is normal. As discussed earlier this is also possible for inpatients, but in the community such opportunities are increased and choices made may have especially damaging consequences. At work the individual may behave inappropriately and their performance may deteriorate, however, some people with mania feel that they are at their most productive and creative. They may make impulsive purchases or be less concerned about credit-card debts, as discussed earlier. The principle difficulty faced by community-based nurses is that as the individual is being cared for in the community they are usually deemed competent to make decisions and be responsible for their own actions. The nurse is in a paradoxical situation; the individual's freedom and rights must be respected in spite of the fact that they may be damaging their interests and those of their family. If an individual is too ill to work and is declared sick, they can then be asked to leave the workplace. However, limiting negative consequences in other areas of life is often more difficult. The nurse's role is to encourage the person to reflect carefully on their decisions and consult their family.

Another relevant consideration when caring for people suffering from mania living in the community is their fitness to drive. A person with mania may drive dangerously, they may ignore speed limits or not realize the speed they are travelling at. They may misjudge distances and fail to notice obstacles because their attention is distracted. Individuals with mania can disregard their personal safety and that of others owing to grandiose mood and feelings of invulnerability. Therefore it is preferable that people suffering from mania do not drive and if they insist, the nurse should consider the possibility of restricting their freedom of action under the provisions of the Mental Health Act (1983).

Boxes 14.2 and 14.3, present case studies of two individuals with different courses of bipolar disorder to illuminate the features of the disorder described.

Mark's case (in Box 14.2) shows that bipolar disorder can have a very gradual onset and that it might not be recognized quickly. Other health professionals, with whom Mark worked, missed his change in mood until he was experiencing a very significant degree of mania. This case study illustrates also the importance of interagency cooperation, which meant that although Mark's first key interaction was with the criminal justice system, he was quickly diverted into the health system. The case study demonstrates also that with adequate care and support it is possible for an individual to recover from mania and return to a demanding and responsible job.

Although Amanda's case (Box 14.3) shows that deterioration in her mood was not prevented, training Amanda and her family to spot her symptoms early facilitated early assessment by the community psychiatric nurse. Good multi-disciplinary team-work enabled early intervention which limited the duration of mania and Amanda was able to leave hospital after only four weeks. It was also possible to treat Amanda as a voluntary patient without needing to detain her under the Mental Health Act (1983).

Conclusion

In summary the main points of this chapter are:

- Mood disorders are the most common of the psychiatric disorders, particularly depression, which has been described as the common cold of psychiatry.
- There are effective evidence-based treatments for both depression and mania.
- The role of the nurse is crucial in ensuring the safety and well-being of people experiencing depression and mania both in inpatient and community-care settings.

Box 14.2 Case study: Mark – a 24-year-old with first onset of bipolar disorder

Mark was a final-year medical student when he experienced his first and, to date, only episode of mania. He was 24 years of age and was studying for his final examinations. As Mark approached his finals, he began working longer and longer hours on his revision while sleeping less and less. He had always been a confident person but he began to feel that he could accomplish anything. He had no concerns about his forthcoming examinations or the other final-year work that he had to complete. He also began to have periods where he was not sleeping for several days at a time. His friends began to notice that his speech was pressured and the content of his conversation became less and less rational and based in reality. Although Mark felt that he was doing 'the best work of his life' his tutors began to express concern about his falling academic standard. He submitted several essays which were overlength, inadequately referenced, rambling and which contained many factual errors. When Mark was confronted with this work he became angry and blamed the markers for not appreciating his 'special knowledge'.

Soon after this confrontation on a Friday night after spending an evening drinking with his friends Mark was arrested by the police after becoming involved in a fight in a pub. While in police custody the custody sergeant became concerned at Mark's behaviour as he was constantly pacing his cell showing aggression towards police officers and speaking, or rather babbling, incoherently at a very fast pace. The content of his speech was almost non-sensical. The custody sergeant was not sure that Mark had understood the charge against him, and so notified the police surgeon. The police surgeon was concerned about Mark's psychiatric condition and called the on-call psychiatrist who arranged for Mark to be transferred to the local psychiatric acute admissions unit. When Mark stated that he did not wish to go and that he wanted to be either set free or to be retained in custody it was decided to admit him to hospital under Section 2 of the Mental Health Act (1983).

Mark was treated with a mood stabilizer (lithium) and gradually his mood began to become less manic and less thought disordered. However, Mark's mood drifted over a period of a month from mania to a severe depression with suicidal thoughts. He was then treated with an anti-depressant SSRI (fluoxetine) while the lithium was continued. During this time the magistrates' court gave Mark a conditional discharge.

Mark's mood lifted and after seven weeks in hospital his mood had stabilized to the extent where it was felt that he could be discharged to stay with his parents. Mark received community support from a community psychiatric nurse while he was staying at his parents' home. Mark was finally judged as fit to continue his medical career and he returned to university to repeat his final year. During this time he continued to take lithium and eventually graduated.

Box 14.3 Case study: Amanda – a 42-year-old with recurrence of a manic episode

Amanda is a 42-year-old lady who has suffered from bipolar disorder since she was 22 years of age, and has had five acute episodes. Her bipolar disorder usually manifests itself as a manic episode although she did have one instance of severe depression during which time she attempted to take her own life. Amanda was prescribed lithium as a mood stabilizer since her first episode which has helped her to be symptom free for several periods, and so function as a full-time mother to two small children and hold down a part-time job. Amanda, who had been taught to monitor her mood, noticed that it had started to become manic. Her family had also noticed marked pressure of speech and that she appeared to be spending a large amount of money on presents for the children, for her sister's children and on goods for the house. As a consequence of this she accumulated considerable debt on her credit card. Acting on a prior agreement with Amanda, and her previously agreed authority with the credit card company, Amanda's husband arranged for her credit card to be suspended and for some of the goods to be returned.

Amanda herself recognized these as her usual symptoms of mania and contacted her community psychiatric nurse who referred her for psychiatric treatment. Amanda's lithium dose was increased. However, her mood continued to deteriorate and she became very manic and also to show signs of psychotic episodes. The multi-disciplinary community mental health team in consultation with Amanda and her family decided that Amanda would be better treated in hospital. In hospital, Amanda's mood stabilizer was changed from lithium to carbamazepine and she was treated also with anti-psychotic medication. As her manic state decreased and her psychotic symptoms resolved she was also supported with cognitive behavioural therapy which she has found useful in the past. As her mood stabilized Amanda developed some symptoms of mixed mood, notably depressed psychomotor activity, while her thoughts continued to race as evidenced by her pressure of speech. However, these symptoms resolved as her mood stabilized.

Questions for reflection and discussion

1   DSM IV states that feelings of sadness and grief are part of everyday life and should not be pathologized. What do you think of this statement?

2   How do we decide when sadness and grief are a 'normal' part of everyday life or are an illness? Do you think it feels any different to the person experiencing the low mood?

3   Sometimes when an individual is severely depressed and is at a high risk of self harm, electro-convulsive therapy (ECT) may be prescribed against their will. What do you think of this practice?

4   Mental health professionals have a duty to balance an individual's freedom against the need to protect them, even from themselves. Given this, how would you support an individual facing involuntary treatment?

5   A family member of a woman suffering from bipolar disorder recently said, 'It's all right for her when she's high – she's having a wonderful time, it's the family which has the problems.' What do you think of this statement? How would you support an individual experiencing bipolar disorder and how would you balance their needs with those around them, especially family members?

▌ Annotated bibliography

- Hale, A.S. (1997) Depression, *British Medical Journal* **315**: 43–5. Porter, R. and Ferrier, N. (1999) Emergency treatment of depression, *Advances in Psychiatric Treatment* **5**: 3–10. These two papers provide an overview of current thinking on depression and its treatment from a medical perspective. They are useful sources of reference for students from a range of health care disciplines and Hale's paper, in particular, is also accessible to the lay reader.
- Kingdom, D.G. (1998) Cognitive behaviour therapy for severe mental illness, in C. Brooker and J. Repper, *Serious Mental Health Problems in the Community. Policy Practice and Research*. London: Bailliere Tindall. This chapter provides a good introduction to cognitive behavioural therapy. It sets the therapy within the policy context of the NHS and so provides useful pointers to planning and implementing care.
- Barker, P.J. (1997) *A Self-help Guide to Managing Depression*. London: Nelson Thornes. This book is a useful guide to depression. It is written to be read as a series of step-by-step sections by an individual experiencing depression and is, therefore, accessible and easy to read. Although primarily for service users, its focus on the daily living problems caused by depression provides some useful pointers for planning nursing care.

▌ References

American Psychiatric Association (1990) *The Practice of ECT: Recommendations for Treatment, Training and Privileging*. Washington, DC: American Psychiatric Press.

American Psychiatric Association (1994) *Diagnostic and Statistical Manual of Mental Disorders*, 4th edn. Washington, DC: American Psychiatric Press.

Baldessarini, R.J., Tondo, L., Hennen, J. and Viguera, A.C. (2002) Is lithium still worth using? An update of selected recent research, *Harvard Review of Psychiatry* **10**(2): 59–75.

Department of Health (1999) *National Service Framework for Mental Health.* London: The Stationery Office.

Fava, G.A., Ruini, C., Rafanelli, C. and Grandi, S. (2002) Cognitive behavior approach to loss of clinical effect during long-term antidepressant treatment: a pilot study, *American Journal of Psychiatry* **159**(12): 2094–5.

Goodwin, F.K. and Jamison, K.R. (1990) *Suicide in Manic Depressive Illness.* New York: Oxford University Press.

Hale, A.S. (1997) Depression, *British Medical Journal* **315**: 43–5.

Kraepelin, E. (1896) Leipzig (ed) Ambr. Abel. Die psychologische Versuche in der Psychiatrie. Emil Kraepelin (Hg.): *Psychologische Arbeiten* Bd. 1, S. 1–91.

McIntyre, R. (2002) Psychotropic drugs and adverse events in the treatment of bipolar disorders revisited, *Journal of Clinical Psychiatry* **63** Suppl. 3: 15–20.

Porter, R. and Ferrier, N. (1999) Emergency treatment of depression, *Advances in Psychiatric Treatment* **5**: 3–10.

Rizley, R. (1978) Depression and distortion in the attribution of causality, *Journal of Abnormal Psychology* **87**(1): 32–48.

Rothenberg, A. (2001) Bipolar illness, creativity, and treatment, *Psychiatric Quarterly* **72**(2): 131–47.

Royal College of Psychiatrists (1995) *The ECT Handbook* (Council Report CR39).

Scott, C., Tacchi, M.J., Jones, R. and Scott, J. (1997) Acute and one year outcome of a randomised controlled trial of brief cognitive therapy for major depressive disorder in primary care, *British Journal of Psychiatry* **17**: 131–4.

Scott, J., Garland, A. and Moorhead, S. (2001) A pilot study of cognitive therapy in bipolar disorders, *Psychological Medicine* **31**(3): 459–67.

Seligman, M.E.P. (1975) *Helplessness: on Depression, Development and Death.* San Francisco: W.H. Freeman.

Thornicroft, G. and Sartorius, N. (1993) The course and outcome of depression in different cultures: 10-year follow-up of the WHO Collaborative Study on the Assessment of Depressive Disorders, *Psychological Medicine* **23**(4): 1023–32.

Yatham, L.N. (2002) The role of novel antipsychotics in bipolar disorders, *Journal of Clinical Psychiatry* **63** Suppl 3: 10–14.

15

The person with an anxiety disorder

Paul Rogers, Joe Curran and Kevin Gournay

Chapter overview

Anxiety disorders fall within the remit of primary care. Today, it is rare for people with a primary diagnosis of anxiety disorder to require hospitalization. The English National *Service Framework (NSF) for Mental Health* notes that: 'Around 90 per cent of mental health care is provided solely by primary care. . . . The most common mental health problems are depression, eating disorders and anxiety disorders' (DH 1999: 29). However, outside of primary diagnosis, it is important to note that anxiety symptoms and anxiety disorders are not merely the realms of primary care. Anxiety symptoms and disorders are prevalent and co-morbid within a range of mental health disorders and people with anxiety symptoms and disorders can be found within the full range of service provisions.

This chapter examines the history of anxiety disorders and the development of cognitive behaviour therapy (CBT), and focuses on the care and treatment of people suffering from common anxiety disorders: phobias (specific, agoraphobia and social phobia); obsessive-compulsive disorder; post-traumatic stress disorder; panic disorder; health anxiety; and generalized anxiety disorder. Body dysmorphic disorder is included also (due to the known high levels of anxiety that people experience). For each disorder, the background and prevalence, definition and diagnosis, treatment effectiveness and a case illustration(s) are provided. Thereafter, the impact on functioning is examined. Following on, a discussion of the main treatment measures and an overview of behavioural and cognitive behavioural treatment are provided. Finally, a discussion of nurse therapy and self-help is provided. This chapter covers:

- Anxiety disorders and CBT;
- Specific disorders;
- Impact on lifestyle and social functioning;

- Assessment and treatment measures;
- Nurse-led psychological treatment;
- Principles and practice of exposure;
- Principles and practice of CBT;
- Self-help.

Anxiety disorders and CBT: A historical perspective

Fear is one of the universal basic emotions that are not learned and occur across cultures (for example, Ekman 1992). The fear/anxiety response is a basic survival response that is utilized to help an organism deal with threat or danger. This process has become known as the 'fight-or-flight' response after Cannon's (1929) account of the 'emergency response' or 'alarm reaction'. Later writers have suggested additions to the basic 'fight-flight' description to take into account other observed reactions during the fear response, for example, 'fight-flight-freeze-faint' (Beck *et al.* 1985: 48) and 'withdrawal, immobility, aggressive defence, or deflection of attack' (Marks 1987: 81). Overall, the anxiety response is a necessary and normal response that not only serves a useful purpose in response to current threat, but also helps the evolutionary survival of the species (Stein and Bouwer 1997; Barlow 2002). The three main physiological systems that are involved in the anxiety/fear response are the motor system, autonomic nervous system and the neuroendocrine system (Marks 1987).

Definitions of anxiety and related concepts

Marks (1987: 5) suggests that fear can be seen as a 'usually unpleasant response to realistic danger', whereas anxiety is 'similar to fear but without objective source of danger'. A phobia is fear of a situation, which is out of proportion to the actual danger and cannot be explained or reasoned away. Panic is a sudden upsurge of acute intense fear, often associated with frantic attempts to escape. These definitions give a useful indication that a distinction is made between realistic and unrealistic responses to situations. These characteristics are important to note as fear and anxiety are sometimes referred to in alternative ways (for example, Beck *et al.* 1985), or may be used synonymously. The important thing to recognize is that sources of danger (that may or may not be realistic), give rise to a set of unpleasant responses. Beck *et al.* (1985) have listed the following main physical, behavioural, cognitive and affective responses (symptoms) that comprise the anxiety response.

Physiological symptoms

- *Cardiovascular*: Palpitations, heart racing, increased blood pressure, faintness (and/or actual fainting);

- *Respiratory*: rapid breathing, shortness of breath, shallow breathing, lump in throat, choking sensation;

- *Neuromuscular*: Increased reflexes, muscle spasms, tremors, rigidity, fidgeting, wobbly legs;

- *Gastrointestinal*: abdominal discomfort, nausea, vomiting;

- *Urinary tract*: Pressure to urinate, frequency of urination; and

- *Skin*: Face flushed or pale, localized and/or generalized sweating, itching, 'hot and cold spells'.

Behavioural symptoms

These include: Inhibition, tonic immobility, flight, avoidance, restlessness, impaired coordination, speech dysfluency (for example, stammering) and hyperventilation.

Cognitive symptoms

- *Sensory-perceptual*: hazy, cloudy, foggy 'mind', feelings of unreality, hypervigilance;

- *Thinking difficulties*: confusion, difficulty concentrating, distractibility, unable to control thinking; and

- *Conceptual*: fear of losing control, fear of mental disorder, repetitive fearful ideation.

Descriptions of behaviour similar to anxiety have a long history (detailed in Berrios 1999). It was not until the second half of the seventeenth century that the term 'anxiete' developed a psychological meaning, although symptoms of anxiety continued to be treated as physical problems until the middle of the nineteenth century (Berrios 1999). Psychological approaches to understanding the nature of anxiety were initially developed by the observations of Sigmund Freud (1977) who described the psychoanalytic treatment of a phobia in a 5-year-old boy: 'Little Hans'. In the late nineteenth and early twentieth centuries Freud, through observation of patients presenting for therapy, developed his theory of the unconscious. His view was that anxiety was largely due to the presence of unconscious conflicts taking place within the individual. The presence of anxiety at any given time was due to the patient's usual *defence mechanisms* being insufficient to deal with the conflict. In 1927, the Russian physiologist Ivan Pavlov published a series of experiments on dogs that, initially, were aimed at measuring secretions of bile. While conducting these experiments Pavlov observed that the dogs started salivating prior to the introduction of the food into the experimental chamber. This led to laboratory-based experiments that are today termed as classical conditioning. Applying this process to fear, Watson and Rayner (1927) deliberately paired the stimulus of a white rat with a loud noise in a 2-year-old child, identified in the original study as 'Albert B' but who has come to be known as 'Little Albert'. Subsequent presentation of the rat, a rabbit, cotton wool and the experimenter's white hair induced the fear response in the child. In addition to demonstrating the acquisition of the fear response to the original stimulus, this study also demonstrates the process of *generalization*, where objects that resemble the initially trained stimulus become associated with fearful responding.

Thereafter, based on earlier theories from Thorndike, Hull Guthrie, and his own experimental procedures conducted on rats or pigeons, B.F. Skinner categorized the behaviour of organisms into two types – *respondent* (similar to Pavlov's description of reflexes), and *operant* – usually defined as anything the organism does that has an effect. Skinner generally focused his work on operant behaviour and in particular the factors that 'maintain' behaviours. Several principles were derived, the most commonly known of these related to the process of reinforcement (for example, Skinner 1938). With regard to anxiety the principle of *negative reinforcement*, or the principle that any behaviour that leads to the removal or cessation of a stimulus strengthens the behaviour, is most readily applied. Thus, the behaviours of escape, avoidance, checking, cleaning, taking anxiolytic medication, etc., often seen in anxiety disorders are more likely to reoccur if they are successful at reducing the anxiety response. In 1960, an attempt was made to account for the acquisition and maintenance of fearful responding that utilized both classical conditioning and operant conditioning principles (Mowrer 1960). This is known as *two-factor learning theory*.

The late 1950s and early 1960s saw the development of more cognitively based accounts of human psychopathology by Albert Ellis (1962) and Aaron Beck (1961). Ellis's approach (Rational Emotive Behaviour Therapy), works with clients to help identify various irrational beliefs that, if held with a strong degree of conviction, are hypothesized to be associated with higher degrees of distress. Beck's original focus was depression – a disorder that at the time was largely unresponsive to psychological treatment approaches (for example, Eysenck 1952). The basic premise of Beck's approach is that it is the appraisal of a situation, or the meaning one applies to it, that is important in its development and, more importantly maintenance. It is important to examine appraisals (or thoughts) in three areas – thoughts about oneself, thoughts about the world and other people, and thoughts about the future. In anxiety disorders appraisals are often made that reflect themes of threat or danger, personal vulnerability and ability to cope, and controllability. The development of cognitive accounts of psychological problems, by people such as Meichenbaum, Mahoney, Bandura in addition to Beck and Ellis was sufficient to be labelled a 'cognitive revolution' (Mahoney and Thoresen 1974).

Theoretical perspectives on the nature and causes of anxiety disorders vary widely. For example, personality theorists have focused on the differences between individuals' dispositions to respond in particular ways. These approaches are collectively known as *trait theories*, where traits are described as 'personality characteristics that are *stable over time* and *across situations*' (Pervin and John 2001: 224, italics in original). For example, Eysenck's (1947) dimensions of neuroticism and, to some degree, introversion relate to personality factors associated with anxiety or anxious behaviour. Biological theories of anxiety focus on the physiological bases of the anxiety disorders, examining the evolutionary, neurophysiological and physical aspects of: for example, panic disorder, OCD and social phobia (Stein and Bouwer 1997) and the possible adaptive functions of anxiety, stress and depression (Nesse 1999). Finally, although the experience of anxiety/fear is seen to be a universal emotion, it is important to consider cultural factors that are involved in the classification of an individual's experience as disordered and requiring treatment or therapy.

Specific disorders

Phobias

Prevalence studies on phobias suggest that 1–2 per cent of the general population suffer from agoraphobia (for example, Angst and Dobler-Mikola 1983), 1–2 per cent from social phobia (Weissman *et al.* 1985) and 7 per cent from specific phobias (ibid.). Phobia onset varies; specific phobias tend to develop in childhood and may be an exaggerated response of normal childhood developmental fears. For example, it is normal for children to fear heights when aged 2 months, strangers between the ages 6 months and 2 years and animals between the ages of 2 and 4. Agoraphobia usually develops between the ages of 18 and 35 (Marks 1969; Thorpe and Burns 1983). Social phobia usually develops between the ages of 15 and 21 (Amies *et al.* 1983). No singular causal model adequately explains why the age of onset of different phobias differs and also why some people develop phobias and others do not. It is generally agreed that a genetic, biological basis underlies the development of phobia. However, it is also agreed that developmental learning has a role to play through either: direct conditioning, vicarious conditioning (observing another persons fear), and by the transmission of information or instruction (for example, phobias of tuberculosis which became prevalent at the turn of the century following government information policies, later seen in the 1980s with the development of HIV/Aids phobias).

Definition and diagnosis

Phobias were first recognized as separate diagnostic categories using the International Classification of Diseases (ICD; World Health Organization 1992) and the Diagnostic and Statistical Manual in the late 1940s and early 1950s. Presently, DSM-IV (American Psychiatric Association (APA) 1994) has three classifications of phobic disorders:

1   **Agoraphobia.** Defined by DSM-IV (APA 1994) as 'anxiety about, or avoidance of, places or situations from which escape might be difficult (or embarrassing) or in which help may not be available in the event of

having a panic attack or panic-like symptoms'. The important issue within this definition is that there is usually a fear of having panic-like symptoms (a fear of fear) and being unable to or having difficulty obtaining immediate escape where panic may ensue (for example, hairdressers, buses, cinemas).

2 **Social phobia.** A DSM-IV (APA 1994) definition of social phobia is 'clinically significant anxiety provoked by exposure to certain types of social performance situations, often leading to avoidance behaviour'. This can include writing cheques in public, socializing at a party, public speaking, etc. The important issue within this definition is that there is a fear of one's own social performance (for example, saying or doing something embarrassing). As such, a consequential fear of negative evaluation by others naturally follows. This differs from agoraphobia where being unable to escape a specific place causes the anxiety.

3 **Specific phobias.** A DSM-IV (APA 1994) definition of specific phobia is 'clinically significant anxiety provoked by exposure to a specified feared object or situation, often leading to avoidance behaviour'. Specific fears can include: dogs, dental procedures, spiders, thunder and lightening, etc.

Case studies: agoraphobia, social phobia, specific phobia

Agoraphobia

John is a 27-year-old postman, married with three children and has a six-year history of agoraphobia. John recalled having his first panic attack in a crowded shop five years earlier after returning from a two-week summer holiday. At the time of this first panic attack, it started with severe sweating, and then feeling dizzy, followed by increased heartbeat leading him to think he was going to collapse or faint. His fear had gradually worsened and he gradually began to avoid more and more places. The pattern was that he would give up going into places after having a panic attack as he feared further attacks (for example, crowded shops, restaurants, hairdressers, buses, quiet shops and lifts). In addition he always carried a bottle of water, wore shorts and loose clothing, and carried a hand-held fan. Two months earlier he had had a panic attack at work and had been off sick since and worried that he could never return. However, his work attendance had suffered over the preceding year as he disliked walking and delivering post when it was hot, so he asked to begin his round earlier and earlier during summer months.

Social phobia

Steven is a 19-year-old student who was having increasing difficulty continuing with his degree. He had a lifelong history of shyness. However, this never effected his day-to-day functioning and although slightly anxious in situations, never panicked. His problems began when he started his degree course and had to move away from home. Within two weeks of starting university he dropped his tray carrying his dinner in the university dining room and there was a big cheer and some people laughed. He felt very embarrassed and ever since feared a further episode. Soon his fear began to affect other areas, and within two months he was unable to eat or drink in public or sign anything in case his hands shook, and was petrified whenever he had to enter situations where there were large crowds (including giving classroom presentations). He began to avoid these activities and quite soon after began drinking increasing amounts of alcohol to help him to face day-to-day situations. Within four months, he could rarely leave the house without first having had alcohol and began to secretly carry alcohol with him throughout the day.

Specific phobia (illness phobia of HIV/Aids)

Michael was a 23-year-old final-year student nurse who lived at home with his parents. He developed a terrifying fear of 'catching HIV' and dying of Aids. He had intrusive unwanted thoughts and images when at work, that somehow the virus had entered his skin (although there were no cuts and he took appropriate precautions). He stated that when exposed to blood-related stimuli he felt very anxious, and his conviction in this belief that he was infected was 75 per cent, but afterwards he only believed it 15 per cent. On occasions he has panicked and left the ward he was working on until his panic subdued, informing colleagues that he had a problem with asthma and nausea. His fears were worse at work, when giving blood, and in public toilets. He worried excessively about all physical feelings, which he believed were signs and symptoms of HIV/Aids. Because of his fears he constantly checked his whole body for any possible signs, read extensively about HIV/Aids and wore two or three pairs of protective gloves. He avoided all public toilets, thinking about his fears, and had begun to take time off work repeatedly. As a consequence of his time absent from work he was asked to an occupational health review but was considering leaving his training course.

Treatment efficacy: phobias

Roth and Fonagy (1996) in their comprehensive review of anxiety disorders and 'what works for whom?' concluded: 'There is little justification for using anything other than exposure treatments for specific phobias' (1996: 142). Undoubtedly, the most efficacy as demonstrated through randomized controlled treatment trials come from behaviour therapy using exposure and cognitive techniques. Such treatments can vary in length, with on average 8–12 sessions (including assessment) required for agoraphobia and social phobia, and up to 6 sessions for specific phobias. Interestingly, some specific phobias can be successfully treated with only 2 to 4 sessions (for example, dental phobia, see Liddell *et al.* 1994). It is important to note that there is no justification for the use of dynamic or humanistic therapies in the treatment of phobias (see Roth and Fonagy 1996: 144). The NHS Centre for Reviews and Dissemination (2002a) published a critical assessment of treatments for social phobia which found that exposure and cognitive behavioural treatments resulted in 'significant and meaningful reductions in anxiety'. Furthermore, the review noted that the 'combination of psychological and pharmacological treatments was disappointing and did not exceed the effects of psychological treatments alone'.

Obsessive-compulsive disorder

Obsessive-compulsive disorder (OCD) is classed as an anxiety disorder in DSM-IV (APA 1994). OCD has two symptom clusters: Obsessional thoughts (ruminations) and compulsive actions (rituals). Most patients have a mixture of both symptoms. Approximately 1.5 per cent of the population at any given time will suffer from OCD (de Silva and Rachman 1998). The condition affects people irrespective of class, race, culture or gender.

Normal obsessions also occur in the vast majority of people (for example, checking our children at night when newborn). However, such obsessions are generally considered useful or slightly annoying and do not interfere with our day-to-day lives to a significant level or cause significant distress. It is when the obsessions become major preoccupations and have no significant rationale sense that they become pathologized. The most common themes of obsessions are:

1   being contaminated (for example, germs, dirt, diseases; and sufferers will be afraid of touching things for fear of becoming contaminated or passing on contaminants);
2   doubting, whereby, a sufferer may suddenly worry in case they haven't locked their house properly, or may be driving down the street, and suddenly worry that they hit someone or ran over someone;
3   violent thoughts or imagery (for example, thoughts to kill one's own children, partner, or to harm oneself);
4   sexual thoughts or imagery (for example, thoughts to run through the church service naked);
5   orderliness, where objects have to be lined up or arranged in a particular way (for example, at right angles to each other).

Common compulsions include:

1   washing or hygiene rituals (usually in the context of obsessions about cleanliness, germs, etc.);
2   repeated checking (usually in the context of obsessive doubting including seeing if the door is locked; the gas or taps are off; electricity is unplugged, etc.);
3   counting (usually there is a 'magical number' and the person has to do a behaviour a set number of times, for example, washing each finger 7 times then each hand 7 times);

4   Reassurance seeking, whereby the person will constantly seek reassurance from their partner, health care professional, friend, etc., that things are all right (for example, 'Did I lock the door? Are you sure? Did you see me do it? Did I do it properly? Are you sure?').

Definition and diagnosis

A DSM-IV diagnosis of OCD is made if the person exhibits either obsessions or compulsions. Obsessions are indicated by the following:

1   The person has recurrent and persistent thoughts, impulses or images that are experienced, at some time during the disturbance, as intrusive and inappropriate and that cause marked anxiety or distress.
2   The thoughts, impulses or images are not simply excessive worries about real-life problems.
3   The person attempts to ignore or suppress such thoughts, impulses or images or to neutralize them with some other thought or action.
4   The person recognizes that the obsessional thoughts, impulses or images are a product of his or her own mind (not imposed from without as in thought insertion).

Compulsions are indicated by the following:

1   The person has repetitive behaviours (for example, hand washing, ordering, checking) or mental acts (for example, praying, counting, repeating words silently) that the person feels driven to perform in response to an obsession or according to rules that must be applied rigidly.
2   The behaviours or mental acts are aimed at preventing some dreaded event or situation; however, these behaviours or mental acts either are not connected in a realistic way with what they are designed to neutralize or prevent or are clearly excessive.

Additionally, at some point during the course of the disorder, the person should have recognized that the obsessions or compulsions were excessive or unreasonable (however, this does not apply to children). Finally, the obsessions or compulsions cause marked distress, are time consuming (take more than 1 hour a day), or significantly interfere with the person's normal routine, occupational/academic functioning or usual social activities or relationships.

Case study: obsessive compulsive disorder

Sarah is a 63-year-old widow who was recently referred by her GP after he was contacted by an environmental health agency. Sarah was primarily obsessed that she would lose her wedding ring and this led her to not throw anything away (in case her ring slipped off and she couldn't find it). She also feared that she would throw away important letters, bills, receipts, etc.

Consequently, she retained all rubbish bags in the upstairs bedrooms as an added safety precaution. She avoided bathing and washing for fear that her wedding ring would slip off down the plughole, leaving the house and opening letters (in case she lost the contents). Due to the obvious smell, her neighbours called in environmental health to investigate. She had had the problem for 30 years, but her husband and son would invariably help her and would not allow her behaviours to become so severe. However, the problem worsened five years earlier when her husband died unexpectedly, and a year ago her only son emigrated to Australia.

Treatment efficacy: obsessive compulsive disorder

The NHS Centre for Reviews and Dissemination published a quantitative review of effectiveness of psychological and pharmacological treatments for obsessive-compulsive disorder (2002b). This review found that 'exposure with response prevention was highly effective in reducing obsessive compulsive disorder symptoms. Cognitive approaches were also found to be at least as effective as exposure procedures. Serotonergic medication, particularly chlomipramine, also substantially reduce obsessive compulsive symptoms.'

Post-traumatic stress disorder

Post-traumatic stress disorder (PTSD) has only existed as a diagnosis since 1980 (American Psychiatric Association 1980), and since 1992, using the International Classification of Diseases (World Health Organization 1992). However, the psychological and social effects of being exposed to a traumatic event have been recognized throughout history with 'shell shock' (Southard 1919), 'traumatic neurosis' (Kardiner 1941) and rape trauma syndrome (Burgess and Holstrom 1974) being earlier means of describing the individual effects of specific traumas. Not everyone who is exposed to a trauma develops PTSD. However, the previous belief that the response was a reaction to a 'rare event' has been dismissed as US research shows that 75 per cent of the general population have been exposed to a traumatic event which is significant enough to cause PTSD (Green and Lindy 1994). While Breslau *et al.* (1998), in a US prevalence study in Detroit of 2181 people showed that 89.6 per cent of respondents had been exposed to an event once in their life which met DSM-IV criteria for the stressful traumatic event. However, only 25 per cent of these people will develop PTSD, and it is estimated that 12.5 per cent will continue to have PTSD for decades afterwards. Approximately 1 per cent of the general population will have PTSD at any one time (Helzer *et al.* 1987). However, prevalence varies following trauma according to the trauma type: 22–50 per cent of combat veterans; 75 per cent of shipwreck survivors; 50 per cent of bomb survivors; 37 per cent of hijack survivors; 22 per cent of air-crash survivors; 49 per cent of rape survivors; 21 per cent of survivors of assaultative violence; 24 per cent for sexual assault other than rape; and 10 per cent following a child's life-threatening illness. The reason why traumas affect some people more than others has not been fully explained. Certain factors are known to affect a person's response. These include: previous unresolved traumatic experiences, the traumatizing event, what happened to the person after the trauma experience (short term and long term), the amount of stress in the person's life at the time of the trauma, and gender of trauma victim. In the Detroit study by Breslau *et al.* (1998), results suggested that when all factors were controlled for, that sex was a significant risk factor for developing PTSD, with the rate for women being two-fold higher than men.

Definition and diagnosis

PTSD is diagnostically classed as an anxiety disorder. A DSM-IV (APA 1994) diagnosis of PTSD is made after a person has been exposed to an extreme traumatic stressor involving direct personal experience of an event that involves actual or threatened death or serious injury, or a threat to the physical integrity of self or others. Also, at the time of the trauma the person felt intense fear, helplessness or horror. The person then later develops three persistent clusters of symptoms: one symptom of re-experiencing the trauma, three symptoms of avoidance of trauma-related stimuli and two symptoms of increased arousal. The symptoms must be present for more than one month and cause significant impairment of functioning.

Case study: post-traumatic stress disorder

Sean is a 37-year-old lorry driver in the army, who was involved in a civilian rescue following a coach crash. He was the first rescuer on the scene and climbed into the crashed coach when it was still unstable and when petrol was pouring out of the tank. While climbing in he saw one person who was dead and her limbs were grotesquely twisted around her. He gave immediate first aid to as many people as he could and remembers holding one man's hand while he died only to notice afterwards that the hand had been completely severed. There were people screaming and crying for help who were trapped and many died within 10 minutes of the crash. Later, other passers-by assisted before the emergency services arrived 20 minutes later. Five years later, he still could not drive. He had been sacked and was drinking a bottle of whisky a day, taking 30 mgs valium daily as well as sleeping tablets, night sedation and approximately five to six cannabis 'joints'. He was terrified of sleeping as his nightmares woke him up. He had intrusive thoughts about the 'hand' constantly and his nightmare involved seeing the woman who had died and whose limbs were twisted suddenly opening her eyes and screaming 'help me'. He was hypersensitive to noise, and avoided anything which reminded him of his trauma. He felt 'guilty' all the time and regularly had thoughts, 'If only I had . . .' or 'I should have . . .' These thoughts made him feel he could have saved more people, and because he did not, he felt responsible. He was severely depressed and had twice attempted suicide by overdose.

Treatment efficacy: post-traumatic stress disorder

The NHS Centre for Reviews and Dissemination's (2002c) meta-analysis of the comparative efficacy of treatments for post-traumatic stress disorder supports the use of behaviour therapy, eye-movement desensitization, reprocessing, and selective seretonin reuptake inhibitors. However, it noted also that 'it remains to be seen whether the efficacy of treatment can be improved by using these interventions in combination'.

Panic disorder

Panic attacks occur in a number of anxiety disorders and may be a response to various external situations or triggers, as in specific phobias. Where the occurrence becomes the central cause for concern, panic disorder is said to develop. Unlike other anxiety disorders, where the situations that trigger panic attacks can be easily identified, panic disorder is characterized by episodes of intense anxiety that occur 'out of the blue' – including at night while asleep – making it difficult for an individual to predict their occurrence. A consequence of this is that people become hypervigilant to bodily changes in their level of physiological arousal that results in an increased perception to changes in bodily arousal (Barlow 2002). This body vigilance was observed to be elevated in panic disorder patients compared to social phobia patients and non-anxious controls by Schmidt *et al.* (1997), who also noted that body vigilance is related to a history of spontaneous panic attacks. Similarly, Ehlers (1993) suggested that heightened symptom perception in panic disorder patients may be explained by three factors;

1   greater physiological reactivity;

2   enhanced ability to perceive physiological sensations;

3   increased attention.

Panic disorder may be associated with avoidance of places or situations in which panic attacks may occur, in which case the term panic with agoraphobia is used. The lifetime prevalence of panic disorder with or without agoraphobia is between 1.5 per cent and 3.5 per cent of the populations studied. Panic disorder with agoraphobia occurs in twice as many women as men (Eaton *et al.* 1991), with panic disorder without agoraphobia showing a female to male gender ratio of 3:1.

Panic disorder is also associated with impaired quality of life (Markowitz *et al.* 1989) and an increased risk of suicidal ideation and attempts when compared with other psychiatric disorders (Weissman *et. al.* 1989). An important feature of panic disorder is the cognitive interpretation that people make of their symptoms. Clark's (1986) cognitive model of panic disorder proposed that panic attacks result from a catastrophic misinterpretation of bodily sensations (i.e. that sensations are perceived as more dangerous than they really are). Examples of such misinterpretations include palpitations being interpreted as a sign of an impending heart attack, breathlessness indicating impending suffocation and dizziness as a sign that someone is about to faint. A further feature of panic disorder with and without agoraphobia is the presence of *safety behaviours* (Salkovskis 1991). Three main types of safety behaviours have been suggested by Salkovskis *et al.* (1996) as:

- avoidance,
- escape,
- subtle avoidance behaviours.

All three types of safety behaviours are seen to maintain the presence of panic attacks and panic disorder as they prevent the client from learning that the feared catastrophe does not happen. Salkovskis *et al.* (1996) identified a number of safety behaviours that people engaged in that were associated with the type of catastrophe they feared. For example, where people feared having a heart attack, common responses were to sit down, keep still and ask for help. Similarly, where people feared losing control, common responses were making deliberate attempts to control behaviour, slowing down and looking for an escape route. The identification of safety behaviours forms an important part of treatment.

Definition and diagnosis

Panic disorder is classified as an anxiety disorder in DSM-IV (APA 1994). For panic disorder to be present, unexpected panic attacks must occur. Panic attacks are defined as 'a discrete period of intense fear and discomfort, in which four (or more) of the following symptoms developed abruptly and reached a peak within 10 minutes (DSM-IV, APA 1994: 432): palpitations, pounding heart or accelerated heartrate; sweating; trembling or shaking; sensations of shortness of breath or smothering; feeling of choking; chest pain or discomfort; nausea or abdominal distress; feeling dizzy, unsteady, light-headed or faint; derealization (feelings of unreality) or depersonalization (being detached from oneself); fear of losing control or going crazy; fear of dying; paraesthsias; and chills or hot flushes.

In diagnosing panic disorder, Criterion A states that both panic attacks must occur and at least one of the attacks has been followed by one month (or more) of one (or more) of either persistent concern about additional attacks, and/or worry about the implications of the attack or its consequences (for example, losing control, having a heart attack, 'going crazy') and/or a significant change in behaviour related to the attacks. Criterion B relates to the presence or absence of agoraphobia (see above) and determines whether the problem is classified as panic disorder with agoraphobia or panic disorder without agoraphobia.

Case study: panic disorder

Sharon was a 26-year-old single woman with a history of panic attacks that occurred out of the blue, including at night. Her first panic attack occurred some five years earlier while she was studying for her final exams at university. At that time she experienced intense symptoms of a pounding heart, trembling and shaking, tightness in her chest, shortness of breath, feelings of unreality (derealization) and dizziness. As she was alone at home at the time she immediately called an ambulance and was admitted to hospital via the Accident and Emergency department for 24-hour cardiac monitoring. She was discharged the following day with no abnormal cardiac symptoms detected. At the time of the initial panic attack she reported thinking she was having a heart attack and was about to die. Despite the hospital report she became increasingly concerned about the episode and in particular about the possibility of having future attacks and dying as a consequence of one. Her panic attacks persisted and occurred in a variety of situation, most notably when she was alone, when she was tired, or when she was 'wound up'. Over time, she became particularly adept at monitoring her heartrate and pulse, and became very aware of any altered sensations in her chest, left arm and fingertips. If she noticed any symptoms in these areas she experienced an increase in her symptoms that she interpreted as indicating that there was something seriously wrong with her heart and that death was imminent. In an effort to reduce and control her symptoms she avoided any situation in which they occurred, specifically exercising, crowded places, funfairs, standing up quickly, and driving. These were all situations in which she had previously experienced her feared symptoms. In addition, she always carried her mobile phone with her to enable her to summon help in the event of an attack, avoided going out alone to strange places preferring to go out with a trusted friend, and sat down trying to think 'positive thoughts' if she noticed any symptoms.

Treatment efficacy: panic disorder

Unfortunately, neither The NHS Centre for Reviews and Dissemination nor the Cochrane Database of Systematic Reviews (2nd quarter 2002) databases have examined panic disorder whether it is with or without agoraphobia. However, the NHS Centre for Reviews and Dissemination (2002d) has published a review of the efficacy and cognitive processes of cognitive behaviour therapy in the treatment of panic disorder with agoraphobia, which concludes that CBT is an effective treatment.

Health anxiety

Anxiety about one's own health is a common phenomenon, which affects everyone. Such anxiety drives us to seek medical assistance when we are concerned. Medical assistance in turn enables early detection and therefore early treatment of disease and illness or reassurance that our fear and concerns are unwarranted and that everything is well. When reassured that all is well, most people's fears will reduce and they will pay decreased attention to their complaint/symptom and resume normal day-to-day functioning. However, what happens if the reassurance does not work? What if the test was not completed correctly? What if the tests are not sensitive enough? What if the doctor doesn't even commission the tests, how can he be so sure? Such thoughts can develop in many people and should the 'triggering problem/symptom' continue we will most likely return to our doctor and seek clarification, further reassurance or appropriate tests. Such cycles can continue until one of the following occurs: the triggering problem/symptom dissipates by itself; we are happy with the doctor's competence and the reassurance provided; a condition is found, diagnosis made and treatment begins; or we undergo a full range of tests which rule out all possible causes.

For some people their fears persist, they repeatedly seek medical assessment from health professionals. Additionally, their feared illness may change, so that on one occasion they fear they have cancer, and on another occasion they fear having a stroke. At what point someone's concerns are labelled as 'psychological' is a matter of opinion and conjecture and is a far cry from being an 'exact science'. However, such health anxiety can be extremely disabling for the sufferer but also can create excessive demands on medical services.

Definition and diagnosis

Diagnosis using DSM IV (APA 1994) is often through the use of hyponchondriasis, a somatoform disorder. A pattern of recurring, clinical complaints, which result in clinical assessment and intervention or cause significant impairments in social, occupational or other areas of functioning occur. DSM IV diagnostic criteria for hyponchondriasis requires six criteria to be present:

1   The person is preoccupied with fears of having, or the idea of having, a serious disease based on the person's misinterpretation of bodily symptoms;

2   The preoccupation persists despite appropriate medical evaluation and reassurance;

3   The belief is not of delusional intensity and is not restricted to a concern about appearance (i.e. BDD);

4   The preoccupation causes clinically significant distress or impairment in social, occupational or other important areas of functioning;

5   The duration of the disturbance is at least six months;

6   The preoccupation is not better accounted for by GAD, OCD disorder, a major depressive episode, separation anxiety or another somatoform disorder.

An alternative diagnosis is illness phobia. Illness phobia falls under the category of a specific phobia (other subtype) and is made when a person has a fear and significant avoidance of contracting an illness. The feared illness will usually be consistent, and the feared illness and avoidance of possible stimuli that may cause such an illness does not fluctuate over time (for example, avoidance of asbestos or possible asbestos materials for fear of developing cancer). A range of current societal fears regarding specific or 'new' illnesses can influence such illness phobias. Marks (1987) suggests that phobias of specific illnesses reflect those worries, which are fashionable either in the culture at large or in the family subculture. Illness-related fears cause many diagnostic problems and there are a number of differing views regarding whether it is a separate disorder (illness phobia) or part of a hypochondriachal disorder. Marks (1987) distinguishes between illness phobia and hypochondriasis: 'Where the fears concern multiple bodily symptoms and a variety of illnesses we speak of hypochondriasis. When the fear persistently focuses on a single symptom or illness in the absence of another psychiatric disorder the term illness phobia is appropriate: it is the focal form of hypochondriasis' (1987: 410).

Case study: hypochondriasis

Terry is a 37-year-old married bank manager. He had developed a range of symptoms which caused him to fear that he had a brain tumour as he was having 'migraine attacks', blurred vision, dizziness, nausea and panic. Over time and following a range of investigations (CT scan, pathology tests, EEG) his beliefs changed and he worried about having a stroke. His strength of belief that he had a brain tumour was 60 per cent and that he would have a stroke in the next year was 90 per cent. His fears about tumour and stroke were triggered by headache, blurred vision, dizziness, being out of breath following exertion, and reading or hearing about illness on the television or in newspapers. He had a comprehensive knowledge and had purchased approximately £500 worth of medical texts as well as surfing the internet daily for medical information. Despite repeated reassurance, he was worried that 'something had been missed'. He visited his GP on a weekly basis, with each consultation taking on average 20 minutes before he was suitably reassured. He had a premorbid history of being anxious and had a family history of cancer and stroke.

Treatment efficacy: health anxiety

Unfortunately, neither The NHS Centre for Reviews and Dissemination nor the Cochrane Database of Systematic Reviews (2nd quarter 2002) databases have examined the efficacy of treatments for health anxiety. However, a review of the clinical trials registered on the Cochrane Controlled Trials Register suggests that CBT approaches are effective. Two recent clinical trials (Bouman and Visser 1998; Visser and Bouman 2001) found that exposure plus response prevention and cognitive therapy were both equally as effective in treating hypochondriasis.

Generalized anxiety disorder

Generalized anxiety disorder (GAD) is characterized by apprehensive worry and physical symptoms of restlessness, fatigue, impaired concentration, irritability, muscle tension and/or insomnia (APA 1994). The main cognitive symptom of worry is defined by Wells and Butler (1997): 'Worry occurs as a chain of thoughts, which have a negative affect component. It is concerned with future events where there is uncertainty over outcome' (1997: 161). While worrying can be the cause of clinical concern it is important to recognize that it may be seen to serve a useful purpose, such as adaptive, problem-focused coping and information seeking (Davey *et al.* 1992). Some evidence for the adaptive functions of worry was found by Borkovec and Roemer (1995) who, studying college students, found that motivational, preparation for the worst and avoidance/prevention of negative outcomes statements were rated as functions of worry across both GAD and non-GAD groups. The GAD group differed in their ratings of worrying as serving a function of distraction from more emotional topics.

Barlow's definition of anxiety includes 'anxious apprehension' (2002: 64), which incorporates the idea that anxiety is a 'future-oriented' mood state and clearly differentiates anxiety from panic or fear. From this perspective the type of thinking that characterizes GAD is seen as the core cognitive processes across many of the anxiety disorders. GAD has a lifetime prevalence of 3.8–5.1 per cent (Blazer *et al.* 1991; Wittchen *et al.* 1994) and is twice as common among women as men (Wittchen *et al.* 1994). The course of GAD is generally persistent (Noyes *et al.* 1992) and is associated with impairments in role functioning, social life and life satisfaction (Massion *et al.* 1993).

Definition and diagnosis

Generalized anxiety disorder is diagnosed using DSM IV (APA 1994) criteria if the following are seen:

1   Excessive anxiety and worry (apprehensive expectation), occurring more days than not for at least six months, about a number of events or activities (such as work or school performance).
2   The person finds it difficult to control the worry.
3   The anxiety and worry are associated with three (or more) of the following symptoms: restlessness or feeling keyed up and on edge, easily fatigued, difficulty concentrating or mind going blank, irritability, muscle tension and sleep disturbance (difficulty falling or staying asleep, or restless unsatisfying sleep).
4   The focus of the worry is not confined to another 'Axis I' disorder, for example, worry is not about having a panic attack as in panic disorder, being contaminated as in obsessive-compulsive disorder, or being embarrassed in public as in social phobia.
5   The anxiety or worry should cause clinically significant distress or impairment in social, occupational or other important areas of functioning.
6   The anxiety or worry is not due to the physical effects of a substance or general medical condition.

Wells (1997) suggests that GAD should be seen primarily as a disorder of worrying and that two types of worry should be distinguished: Type 1 worries and Type 2 worries. Type 1 worries are those that may be seen to reflect normal concerns, that may be voluntarily initiated and may have some value in helping solve problems. Type 2 worry is seen as 'worry about worry' (Wells 1997: 202), and reflects an individual's appraisal of the process of worrying itself. Examples given include, 'My worries are uncontrollable', 'Worrying is harmful', 'I could go crazy with worrying' (ibid.).

Case study: generalized anxiety disorder

Andrew was a 49-year-old tradesman who reported feeling worked up, tense and worried for most of his waking day. He had difficulty sleeping, particularly getting off to sleep. His chief complaint was that he was unable to stop worrying about 'stupid little things' that, he considered, most people would take in their stride. Examples of current worries were his ability to do his job properly, where he should go on holiday, and whom he should invite to his 50th birthday party. He reported thinking things over and over in his head to try and plan and prepare but he always found that he couldn't stop the process once started. In addition he reported feeling low and sad at the impact his inability to stop worrying had had on his and his family's life. When he noticed these emotions he would try to think of ways of making things up to them, by attempting to plan special events or outings, but found that he was never able to settle on a suitable solution. Although his predominant emotion was anxiety he did experience episodes of irritability and annoyance with himself. His characteristic thinking process was reported as consisting of many 'What ifs', for example, 'What if I don't get this job done on time?', 'What if they (my family) don't like what I've done for them?' More detailed examination of his thinking suggested that he was particularly concerned that he would get things wrong, that he would not cope, or that he would never be able to switch his thoughts off.

Treatment efficacy: generalized anxiety disorder

The NHS Centre for Reviews and Dissemination's meta-analysis of the comparative efficacy of treatments for generalized anxiety disorder (2002e) found that both CBT and pharmacotherapy (predominantly drugs classed as benzodiazepines) are 'effective treatments for GAD and that both yielded relatively large effect sizes on measures of anxiety severity at post-treatment'. Additionally, there was some evidence suggesting that CBT was 'better at eliminating the symptoms of depression that are often seen in GAD'.

Body dysmorphic disorder

Body image has been defined as the 'picture we have in our minds of the size, shape and form of our bodies and to our feelings concerning these characteristics and our constituent body parts' (Slade 1994: 498). Body image is important to everyone and can be dramatically altered following a life event (for example, facial disfigurement following trauma or breast changes following mastectomy). Some people develop a prevailing preoccupation with a part of their appearance. Such preoccupations may have been effected by familial and peer views and norms or media stereotypes. It has been suggested that 'an extreme of this preoccupation may be manifest in very common eating disorders. There are ... many variants of these disturbances of body image, although as yet no systematic taxonomy to cover them comprehensively' (Gournay *et al.* 1997: 39). Body dysmorphic disorder (BDD) was earlier known as dysmorphophobia and has been reported on as early as 1886: 'Dysmorphophobia is a persistent complaint of a specific body defect that is not noticeable to others' (Morselli 1886: 112).

Marks (1987) suggested that: 'Occasionally (in dysmorphophobia) several parts of the body are involved. The fixity of the idea can amount to a delusion and in some cases can have additional schizophrenic or organic features' (1987: 370). Furthermore, Marks provides an account of typical features based on referrals to the Behavioural Psychotherapy Unit at the Maudsley Hospital: Specific fears may involve '. . . the face, penis, breasts, or hips: of body or limbs being wrinkled, misshapen, or too large or small: or of bad odours coming from sweat in the axilla or from the breath, genitals or rectum' (ibid.). DSM-IV (APA 1994) notes that: 'some individuals use special lighting or magnifying glasses to scrutinise their "defect". There may be excessive grooming behaviour (for example, excessive hair combing, hair removal, ritualised make-up application or skin picking)' (1994: 468).

Very little is truly known about the causes, predisposing factors and prevalence of the disorder. Indeed, DSM-IV (APA 1994) notes that reliable information on prevalence is lacking. Incidence in the cosmetic surgery population is approximately 7 per cent (Sarwer *et al.* 1998) and 11 per cent for dermatological patients (Phillips *et al.* 2000). There is little doubt that sufferers tend to not seek psychological help for their distress as they feel too ashamed. DSM-IV suggests that the onset of the disorder is usually in adolescence but may not be diagnosed for many years, often because individuals with the disorder are reluctant to reveal their symptoms. Furthermore, it seems likely that BDD sufferers continue to suffer long term with few symptom-free periods, although the symptom intensity may vary over time.

Definition and diagnosis

Body dysmorphic disorder is categorized as a somatoform disorder in the fourth edition of the *Diagnostic and Statistical Manual* (DSM-IV: American Psychiatric Association (APA) 1994). There are three DSM-IV criteria that must be met before a diagnosis of BDD can be made:

1   There is a preoccupation with an imagined defect in appearance. If a slight physical anomaly is present, the person's concern is markedly excessive.

2   The preoccupation causes clinically significant distress or impairment in social, occupational or other important areas of functioning.

3   The preoccupation is not better accounted for by another mental disorder (for example, dissatisfaction with body shape and size in anorexia nervosa).

Differential diagnosis is important and a diagnosis of BDD should not be made if the preoccupation is specific to 'fatness' (for example, anorexia nervosa) or sexual identity (for example, gender identity disorder). It is also important to differentiate between BDD and social phobia. In BDD the fear is of negative evaluation due to appearance while in social phobia the fear is due to negative evaluation because of behaviour. It is also important to distinguish BDD from obsessive-compulsive disorder (OCD), due to the obsessive and compulsive qualities involved in both (for example, long periods of time ruminating, excessive checking behaviours. In some cases the preoccupation and intensity of belief can be such that it is of a delusional-like intensity. In such cases it is common for a diagnosis of delusional disorder (somatic type) to be made. Veale *et al.*'s (1996) survey of 50 people with BDD (excluding those with body image disturbances due to an eating disorder), found that BDD has a high co-morbidity with social phobia and depression and that a large proportion of the participants had attempted suicide.

Case study: body dysmorphic disorder

Susan is a 33-year-old hairdresser who attended her GP following a recent bout of ill-health involving panic attacks, low mood, attempted suicide and avoidance of leaving the house. The problem began six weeks earlier when she developed a light rash (which she called spots) over her neck area. She believed that she was 'smelly, disgusting, ugly, revolting and hideous' as a consequence. She took sick leave for three weeks until it cleared up and did not leave the house or let anyone see her during this period except her boyfriend who lived with her. She constantly asked him for reassurance, and she estimated the frequency of this as approximately every 15 minutes. The consequence was that her boyfriend could not cope and moved out, which she said reinforced her belief in being hideous. She said that she woke up one morning and when she looked in the mirror noticed the problem. She had an immediate panic attack (breathlessness, palpitations, shaking) and remembers thinking, 'Oh my God what has happened to me?' Since the 'outbreak' she was constantly in fear of a re-occurrence and developed a number of coping behaviours. She washed her neck hourly with perfume-free soap (including bed-time, setting her alarm clock), constantly mirror-checked (for example, at work, when shopping), constantly asked her boyfriend (who had returned to their home) to check her skin, washed her bed sheets and pillowcase daily. Furthermore, she could not allow any piece of clothing to touch her neck for fear of a reaction. She avoided all make-up and perfume and began to eat only plain foods and also avoided eating out.

Furthermore, she became panicky when in smoky environments and ceased all socializing. Any sign of a spot/blemish would immediately result in a panic attack and thoughts of being disgusting.

Treatment efficacy: body dysmorphic disorder

No NHS guidance is currently available of treatment efficacy for trichotillomania, due to the few trials available. Although many single case or case series cognitive behavioural treatments (CBT) had been described (for example, Munjack 1978). It is only more recently that a systematic and controlled study of the effectiveness of CBT has been undertaken (Veale *et al.* 1996). In all the salient treatment literature, exposure therapy as part of CBT has been the prerequisite for all successful treatment outcomes.

▌ Impact on lifestyle and social functioning

The NSF for Mental Health notes:

> Panic attacks, phobias, or persistent generalised anxiety can impede a person's ability to work, form relationships, raise children, and participate fully in life. GPs often see anxiety, mixed anxiety and depressive disorders, which may be associated with high levels of disability. People who have anxiety symptoms usually smoke more, and may drink more alcohol too, increasing their risk of physical ill health.
>
> (DH 1999: 30)

The experience of any anxiety disorder usually has significant consequences for a person's lifestyle and social functioning. For example, someone who suffers from either agoraphobia or social phobia can have a very restricted social life as places where there are lots of people can cause anxiety. Some anxiety disorders can effect travelling (for example, PTSD following a road traffic accident; agoraphobia as the person is a long way from home). Due to the incapacitating effects, a person's mood can also suffer as they are no longer independent, in control and confident. Furthermore, the sufferer will often avoid and reduce their activity levels which can reduce mood. The evidence for the co-morbidity of anxiety disorders with depression is extensive. For example, Rapaport and Maser (1992) estimate that between 15 and 50 per cent of sufferers with agoraphobia also have a coexisting depressive disorder (see Roth and Fonagy 1996 for further details). Consequently, it is important to routinely assess mental state for possible depression and suicide risk in all clients.

Some anxiety disorders can at times be life-threatening. For example, blood-injection-injury phobia often affects a person's ability to receive urgent medical procedures. Marks (1987) notes that 'emergency is not an uncommon reason for referral, although even then some sufferers would rather literally die than have a venepuncture or operation' (1987: 377).

Assessment and treatment measures

Measurement is an important aspect of all interventions as it often allows for an assessment of the problem when comparing to other sufferers and also aids single case-study evaluation. There are two types of measures: case-specific measures and validated questionnaires, of which both have their advantages and disadvantages. Case-specific measures are problem- as opposed to disorder-focused, which are individualized to reflect the client's problems, and provide specific feedback on an individual's progress over time. In contrast validated questionnaires allow a comparison of the disorder for an individual with a given population.

Case-specific measures

Problem ratings (Marks 1986)

An explicit definition of the problem is collaboratively (client and therapist) developed and agreed from the assessment. The core components of any problem statement are: the problem, the feared consequence, the antecedent, the coping behaviour, and the impact on daily living; an example being: 'nightmares, fear of travelling and thinking about my accident due to panic whenever I am reminded about my car crash, leading to avoidance of all trauma reminders affecting my mood, independence and work life'. Problem ratings are case-specific measures of the distress and impact caused by the problem in given situations, which the client rates on a 9-point scale.

Target ratings (Marks 1986)

Treatment targets are collaboratively agreed and specified by client and therapist and are recorded in behavioural terms. These targets are behavioural goals, which the client is currently unable to achieve, but wishes to do so by the completion of therapy. Usually, two to four targets are agreed. Targets are: precise, positively stated, client centred, realistic and measurable; an example being: 'daily travel to and from work alone, past the accident scene'. Target ratings are case-specific measures of discomfort and success at achieving the behaviour, which the client rates on a 9-point scale.

Work and social adjustment scale (Marks 1986)

The work and social adjustment scale takes client ratings of how the problem affects work, home management, social leisure, private leisure and relationships, using a 0–8 scale.

Validated questionnaires for all cases

The fear questionnaire (Marks and Mathews 1979)

This is a useful measure for all anxiety disorders. This is rated by the client and yields three scores (a) total avoidance, (b) main phobia and (c) anxiety-depression.

The Beck anxiety inventory (Beck *et al.* 1988)

Patients respond to 21 items rated on a scale from 0 to 3. Each item is descriptive of subjective, somatic or panic-related symptoms of anxiety.

The Beck depression inventories (Beck 1961; Beck *et al.* 1996)

Patients respond to 21 items on a scale from 0 to 3 to assess the intensity of depression.

Disorder-specific validated questionnaires

Disorder-specific questionnaires are useful for the specific disorder being assessed. The main specific measures used for all the disorders discussed in this chapter are presented in Table 15.1.

Nurse-led psychological treatment

Over the past 30 years nurse-delivered CBT has become recognized as a specialist area of nursing. Traditionally the application of specific therapies has been considered as being the sole domain of psychologists. However, with the development of multi-professional training courses, there has been a shift away from therapy ownership determined by profession towards a pragmatic multi-professional approach to therapy provision. CBT has been one of the main therapies where this trend is evident. The training of nurses to use behavioural and cognitive behavioural approaches has been delivered through the English National Board (ENB) Course No. 650. Professor Isaac Marks set up this 18-month course at the Maudsley Hospital in 1972, with additional sites springing up across the UK and Eire. Therapeutic outcomes of those nurses trained on the ENB 650 course have been rigorously evaluated. It is known that the therapeutic outcomes of clients treated by nurse therapists compares equally to those treated by psychologists and psychiatrists (Marks *et al.* 1975, 1978; Marks 1985), and their selection and management decisions match those of psychiatrists (Marks *et al.* 1977). Furthermore, clients treated by nurse therapists use less health care resources after one year, compared with an increased use of resources by those treated by GPs (Ginsberg *et al.* 1984). A recent follow-up study by Gournay *et al.* (2000) identified that to date 274 nurses have undergone this training since 1972.

Table 15.1 Specific measures used for disorders and Internet self-help resources

Disorder	Specific measures	Self-help resources
All phobias	The fear questionnaire (Marks and Mathews 1979)	www.triumphoverphobia.com www.phobics-society.org.uk www.no-panic.co.uk
Agoraphobia	The mobility inventory for agoraphobia (Chambless et al. 1985) The agoraphobic cognitions questionnaire (Chambless et al. 1984)	www.triumphoverphobia.com www.phobics-society.org.uk www.no-panic.co.uk
Social phobia	Fear of negative evaluation scale (Watson and Friend 1969) Social phobia and anxiety inventory (Beidel et al. 1994) Social interaction anxiety scale and social phobia scale (Brown et al. 1997)	www.triumphoverphobia.com www.phobics-society.org.uk www.no-panic.co.uk
Specific phobias	Dental fear survey (McGlynn et al. 1987) Spider phobia beliefs questionnaire (Arntz et al. 1993)	www.needlephobia.co.uk/ (needle) www.beyondfear.org/ (dental)
Obsessive-compulsive disorder	Yale-Brown obsessive-compulsive scale (McKay et al. 1995) Maudsley obsessional-compulsive inventory (Hodgson and Rachman 1977) The Padua Inventory (Sanavio 1988)	www.obsessive-action.demon.co.uk www.ocfoundation.org www.no-panic.co.uk
Post-traumatic stress disorder	The clinician-administered PTSD scale (CAPS 2) (Blake et al. 1995) Impact of event scale (IES) (Horowitz et al. 1979) PTSD diagnostic scale (PDS) (Foa et al. 1997)	www.ncptsd.org/index.html
Panic disorder	The fear questionnaire (Marks and Mathews 1979) The automatic thoughts questionnaire (Wells 1997)	http://mentalhelp.net www.cyberpsych.org/anxieties www.panicdisorder.about.com www.no-panic.co.uk
Health anxiety	Symptom interpretation questionnaire (Robbins and Kirmayer 1991) The illness attitude scale (IAS) (Kellner 1994)	http://healthanxiety.com
Generalized anxiety disorder	Penn State worry questionnaire, the worry and anxiety questionnaire (Meyer et al. 1990)	http://mentalhelp.net www.cyberpsych.org/anxieties www.no-panic.co.uk
Body dysmorphic disorder	The Body Dysmorphic Disorder Examination (BDDE) (Rosen et al. 1995) Modified Yale-Brown obsessive compulsive scale (YBOCS) for BDD (Hollander et al. 1994)	www.worldcollegehealth.org/031199.htm http://mentalhelp.net

Standard 2 of the *National Service Framework for Mental Health* states that: 'Any service user who contacts their primary health care team with a common mental health problem should . . . be offered effective treatments, including referral to specialist services for further assessment, treatment and care if they require it' (DH 1999: 28). However, the 274 nurses trained in CBT is woefully inadequate to meet this target. We have suggested in other papers (for example, Gournay 1998; Rogers and Liness 1999; Rogers and Gournay 2000) that there is a dramatic shortage of appropriately trained and accredited CBT therapists across the UK (for example, 1000 in total incorporating psychologists and nurses). These numbers are not sufficient to meet the needs of those clients referred and it is not unusual for clients to have to wait more than a year and up to two years in some instances for adult outpatient CBT in some areas.

Implementation of the standards is non-negotiable. The *NSF for Mental Health* clearly states:

> Local health and social care communities must translate the national standards and service models into local delivery plans . . . (and) . . . It will require systematic and sustained system changes, harnessing the skills and capabilities that already exist in mental health services, and sharing learning across and between organisations.
>
> (DH 1999: 83)

while the workforce planning, education and training within Standard 5 aims: 'to enable mental health services to ensure that their workforce is sufficient and skilled, well led and supported, to deliver high quality mental health care, including secure mental health care (1999: 108). Furthermore, the standard specifically identified that the position in 1999 was such that: 'Not all mental health service staff, even those trained relatively recently, have the skills and competencies to deliver modern mental health services. For example, psychological interventions, such as cognitive behaviour therapy, and complex medication management' (ibid.).

However, five years after the publication of the *NSF for Mental Health* access to CBT training for nurses had not improved. Applications to CBT training centres in London and Sheffield have, in fact, decreased and service managers repeatedly report that they are either unable to fund the training costs out of limited budgets or are unable to cover the replacement costs of staff training. Unless greater investment is available both to release nurses and to improve accessibility to training, this situation will undoubtedly worsen over time.

CBT interventions are developing a greater evidence base and the number of disorders that the limited number of trained nurse therapists are required to see is ever increasing. Two available solutions are refining and reducing therapy training to ensure that

- only those 'active ingredients' which are necessary for a successful outcome are provided;
- greater use of self-help is encouraged and facilitated.

However, these solutions are merely short-term and cannot replace equitable access to evidence-based treatment.

Principles and practice of exposure

Exposure has been defined as: 'facing something that has been avoided because it provokes anxiety' (Hawton *et al.* 1989: 102). The term 'exposure' covers a number of different processes that may be applied in practice. *In-vivo* exposure refers to exposure 'in real life', where the client is actually in the presence of the feared stimulus or situation. *Flooding* is used to denote the process in which the client faces the stimulus or situation that is the most anxiety-provoking. Imaginal exposure is where the client is asked to produce mental images of the feared stimulus, situation or object. *Implosion* techniques are the imaginal equivalent of *flooding*, where the client is asked to produce an image or mental description of the most feared situation. *Interoceptive* exposure techniques are used where the feared or avoided stimuli are internal physical sensations perceived by the client. *Virtual reality* exposure uses technology that provides stimuli that may be perceived as similar or equivalent to real-life situations but where *in-vivo* exposure methods may be impractical – as in the case of flying phobias. *Systematic desensitization* (Wolpe 1958, 1990) is a term used to describe a particular therapeutic procedure that is based on Wolpe's theory of 'reciprocal inhibition', that states that one cannot be anxious and relaxed at the same time. *Modelling procedures* (Bandura 1969) are those in which the therapist demonstrates the exposure task in front of the client.

The majority of the exposure-based treatments discussed in this section are those that involve *in-vivo* exposure, imaginal exposure and modelling techniques. As can be seen from the range of anxiety disorders identified in DSM-IV (APA 1994), a wide range of situations or stimuli can trigger an anxiety response. Some of these may be external, such as specific objects or places, and some may be internal, such as specific thoughts, physical symptoms or memories. When planning an exposure programme, careful assessment will reveal the range of internal and external stimuli that reliably elicit an anxiety response.

Purpose of exposure

The purpose of exposure-based treatments is to produce a reduction or removal of the anxiety response in the presence of the formerly anxiety-evoking stimulus, situation or thought. As such, the goal of therapy is to produce *habituation* of the anxiety response. Habituation is a general term used in biological and behavioural sciences that is defined as: 'a decrement in response as a result of repeated stimulation under normal circumstances, excluding response decrements due to injury, drugs, or other abnormal conditions' (APA 2000: 47).

Another term commonly used in the behavioural literature is 'extinction' that is used to describe the process of reduction or decline in a previously learned response. Exposure-based treatments were derived from behavioural learning theories that attempted to account for the acquisition and maintenance of anxiety responses. Initially, the well-known theory of classical conditioning (Pavlov 1927; Watson and Rayner 1927) was thought to account for the acquisition of anxiety and fear. More recently Davey (1997) has reformulated the classical conditioning model to take into account the process of 're-evaluation of the UCS', where UCS stands for 'unconditioned stimulus'. In practice, the terms habituation and extinction tend to be used synonymously (Marks and Dar 2000). Some attention has been given to the processes through which exposure works. One such formulation is that of 'emotional processing' (Foa and Kozak 1986) in which it is hypothesized that exposure-based treatments have their effect through the modification of an internal fear structure, in which cognitive, affective and behavioural information about the feared stimulus is contained.

Implementing exposure

Marks summarized the key principles of conducting exposure-based therapy as: live exposure is preferable to 'fantasy exposure', although the latter could be used 'when the real stimuli evoking fear are not readily accessible for live exposure' (1987: 462). Self-exposure (or self-directed exposure) is, generally, of equivalent value to therapist-aided exposure; longer exposure periods reduce fear more than shorter ones – 50-minute sessions are recommended; practice between treatment sessions should occur; in OCD completing the ritual was not a problem as long as the ritual did not terminate the exposure session; response prevention was better if self-imposed; rapid exposure (flooding) can yield better gains than graded exposure although it is important to go at the pace of the client; response-induction aids such as grading and varying the tasks, attending to all fear cues, modelling when necessary may be of value; modelling is of use to demonstrate tasks but is not necessary for all; praise for progress motivates the patient. Clients are asked to maintain a diary of their anxiety rating before, during (at its worst) and after (just as the exposure is finishing) on a weekly basis. These serve to give both the client and therapist objective self-ratings of anxiety over time without having to rely on memory (Figure 15.1). Given these principles it is necessary to determine how they may be applied in practice.

How to conduct exposure

Prior to conducting an exposure programme it is important that the client understands what is involved and the reasons for treatment. At this stage it is often useful to use examples from the client's own life experience to illustrate the principle that 'the more you do something the easier it gets'. Such an example might include learning to drive.

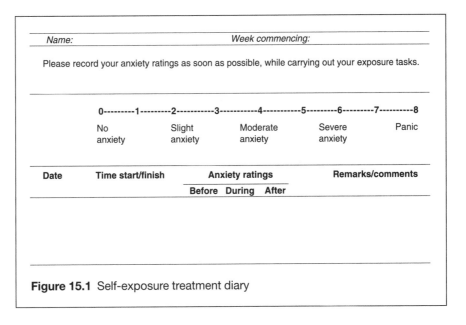

Figure 15.1 Self-exposure treatment diary

A careful assessment is conducted in which all situations that elicit anxiety are identified. In addition, all situations that the client avoids as a result of their fear are detailed. From this a detailed hierarchy of feared or avoided situations is compiled. Wolpe (1990) suggests identifying around ten steps when compiling a fear hierarchy, and also identifies two main types of hierarchy – *conventional* and *idiosyncratic*. Conventional hierarchies are those that may reflect typical behaviours common to the problem, for example, height in feet for someone with a height phobia or distance from home for someone with an agoraphobic problem. Idiosyncratic hierarchies on the other hand vary according to the individual, for example, 'degree of hairiness of spider' or 'dirtiness of door handles' in OCD.

Once the hierarchy is complete the client is then asked to enter the feared situations or remain in the presence of the feared stimulus, situation or thought until their initial anxiety rating on entering the situation is reduced by 50 per cent. In practice, this generally takes around 50 minutes to one hour (Marks 1987), but may vary according to individuals and the type of problem (for example, OCD problems may require sessions of up to two hours). It is important to select a stimulus that is rated as moderately anxiety provoking for the first set of exposure tasks, to help ensure that the client will habituate within the first session and to help demonstrate that anxiety does go away without escaping or avoiding the triggers. Earlier exposure sessions may be *therapist assisted*, so that the therapist can be on hand to prompt the client to attend to the stimulus without distracting, help collect anxiety ratings, reinforce progress and, where necessary, model approach behaviours to the stimulus. Once the client has gained experience, understanding and some confidence in the process *homework* tasks are devised. Homework involves the client engaging in *self-directed* exposure tasks on a daily basis to stimuli or situations identified on the hierarchy. Homework tasks should be clearly agreed and planned, and be done at a less stressful time of day when the client will be free from interruptions. Self-directed exposure tasks are generally as effective as therapist-assisted sessions, and have the additional benefits of ensuring that the therapist doesn't become a safety signal for fear reduction and will enhance the client's confidence or 'self-efficacy' (Bandura 1997).

The role of the mental health practitioner in exposure-based treatments is to help the client work through the process of treatment for themselves, while providing guidance and support. It is important that the practitioner is able to let the client work at their own pace, while being aware that some prompting and encouragement may be necessary if clients are to achieve their desired aims. It is also important to monitor the client's progress by looking for evidence of habituation within exposure sessions (i.e. did the client's anxiety reduce from beginning to end?) and across sessions (i.e. does the same stimulus produce less initial anxiety each time it is faced?). This can usually be done by asking the client to complete homework diaries that detail the stimulus exposed to, the length of the session, and anxiety ratings and the beginning, middle and end of the session.

Principles and practice of cognitive behaviour therapy

The cognitive theories and treatments in use today have generally followed on from Beck's original theories. Broadly speaking, cognitive approaches to emotional disorders focus on two main areas of a person's experience; the *appraisals* a person makes while in a situation, and the *information-processing biases* that occur (McNally 2001). In anxiety, appraisals that are made generally reflect themes of danger and vulnerability. Information-processing biases are seen where certain types of information is noticed (or processed) over other types of information, for example, selective attention to threat cues (Mathews 1997).

The initial assessment and focus of therapy is on the person's *automatic thoughts* that reflect their ongoing appraisals of events in their lives. This is aided by the use of an assessment diary, whereby the person is taught and assisted to begin self-monitoring their emotional changes, allowing identification of the negative thoughts that preceded them (Figure 15.2).

Two other areas of cognition play an important part: *assumptions* and *schema*. Assumptions are those underlying beliefs that a person has that are activated at times of emotional distress and are seen as more enduring than automatic thoughts and reflect more general themes of danger and vulnerability. Wells (1997) describes assumptions as conditional in that they have an 'If . . . then' characteristic to them, for example, 'If I feel anxious then that means there's something wrong with me.' An additional view of assumptions is that they reflect general attitudes or rules, for example, 'Anxiety is dangerous.' Schema are seen as more stable and rigid underlying

COMMENCING:............................ NAME:.. WEEK ....

Emotion rating scale

0 per cent   100 per cent

My experience of this emotion was nil   *My experience of this emotion was the worst ever*

Conviction rating scale

0 per cent   100 per cent

I absolutely do not believe this thought is true   *I am absolutely convinced that this thought is true*

As shown and discussed by your nurse or therapist, please record and rate your emotions and negative thoughts as soon as possible after they have occurred. If you are in doubt please try and record what you think is correct.

Date & time	Emotion	Trigger	Negative thoughts	Conviction	Coping
	What was the negative emotion? (for example, depressed, sad, angry) How intense was this emotion using the 0–100 per cent scale?	What was the trigger? (for example, internal thoughts, images, memories or external triggers)	What did you think when this happened? What did this mean about you? (for example, I failed, It was my fault, I'll never do this, it's hopeless)	When you had these negative thoughts, how strongly did you belief each thought was true using the 0–100 per cent scale?	What did you do to cope with these thoughts? (for example, I did nothing, I argued with myself, I asked a friend, I ignored them, I took medication)

Figure 15.2 Cognitive assessment diary

cognitive structures that reflect a person's early experience and are stated in very concrete terms, for example, 'I'm inadequate' or 'I'm vulnerable.' It should be noted here that the terms 'assumption' and 'schema' may be used to mean the same thing by some writers (for example, Padesky 1994).

Practice of therapy

In a review, Clark (1999) has identified the active ingredients of cognitive therapy for anxiety disorders as: education, verbal discussion techniques, imagery modification, attentional manipulation, exposure to feared stimuli, manipulation of safety behaviours and other behavioural experiments. These therapeutic activities are directly used to address distorted thoughts and beliefs. For more detailed descriptions of the principles and practice of cognitive therapy the reader is referred to Beck (1995), Wells (1997) and Curwen, Palmer and Ruddell (2000). CBT is considered also in Chapter 10 of this book.

Education

Education involves explaining the cognitive model of anxiety to the client, using the client's own material and experience where possible. This process of socialization aids collaboration and begins to demonstrate the collaborative nature of therapy. At other times education may be quite didactic, particularly in relation to the treatment components (McGinn and Sanderson 2001). Reading materials, such as pamphlets and self-help books are used to assist socialization and provide opportunity for education to continue outside the session (Wells 1997; McGinn and Sanderson 2001).

Verbal discussion techniques

Verbal techniques are central to the practice of cognitive therapy and involve questioning, Socratic dialogue and guided discovery. Socratic dialogue (or *Socratic questioning*) is a method of questioning derived from Plato's accounts of the Greek philosopher Socrates' style of discussion when helping people understand philosophical points. Guided discovery (Beck 1995) refers to the process that involves the therapist helping the client identify the meaning underlying their appraisals and often utilizes the 'downward arrow technique' (Burns 1980). Specific verbal techniques are used to help the client identify patterns in their thinking and to facilitate the client challenging their own thoughts. This process requires particular care and skill as it important that the client is encouraged to be aware of and challenge their own thoughts and does not feel belittled or ridiculed by the therapist.

Imagery modification

Given that automatic thoughts can occur in image form as well as verbal (Wells 1997), it is useful to assess the presence of past or future images relevant to anxiety. Where images form a significant part of cognitive content, asking clients to change or modify the content of the image may be associated with a change in meaning.

Attentional manipulation

From an information-processing perspective, the process of selective attention to threat cues, or *attentional bias*, is present in a number of anxiety disorders (Wells and Matthews 1994), although what is attended to and the perspective taken may differ among disorders (Wells and Papageorgiou 1999). Attentional manipulation aims to redirect attention away from the self and onto external sources.

Exposure to feared stimuli

Exposure may be practised as detailed above. However, in cognitive therapy exposure is used in the context of helping to modify thoughts and beliefs. For example, in panic disorder with agoraphobia a client may be asked to enter an avoided situation and remain until anxiety has reduced by 50 per cent. The therapist's focus at the end of this task is then on the client's thoughts before, during and after the exercise to see if initial predictions (for example, 'I'll never stop panicking') were valid.

Manipulation of safety behaviours

Safety behaviours are the acts that people carry out which are designed to prevent a feared catastrophe or outcome (Salkovskis 1991). The client may also see them as things that help them cope in a situation. Salkovskis *et al.* (1996) conducted a survey of the types of safety behaviours people employed. Examples of safety behaviours in panic disorder include carrying a mobile phone to enable help to be summoned quickly, carrying medication in case of a sudden panic, sitting near a door to enable a quick escape. Where safety behaviours are observed, the role of the clinician is to give up the safety behaviour to find out if the feared outcome does, in fact, occur. This may be introduced through verbal discussion (for example, 'You seem to be saying that carrying a mobile phone actually prevents you from panicking') before going to test out the client's hypothesis in a *behavioural experiment*.

Behavioural experiments

Behavioural experiments generally involve testing predictions about physical, social or psychological danger that involve a combination of exposure plus disconfirmatory manoeuvres or survey-based techniques (Wells 1997). As with all cognitive techniques the principal focus is belief change, so experiments should be designed that specify a clear hypothesis from the client, followed by a task that tests out the belief in an appropriate setting. An example relevant to OCD might involve a client expressing the hypothesis: 'If I don't wash all my food thoroughly I'll get food poisoning.' Here the experiment would involve not washing a certain amount of food sufficient to activate the thoughts, eating and 'waiting to see what happens'.

Self-help

Recent developments in the delivery of mental health services have led to the increasing importance of self-help packages for health professionals involved in the treatment of anxiety problems. A look in any bookshop or a brief internet search will demonstrate that a large number of resources are available to someone looking for information on how to deal with anxiety. Given the NSF for Mental Health standards it is imperative that clinicians understand what opportunities exist to facilitate a client to help himself or herself, and can make informed judgements on the types of materials to offer or recommend to clients. A good example of a model of service delivery that relates to the principles of 'stepped care' and considers the needs of the client is the Multiple Access Point Level Entry (MAPLE) approach (Lovell and Richards 2000). Here it is recommended that self-help materials be utilized early in the process of treatment to enable clients to access effective treatments.

When selecting self-help materials, Williams (2002) suggests that the following factors should influence how we choose and use them with patients:

- selection of patients/clients;
- how do the materials fit in with how we work with patients/clients;
- the evidence-base;
- the structure of the materials.

There are several methods of delivering self-help materials, including books, audio-cassettes, videos and computer programs. These resources may be utilized at any stage in the treatment process. Before coming into contact with a health professional the person may have consulted, attended or used one or a number of resources aimed at helping them reduce their anxiety or cope with their problem. These may include the following:

- internet resources (Table 15.1);
- off-the-shelf books (for example, *Feel the Fear and Do It Anyway*, Jeffers 1988);
- self-help groups (for example, Triumph Over Phobia);
- over-the-counter medication (for example, St John's Wort, Kalms, Nytol);
- homeopathic remedies (cf. Chapter 12);
- information derived from others' experiences or cultural factors.

It is not possible here to provide a comprehensive review and recommendation of self-help in all its forms. However, Norcross *et al.* (2000) have produced a guide to self-help resources in mental health. This is the product of five studies in the USA, in which clinical and counselling psychologists were surveyed, and sets about identifying and rating a variety of self-help materials and organizations across a range of clinical problem areas. Subject areas include: anger, anxiety disorders, assertiveness, eating disorders, schizophrenia, stress management and relaxation, and communication and people skills. The range of material covered includes books, films and internet resources. The book also provides strategies for selecting self-help resources offers some useful guidance on factors to consider when approaching the area.

Conclusion

This chapter has examined the history of anxiety disorders and provided an insight into phobias, obsessive-compulsive disorder, post-traumatic stress disorder, panic disorder, health anxiety and generalized anxiety disorder and body dysmorphic disorder. A current review of the evidence has been provided which invariably involves CBT. We have given insights into the processes and practices of CBT and where to access self-help. Although often seen as 'non-severe', anxiety disorders can be extremely disabling and have significant effects on a person's life and relationships. The last 30 years have seen great leaps in both the development of evidence-based treatments for anxiety disorders and in nurse-delivered CBT. The issue of accessibility to such treatments, workforce planning and staff training remain a significant challenge for policy makers and the NHS. We argue that significant rethinking of service provision and professional roles are required if we are ever going to truly meet the NSF guidance in delivering evidence-based interventions for sufferers of anxiety disorders.

In summary the main points in this chapter are:

- Although often seen as 'non-severe', anxiety disorders can be extremely disabling and have significant effects on a person's life and relationships.
- Accessibility to CBT, workforce planning and staff training remain significant challenges for policy makers and the NHS.
- Significant rethinking of service provision and professional roles are required if we are ever to truly meet the NSF guidance in delivering evidenced-based interventions for sufferers of anxiety disorders.

Acknowledgement

This chapter draws in part on material published in a series of continuing professional development articles in *Mental Health Practice*.

▌Questions for reflection and discussion

1   Following the treatment efficacy evidence for CBT that has been offered in this chapter, consider the last five patients that you have seen with an anxiety disorder and ask yourself:

    • Did they have access to CBT?
    • What local services are on offer?
    • What could be done to improve CBT access in your clinical area for this often neglected population?

2   Consider the anxiety measures that we have highlighted. Do you routinely use these measures in your practice? If not, then could you improve your measurement and assessment of anxiety disorders in your practice and in the practice of others?

3   Consider the skills required within the core components of exposure and CBT. Do you have these skills as core components of your nursing knowledge and experience? If so, what relevance do they have for your current working practices and what areas of learning need can you identify for further professional development?

4   Considering the lack of trained therapists who can provide CBT, what improvements can you instigate to improve patients' access to self-help resources for your own practice and the practice of others?

▌Annotated bibliography

• Marks, I.M. (1987) *Fears, Phobias and Rituals: Panic, Anxiety and their Disorders*. Oxford: Oxford University Press. A classic text, which although in need of update in regards to the analyses of the clinical trials that are reviewed, still contains arguably the best psychopathological review of the field. Professor Marks was one of the main researchers/clinicians who was responsible for exposure therapy as it is practised today and a great supporter of nurse-led therapy.
• Wells, A. (1997) *Cognitive Therapy of Anxiety Disorders: A Procedural Manual and Conceptual Guide*. Chichester, West Sussex: Wiley. An excellent, pragmatic text, which provides an invaluable theoretical and clinical review. Wells provides a number of questionnaires and measures which readers are free to use. Predominantly CBT in focus, and includes exceptional chapters on interventions for panic and worry which are hard to find.
• Rachman, S. (1998) *Anxiety*. Hove: Psychology Press. Written by a leading researcher and clinician in the field of anxiety disorders this book provides a detailed, yet concise, account of the nature of anxiety, the main theoretical approaches and the clinical presentations seen in practice. The book is thoroughly referenced throughout, summarizing

the research to date. Specific attention is given to panic and anxiety, agoraphobia, obsessions and compulsion, social anxiety and generalized anxiety disorder. The book is relatively easy to read and is likely to be useful to student mental health practitioners.

- Leahy, R.L. and Holland, S.J. (2000) *Treatment Plans and Interventions for Depression and Anxiety Disorders*. New York: Guilford Press. As the title suggests this book's main emphasis is on treatment, although each chapter contains descriptive and diagnostic information for all of the disorders covered. The book is rich in practical detail and advice, including flow-charts to aid diagnosis, session-by-session treatment options to the 'Information for Patients' handouts. All forms and supplementary information, which are contained on an accompanying CD-ROM, can be printed by purchasers for their, and their clients', use. The treatment approaches are specifically cognitive-behavioural and written for practising clinicians. Being American, occasional reference is made to the 'managed care' system, although this does not affect the relevance of the text to the practising (or soon to be practising) UK mental health practitioner.
- Steketee, G. (1993) *Treatment of Obsessive Compulsive Disorder*. New York: Guilford Press. Although slightly dated and, therefore, not including recent accounts of cognitive treatments of OCD, this book provides one of the most accessible accounts of exposure and response prevention available. Separate chapters are provided for assessment, implementing direct exposure, implementing imaginal exposure, preventing rituals and managing complications and maintaining treatment gains. The appendices contain a number of the major assessment instruments that purchaser's can use in their work with clients.

References

American Psychiatric Association (1980) *Diagnostic and Statistical Manual of Mental Disorders* (3rd edn). Washington, DC: American Psychiatric Association.

American Psychiatric Association (1994) *Diagnostic and Statistical Manual of Mental Disorders* (4th edn). Washington, DC: American Psychiatric Association.

American Psychological Association (2000) *Encyclopedia of Psychology*. Washington, DC and Oxford: American Psychological Association and Oxford University Press.

Amies, P.L., Gelder, M.G. and Shaw, P.M. (1983) Social phobia: A comparative clinical study, *British Journal of Psychiatry* **142**: 174–9.

Angst, J. and Dobler-Mikola, A. (1983) Anxiety states, panic and phobia in a young general population, in World Psychiatry Congress Proceedings, New York: Vienna Plenum.

Arntz, A., Lavy, E., van den Berg, G. and van Rijsoort, S. (1993) Negative beliefs of spider phobics: A psychometric evaluation of the Spider Phobic Beliefs Questionnaire, *Advances in Behaviour Research and Theory* **15**: 257–77.

Bandura, A. (1969) *Principles of Behavior Modification.* New York: Holt, Reinhart and Winston.

Bandura, A. (1997) *Self-efficacy: The Exercise of Control.* New York: W.H. Freeman and Co.

Barlow, D.H. (2002) *Anxiety and its Disorders* (2nd edn). New York: Guilford Press.

Beck, A.T. (1961). An inventory of measuring depression, *Archives of General Psychiatry* **4**: 561–71.

Beck, A.T., Emery, G. with Greenberger, R.L. (1985) *Anxiety Disorders and Phobias: A Cognitive Perspective.* New York: Basic Books.

Beck, A.T., Epstein, N., Brown, G. and Steer, R.A. (1988) An inventory for measuring clinical anxiety: psychometric properties, *Journal of Consulting and Clinical Psychology* **56**: 893–7.

Beck, A.T., Steer, R.A. and Brown, G.K. (1996) *BDI-II Manual.* San Antonio: The Psychological Corporation.

Beck, J.S. (1995) *Cognitive Therapy: Basics and Beyond.* New York: Guilford Press.

Berrios, G. (1999) Anxiety disorders: a conceptual history, *Journal of Affective Disorders* **56**: 83–94.

Blake, D.D. *et al.* (1995) The development of a clinician-administered PTSD scale, *Journal of Traumatic Stress* **8**: 75–90.

Blazer, D.G., Hughes, D., George, L.K., Swartz, M. and Boyer, R. (1991) Generalized anxiety disorder, in L.N. Robins and D.A. Reiger (eds) *Psychiatric Disorders in America: The Epidemiolocal Catchment Area Survey.* New York: Free Press.

Borkovec, T.D. and Roemer, L. (1995) Perceived functions of worry among generalized anxiety disorder subjects: distraction from more emotionally distressing topics?, *Journal of Behavior Therapy and Experimental Psychiatry* **26**(1): 25–30.

Bouman, T.K. and Visser, S. (1998) Cognitive and behavioural treatment of hypochondriasis, *Psychotherapy and Psychosomatics* **67**(4–5): 214–21.

Breslau, N., Kessler, R.C., Chilcoat, H.D. *et al.* (1998) Trauma and post-traumatic stress disorder in the community: The 1996 Detroit area survey of trauma, *Archives of General Psychiatry* **55**: 626–32.

Burgess, A.W. and Holstrom, L.L. (1974) Rape Trauma Syndrome. *American Journal of Psychiatry* **131**(9): 981–5.

Burns, D.D. (1980) *Feeling Good: The New Mood Therapy.* New York: Signet.

Cannon, W.B. (1929) *Bodily Changes in Pain, Hunger, Fear, and Rage* (2nd edn). New York: Appleton-Century-Crofts.

Chambless, D.L., Caputo, G.C., Bright, P. and Gallager, R. (1984) Assessment of 'fear of fear' in agoraphobics: The Body Sensations Questionnaire and the Agoraphobic Cognitions Questionnaire, *Journal of Consulting and Clinical Psychology* **52**: 1090–7.

Chambless, D.L., Caputo, G.C., Jasin, S.E., Gracely, E.J. and Williams, C. (1985) The Mobility Inventory for Agoraphobia, *Behaviour Research and Therapy* **23**(1): 35–44.

Clark, D.M. (1986) A cognitive approach to panic, *Behaviour Research and Therapy* **24**: 461–70.

Clark, D.A. (1999) Anxiety disorders: why they persist and how to treat them, *Behaviour Research and Therapy* **37**: S5–S27.

Cochrane Database of Systematic Reviews (2002) Cochrane Collaboration, Issue 2. Oxford: Update Software.

Curwen, B., Palmer, S. and Ruddell, P. (2000) *Brief Cognitive Behaviour Therapy.* London: Sage.

Davey, G.C.L. (1997) A conditioning model of phobias, in G.C.L. Davey (ed.) *Phobias: A Handbook of Theory, Research and Treatment*, Ch. 15, pp. 301–22. Chichester: Wiley.

Davey, G.C.L., Hampton, J., Farrel, J. and Davidson, S. (1992) Some characteristics of worrying: evidence for worrying and anxiety as separate constructs, *Personality and Individual Differences* **13**: 133–47.

Department of Health (1999) *A National Service Framework for Mental Health*. London: The Stationery Office.

de Silva, P. and Rachman, S. (1998) *Obsessive-Compulsive Disorder – The Facts*. Oxford: Oxford Medical Publications.

Eaton, W.W., Dryman, A. and Weissman, M.M. (1991) Panic and phobia, in L.N. Robins and D.A. Reiger (eds) *Psychiatric Disorders in America: The Epidemiolocal Catchment Area Survey*. New York: Free Press.

Ekman, P. (1992) An argument for basic emotions, *Cognition and Emotion* **6**: 169–200.

Ehlers, A. (1993) Interoception and panic disorder, *Behaviour Research and Therapy* **15**: 3–21.

Ellis, A. (1962) *Reason and Emotion in Psychotherapy*. New York: Lyle Stuart.

Eysenck, H.J. (1947) *Dimensions of Personality*. London: Trubner and Co. Ltd.

Eysenck, H.J. (1952) The effects of psychotherapy: an evaluation, *Journal of Consulting Psychology* **16**: 319–24.

Foa, E.B. and Kozak, M.J. (1986) Emotional processing of fear: exposure to corrective information, *Psychological Bulletin* **99**: 20–35.

Foa, E.B., Cashman, L.A., Jaycox, L. and Perry, K. (1997) The validation of a self-report measure of posttraumatic stress disorder: The Posttraumatic Diagnostic Scale, *Psychological Assessment* **4**: 445–51.

Freud, S. (1977) Analysis of a phobia in a five-year-old boy, *Pelican Freud Library*, Volume 8, Case Histories 1. Harmondsworth: Penguin.

Ginsberg, G., Marks, I.M. and Waters, H. (1984) Cost benefit analysis of a controlled trial of nurse therapy for neurosis in primary care, *Psychological Medicine* **14**: 683–90.

Gournay, K. (1998) Obsessive Compulsive Disorder: Nature and Treatment, *Mental Health Practice* **1**(8): 35–43.

Gournay, K., Veale, D. and Walburn, J. (1997) Body dysmorphic disorder: pilot randomised controlled trial of treatment; implications for nurse therapy research and practice, *Clinical Effectiveness in Nursing* **1**: 38–46.

Gournay, K., Denford, L., Parr, A.M. and Newell, R. (2000) British nurses in behavioural psychotherapy: a 25-year follow-up, *Journal of Advanced Nursing* **32**(2): 1–9.

Green, B.L. and Lindy, J.D. (1994) Post-traumatic stress disorder in victims of disaster, in D.A. Tomb (ed.) *The Psychiatric Clinics of North America* **8**: 301–10.

Hawton, K., Salkovskis, P., Kirk, J. and Clark, D. (eds) (1989) *Cognitive Behaviour Therapy for Psychiatric Problems: A Practical Guide*. Oxford: Oxford University Press.

Helzer, J.E., Robins, L. and McElvoy, L. (1987) Post-traumatic stress disorder in the general population, *New England Journal of Medicine* **317**: 1630–4.

Hodgson, R.J. and Rachman, S. (1977) Obsessive-compulsive complaints, *Behaviour Research and Therapy* **15**: 389–95.

Horowitz, M., Wilner, N. and Alvarez, W. (1979) Impact of Event Scale: A measure of subjective stress. *Psychosomatic Medicine* **41**: 209–18.

Jeffers, S. (1988) *Feel the Fear and Do It Anyway*. New York: Fawcett Columbine.

Kardiner, A. (1941) *The Traumatic Neurosis of War*. New York: Hoeber.

Kellner, R. In: Fischer, J. and Corcoran, K. (1994) *Measures for Clinical Practice: A Sourcebook*, 2nd edn (2 vols). New York: Free Press, vol. 2, pp. 264–7.

Liddell, A., Di Fazio, L., Blackwood, J. and Ackerman, C. (1994) Long-term follow-up of treated dental phobics, *Behavior Research and Therapy* **32**: 605–10.

Lovell, K. and Richards, D. (2000) Multiple access points and levels of entry (maple): ensuring choice, accessibility and equity for CBT services, *Behavioural and Cognitive Psychotherapy* **28**(4): 379–91.

Mahoney, M. and Thoresen, C. (1974) *Self-control: Power to the Person*. Monterey, CA: Brooks-Cole.

Markowitz, J.S., Weissman, M.M., Ouelette, R., Lish, J.D. and Klerman, G.L. (1989) Quality of life in panic disorder, *Archives of General Psychiatry* **46**: 984–92.

Marks, I.M. (1969) *Fears and Phobias*. New York: Academic Press.

Marks, I.M. (1985) Psychiatric nurse therapists in primary care, *Royal College of Nursing Research Series*, London: RCN.

Marks, I.M. (1986) *Behavioural Psychotherapy: Maudsley Pocket Book of Clinical Management*. Bristol: Wright.

Marks, I.M. (1987) *Fears, Phobias and Rituals: Panic, Anxiety and their Disorders*. Oxford: Oxford University Press.

Marks, I.M. and Dar, R. (2000) Fear reduction by psychotherapies: recent findings, future directions, *British Journal of Psychiatry* **176**: 507–11.

Marks, I.M. and Mathews, A.M. (1979) Brief standard self-rating for phobic patients, *Behaviour Research and Therapy* **17**: 59–68.

Marks, I.M., Hallam, R.S. and Connolly, J.C. (1975) Nurse therapists in behavioural psychotherapy, *British Medical Journal* **19**(3): 144–8.

Marks, I.M., Hallam, R.S., Connolly, J.C. and Philpott, R. (1977) *Nursing in Behavioural Psychotherapy. An Advanced Clinical Role for Nurses*. London: Royal College of Nursing.

Marks, I.M., Bird, J. and Lindley, P. (1978) Behavioural nurse therapists: developments and implications, *Behavioural Psychotherapy* **6**: 25–6.

Massion, A., Warshaw, M. and Keller, M. (1993) Quality of life and psychiatric comorbidity in panic disorder versus generalized anxiety disorder, *American Journal of Psychiatry* **150**: 600–7.

Mathews, A. (1997) Information processing biases in emotional disorders, in D.M. Clark and C.G. Fairburn (eds) *Science and Practice of Cognitive Behaviour Therapy*, Ch. 3, pp. 47–66. Oxford: Oxford University Press.

McGinn, L.K. and Sanderson, W.C. (2001) What allows cognitive behavioural therapy to be brief: overview, efficacy and crucial factors facilitating brief treatment, *Clinical Psychology: Science and Practice* **8**(1): 23–37.

McNally, R.J. (2001) On the scientific status of cognitive appraisal models of anxiety disorder, *Behaviour Research and Therapy* **39**: 513–21.

Meyer, T.J., Miller, M.L., Metzger, R.L. and Borkovec, T.D. (1990) Development and validation of the Penn State worry questionnaire, *Behaviour Research and Therapy*, **28**: 487–95.

Morselli, E. (1886) Sulla dismorfofobia e sulla tafefobia, *Bolletinno della R accademia di Genova* (Genova) VI, 110–19.

Mowrer, O.A. (1960) *Learning Theory and Behaviour*. New York: Wiley.

Munjack, D. (1978) Behavioural treatment of dysmorphophobia, *Journal of Behavioural Therapy and Experimental Psychiatry* **134**: 382–9.

Nesse, R.M. (1999) Proximate and evolutionary studies of anxiety, stress and depression: synergy at the interface, *Neurosciences and Biobehavioral Reviews* **23**: 895–903.

NHS Centre for Reviews and Dissemination Reviewers (2002a) The treatment of social phobia: a critical assessment, *Database of Abstracts of Reviews of Effectiveness, University of York*, Vol. 2, June 2002. http://gateway2.ovid.com/ovidweb.cgi (accessed 28 August 2002).

NHS Centre for Reviews and Dissemination Reviewers (2002b) Effectiveness of psychological and pharmacological treatments for obsessive-compulsive disorder: a quantitative review, *Database of Abstracts of Reviews of Effectiveness, University of York*, Vol. 2, June 2002. http://gateway2.ovid.com/ovidweb.cgi (accessed 28 August 2002).

NHS Centre for Reviews and Dissemination Reviewers (2002c) Comparative efficacy of treatments for post-traumatic stress disorder: a meta-analysis, *Database of Abstracts of Reviews of Effectiveness, University of York*, Vol. 2, June 2002. http://gateway2.ovid.com/ovidweb.cgi (accessed 28 August 2002).

NHS Centre for Reviews and Dissemination Reviewers (2002d) The efficacy and cognitive processes of cognitive behaviour therapy in the treatment of panic disorder with agoraphobia, *Database of Abstracts of Reviews of Effectiveness, University of York*, Vol. 2, June 2002. http://gateway2.ovid.com/ovidweb.cgi (accessed 28 August 2002).

NHS Centre for Reviews and Dissemination Reviewers (2002e) Cognitive behavioural and pharmacological treatment of generalized anxiety disorder: a preliminary meta-analysis, *Database of Abstracts of Reviews of Effectiveness, University of York*, Vol. 2, June 2002. http://gateway2.ovid.com/ovidweb.cgi (accessed 28 August 2002).

Norcross, J., Santrock, J., Campbell, L. and Smith, T. (2000) *Authoritative Guide to Self-Help Resources in Mental Health*. New York: Guilford Press.

Noyes, R., Woodman, C., Garvey, M.J. *et al.* (1992) Generalized anxiety disorder versus panic disorder: Distinguishing characteristics and patterns of comorbidity, *Journal of Nervous and Mental Disease* **180**: 369–70.

Padesky, C. (1994) Schema change processes in cognitive therapy, *Clinical Psychology and Psychotherapy* **1**(5): 267–78.

Pavlov, I.P. (1927) *Conditioned Reflexes* (trans. G.V. Anrep). London: Oxford University Press.

Pervin, L.A. and John, O.P. (eds) (2001) *Personality: Theory and Research* (8th edn). New York: John Wiley and Sons.

Phillips, K.A., Dufresne, R.G., Wilkel, C.S. and Vittorio, C.C. (2000) Rate of body dysmorphic disorder in dermatology patients, *Journal of the American Academy of Dermatology* **42**(3): 436–41.

Rapaport, M.H. and Maser, J.D. (1992) Secondary depression: Definition and treatment, *Pharmacology Bulletin* **28**: 27–33.

Rogers, P. and Gournay, K. (2000) Phobias: nature, assessment and treatment (RCN Continuing Education), *Mental Health Practice* **3**(8): 30–5.

Rogers, P. and Liness, S. (1999) Post-traumatic stress disorder: nature, assessment and treatment (RCN Continuing Education), *Mental Health Practice* **2**(5): 27–37.

Rosen, J.C., Reiter, J. and Orosan, P. (1995) Assessment of body image in eating disorders with the body drymorphic disorder examination, *Behaviour Research and Therapy* **33**(1): 77–84.

Roth, A. and Fonagy, P. (1996) *What Works for Whom: A Critical Review of Psychotherapy Research*. London: Guilford Press.

Salkovskis, P.M. (1991) The importance of behaviour in the maintenance of anxiety and panic: a cognitive account, *Behavioural Psychotherapy* **19**: 6–19.

Salkovskis, P.M., Clark, D.M. and Gelder, M.G. (1996) Cognition-behaviour links in the persistence of panic, *Behaviour Research and Therapy* **32**: 1–8.

Sarwer, D.B., Wadden, T.A. and Pertschuk, M.J. (1998) Body image dissatisfaction and body dysmorphic disorder in 100 cosmetic surgery patients, *Plastic and Reconstructive Surgery* **101**(6): 1644–9.

Schmidt, N.B., Lerew, D.R. and Trakowski, J.H. (1997) Body vigilance in panic disorder: evaluating attention to bodily perturbations, *Journal of Consulting and Clinical Psychology* **65**(2): 214–20.

Skinner, B.F. (1938) *The Behavior of Organisms*. New York: Appleton-Century-Crofts.

Slade, P.D. (1994) What is body image?, *Behaviour Research and Therapy* **32**: 497–502.

Southard, E.E. (1919) *Shell Shock and Neuropsychiatric Problems*. Boston: Leonard.

Stein, D.J. and Bouwer, C. (1997) A neuro-evolutionary approach to the anxiety disorders, *Journal of Anxiety Disorders* **11**(4): 409–29.

Thorpe, G.K. and Burns, L.E. (1983) *The Agoraphobic Syndrome*. Wiley: New York.

Veale, D., Gournay, K., Dryden, W. *et al.* (1996). Body dysmorphic disorder: a cognitive behavioural model and pilot randomised controlled trial, *Behaviour Research and Therapy* **34**: 717–29.

Visser, S. and Bouman, T.K. (2001) The treatment of hypochondriasis: exposure plus response prevention vs cognitive therapy. [Clinical Trial. Journal Article. Multicenter Study. Randomized Controlled Trial], *Behaviour Research and Therapy* **39**(4): 423–42.

Watson, B. and Friend, R. (1969) Measurement of social-evaluate anxiety, *Journal of Consulting and Clinical Psychology* **33**: 448–57.

Watson, J.B. and Rayner, R. (1927) Conditioned emotional reactions, *Journal of Experimental Psychology* **3**(1): 1–14.

Weissman, M.M., Leaf, P.J., Holzer, C.E. and Merikangas, K.R. (1985) Epidemiology of anxiety disorders, *Psychopharmacology Bulletin* **26**: 543–5.

Weissman, M.M., Klerman, G.L., Markowitz, J.S. and Ouellette, R. (1989) Suicidal ideation and suicide attempts in panic disorder and attacks, *New England Journal of Medicine* **321**: 1209–14.

Wells, A. (1997) *Cognitive Therapy of Anxiety Disorders: A Procedural Manual and Conceptual Guide*. Chichester: Wiley.

Wells, A. and Butler, G. (1997) Generalized anxiety disorder, in D. Clark and C. Fairburn (eds) *Science and Practice of Cognitive Behaviour Therapy*. Oxford: Oxford Medical Publications, ch. 7, pp. 155–78.

Wells, A. and Matthews, G. (1994) *Attention and Emotion: A Clinical Perspective*. Hove: Psychology Press.

Wells, A. and Papageorgiou, C. (1999) The observer perspective: biased imagery in social phobia, agoraphobia, and blood injury phobia, *Behaviour Research and Therapy* **37**: 653–8.

Williams, C. (2002) Choosing and using self-help materials, *Behavioural and Cognitive Psychotherapy* **30**: 243–5.

Wittchen, H.U., Zhao, S., Kessler, R.C. and Eaton, W.W. (1994) DSM-III-R generalized anxiety disorder in the National Comorbidity Survey, *Archives of General Psychiatry* **51**: 355–64.

Wolpe, J. (1958) *Psychotherapy by Reciprocal Inhibition*. Stanford, CA: Stanford University Press.

Wolpe, J. (1990) *The Practice of Behavior Therapy* (4th edn). New York: Pergamon Press.

World Health Organization (1992) *International Classification of Diseases and Related Health Problems* (10th edn). Geneva: World Health Organization.

16

The person with an eating disorder

Janet Treasure, Alison Carolan and Gill Todd

Chapter overview

In this chapter we have chosen not to follow the usual medical model of describing an illness (in terms of history, aetiology, diagnosis, clinical features, treatment and prognosis) nor have we used Leventhal's illness perception model (a lay conceptualization of illness identity, causal attributions, illness timescale, illness consequences) (Leventhal *et al.* 1984). Instead we have chosen to structure our consideration of treatment and care for a person suffering from an eating disorder around the standards of the *National Service Framework (NSF) for Mental Health* (DH 1999). We have therefore tailored our presentation of the knowledge base related to eating disorders into a structure, which was developed to organize and to ensure quality in services.

This chapter covers:

- Standard 1: mental health promotion. Here we cover demographic features and aetiology of eating disorders.
- Standards 2 and 3: primary care and access to services. This section covers aspects of diagnosis and engagement into treatment.
- Standards 4 and 5: effective services for people with severe mental illness. This section addresses the evidence base for treatment.
- Standard 6 pertains to individuals who care for people with mental health problems. This is a new element that is extremely important for people with eating disorders.
- Standard 7: action necessary to reduce suicides. This includes a synopsis of prognostic features and outcome of eating disorders.

So what is missing from such an approach? Well, we do not have any history and there is less of focus on clinical features – although these are covered by Basu in Chapter 18. However, nurses work in all areas of the NHS and we argue that it is important to think in terms of this wider framework. Writing this chapter in the context of the *NSF for Mental Health* has been a refreshing experience. It has allowed us to see the care and treatment of people suffering from eating disorders from a different perspective and we hope that this format will allow readers to do so, too.

Standard 1: Mental health promotion – aetiology and demographic features

Health promotion is the focus of Chapter 1 of this book. As in many other psychiatric conditions, it is unlikely that there is one causal factor but rather a host of variables which interact to produce the eating disorder. Then, once the illness has emerged, an array of factors act to maintain the disorder. It is generally agreed that there are two domains of risk factors. The first is the dieting/weight/eating domain and the second includes factors which are general to all forms of psychopathology. These are outlined in Table 16.1.

Our confidence in the risk factors evidence base for the bulimic disorders is much stronger than that for anorexia nervosa as several of them have been validated in prospective studies or in randomized trials. However, we argue that primary prevention is of most relevance for the bulimic disorders rather than for anorexia nervosa. Bulimia nervosa is a disease with a recent history, which suggests that some novel environmental exposure has been an important causal element. The illness emerged in the later half of the twentieth century. The risk has gradually increased with each birth cohort born since 1950 (Kendler *et al.* 1991). Bulimia nervosa was first described clinically by Russell in 1979 (Russell 1979). There is much less evidence of an increased incidence of anorexia nervosa and so the attributable risk to environmental factors is probably less. Also because anorexia nervosa is less common, a population-based prevention programme is less efficient. However, anorexia nervosa is the ideal candidate for a secondary prevention strategy because it is an overt condition. Thus it should be amendable to early detection and treatment.

To whom and where should prevention work be targeted?

The incidence and prevalence and demographic features associated with eating disorders are shown in Tables 16.2, 16.3 and 16.4. These show that for maximum impact primary prevention work for bulimia nervosa should be focused on adolescent females in urban settings. The most effective strategy for prevention in anorexia nervosa would be early intervention (secondary prevention) in which schools and colleges are able to recognize the problem and use appropriate means to engage the individual into a plan of management. In the case of bulimia nervosa dentists can detect signs. Thus prevention merges into early intervention and Standards 2 and 3 of the *NSF for Mental Health* (DH 1999).

Table 16.1 Risk factors in eating disorders

Specific factors related to dieting, weight and eating

- There is a family history of obesity in the binge-eating disorders (Fairburn *et al.* 1997, 1998). In contrast there is a family history of leanness in anorexia nervosa (Hebebrand and Remschmidt 1995).
- There is a tendency to premorbid obesity in bulimic disorders (Fairburn *et al.* 1997) and to leanness in anorexia nervosa (Hebebrand and Remschmidt 1995).
- There is often teasing about weight and shape from family and peers in bulimic disorders (Fairburn *et al.* 1997, 1998).
- There is more exposure to dieting in bulimic disorders (Fairburn *et al.* 1997, 1998).
- Body dissatisfaction, dieting/overeating, drive for thinness, internalization of thin ideal are risk factors for bulimic disorders (Stice 2002).

General risk factors

Predisposing factors

- There is increased number of cases of eating disorders within families (Strober *et al.* 2000). Twin studies suggest that over 50 per cent of the variance is attributed to genetic factors (Bulik *et al.* 2000).
- There is an increased risk of perinatal stress or trauma in anorexia nervosa (Cnattingius *et al.* 1999; Shoebridge and Gowers 2000).
- There is insecure attachment: avoidant in anorexia nervosa (Ward *et al.* 2001) and ambivalent in bulimia nervosa (Ward *et al.* 2000).
- There is increased risk of adverse environmental exposures (sexual and physical abuse and neglect) in particular for bulimia nervosa (Johnson *et al.* 2002).

Precipitating factors

- puberty for anorexia nervosa;
- life events (Schmidt *et al.* 1997).

Perpetuating (maintaining factors) (Stice 2002)

- culture of thinness, internalization of thin ideal, body dissatisfaction;
- perfectionism (Stice 2002);
- emotional regulation;
- interpersonal difficulties.

Perinatal complications and stress during pregnancy: anorexia nervosa (AN)

- A quarter of parents had experienced severe obstetric difficulty and loss, compared to only 7.5 per cent of matched comparison parents (Shoebridge *et al.* 2000).
- The incidence of prematurity and birth trauma is elevated by 2–3 fold in the birth histories of those with AN (Cnattingius *et al.* 1999).
- Pregnancy complications were noted more often (Foley *et al.* 2001; Schmidt *et al.* 1997).
- There is a trend for people with anorexia nervosa to be born in the spring months, which opens the possibility that exposure to viral infection *in utero* may increase the risk (Rezaul *et al.* 1996; Eagles *et al.* 2001).

Table 16.2 Incidence of anorexia nervosa per year per 100,000 population

Region	Source	Period	Incidence	Author
Netherlands	General practitioners	1985–89	8.1	(Hoek *et al.* 1995)
England, Wales	General practitioners	1993	4.2	(Turnbull *et al.* 1996)

Table 16.3 Two-stage surveys of prevalence of anorexia nervosa and bulimia nervosa in young females

Source	Age	N	Screening	Criteria	Prevalence	Authors
Household census	18–24		DIS	DSM-III	4.5	BN (Bushnell *et al.* 1990)
	25–44				2.0	
	(18–44)	(777)			(2.6)	
General practice	16–35	540	questionnaire	DSM-IIIR	1.5	BN (Whitehouse *et al.* 1992)
General practice	16–35	540	questionnaire	DSM-IIIR	0.2	AN (Whitehouse *et al.* 1992)

Table 16.4 Demographic features associated with eating disorders

Anorexia nervosa

- Incidence rates of anorexia nervosa are highest for females 15–19 years old (Turnbull *et al.* 1996).
- The risk in women 10× that of men (Turnbull *et al.* 1996).
- Upward trend in the incidence of anorexia nervosa since the 1950s especially in females 15 to 24 years of age (Lucas *et al.* 1999).
- Social class? increase in higher socioecomomic groups (McClelland and Crisp 2001).

Bulimia nervosa

Incidence rates highest females 20–24 (Turnbull *et al.* 1996; Hoek *et al.* 1995).
The risk in women 20× that of men (Turnbull *et al.* 1996).
Bulimia nervosa increase risk cohorts born after 1950 (Kendler *et al.* 1991).
All social classes (Gard and Freeman 1996).
Three-fold increase in urban (Hoek *et al.* 1995).
Occupation: e.g. ballet (Vandereycken and Hoek 1993).

What should be the focus of any prevention work?

Many risk factors are not modifiable and so they cannot be targets of any health promotion programme. Moreover there is controversy as to the effectiveness of prevention packages which have had eating disorders as their focus as some have appeared to be ineffective (irrelevant to the majority) or dangerous as there is a risk that unhealthy ideas are implanted into vulnerable people (Rosenvinge and Borrenson 1999). (The popularity of pro-anorexia websites attest to this danger.) Thus, programmes have to be more sophisticated and have a focus on the complex mix of risk and resilience factors. This will include giving information and counselling: to parents about good parenting, to teachers about how to become good role models, and to adolescents directly.

Standards 2 and 3: Primary care and access to services

The *NSF for Mental Health* (DH 1999) has specified that each health authority has to implement guidelines for the treatment and referral pathways for eating disorders. However, general practitioners (GPs) do not appear to have the skills/resources to detect and diagnose eating disorders. There is usually a considerable delay (on average 7.4 months) between the time parents first seek help from primary care for their child's eating problem and the point where diagnosis is made and there is a referral to a specialist service (Fosson *et al.* 1987). Indeed carers in the UK were dissatisfied with management in primary care (Haigh and Treasure 2002).

Detection and diagnosis

The criteria on which the diagnoses are made are shown in Tables 16.5 and 16.6.

Table 16.5 Criteria for diagnosis of anorexia nervosa

Current classification and definition (the main points of ICD10 (WHO 1992) and DSM-IV (APA 1994) combined)

- body weight at least 15 per cent below that for normal/expected age and height: in children this is weight below the second percentile;
- weight loss is self-induced;
- self-perception of being too fat;
- absence of three consecutive menstrual cycles when otherwise expected;
- denial of the seriousness of low body weight.

Table 16.6 Criteria for diagnosis of bulimia nervosa

Current classification and definition (the main points of ICD10 (WHO 1992) and DSM-IV (APA 1994) combined)

- A persistent compulsion to overeat accompanied by a sense of lack of control. The overeating consists of more than 1000 calories – more than others would eat during a similar 2-hour period.
- These bouts of overeating occur at least twice a week over a 3-month period.
- A variety of strategies are used to compensate for weight gain, e.g. self-induced vomiting, laxatives, diuretics, fasting, drugs to stimulate metabolism, appetite suppressants, and over-exercise.
- Over-concern about weight and shape.
- Self-perception of being too fat.

Binge-eating disorder

In this condition there is recurrent and persistent episodes of binge eating at least 2 days a week for 6 months, marked distress, and absence of regulatory controls. Also self-worth is defined through shape and weight.

Another eating disorder, night-eating syndrome first described by Albert Stunkard in 1954 has been recently described to occur in obesity. In this condition at least 50 per cent of daily calories are consumed after evening meal (Stunkard 2000).

The primary-care hurdle

Epidemiological research from different European countries highlights how eating disorders are under-diagnosed in primary care (Whitehouse *et al.* 1992; Hoek 1993). A number of different reasons seem to present potent barriers to early diagnosis and intervention. These include:

- patient delay in presenting their eating problems;
- doctor delay in diagnosing eating disorders at an early stage;
- communication difficulties between doctors and eating-disorder patients;
- attitudinal biases of general practitioners towards these patients;
- gender differences between general practitioners and eating-disorder patients; and
- inadequate interventions by general practitioners including referrals to other specialists.

It is important that all of these barriers are overcome in order to facilitate secondary prevention by early intervention.

Engagement in primary care: general practitioner/school nurse

Anorexia nervosa

Arguably this is one of the most difficult phases to bridge in the management of anorexia nervosa. The first hurdle usually is for carers, friends, teachers and colleagues to express their concerns for the individual's health and to suggest that it is important to seek help. The interpersonal process of the meeting is a critical factor, which can have a profound impact on the process of diagnosis and management. Diagnosis should not be too difficult a process especially if a corroborative history is taken from informants. The differential diagnosis includes rarer conditions such as brain tumours in children, and thyroid disease and inflammatory bowel disease. Thus simple investigations such as the erythrocyte sedimentation rate and thyroid function test and a physical examination are sufficient.

However, delivering the diagnosis to the individual and negotiating a plan of management is a delicate procedure. The therapeutic alliance is critical. First the individual needs to engage in the process of change. It is usual in the first medical encounter for the patient to have recognized a health problem and to come to the health professional for help. This rarely occurs in anorexia nervosa. Instead in the classical case there is a rejection of the sick role and denial of disease. Lasegue illustrated this by one of his patient's remarks 'I do not suffer therefore I am well' (Lasegue [1873] 1964). Thus if we use the concepts of the transtheoretical model of change we find that people with anorexia nervosa coming to a health professional are usually in the precontemplation or contemplation stage of readiness to change (Blake 1997). That is they do not want to change (precontemplation) or they are in two minds about the need to change (contemplation). Figure 16.1 illustrates the various stages of change that are common in anorexia nervosa and also indicates what type of therapeutic approach might be helpful. The exchange of information, the assessment of risk and the development of a management plan need to be mapped onto this template. People with anorexia nervosa present to a health professional to appease close others who are all too aware of the signs of overt signs of illness. It is the carers who are concerned. These divergent views between the person with anorexia nervosa and those of her family and professional helpers have to be negotiated in order to attain a satisfactory outcome of treatment rather than a protracted tug of war.

The interpersonal process within the first encounter needs to take this ambivalence or indeed resistance into account. The skills of motivational interviewing are invaluable for such an exchange (Miller and Rollnick 1991). The theoretical concepts included in models of health behaviour can inform the exchange. Two elements are common to most of these models. The first is the importance of change to the individual and the second is confidence that change is possible. The importance of change relates to the decisional balance of the pros and cons about change. People with anorexia nervosa usually have some form of positive reinforcement (extrinsic or intrinsic) or avoid aversive situations by maintaining their illness. They also have little confidence in their ability to find other solutions to their problems, other

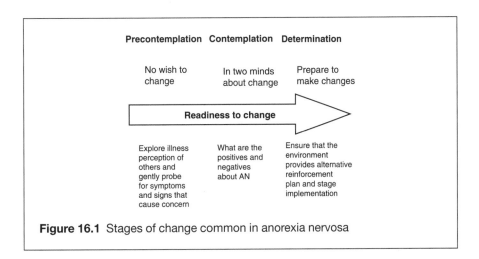

Figure 16.1 Stages of change common in anorexia nervosa

than restricting their life. It is useful to acknowledge and elicit these maintaining factors in the first phase of information exchange. The meta beliefs about anorexia nervosa include the reinforcing features described above. However, starvation itself results in secondary consequences that can maintain the illness. Thus, starvation itself can lead to a loss of hunger and a drive for overactivity as exemplified by animal models. The negative mood state can start a vicious circle in which not eating is seen as a solution to this stress. The switch of thought content from problems to food can be reinforcing for those who use avoidance strategies as a coping reaction to stress. In some cases the social consequences can merely exaggerate the type of stress that triggered the onset of the illness.

Bulimia nervosa

In bulimia nervosa there may also be ambivalence about getting help but the source of these mixed feelings differs. It is less usual for the person with bulimia nervosa to be encouraged to seek help by others. This is because the symptoms can be less overt and the most common time of onset is after leaving home. The individual herself is aware that her behaviour is atypical but is ashamed to talk about it and fears humiliation. People with bulimia nervosa are usually eager to stop the binge eating but they may be reluctant to give up the weight-control strategies. This is because such strategies may be the first effective solution in a lifetime's battle with body dissatisfaction.

Treatment in primary care and pathways of care

In the *NSF for Mental Health* there is the suggestion that some eating disorders might be treated in primary care. However, there is very little evidence to support the efficacy of interventions in primary care. Indeed, such interventions may serve to maintain the disorder. A Dutch survey of 108 patients with eating disorders showed that 38 per cent of the patients received medication from their general practitioners. This was usually to palliate symptoms, e.g. vitamins, laxatives, hormones (to induce menses) and drugs to stimulate or suppress the appetite (Noordenbos 1992). In the UK, 45 per cent of people with bulimia nervosa were prescribed an anti-depressant by their general practitioner (Turnbull *et al.* 1996). It is unusual for people within primary care to have the expertise or resources to provide evidence-based psychotherapeutic approaches such as CBT. In the UK, 80 per cent of cases of anorexia nervosa and 60 per cent of cases of bulimia nervosa are referred on for specialized help (Turnbull *et al.* 1996).

It is possible that standards of care for the primary care of eating disorders will improve. For example, following the publication of the *NSF for Mental Health* many health authorities have produced care pathways for eating disorders (Figure 16.2 shows such as pathway developed in Croydon with our team). Also new technology such as cognitive behaviour therapy (CBT) administered by CD-ROM holds promise as an intervention that

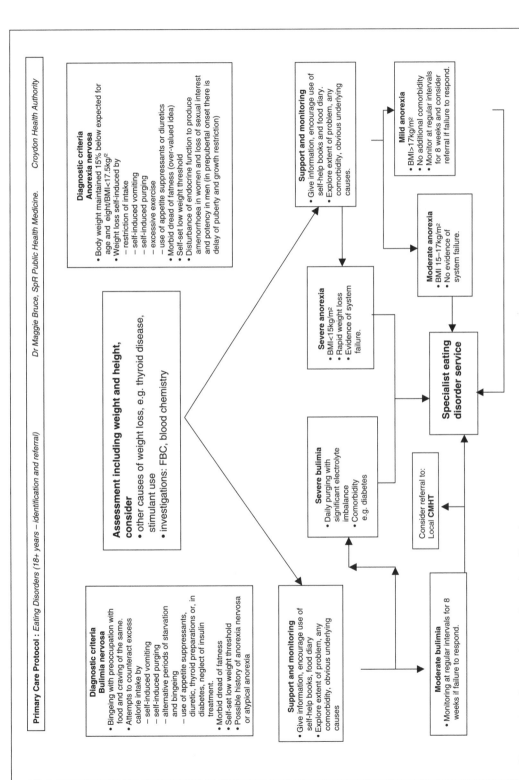

Primary Care Protocol : *Eating Disorders (18+ years – identification and referral)*   *Dr Maggie Bruce, SpR Public Health Medicine.*   *Croydon Health Authority*

**Diagnostic criteria
Anorexia nervosa**
- Body weight maintained 15% below expected for age and eight/BMI<17.5kg/²
- Weight loss self-induced by
  – restriction of intake
  – self-induced vomiting
  – self-induced purging
  – excessive exercise
  – use of appetite suppressants or diuretics
- Morbid dread of fatness (over-valued idea)
- Self-set low weight threshold
- Disturbance of endocrine function to produce amenorrhoea in women and loss of sexual interest and potency in men (in prepubertal onset there is delay of puberty and growth restriction)

**Diagnostic criteria
Bulimia nervosa**
- Bingeing with preoccupation with food and craving of the same.
- Attempts to counteract excess calorie intake by
  – self-induced vomiting
  – self-induced purging
  – alternative periods of starvation and bingeing
  – use of appetite suppressants, diuretic, thyroid preparations or, in diabetes, neglect of insulin treatment.
- Morbid dread of fatness
- Self-set low weight threshold
- Possible history of anorexia nervosa or atypical anorexia

Assessment including weight and height, consider
- other causes of weight loss, e.g. thyroid disease, stimulant use
- investigations: FBC, blood chemistry

Support and monitoring
- Give information, encourage use of self-help books and food diary.
- Explore extent of problem, any comorbidity, obvious underlying causes.

Support and monitoring
- Give information, encourage use of self-help books, food diary
- Explore extent of problem, any comorbidity, obvious underlying causes

Severe anorexia
- BMI<15kg/m²
- Rapid weight loss
- Evidence of system failure.

Severe bulimia
- Daily purging with significant electrolyte imbalance
- Comorbidity e.g. diabetes

Moderate anorexia
- BMI 15–17kg/m²
- No evidence of system failure.

Mild anorexia
- BMI>17kg/m²
- No additional comorbidity
- Monitor at regular intervals for 8 weeks and consider referral if failure to respond.

Specialist eating disorder service

Consider referral to: Local **CMHT**

Moderate bulimia
- Monitoring at regular intervals for 8 weeks if failure to respond.

Figure 16.2 Care pathways for eating disorders

could be delivered in schools, colleges or in primary care settings (Murray *et al.* 2003).

Standards 4 and 5: Effective services for people with severe mental illness: evidence-based eating disorders treatment

It is hoped that the interest in evidence-based medicine and guidelines for medical care will facilitate the development of services that are of high quality, acceptable and effective. Tables 16.7 and 16.8 summarize findings of treatment efficacy for eating disorders. The National Institute for Clinical Excellence (NCMH 2004) guidelines should be available by the time this chapter is published but meanwhile there are the American guidelines (American Psychiatric Association 2000).

Matching treatment to need and acceptability

In spite of what we know about the effectiveness of treatments for eating disorders overall, there remain many questions of what is cost effective and/or acceptable for individual patients. The broad clinical presentation of anorexia nervosa over age and severity, and the paucity of evidence, means that there is great uncertainty whether any of the findings can be generalized. There needs to be a careful evaluation of the risks and resources and hence prognosis for individual patients. Matching the intensity and type of treatment to need involves a careful risk assessment of medical, clinical and psychosocial factors. There is a need to balance the severity of the weight loss against the resources that the patient has to implement renutrition and to judge whether starvation requires acute management. Inpatient treatment was regarded as standard, as reflected in the American Psychiatric Association guidelines (APA 2000). Indeed it is highly effective in correcting malnutrition in the short term although the long-term outcome is less certain. A wider range of management strategies may be more cost effective and acceptable. For example, the management plan may include day and outpatient care with complex mixes of types of therapy, and number of hours, over a variety of durations and with an individual and various members of the patient's family. If there is less of a need for urgent attention to nutrition then it is possible to consider various forms of outpatient psychotherapy.

Risk assessment

Decisions on short-term risk involve a combined assessment of the medical risk and the person's psychological capacity to consent to treatment, taking into account the possible resources of motivation and psychosocial support. Features in the history that indicate a high medical risk are shown in Table 16.9. The clinical examination should include body mass index

Table 16.7 Summary of evidence on treatment efficacy for anorexia nervosa

Setting of service

Limited evidence from one small RCT found that outpatient treatment was as effective as inpatient treatment in increasing weight and improving Morgan Russell scale global scores at one, two and five years in those individuals who do not warrant emergency intervention (Crisp *et al.* 1991; Gowers *et al.* 1994).

Types of psychotherapy

- One small RCT found limited evidence that focal analytical therapy or family therapy versus treatment as usual significantly increased the number of people recovered or improved as assessed by the Morgan Russell scale at one year (Dare *et al.* 2001).
- One small RCT found no significant difference in outcomes between psychotherapy and dietary counselling at one year (Hall and Crisp 1987). A second RCT comparing cognitive therapy versus dietary counselling found a 100 per cent failure to take-up/withdrawal rate with dietary counselling (Serfaty 1999).
- Six small RCTs found no significant difference between different psychotherapies (Russell *et al.* 1987; Treasure *et al.* 1995; Eisler *et al.* 1997, 2000; Robin *et al.* 1999; Wallin *et al.* 2000). However, all the RCTs were small and were unlikely to have been powered to detect a clinically important difference between treatments.

Pharmacotherapy

Drug	Method (n>30)	Effect	Comments	Authors
Cisapride	1 RCT	0	Withdrawn Care re QT interval	
Cyproheptadine	3 RCT	0		(Vigersky and Loriaux 1977; Goldberg *et al.* 1979; Peterson *et al.* 1986)
Oestrogen	1 RCT, 1 other	0		(Klibanski *et al.* 1995)
Neuroleptics	0		Care re QT interval	
SSRI	2 RCT	0-acute +-Relapse prevention		(Attia *et al.* 1998; Kaye *et al.* 2001)
Tricyclic	2 RCT	0	Care re QT interval	(Biederman *et al.* 1985; Peterson *et al.* 1986)
Zinc	1 RCT	0		(Birmingham *et al.* 1994)

(BMI), muscle strength and blood pressure, pulse rate, temperature and circulation. An examination of the skin and temperature is important for those at high risk.

Opinions on how risk should be managed vary between countries, centres and clinicians. The APA guidelines recommend admitting to hospital when body mass index < 16 kg/m^2 or weight loss > 20 per cent) (DSM-IV practice guidelines, APA 2000). In the UK, outpatient, psychotherapeutic

Table 16.8 Summary of evidence on treatment efficacy for bulimia nervosa

Psychotherapy

- Systematic reviews have found that CBT versus remaining on waiting list reduces specific eating disorder symptoms and non-specific symptoms, for example, depression (Hay and Bacaltchuk 2000).
- One systematic review (Hay and Bacaltchuk 2000) and one subsequent RCT (Agras *et al.* 2000) have found that other psychotherapy (non CBT) versus waiting list improved symptoms.
- CBT more effective than IPT at 20 weeks but this difference not present at 4 months (Hay and Bacaltchuk 2000).

Anti-depressants

- Systematic reviews have found that anti-depressants reduce bulimic symptoms in the short term but there is less certainty about their role in maintenance (Bacaltchuk *et al.* 2000a).
- There is not enough evidence to compare the different classes of anti-depressants (Bacaltchuk and Hay 2001).
- One systematic review comparing anti-depressants and psychotherapy found no significant difference in bulimic symptoms (Bacaltchuk *et al.* 2001).
- Combinations of anti-depressants and psychotherapy. One systematic review has found that combination treatment versus anti-depressants reduces binge frequency and depressive symptoms but not binge-eating remission rate. Combination therapy versus psychotherapy also showed the same pattern of differential response (Bacaltchuk *et al.* 2000b).

Table 16.9 Features in history that indicate medical risk

- excess exercise with low weight;
- blood in vomit;
- inadequate fluid intake in combination with poor eating;
- rapid weight loss;
- factors which disrupt ritualized eating habits (journey/holiday/exam).

approaches are used for people whose body mass index may be as low as 13 kg/m^2 (Palmer and Treasure 1999). In such cases, there needs to be careful medical risk management and close cooperation between professional and lay carers. The patient's level of motivation and their psychosocial resources can act as a buffer against the medical risks. Measuring the early response to treatment, such as a change in weight, or the arrest of weight loss and the ability to show active involvement in treatment is a good proxy measure of motivation and capacity to respond to outpatient psychotherapy.

Once the decision is made that high intensity treatment (day or inpatient care) is needed, the next question is: What are the goals of this high intensity care? Traditionally the goal was weight restoration to a body mass index within the normal range (with less attention paid to goals for the other aspects of the psychopathology). This often leaves a gap between physical and psychological recovery that can be difficult to bridge (Fennig *et al.* 2002). An alternative position is that admission should be long enough to ameliorate the medical risk, short of restoring weight to normal. This lessens the gap between physical and psychological recovery. In many countries this decision is made pragmatically depending on how services are organized such as whether there is a model of shared care between community resources including carers and specialist services. Evidence from a large naturalistic study suggests that short admissions are more effective for those with a short duration of illness, i.e. adolescents, whereas long admission have a better chance of success in those with a longer duration of illness, i.e. adults (Kachele for the study group MZ-ESS 1999). Unnecessary hospitalization, has obvious disadvantages in terms of health care costs, schooling/career and disruption of social experiences, in addition to which there is some weak evidence that it may have a negative impact on the long-term outcome of the illness (Gowers *et al.* 2000). Thus, the stage at which psychotherapy is started may need to vary depending on the clinical and demographic details of the patient. In young people, outpatient management should start after a shorter time and possibly at a lower weight than for cases with a long duration.

Bulimia nervosa

Matching patients to treatments

In contrast to anorexia nervosa, there is no evidence to support the need to match patients to treatment in bulimia nervosa. Although a number of pre-treatment prognostic indicators have been identified (Keel and Mitchell 1997; Vaz 1998), few of them have been replicated across studies and across different treatments. Hay and Bacaltchuk's (2000) systematic review found no evidence of heterogeneity between studies, which might support treatment-matching. Severity and duration of bulimic symptoms have had an inconsistent link to outcome. There seems to be somewhat more agreement that personality disorder features such as borderline or impulsive features predict a poorer outcome. However, the main conclusion to be drawn with confidence from the literature on pre-treatment outcome predictor variables is that none of the ones identified have any major utility in helping us choose which treatment is most helpful for a particular patient.

Issues of risk management are also less of a priority in the choice of treatment for bulimia nervosa. The need for admission or even daycare is relatively rare and the great majority of patients can be managed safely as outpatients. There are, however, some particular circumstances in which risk issues need to be identified at assessment and taken into account in planning the patients' care, both in the short and longer term. These concern patients with self-harm and suicidality and other high-risk behaviours, those who are pregnant or have small children and those with medical comorbidity such as diabetes mellitus.

Standard 6: Carers

Carers of people with anorexia have high levels of unmet needs. These are illustrated in Table 16.10. The experience of caring is very difficult. Many carers have high levels of distress, which in many cases reaches clearly significant levels. It is perhaps not unexpected that mothers have a higher emotional reaction than fathers who tend to use more cognitive coping strategies. However, our work has illustrated that other carers (siblings and partners) also have high levels of emotional arousal, which may warrant treatment in its own right either by psychotherapy or medication. Many facets of care are problematic. As eating disorders typically develop during adolescence it is usual for the sufferer to be living at home with the family. This can have a profound impact on family life. The domains illustrated in Table 16.10 are particularly relevant.

Services have probably not addressed the needs of carers enough. Carers often perceive themselves to be blamed when they are required to participate in family therapy in child and adolescent services. Alternatively, they may feel marginalized in adult services. There are many ways to deliver these interventions which can fulfil carers' needs and which may also improve the outcome of people with anorexia nervosa. The traditional approach is to use psycho education, books and workbooks for the family (Treasure 1997) and incorporate them into family meetings or in groups for carers. A more recent method has been to use multi-family group interventions (Dare and Eisler 2000; Scholtz and Asen 2001; Colahan and Robinson 2002). In a pilot study we found that such an approach (summarized in Table 16.11) in severe, chronic anorexia nervosa leads to a reduction in levels of carers' distress, levels of expressed emotion fall and the perception of burden diminishes. There is also evidence that this approach can improve the outcome in people with anorexia nervosa.

In addition, some services are adapting to include community outreach workers who can conduct emergency assessments and initiate home-feeding where appropriate and provide primary care, school and carer liaison. It is to be hoped that newer technologies such as web-based information resources (see, for example, www.eatingresearch.com) may address carers' needs for information.

Standard 7: Suicide

Unlike most other psychiatric illness the mortality linked to eating disorders is not predominately associated with suicide but with malnutrition and methods of weight control. Both crude and standardized mortality rates reported from a meta analysis of studies of outcome are shown in Table 16.12. Thus people with anorexia nervosa have an almost ten-fold risk

Table 16.10 Needs of carers of people with anorexia nervosa

Dimension of difficulty	Carers needs/difficulties	Methodology
Not enough information	Need for pragmatic details such as information about what treatment is available, information about the prognosis and plans for future treatment. Help with management and coping strategies. Need to meet other carers and share experiences	Carers' Needs Assessment Measure (CaNAM) (Haigh and Treasure 2002)
Not enough support from professionals	Practical and emotional help in dealing with the eating disorder, both in the present and in terms of the prognosis and plans for the future. Practical support, such as help with meal times and skills to manage difficult behaviours	
Negative symptoms	Difficult to deal with withdrawal, not talking	Experience Care Inventory (Treasure *et al.* 2001)
Difficult behaviour	Irritability, food, vomit, stealing	
Dependency	At home, unable to work, no social life	
Loss	Sadness at poor quality of life	
Stigma	Illness so overt. Others unable to understand	
Need to back up	Financial and social dependence	
Difficulties with service	See above	
Emotional representation	Carers experience a great variety of emotions in response to their relative's suffering. These emotions vary from overwhelming sadness and distress to fear, anger and even hostility. Many carers also feel self-blaming emotions such as guilt, failure and inadequacy	Qualitative Analysis Letter 'What it is like to be mother/father/sister of an eating disorder individual?' (Whitney *et al.* 2004)
Cognitive reaction	Carers primarily try to block out bad experiences and be hopeful and optimistic and distract or detach themselves. Carers reconstruct the illness as something separate from their daughter	
Consequences	Carers generally perceive negative effects of the illness on the sufferer's personality and behaviours. As a consequence of the illness, carers perceive the sufferer to be more dependent, demanding, impulsive and selfish. Carers also perceive many physical and mental consequences and the ultimate threat of death from the sufferer's deterioration. Finally, carers express the opportunities that have been lost on account of the illness	
Effect on the family	Carers perceive the illness to contribute to many family problems such as friction in relationships, greater arguments between family members and a stressful atmosphere in the household. The illness also impinges on the family's social life and makes it difficult to makes plans for the future. Carers perceive the illness to have great effects on the carers' and family members' mental and physical functioning, making them feel worn out and negative about themselves	

Table 16.11 Giving carers skills to become more effective helpers (Treasure *et al.* 2002)

- Teaching positive communication skills (good listening, skilful summarizing).
- Helping carers to understand the sufferers perspective on their readiness, willingness and ability to change.
- Exploring the positives of anorexia nervosa and finding solutions for how they can be replaced.
- Understanding models of behaviour change, i.e. reinforcing positive behaviours.
- Giving carers skills for meal supervision.

Table 16.12 Mortality in eating disorders

	Years follow-up	Crude mortality rate (CMR)	Standardized mortality rate (SMR)	Standardized suicide rate
Anorexia nervosa	6–12		9.6 (95% CI 7.8–11.5) (Nielsen 2001)	58 (Herzog *et al.* 2000)
	12–40	5.9% (178 deaths in 3006 patients) (Sullivan 1995)	3.7 (95% CI 2.8–4.7) (Nielsen 2001)	
Bulimia nervosa	5–11	0.4% (11 deaths in 2692 patients) (Keel and Mitchell 1997)	7.4 (95% CI 2.9–14.9) (Nielsen 2001)	
			1.56 (95% CI 0.8 to 2.7) (Nielsen 2001)	
EDNOS			SMR was 2.8 (95% CI 0.8–7.3)	

of dying compared to healthy people the same age and sex. In the studies specifying cause of death, 54 per cent of the subjects died as a result of eating-disorder complications, 27 per cent committed suicide and the remaining 19 per cent died of unknown or other causes.

Reducing suicide rates

In order to decrease the mortality attributed to suicide and to other causes it will be necessary to improve the outcome of current interventions. There has been a recent meta analysis of the factors associated with a poor prognosis in anorexia nervosa and these are shown in Table 16.13. Many of the same factors are linked to high levels of mortality (Zipfel *et al.* 2000).

Many of these features are possibly not modifiable. However, it is possible that prevention work may be able to intervene for those at high risk, for example, those with obsessive-compulsive features and difficulties in childhood, or prevent the development of maladaptive weight control strategies such as vomiting. There are some factors, however, that may be a suitable target for intervention. Thus the fact that an illness of long duration and severe weight loss are associated with a poor prognosis suggests that there should be a focus on early effective interventions. Also it is important that any services have skills in effective weight restoration.

Table 16.13 Factors associated with poor prognosis in anorexia nervosa

The chance of relapse or a poorer outcome is based on the following factors, which include:

- − Age of onset (younger do better)
- + Duration of illness
- + Severity of weight loss
- + Hyperactivity, vomiting
- + Bulimia and purging
- + Obsessive-compulsive symptoms
- − Hysterical personality
- + Difficulty with weight gain in the ward environment/short duration inpatient treatment
- − Ability to get weight into the normal range
- + Pretoria developmental or clinical abnormalities
- − Good parent–child relationship
- + High socio-economic status

After Steinhausen 2002

There is less information about the factors associated with poor prognosis and increased mortality in bulimia nervosa.

Conclusion

In summary, what has emerged from this review of eating disorders in the context of the *NSF for Mental Health* is how many gaps and uncertainties there are. Thus:

- There is no prevention strategy in place.

- There are deficiencies in recognition, diagnosis and management within primary care.

- There is an impressive portfolio of research into treatment of bulimia nervosa but very little research into the management of anorexia nervosa.

- From the carers' perspective there are many deficiencies with current services. Carers of people with eating disorders are far more dissatisfied with professional help than are the carers of people with a psychotic illness (Treasure *et al.* 2001). Bloch *et al.* (1995) argue that it is a fundamental right of all carers for professionals to give them an account of the illness and guidance about how to deal with the patient's problems in so far as they impinge on the carer's life. Carers do not think that they are given enough information and practical advice.

- Users have not been included in treatment planning and service development. There have been many books written by users describing their experiences of treatment but this has not been fed back directly into service planning. However, there is user input into the NICE guideline group.

- Finally, the mortality rate from anorexia nervosa is the highest of any psychiatric illness.

By following the structure outlined in the *NSF for Mental Health* there could be improvements in care and service.

Questions for reflection and discussion

1 Reflect on your lifetime relationship with food. Consider how much time is spent meeting this basic human need. How does your relationship with food influence your approach to working with this client group and the difficulties that they face?

2 Consider how your emotions affect your therapeutic practice, your professional and personal relationships. Imagine how complex this becomes for someone whose core beliefs and emotional states are constantly linked to food.

3 What are the key ingredients of research that have enhanced your body of knowledge in this field? Can you think of useful research topics to develop and inform treatment for eating disorders?

Annotated bibliography

- Treasure J., Schmidt, U. and Van Furth, E. (eds) (2003) *Handbook of Eating Disorders*. Chichester: John Wiley & Sons Ltd. Comprehensive reviews of anorexia nervosa and bulimia nervosa, models and hypotheses are examined critically by internationally known experts, all of whom have been influenced by the work of Professor G.F.M. Russell. The book provides detailed coverage of historical development of ideas about eating disorders, aetiological models, consequences and maintaining factors, review of treatment options, prevention and research.
- Hoek, H.W., Treasure, J.L. and Katzman, A. (eds) (1998) *Neurobiology in the Treatment of Eating Disorders*. Chichester: John Wiley & Sons Ltd. This book incorporates recent advances in biological sciences with concepts of the aetiology and treatment of eating disorders. Part 1 offers an overview of epidemiology, aetiology, biological, psychological and social models. Part 2 focuses on advances in neurobiolology research. Part 3 describes evidence-based treatment in anorexia nervosa, bulimia nervosa and binge-eating disorder. Useful summary charts are included at the end of the book.
- Schmidt, U. and Treasure, J. (1993) *Getting Better Bit(e) by Bit(e). A Survival Kit for Sufferers of Bulimia Nervosa and Binge Eating Disorders*.

Hove: Lawrence Erlbaum Associates Ltd. A self-help book providing information and advice. Useful for relatives, friends and professionals to gain an understanding of problems faced on a daily basis and the key changes necessary for recovery.

- Treasure, J. (1997) *Anorexia Nervosa: A Survival Guide for Sufferers and those Caring for Someone with an Eating Disorder*. Hove: Psychology Press. This text includes sections for parents and other carers, sufferers and professionals. It provides a useful introduction for those thrown into the mixture of emotions; one of the strongest is fear, caused by the onset of this illness and the questions raised at this time. Carers' contributions to the development of this book have continued to inform our practice and develop the collaborative approach between all those who care for sufferers, that is desperately needed to overcome the power of anorexia.
- Miller, W.R. and Rollnick, S. (2002) *Motivational Interviewing: Preparing People for Change*. New York: Guilford Press. Motivational interviewing is an effective evidence-based approach to working with ambivalence that keeps many people from making desired changes in their lives. We have found that adopting this style has helped us to work with and understand our clients' perspective when suffering from an eating disorder. We actively promote this approach in our training for professionals and carers. This book provides a comprehensive review of the model and its supporting research, along with practical strategies for increasing motivation and confidence.

References

Agras, W.S., Walsh, T., Fairburn, C.G., Wilson, G.T. and Kraemer, H.C. (2000) A multicenter comparison of cognitive-behavioral therapy and interpersonal psychotherapy for bulimia nervosa, *Archives of General Psychiatry* **57**: 459–66.

American Psychiatric Association (1994) *Diagnostic and Statistical Manual of Mental Disorders DSM-IV* (4th ed.) Washington, DC: APA.

American Psychiatric Association (2000) Practice guideline for the treatment of patients with eating disorders (revision), American Psychiatric Association Work Group on Eating Disorders, *American Journal of Psychiatry* **157**: 1–39.

Attia, E., Haiman, C., Walsh, B.T. and Flater, S.R. (1998) Does fluoxetine augment the inpatient treatment of anorexia nervosa? *American Journal of Psychiatry* **155**: 548–51.

Bacaltchuk, J. and Hay, P. (2001) Antidepressants versus placebo for people with bulimia nervosa, *The Cochrane Database of Systematic Reviews*, CD003391.

Bacaltchuk, J., Hay, P. and Mari, J.J. (2000a) Antidepressants versus placebo for the treatment of bulimia nervosa: a systematic review, *The Australian and New Zealand Journal of Psychiatry* **34**: 310–17.

Bacaltchuk, J., Trefiglio, R.P., Oliveira, I.R. *et al.* (2000b) Combination of antidepressants and psychological treatments for bulimia nervosa: a systematic review, *Acta Psychiatrica Scandinavica* **101**: 256–64.

Bacaltchuk, J., Hay, P. and Trefiglio, R. (2001) Antidepressants versus psychological treatments and their combination for bulimia nervosa, *The Cochrane Database of Systematic Reviews*, CD003385.

Biederman, J., Herzog, D.B., Rivinus, T.M. *et al.* (1985) Amitriptyline in the treatment of anorexia nervosa: a double-blind, placebo-controlled study, *Journal of Clinical Psychopharmacology* **5**: 10–16.

Birmingham, C.L., Goldner, E.M. and Bakan, R. (1994) Controlled trial of zinc supplementation in anorexia nervosa, *International Journal of Eating Disorders*, **15**: 251–5.

Blake, W., Turnbull, S. and Treasure, J. (1997) Stages and processes of change in eating disorders. Implications for therapy, *Clinical Psychology and Psychotherapy* **4**: 186–91.

Bloch, S., Szmukler, G.I., Herrman, H., Benson, A. and Colussa, S. (1995) Counseling caregivers of relatives with schizophrenia: themes, interventions, and caveats, *Family Process* **34**: 413–25.

Bulik, C.M., Sullivan, P.F., Wade, T.D. and Kendler, K.S. (2000) Twin studies of eating disorders: a review, *International Journal of Eating Disorders* **27**: 1–20.

Bushnell, J.A., Wells, J.E., Hornblow, A.R., Oakly-Browne, M.A. and Joyce, P. (1990) Prevalence of three bulimia syndromes in the general population, *Psychological Medicine* **20**: 671–80.

Cnattingius, S., Hultman, C.M., Dahl, M. and Sparen, P. (1999) Very preterm birth, birth trauma, and the risk of anorexia nervosa among girls. *Archives of General Psychiatry* **56**: 634–8.

Colahan, M. and Robinson, P. (2002) Multifamily groups in the treatment of young eating disorder adults, *Journal of Family Therapy* **24**: 17–30.

Crisp, A.H., Norton, K., Gowers, S. *et al.* (1991) A controlled study of the effect of therapies aimed at adolescent and family psychopathology in anorexia nervosa, *British Journal of Psychiatry* **159**: 325–33.

Dare, C. and Eisler, I. (2000) A multi-family group day treatment for adolescent eating disorder, *European Eating Disorders Review* **8**: 4–18.

Dare, C., Eisler, I., Russell, G., Treasure, J. and Dodge, L. (2001) Psychological therapies for adults with anorexia nervosa: randomized controlled trial of out-patient treatments, *British Journal of Psychiatry* **178**: 216–21.

Department of Health (1999) *National Service Framework for Mental Health: Modern Standards and Service Models*. London: Department of Health.

Eagles, J.M., Andrew, J.E., Johnston, M.I., Easton, E.A. and Millar, H.R. (2001) Season of birth in females with anorexia nervosa in Northeast Scotland, *International Journal of Eating Disorders* **30**: 167–75.

Eisler, I., Dare, C., Russell, G.F. *et al.* (1997) Family and individual therapy in anorexia nervosa. A 5-year follow-up, *Archives of General Psychiatry* **54**: 1025–30.

Eisler, I., Dare, C., Hodes, M. *et al.* (2000) Family therapy for adolescent anorexia nervosa: the results of a controlled comparison of two family interventions [In Process Citation], *Journal of Child Psychology and Psychiatry, and allied disciplines* **41**: 727–36.

Fairburn, C.G., Welch, S.L., Doll, H.A., Davies, B.A. and O'Connor, M.E. (1997) Risk factors for bulimia nervosa. A community-based case-control study, *Archives of General Psychiatry* **54**: 509–17.

Fairburn, C.G., Doll, H.A., Welch, S.L. *et al.* (1998) Risk factors for binge eating disorder: a community-based, case-control study [see comments], *Archives of General Psychiatry* **55**: 425–32.

Fennig, S., Fennig, S. and Roe, D. (2002) Physical recovery in anorexia nervosa:

is this the sole purpose of a child and adolescent medical-psychiatric unit? *General Hospital Psychiatry* **24**: 87–92.

Foley, D.L., Thacker, L.R., Aggen, S.H., Neale, M.C. and Kendler, K.S. (2001) Pregnancy and perinatal complications associated with risks for common psychiatric disorders in a population-based sample of female twins, *American Journal of Medical Genetics* **105**: 426–31.

Fosson, A., Knibbs, J., Bryant-Waugh, R. and Lask, B. (1987) Early onset anorexia nervosa, *Archives of Disease in Childhood* **62**: 114–18.

Gard, M.C.E. and Freeman, C.P. (1996) The dismantling of a myth: A review of eating disorders and socio-economic status. *International Journal of Eating Disorders* **20**: 1–12.

Goldberg, S.C., Halmi, K.A., Eckert, E.D., Casper, R.C. and Davis, J.M. (1979) Cyproheptadine in anorexia nervosa. *British Journal of Psychiatry* **134**: 67–70.

Gowers, S., Norton, K., Halek, C. and Crisp, A.H. (1994) Outcome of outpatient psychotherapy in a random allocation treatment study of anorexia nervosa, *International Journal of Eating Disorders* **15**: 165–77.

Gowers, S.G., Weetman, J., Shore, A., Hossain, F. and Elvins, R. (2000) Impact of hospitalisation on the outcome of adolescent anorexia nervosa, *British Journal of Psychiatry* **176**: 138–41.

Haigh, R. and Treasure, J.L. (2002) Investigating the needs of carers in the area of eating disorders: Development of the Carers' Needs Assessment Measure (CaNAM). *European Eating Disorder Review* **11**(2): 125–41.

Hall, A. and Crisp, A.H. (1987) Brief psychotherapy in the treatment of anorexia nervosa, Outcome at one year, *British Journal of Psychiatry* **151**: 185–91.

Hay, P.J. and Bacaltchuk, J. (2000) Psychotherapy for bulimia nervosa and binging, *The Cochrane Database of Systematic Reviews* 4, CD000562.

Hebebrand, J. and Remschmidt, H. (1995) Anorexia nervosa viewed as an extreme weight condition: genetic implications, *Human Genetics* **95**: 1–11.

Herzog, D.B., Greenwood, D.N., Dorer, D.J., *et al.* (2000) Mortality in eating disorders: a descriptive study, *International Journal of Eating Disorders* **28**: 20–6.

Hoek, H.W. (1993) Review of the epidemiological studies of eating disorders, *International Review of Psychiatry* **5**: 61–74.

Hoek, H.W., Bartelds, A.I.M., Bosveld, J.J.F. *et al.* (1995) Impact of urbanization on detection rates of eating disorders, *American Journal of Psychiatry* **152**: 1272–8.

Johnson, J.G., Cohen, P., Kasen, S. and Brook, J.S. (2002) Childhood adversities associated with risk for eating disorders or weight problems during adolescence or early adulthood, *American Journal of Psychiatry* **159**: 394–400.

Kachele, H. for the study group MZ-ESS (1999) Eine multizentrische Studie zu Aufwand und Erfolg bei psychodynamischer Therapie von Eßstörungen, *Psychotherapie, Psychosomatik, medizinische Psychologie* **49**: 100–8.

Kaye, W.H., Nagata, T., Weltzin, T.E. *et al.* (2001) Double-blind placebo-controlled administration of fluoxetine in restricting- and restricting-purging-type anorexia nervosa, *Biological Psychiatry* **49**: 644–52.

Keel, P.K. and Mitchell, J.E. (1997) Outcome in bulimia nervosa, *American Journal of Psychiatry* **154**: 313–21.

Kendler, K.S., MacLean, C., Neale, M. *et al.* (1991) The genetic epidemiology of bulimia nervosa, *American Journal of Psychiatry* **148**: 1627–37.

Klibanski, A., Biller, B.M., Schoenfeld, D.A., Herzog, D.B. and Saxe, V.C. (1995) The effects of estrogen administration on trabecular bone loss in young women with anorexia nervosa, *The Journal of Clinical Endocrinology and Metabolism* **80**: 898–904.

Lasegue, C. (1873) De l'anorexie hysterique, English translation, M.R. Kaufman and M. Heiman (1964) *Evolution of Psychosomatic Concepts*. New York: International Universities Press.

Leventhal, H., Nerentz, D.R. and Steel, D.J. (1984) Illness representations and coping with health threats, in A. Baum (ed.) *Handbook of Psychology and Health*, Vol 4. Hillsdale, NJ: Erlbaum.

Lucas, A.R., Crowson, C.S., O'Fallon, W.M. and Melton, L.J. (1999) The ups and downs of anorexia nervosa, *International Journal of Eating Disorders* **26**: 397–405.

McClelland, L. and Crisp, A. (2001) Anorexia nervosa and social class, *International Journal of Eating Disorders* **29**: 150–6.

Miller, W. and Rollnick, S. (1991) *Motivational Interviewing: Preparing People to Change Addictive Behaviour*. New York: Guilford.

Murray, K., Pombo-Caril, M.G., Bara-Carill, N. *et al.* (2003) Factors determining uptake of a CD-ROM-based CBT self-help treatment for bulimia: Patient characteristics and subjective appraisals of self-help treatment, *European Eating Disorders Review* **11**(3): 243–60.

NCMH, National Collaborating Centre (2004) *National Clinical Practice Guideline: Eating Disorders: Core Interventions in the Treatment and Management of Anorexia Nervosa, Bulimia Nervosa, and Related Eating Disorders*. London: NICE. www.nice.org.uk/CG009NICEguideline

Nielsen, S. (2001) Epidemiology and mortality of eating disorders, *Psychiatric Clinics of North America* **24**(2): 201–14.

Noordenbos, G. (1992) Important factors in the process of recovery according to patients with anorexia nervosa, in W. Herzog, H.C. Deter and W. Vandereycken (eds) *The Course of Eating Disorders. Long-Term Follow-up Studies of Anorexia and Bulimia Nervosa*. Springer Verlag: Berlin-Heidelberg.

Palmer, R.L. and Treasure, J. (1999) Providing specialized services for anorexia nervosa, *British Journal of Psychiatry*, **175**: 306–9.

Peterson, M.E., Orth, D.N., Halmi, N.S. *et al.* (1986) Plasma immunoreactive proopiomelanocortin peptides and cortisol in normal dogs and dogs with Addison's disease and Cushing's syndrome: basal concentrations, *Endocrinology* **119**: 720–30.

Rezaul, I., Persaud, R., Takei, N. and Treasure, J. (1996) Season of birth and eating disorders, *International Journal of Eating Disorders* **19**: 53–61.

Robin, A.L., Siegel, P.T., Moye, A.W. *et al.* (1999) A controlled comparison of family versus individual therapy for adolescents with anorexia nervosa, *Journal of the American Academy of Child and Adolescent Psychiatry* **38**: 1482–9.

Rosenvinge, J.H. and Borrenson, R. (1999) Prevention of eating disorders: Time to change programmes or paradigms? Current update and future recommendations, *European Eating Disorders Review* **7**: 6–16.

Russell, G. (1979) Bulimia nervosa: an ominous variant of anorexia nervosa, *Psychological Medicine* **9**: 429–48.

Russell, G.F., Szmukler, G.I., Dare, C. and Eisler, I. (1987) An evaluation of family therapy in anorexia nervosa and bulimia nervosa, *Archives of General Psychiatry* **44**: 1047–56.

Schmidt, U., Tiller, J., Blanchard, M., Andrews, B. and Treasure, J. (1997) Is there a specific trauma precipitating anorexia nervosa? *Psychological Medicine* **27**: 523–30.

Scholtz, M. and Asen, E. (2001) Multiple family therapy with eating disordered adolescents, *European Eating Disorders Review* **9**: 33–42.

Serfaty, M.A. (1999) Cognitive therapy versus dietary counselling in the outpatient treatment of anorexia nervosa: Effects of the treatment phase, *European Eating Disorders Review* **7**: 334–50.

Shoebridge, P. and Gowers, S.G. (2000) Parental high concern and adolescent-onset anorexia nervosa. A case-control study to investigate direction of causality, *British Journal of Psychiatry* **176**: 132–7.

Steinhausen, H.C. (2002) The outcome of anorexia nervosa in the 20th century, *American Journal of Psychiatry* **159**: 1284–93.

Stice, E. (2002) Risk and maintenance factors for eating pathology: A meta-analytic review (personal communication).

Strober, M., Freeman, R., Lampert, C., Diamond, J. and Kaye, W. (2000) Controlled family study of anorexia nervosa and bulimia nervosa: evidence of shared liability and transmission of partial syndromes, *The American Journal of Psychiatry* **157**: 393–401.

Stunkard, A. (2000) Two eating disorders: binge eating disorder and the night eating syndrome, *Appetite* **34**: 333–4.

Sullivan, P.F. (1995) Mortality in anorexia nervosa, *The American Journal of Psychiatry* **152**: 1073–4.

Treasure, J. (1997) *Anorexia Nervosa. A Survival Guide for Sufferers and Those Caring for Someone with an Eating Disorder*. Hove: Psychology Press.

Treasure, J., Todd, G., Brolly, M. *et al.* (1995) A pilot study of a randomized trial of cognitive analytical therapy vs educational behavioral therapy for adult anorexia nervosa, *Behaviour Research and Therapy* **33**: 363–7.

Treasure, J., Murphy, T., Todd, G. *et al.* (2001) The experience of care giving for severe mental illness: A comparison between anorexia nervosa and psychosis, *Social Psychiatry and Psychiatric Epidemiology* **36**: 343–7.

Treasure, J., Gavan, K., Todd, G. and Schmidt, U. (2002) Changing the environment in eating disorders: Working with carers/families to improve motivation and facilitate change, *European Eating Disorder Review* **11**(1): 25–37.

Turnbull, S., Ward, A., Treasure, J., Jick, H. and Derby, L. (1996) The demand for eating disorder care. An epidemiological study using the general practice research database, *British Journal of Psychiatry* **169**: 705–12.

Vandereycken, W. and Hoek, H.W. (1993) Are eating disorders culture-bound syndromes? in K.A. Halmi (ed.) *Psychobiology and Treatment of Anorexia Nervosa and Bulimia Nervosa*. Washington, DC: American Psychopathological Association, pp. 19–36.

Vaz, F.J. (1998) Outcome of bulimia nervosa: prognostic indicators. *J. Psychosom. Res.* **45**: 391–400.

Vigersky, R.A. and Loriaux, L. (1977) The effect of cyproheptadine in anorexia nervosa: a double blind trial, in R.A. Vigersky (ed.) *Anorexia Nervosa*. New York: Raven Press.

Wallin, U. and Per Kronovall, M.M. (2000) Body awareness therapy in teenage anorexia nervosa: outcome after 2 years, *European Eating Disorders Review* **8**(1): 19–30.

Ward, A., Ramsay, R. and Treasure, J. (2000) Attachment research in eating disorders, *British Journal of Medical Psychology* **73**(1): 35–51.

Ward, A., Ramsay, R., Turnbull, S. *et al.* (2001) The adult attachment interview in anorexia nervosa: A transgenerational perspective, *British Journal of Medical Psychology* **74**(4): 497–505.

Whitehouse, A.M., Cooper, P.J., Vize, C.V., Hill, C. and Vogel, L. (1992) Prevalence of eating disorders in three Cambridge general practices: hidden and conspicuous morbidity, *The British Journal of General Practice* **42**: 57–60.

Whitney, J.B., Murray, J., Gavan, K., Todd, G.E., Whitaker, W. and Treasure, J. (in press). The experience of caring for someone with anorexia nervosa: a qualitative study, *British Medical Journal* (accepted 2004).

World Health Organization (WHO) (1992) *The ICD-10 Classification of Mental and Behavioural Disorders: Clinical Descriptions and Diagnostic Guidelines.* Geneva: World Health Organization.

Zipfel, S., Lowe, B., Reas, D.L., Deter, H.C. and Herzog, W. (2000) Long-term prognosis in anorexia nervosa: lessons from a 21-year follow-up study, *Lancet* **355**: 721–2.

17

The person who misuses drugs or alcohol

Cheryl Kipping

Chapter overview

Drug and/or alcohol use among people with mental health problems can pose significant challenges for the individuals themselves and for those who provide treatment and care. To date, the literature paints a picture of UK provision that is poorly equipped to manage this dual condition. However, innovative practices have been reported and treatment guidelines have been published. This chapter builds upon these developments and begins with an examination of the terms and concepts associated with substance misuse and dual diagnosis. The possible relationships between substance misuse and mental illness are examined, as are the clinical difficulties encountered by clients and the subsequent challenges faced by services. Detailed descriptions of commonly misused substances, assessment methods and treatment models provide a template for clinical application.

This chapter covers:

- Introduction and overview of substance misuse and dual diagnosis.
- Commonly misused substances, modes of use, effects and complications.
- Assessment methods.
- Approaches to treatment and care.
- The needs of older people.

Introduction

Traditionally substance misuse has been thought of as a specialist area of mental health practice but there is growing acceptance that *all* mental health professionals need to have knowledge and skills in this area. This is because substance misuse, both drugs and alcohol, is common among people with mental health problems. Regardless of the setting in which mental health professionals work they will inevitably come into contact with people who are misusing substances. This chapter deals with drug and alcohol use within this context. Although substance misuse tends to be seen as a problem this is not always the case. Moreover, substance use is widespread within society. Something of this broader perspective will be highlighted.

Concepts and terminology

There tends to be a lack of clarity and consistency in the terminology related to substance use and the problems associated with it. Furthermore, as terms acquire negative and stigmatizing connotations (for example substance abuse, addict and addiction) they tend to fall out of usage. Substance use is a broad concept. Use in itself may not be problematic, however, adverse physical, psychological, psychiatric, interpersonal, social or legal consequences are often experienced. The 'problem', however, may not be perceived as such by the user but only by those close to her or him. Substance misuse can be thought of as use that is not socially or medically approved, or which is illegal. It should be noted, however, that what is socially acceptable, medically approved or illegal in one culture, or at one point in time, may not be in another culture or at another time. Although a distinction has been made between drugs and alcohol in the title of this chapter, alcohol is a drug, which happens to be legal. Other widely used, legal drugs include tobacco and caffeine – while caffeine is socially acceptable, smoking tobacco is becoming less so.

Dependence has a more precise meaning, suggesting that a person has developed a compulsion to continue taking a substance on a regular, repetitive basis. Physical dependence indicates that the person's body has adapted to repeated doses of the drug and withholding it will result in withdrawal symptoms. Some substances do not create a physical dependence but do create a powerful psychological dependence. Specific criteria for a diagnosis of substance dependence are identified in the DSM-IV (Diagnostic and Statistical Manual of Mental Disorders) (American Psychiatric Association 1994) and ICD-10 (International Classification of Diseases) (World Health Organization 1992). Criteria for a diagnosis of 'substance abuse' (DSM-IV) and 'harmful substance use' (ICD-10) have also been identified.

This consideration of terms and attitudes to substances may seem unnecessary preamble but thinking about these issues can facilitate reflection on one's own views. Negative attitudes to substance misuse and people who misuse substances have been identified as a potential barrier to working effectively with this group.

Although 'substance misuse' has some negative connotations the term is commonly used and will be adopted in this chapter. Following the approach generally taken in substance misuse services, the term 'client' will be used in preference to patient or service user. 'Users' will be referred to, but in this context users are people who misuse substances.

Overview of dual diagnosis

Dual diagnosis, the coexistence of mental health and substance misuse disorders, is widely seen as a major challenge to mental health services and the staff working in them (for example, Krauz 1996; Gournay *et al.* 1997; Ryrie 2000; Department of Health 2002a). While this definition may seem straightforward, the range of people who might be categorized in this way is very diverse. The Department of Health (DH 2002a) has suggested that the scope of dual diagnosis can be conceptualized as two intersecting continua, where one represents the severity of mental illness and the other the severity of substance misuse (Figure 17.1). Personality disorder is conceptualized as a separate dimension, which can coexist with a mental illness, a substance misuse problem, or both.

Further complexity is added to the dual diagnosis concept when the relationship(s) between mental illness and substance misuse is considered. Crome (1999) has suggested that:

- substance use or withdrawal can produce psychiatric symptoms or illness;

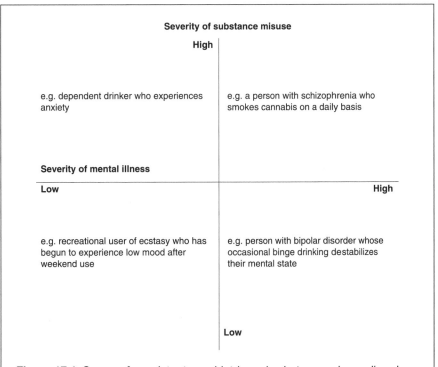

Figure 17.1 Scope of coexistent psychiatric and substance misuse disorder

(After Department of Health 2002a)

- dependence, intoxication or withdrawal can produce psychological symptoms;
- psychiatric disorder can lead to a substance misuse disorder; and
- substance misuse may exacerbate a pre-existing psychiatric disorder.

In clinical practice it can be difficult to identify which of these mechanisms is operating.

A lack of consistency in definitions, sample selection, measurement tools and timeframes in research studies makes it difficult to establish prevalence rates. It is generally accepted that 30–50 per cent of people with a severe mental illness also have problems with substances. This figure is thought to be higher in inner city areas and increasing. The Department of Health (DH 2002a) has argued that substance misuse should be considered usual rather than exceptional in people with severe mental illness.

Dual diagnosis is associated with a range of difficulties. In comparison to people with a mental illness alone, people who also use substances have:

- higher rates of homelessness;
- increased rates of suicidal behaviour;
- increased rates of violence;
- worsening of their psychiatric symptoms;
- poorer adherence with medication;
- increased rates of HIV infection;
- greater contact with the criminal justice system; and
- make increased use of institutional services.

(Banerjee *et al.* 2002; DH 2002a)

Despite growing concern about dual diagnosis, services have been slow to respond. Two main reasons have been identified for this. First, the way in which mental health and substance misuse services have traditionally operated. They have been separate parts of organizational structures and had different expectations and ways of working with clients. Second, staff in both types of service lack the knowledge and skills for working with people with a dual diagnosis. People in mental health services lack the knowledge and skills for working with people with substance misuse problems and vice versa.

Three service models have been identified for working with people with a dual diagnosis: serial, parallel and integrated. The serial model, where mental health and substance misuse disorders are treated consecutively by different services, has been discredited. Each service has expected the client to deal with the other 'problem' first and as a consequence people have fallen through the net of care provision. Rorstad and Checkinski describe the experience of one client. 'I was pushed around like a tennis ball. The alcohol people said I had a mental illness and the mental illness group said I had a drink problem. Neither of them did very much for me' (1996: 9).

In the parallel model, mental health and substance misuse interventions are provided by the two services concurrently. While this model has its critics (for example, Drake *et al.* 1993, 1995) some projects in the UK have developed services in this way and appear to have provided benefits to clients (for example, Kipping 1999; DH 2002a).

In the USA, services have developed using an integrated model, where mental health and substance misuse interventions are provided concurrently in the same setting by one specialist team. There has been considerable enthusiasm for this approach. Ley *et al.* (2002), however, following a systematic review of studies evaluating programmes designed to meet the needs of people with a severe mental illness and a substance misuse problem, concluded that there was no clear evidence supporting one approach over another.

Policy guidance from the Department of Health (DH 2002a) has now set the agenda for the development of UK services. For people with a severe mental illness and a substance misuse problem an integrated approach to care provision is to be provided within mainstream mental health services. It is likely that people with less severe mental disorders and substance misuse problems will be the responsibility of substance misuse and/or primary care services. However, many different services are likely to be involved and finding ways of working together across traditional boundaries will be essential if the diverse and complex needs of people with a dual diagnosis are to be met.

Reasons for substance misuse

Regardless of whether or not people have mental health problems, their reasons for misusing substances are likely to be many and varied. These include the following: the 'buzz', it is the norm in the person's social circle, to give energy, to unwind and aid relaxation, to alleviate boredom, to block out painful thoughts and negative feelings (for example anger, anxiety), to boost confidence, and to avoid withdrawal symptoms.

In people with mental health problems the notion of 'self-medication' has received particular attention. A literature review conducted by Phillips and Johnson (2001) found evidence of people with severe mental illness using drugs to self-medicate negative symptoms, mood problems, anxiety and insomnia. Although it has been suggested that drugs are also used to deal with positive symptoms and the side effects of medication, Phillips and Johnson report that the findings are inconsistent.

Commonly misused substances

This section identifies commonly misused substances and describes how they are used, their effects and complications. If staff in mental health services are to work effectively with people with a dual diagnosis it is essential that they have this knowledge which will underpin assessment, subsequent care planning and treatment interventions. Having an understanding of the language associated with substance misuse can also be important. Some drug users' jargon is included, indicated by the word being presented in italics and inverted commas (for example, '*gear*').

Alcohol

Alcohol is legal, widely available and socially acceptable. Over 90 per cent of adults drink. Alcoholic drinks come in different strengths, indicated by the 'alcohol by volume' (ABV), the percentage of the total liquid that is alcohol. Alcohol consumption can be measured in units. One unit is the equivalent of half a pint of standard strength beer (3–4 per cent ABV), a pub measure of spirits (around 40 per cent ABV) or a small (125ml) glass of wine (8–10 per cent ABV). Recommended 'safe' drinking levels are 3–4 units daily for a man and 2–3 for a woman. However, consistently drinking at the upper levels (i.e. 4 units daily for a man and 3 for a woman) is not advisable suggesting that some days each week should be alcohol free (DH 1995).

The effects of alcohol will depend on how much the person is used to drinking. Tolerance develops (i.e. more is needed to gain the same effect). With small amounts of alcohol the person is likely to feel less inhibited and more sociable and relaxed. Their heart rate will increase and they may appear flushed (due to vasodilation). As consumption increases slurred speech and a lack of coordination may be evident. The drinker's emotions may become labile. With heavy use the person may experience double vision, stagger, lose balance and lose consciousness. Severe intoxication may result in vomiting which can prevent fatal overdose. However, impaired consciousness can lead to death if the drinker inhales his or her vomit.

With regular, heavy use some people become physically dependent and, in the absence of alcohol, experience withdrawal symptoms, typically in the morning, when the level of alcohol in their body has fallen. Sweatiness, shaking, nausea and vomiting are common symptoms. Delirium tremens, a state characterized by rapid pulse, raised blood pressure, feverishness, sweating, shaking, disorientation, agitation, hallucinations, and sometimes also paranoid delusions is experienced by some people. Seizures are another possible complication of alcohol withdrawals. These can occur from 7 to 48 hours after stopping drinking. Both delirium tremens and withdrawal seizures can be fatal.

While some people will drink heavily every day, others will drink in binges. The pattern of these varies, for example, some people will drink heavily for a number of weeks and then remain abstinent for several months, others drink heavily for 2- or 3-day periods and remain abstinent throughout the remainder of the week. Even this latter pattern can pose risks to the person's physical health.

A range of mental and physical health problems are associated with heavy alcohol use. Depression is common, but it can be difficult to assess whether the depression is independent of, or secondary to, alcohol use. If abstinence is achieved and the depression is secondary to drinking, symptoms should begin to improve after 2–3 weeks. A similar picture exists with anxiety and many drinkers experience problems with both depression and anxiety.

Risk of suicide is particularly high in people with alcohol problems. The depressive symptoms associated with drinking are a trigger, and, when intoxicated, the person's inhibitions are likely to be reduced, making them more likely to act on suicidal thoughts. To add to these risks, a range of factors which can be typical of the lifestyles of people with drink problems are associated with suicidal thoughts: having major financial problems (spending money on alcohol can become the priority); difficulties with the police or courts (through alcohol-related convictions); problems with close friends or relatives (due to the impact of the person's drinking on them and the tensions and arguments that may follow); and a lack of social support (as relationships break down) (Meltzer *et al.* 2002). Alcohol, used in combination with other drugs which are central nervous system (CNS) depressants, significantly increases the risk of intentional and accidental overdose.

Alcoholic hallucinosis is a condition where auditory or visual hallucinations occur during or after a period of heavy drinking. Delusions, ideas of reference and an abnormal affect may also be present. Typically the symptoms abate after a few weeks.

Other health problems associated with heavy drinking include: brain damage (which may be irreversible), gastritis, pancreatitis, ulcers, oesophageal varices, peripheral neuropathy, liver damage (for example, alcoholic hepatitis, cirrhosis), Wernicke's encephalopathy and Korsakoff's syndrome. 'Black outs', transient memory loss induced by intoxication, can be experienced by both dependent and non-dependent drinkers. Some people have total memory loss for a period of time, which may last from a few hours to several days.

Because alcohol affects judgement and coordination, drinkers may be particularly prone to accidents, potentially putting themselves and others at risk of harm. Driving, operating machinery and working at heights should be avoided. Older people may be especially susceptible to falling.

Some of the social consequences of drinking have been highlighted above. Others include: school exclusion, lost employment, violence (within and outside the home), neglect of children, engaging in unsafe sex, drinking and driving, homelessness (see Alcohol Concern 2000). Women who drink when they are pregnant risk complications and damage to their unborn child.

Opiates

Opiates are a group of drugs derived from the opium poppy. Synthetically produced opiates are known as opioids. Therapeutically these drugs can be used as painkillers (for example morphine, pethidine, dihydrocodeine), cough suppressants (for example, codeine linctus) and anti-diarrhoea agents (for example kaolin and morphine mixture). Methadone and buprenorphine are opioids used in the treatment of opiate dependency.

Although all opiates have misuse potential, heroin is the most widely misused and will be the focus here. Heroin ('*gear*', '*smack*', '*brown*', '*scag*') is a brownish white powder that can be snorted, smoked or injected. Smoking ('*chasing*', '*booting*') involves placing heroin on aluminium foil and heating it. The vapours given off are then inhaled through a tube. Occasionally heroin is mixed with tobacco and smoked in a cigarette. To prepare heroin for injection it is mixed in a spoon with water and citric acid (to help dissolve the powder) and heated. The liquid preparation is then drawn up into a syringe through a filter, usually a cigarette filter, which removes undissolved material. Heroin can then be injected into the tissue under the skin ('*skin-popping*'), into muscle, or into a vein (intravenous use). Many heroin users never inject. Of those that do, it is common to start by smoking and move to injecting as tolerance develops. Injecting is a more cost-effective way of using; less of the drug is needed to create the desired effect.

Heroin is usually bought in '*bags*'. It induces feelings of well-being, warmth and relaxation. People describe feeling as if they have been wrapped in cotton wool. The initial euphoria ('*buzz*'), particularly following intravenous use, is intense. When intoxicated, the person is likely to have small '*pinned*' pupils, heavy eyelids, and appear drowsy – a state described as '*gouching*'.

With regular, repeated use physical and psychological dependence develop. Heroin is then needed to stave off withdrawal symptoms: dilated pupils, watery eyes, sneezing, runny nose, yawning, goose flesh, feeling cold and shivery, muscle aches and cramps, and diarrhoea and vomiting. Symptoms are likely to begin 6–8 hours after the drug was last used. While they can be very distressing, they are not life-threatening but the discomfort experienced can be a strong motivator to use again. Not all heroin users become physically dependent, but for many, using heroin becomes the focus of their life. Everything else (for example, relationships, possessions, paying bills, self-care, eating) becomes less important than acquiring the money to obtain heroin. Borrowing, stealing from family and friends, selling possessions, getting involved in prostitution, drug dealing, and a range of other criminal activities from shoplifting to armed robbery are all ways in which money may be raised.

Although heroin itself does not have an adverse effect on mental state, psychological and psychiatric symptoms are common in opiate misusers. The National Treatment Outcome Research Study (Gossop *et al.* 2001), which followed the progress of 1075 primarily opiate users, reported that, at the point of entering the study, anxiety and depressive mood were 'common'. Furthermore, 29 per cent of the sample had thought about suicide in the previous three months, 10 per cent had received psychiatric inpatient treatment (for a problem other than drug dependence) in the past two years and 14 per cent had received community psychiatric treatment. Lifestyle factors such as those outlined above may contribute, as may underlying problems, for example, childhood sexual abuse which is common in substance misusers (Bear *et al.* 2000), and has been associated with suicidal thoughts and actions (Meltzer *et al.* 2002).

Death from accidental overdose is another possible consequence of heroin use. This risk increases if the person is injecting, is using other CNS depressant drugs (for example, benzodiazepines and alcohol) or has a reduced level of tolerance (for example, after a period of abstinence in a treatment programme). Variability in the purity of illicit heroin means that overdose is always a risk. As with alcohol, other accidents may be precipitated due to slowed reactions.

Intravenous heroin use brings a range of further complications. Sharing injecting equipment (this include spoons, filters and water, as well as needles and syringes) may result in the transmission of blood-borne viruses, such as HIV and hepatitis B and C. Puncturing the skin to inject can introduce bacteria into the body. These may cause local infections (for example abscesses) or systemic infections (for example septicaemia). Damage to the veins and thromboses are further possible complication of intravenous use. In the early stages of use people generally inject into the veins in their arms but as these collapse they move to other sites, for example, hands and feet. It is not uncommon for people to inject into their groin. This can be particularly dangerous as there is a risk of hitting an artery or nerve rather than the vein. Other dangerous sites are the neck, breast and penis.

Smoking heroin can precipitate or exacerbate respiratory problems. Other health concerns associated with opiate use are constipation, reduced libido and amenorrhoea. Women who do become pregnant and continue to use, risk their baby being opiate dependent.

Although methadone (physeptone) and buprenorphine are used in the treatment of opiate dependency both have the potential for misuse. Methadone is available as a liquid, tablet or in injectable form but is most commonly prescribed in its liquid formulation. Complications can arise from injecting liquid and tablet formulations. Buprenorphine comes as a sublingual tablet. Overdose is possible with both drugs, particularly when used in combination with other CNS depressants.

Benzodiazepines

Benzodiazepines are commonly prescribed for their therapeutic effects in relieving anxiety and promoting sleep. They can also be used as a muscle relaxant and an anti-convulsant. Diazepam, temazepam and nitrazepam are examples. Benzodiazepines are most commonly available in tablet form but when misused may be injected (after crushing). Tolerance develops to both therapeutic and non-therapeutic effects. Physical and psychological dependence occur.

Benzodiazepines may be misused by the person to whom they were prescribed, or by others who have obtained illicit supplies. Reasons for use include: the effects they have if used alone (relieving anxiety, inducing feelings of calmness and relaxation, inducing sleep); enhancing the effect of other substances (for example opiates and alcohol); counteracting the effects of stimulant drugs; and as a substitute for, or to help cope with withdrawal symptoms of, other substances.

In excess, benzodiazepines cause drowsiness, slurred speech, poor co-ordination, and a glassy-eyed appearance (with dilated pupils). When taken in high doses some people experience a paradoxical effect, characterized by aggression and hostility. Benzodiazepine withdrawal symptoms include: feelings of anxiety, sweating, tremor, irritability, headache, nausea, insomnia and perceptual distortions. Sudden cessation of benzodiazepines in someone who has used high doses on a regular basis for a lengthy period of time can induce withdrawal seizures.

Anxiety disorders are very common in people who misuse benzo-diazepines. For such clients detoxification can be extremely difficult as anxiety is also a withdrawal symptom and clients are likely to be highly anxious about detoxification.

As with other CNS depressants a risk of accidents is associated with use. Overdose is possible but unlikely to be fatal unless other CNS depressants have been taken. Injecting potentially brings the problems associated with intravenous use outlined above. There is a risk to the foetus if pregnant women continue to use heavily.

Stimulants

Stimulant drugs include amphetamine, cocaine and crack cocaine. Some amphetamine and amphetamine-like drugs are legally produced and used therapeutically. For example, dexamphetamine (dexedrine) and methyl-phenidate (ritalin) are, somewhat controversially, used for the management of children with attention deficit disorder. In the past amphetamine was prescribed as an appetite suppressant and in the treatment of depression but such use is no longer recommended.

Amphetamine sulphate ('*speed*', '*whizz*', '*sulphate*') is illicitly produced amphetamine. It is a whitish (pink/grey) powder that can be snorted, swallowed or injected. Other forms of amphetamine are amphetamine base, which usually comes as a paste which is swallowed or smoked, and methylamphetamine (or methamphetamine), '*ice*', a crystalline form, which is usually smoked in a pipe designed for the purpose.

Amphetamines cause arousal (increasing heart and respiratory rate), and dilate the pupils. Users seek the feelings of alertness, energy, confidence, exhilaration and reduced fatigue which the drug brings. To the observer they are likely to appear excitable, speak rapidly and have poor concentra-tion. Appetite will be diminished. The effects of amphetamine last 3–4 hours. Following repeated use, tolerance and psychological dependence may develop.

Cocaine ('*coke*', '*charlie*') is a white powder that is usually snorted but can also be injected, swallowed or smoked. When cocaine powder is dis-solved in water and heated with baking soda small crystals of crack cocaine ('*rocks*' or '*stones*') about the size of a raisin are produced. Crack is usually smoked using a crack pipe where the rock is heated and the vapours inhaled. It can also be injected.

Like amphetamine, crack and cocaine produce physiological arousal and feelings of well-being, alertness and exhilaration. The effects, however, are much shorter than those of amphetamine. The psychological peak is reached after about 20–30 minutes for cocaine and is almost immediate for crack. This means that it must be used frequently to sustain the effect.

A range of psychological and psychiatric complications are associated with stimulant use. In contrast to the desired effects, users may experience feelings of anxiety, agitation, irritability and restlessness. After a period of regular, repeated use a *'come down'* or *'crash'*, typified by feelings of lethargy, sleepiness and depression, is common as the body adjusts to the absence of the drug. The depression can be severe and suicide is a risk. Webster (1999) found that in a sample of 288 crack users 64 per cent had experienced suicidal thoughts and 37 per cent had attempted suicide.

A drug-induced psychosis may be precipitated; this usually follows high levels of use over several days. This is characterized by hallucinations, feelings of paranoia and delusions. Symptoms resolve as the drug is eliminated from the body.

Crack users who are smoking are prone to respiratory problems due to the build-up of fluids in the lungs. Wheezing, shortness of breath, coughing and chest pains are common, a condition known as 'crack lung'. Cardiovascular problems such as high blood pressure, irregular heartbeat and strokes can occur with both cocaine and crack. Long-term cocaine use can result in damage to the septum of the nose.

Prolonged use of any stimulants can have detrimental effects on the user's general physical health due to lack of food and sleep. When injected the problems associated with intravenous drug use can occur. Use during pregnancy may bring complications for mother and child. For further information about the effect of substance misuse during pregnancy see Siney (1999).

Significant amounts of money may be required to sustain use, particularly of cocaine or crack, and people may engage in a variety of unscrupulous or illegal ways of raising money, such as those described for heroin users.

Cannabis

Although not generally available for therapeutic use research into the various potential medicinal benefits of tetrahydrocannabinols – THC (the psychoactive ingredient in cannabis) is in progress.

Cannabis can come as a green/brown block of compressed resin (*'hash'*, *'blow'*, *'draw'*) or as herbal cannabis, the leaves, stalks and seeds of the plant (*'marijuana'*, *'grass'*, *'weed'*). *'Skunk'* is a particularly strong variety. Cannabis is usually smoked with tobacco in a *'joint'* or *'spliff'*, but can be smoked in a pipe. It can also be eaten. Cannabis is the most commonly used illicit drug in the UK.

The effects of cannabis depend to a large extent on the expectations and mood of the user and the amount taken. Feelings of relaxation, euphoria and a greater appreciation of sensory experiences are commonly described. When intoxicated cognitive and motor skills will be impaired.

Psychological dependence on cannabis can develop and withdrawal symptoms, including restlessness, anxiety, irritability and insomnia, have been documented. Cannabis induces feelings of anxiety and paranoia in some users. Depression may also be experienced. Heavy use can precipitate psychotic episodes but there is no evidence that cannabis use can lead to a psychotic illness which persists after abstinence, nor that cannabis is a causal factor in schizophrenia. However, recent evidence suggests that cannabis use increases the risk of schizophrenia (Arseneault *et al.* 2002; Zammit *et al.* 2002) and it can exacerbate symptoms. See Johns (2001) for a review of the psychiatric effects of cannabis.

The physical health problems are mainly those associated with smoking tobacco. Research into the long-term effects of cannabis use is inconclusive.

Ecstasy ('Es')

Ecstasy usually comes in tablet form and is swallowed. After about 20–30 minutes it produces a relaxed, euphoric state, a heightened perception of surroundings and a feeling of understanding and acceptance of others. This lasts for 2–4 hours. Tolerance does occur but physical dependence is not thought to. Many tablets sold as ecstasy do not contain any of the active ingredient methylendioxmethylamphetamine (MDMA).

If used over several days (for example over a weekend) ecstasy users may subsequently experience feelings of fatigue and depression. Anxiety, panic, confusion, paranoia and psychosis have been reported with high levels of use.

Delirium, convulsions, cardiac arrythmias and coma have all been associated with ecstasy and some deaths have occurred. Little is know about its long-term effects.

This section has identified substances which are commonly misused, their mode of use, effects and complications. While for some people substance misuse brings enjoyment, for others it can have adverse physical, psychological, psychiatric, interpersonal, social and legal consequences which can be devastating for both the person themselves and those close to them. The information presented here provides the background knowledge needed to conduct a substance misuse assessment.

Assessment

Overview

A thorough assessment is essential for the safe and effective care and treatment of people who misuse substances and should be integral to any mental health assessment. Under-detection of substance misuse in people with a severe mental illness could be as high as 50 per cent (Osher and Drake 1996). Substance misuse is also a key factor in assessing risk. The assessment process is important for engaging and developing a therapeutic relationship with the client, gaining an understanding of the person and his or her circumstances, identifying goals, and deciding on the most appropriate treatment interventions.

The nurse's attitude can be a significant factor in the assessment process, and, indeed, in subsequent work with the client. If disapproval is detected clients may not be honest about their circumstances. Concerns about the sharing of information, and the impact such information might have on treatment decisions, may also influence the extent to which an accurate account is given. For example, people may be worried that the police will be informed about their drug use or the activities which fund it. Women with children may be afraid that social services will be notified of their use and their children taken into care. It is important to explain the organization's confidentiality policy to the client and the circumstances in which confidentiality may be broken.

Substance misuse assessment can take place in various circumstances (from psychiatric or medical emergency situations to a person approaching services for help in a planned way), and in a range of settings (for example, GP surgery, accident and emergency department, psychiatric ward, community mental health team, substance misuse team, client's home). The assessment procedure will need to be adapted accordingly. The level of assessment will depend on the context in which it is being conducted. Obtaining assessment information can be particularly difficult in people with mental health problems who may not want to engage with services and, even if they do, their ability to participate in the process may be limited by their mental illness and/or substance misuse symptoms. Assessment is an ongoing process. It will take time to build a full picture of the person's use, the way it has developed over time and its impact on various aspects of their life. Furthermore, an individual's needs will change over time.

There are no national standards for assessing people with substance misuse problems (DH 2002b) but it is generally accepted that the key components of a comprehensive assessment are:

- current and recent use;
- past use;
- physical health (including sexual health);
- mental health;
- social situation (including accommodation, family circumstances – especially children, employment, finances);
- legal situation;
- personal and family history;
- risk assessment; and

- client's perception of situation, reasons for using and motivation for change.

Some of these components are common to mental health and substance misuse assessments. The remainder of this section focuses on those which are unique to substance misuse: current and recent use; past use; and the client's perception, reasons for using and motivation for change. Risk assessment will also be included as there are specific risks associated with substance misuse. The physical, mental, social and legal complications which can be associated with substance misuse were identified in the previous section; evidence of these should be sought in the assessment. This information should be integrated with the specific substance misuse information described below and with information that would routinely be obtained in a mental health assessment.

Current and recent use

Information about which substances are being used, the quantity and frequency of use, route of administration and length of time that the person has been using at the current level is needed. They should also be asked about alcohol and drugs – illicit and prescribed. Prompting for specific substances and further questioning to gain clarification (for example, what type/strength of lager is being consumed, whether prescribed medication is being taken as directed) may be necessary. If a person is injecting, information about the site(s) where they are injecting, whether they share equipment, and whether they know where to obtain clean equipment should be obtained. Injection sites should be inspected.

Taking a history of the past five days' use, starting with 'today' and working back provides an indication of whether the person's use is reasonably stable from day to day, or whether there is a more chaotic picture. A more detailed picture of use over the course of the day may also be desirable (for example, finding out how many times someone is injecting, establishing what time alcohol consumption usually begins, whether it continues at a steady rate through the day, or whether there are breaks). Factors which influence patterns of use over a longer time period should also be explored (for example, the client may use heavily on the days immediately after receipt of benefit payments). Other patterns should also be explored, such as whether the client uses one drug to counteract the effects of another.

Details of withdrawal symptoms are needed to establish whether or not the person is physically dependent on any of the substances being used. Previous experiences of withdrawal seizures and delirium tremens should be noted, as should any overdoses (accidental and intentional). Information about how the client is funding their substance use should also be obtained.

Observation of the person's physical appearance and non-verbal communication is an integral part of the assessment. Factors to observe include: whether there are signs of intoxication or withdrawal, whether there is evidence of any injuries, whether the person appears underweight, whether they are dishevelled or unkempt, whether they appear agitated or anxious. Another important source of information is objective tests such as urinalysis, breathalyser readings and blood tests (for example, liver function). Other health care professionals (for example, the GP) and family and friends can also provide supplementary information if the client consents to their involvement.

Throughout the assessment process opportunities for providing health education/harm minimization information (for example, how to inject more safely, advising alcohol-dependent people not to stop drinking immediately because of the risk of withdrawal seizures and delirium tremens) should be taken.

Past use

A substance misuse history will be required. This should establish when the person began taking each of the substances they have used (or are currently using), what prompted use, how use has developed over time, the impact it has had on different aspects of their life (for example, education and employment, relationships, finances, physical and mental health, contact with the criminal justice system), whether there have been any periods of abstinence, how these were achieved and maintained, and details of any previous treatment for substance misuse (what was provided, what was helpful and the outcome). Obtaining a chronological account of a person's substance misuse and mental health history may provide insights into the inter-relationship of the two.

Risk assessment

It is essential that substance misuse is considered when assessing risk. Nurses should have a good understanding of the impact that substance misuse can have on areas of risk such as suicide and violence. In addition there are specific risks associated with substance misuse and the lifestyle which may be associated with it. Table 17.1 summarizes these risks. This information should be seen in conjunction with that provided in Chapter 8 of this book.

Suicide reduction is a *NSF for Mental Health* target (DH 1999a). Recent evidence demonstrating the strong association between substance use and suicide is summarized below.

A survey conducted by the Office of National Statistics (ONS) (Meltzer *et al.* 2002) asked a sample of 8450 16- to 74-year-olds living in Britain about self-harming, and suicidal thoughts and behaviour. The Alcohol Use Disorders Identification Test (AUDIT) (Babor *et al.* 1989) and the Severity of Alcohol Questionnaire (SADQ) (Stockwell *et al.* 1983) were used to determine severity of alcohol use. The researchers found that whereas 4 per cent of people who were not problem drinkers had attempted suicide at some time in their lives, 9 per cent of a moderately dependent group and 27 per cent of a severely dependent group had done so. The corresponding figures

Table 17.1 Risk and substance misuse

	Alcohol	Stimulants (e.g. crack, cocaine, amphetamine)	Opiates (e.g. heroin methadone)	Benzodiazepines	Cannabis	Other factors
Suicide	Can trigger/exacerbate depression Reduces inhibitions Increases risk of death when combined with other CNS depressants May trigger psychotic symptoms (alcoholic hallucinosis, delirium tremens – dts)	Low mood/depression associated with 'come down' May trigger psychotic symptoms	Psychological and psychiatric symptoms are common in opiate users – overdose may be means of suicide, particular risk when combined with other CNS depressants NB Can be difficult to distinguish accidental and deliberate overdose	May be combined with other CNS depressants in suicide attempt	May trigger/exacerbate depression May trigger psychotic symptoms	Lifestyle factors may contribute, e.g. lack of social support, financial problems, difficulties with police/courts, problems in relationships with close friends/relatives, feelings of hopelessness and helplessness Also factors associated with life experiences, e.g. sexual abuse, violence in the home People misusing drugs have access to substances which are lethal in overdose
Violence	Triggers emotional lability/irritability, reduces inhibitions Environmental factors and misperceptions may be a factor May have history of violence when intoxicated or withdrawing (cf. dts)	Heightened state of arousal and excitability, risk of misperception May trigger psychotic symptoms or relapse in mental state producing feelings of paranoia, delusions, hallucinations, hostility	See other factors	Can cause idiosyncratic effect, i.e. agitation, violence	May trigger psychotic symptoms or relapse in mental state	Violent activity may be associated with funding drug use (e.g. mugging, armed robbery). High levels of violence associated with crack scene (often involving firearms) User may be victim of violence, e.g. if has drug debts, if involved in sex work, if in dispute with other users Professionals may be at risk of violence from clients/their associates during home visits
Accidents	Sedating effect/lack of coordination may result in accidents (cf. drink driving, operating machinery, working at heights) – risk may be increased if combination of substances being used. Falls may be when intoxicated or when withdrawing (seizures – 7–48 hours after stopping drinking) Risk of death due to inhaling on vomit	Possible due to poor concentration	As for sedating effect of alcohol and inhaling on vomit – also risk of accidental overdose – risk increased when: injecting; combined with other CNS depressants (e.g. alcohol, benzodiazepines, other opiates), tolerance reduced, if being injected by someone else, uncertainty about strength/purity, if injecting in neck or groin, if using alone	As for sedating effect of alcohol Falls may be associated with withdrawal seizures	Impairment of cognitive and motor skills	Staff may be at risk of needle-stick injury and contracting blood-borne diseases

Physical health	Nutritional deficits (e.g. vitamin B deficiency) Withdrawal seizures, delirium tremens Cognitive impairment Other specific illnesses/health problems associated with alcohol, e.g. pancreatitis, ulcers, liver damage, hypertension, Wernicke's encephalopathy, Korsakoff's syndrome, etc. Engaging in unsafe sex	Injecting risks (see opiates) – also risk of contracting blood-borne viruses when using crack pipes as a result of exposure through cuts or burns Respiratory problems associated with smoking drugs (e.g. 'crack lung') Risk of seizures/fits Cardio-vascular problems associated with crack/cocaine (e.g. heart attack, stroke) Prolonged use produces detrimental effect on general physical health due to lack of sleep and food	Injecting risks – infections (local and systemic), vein damage, deep vein thrombosis, contracting blood-borne diseases (Hep B, C, HIV) by sharing injecting equipment (including spoon, filters, water) and inadequately cleaning surfaces on which injection being prepared Respiratory problems if smoking drugs	Risks associated with crushing and injecting tablets	Respiratory problems associated with smoking	May not be registered with GP or engaged with other health services Some substances (especially opiates) mask pain Sexually transmitted diseases if exchanging sex for drugs and not using condoms
Self-neglect	Not eating, neglect of personal hygiene, lack of basic amenities in accommodation/no accommodation					
Abuse/ exploitation	Engaging in sexual activity – would not choose to when sober	Sex exchanged for substances Benefit book retained by dealers	As for stimulants			Vulnerable people may be coerced into giving/lending money to others Home may be used by others for using/dealing
Deliberate self-harm	Alcohol use often precursor – reduces inhibitions, numbs pain					
Children	Effect of substances on unborn child, non-attendance for ante-natal care, child having access to dangerous substances and injecting equipment – if not stored or disposed of safely, child witnessing substance use/effects of substance use. Child(ren) being neglected (e.g. because parents' priority is substance use, money spent on substances rather than essentials, parent is intoxicated and unable to meet child's needs, parent leaves child unattended, child not taken to school					
Other	Alcohol blackouts (may be transient or last several days) In people with other substance misuse problems – may trigger relapse into use – may become substitute for other substances	Diversion of prescribed drugs which are potentially lethal to people with no/low tolerance				Inadequate care may result from poor communication between services and professionals lack of knowledge/skills Link with offending behaviour, e.g. use of some substances is illegal, means of funding use may involve illegal activity

for people who had experienced suicidal thoughts were 14 per cent, 27 per cent and 57 per cent, respectively.

Drug use was also associated with an increased risk of attempting suicide. Using their own measure for assessing dependence the researchers found that people defined as drug dependent (excluding cannabis) were five times more likely to have attempted suicide than those who were not: 20 per cent of the dependent group compared to 5 per cent of the non-dependent group.

Another source of evidence demonstrating the association between substance use and suicides is 'Safety First', the *National Confidential Inquiry Report into Suicide and Homicide by People with Mental Illness* (DH 2001b). The Inquiry Team received notifications of all suicides committed in England and Wales between April 1996 and March 2000; 5099 of these people had been in contact with mental health services in the year before death. Of these, 9 per cent had a primary diagnosis of alcohol dependence, and alcohol dependence was a common secondary diagnosis. A further 40 per cent had a history of alcohol misuse. In relation to drug use, 4 per cent of those who committed suicide had a primary diagnosis of drug dependence, and drug dependence was a common secondary diagnosis. A further 28 per cent of people who committed suicide had a history of drug misuse and 19 per cent a history of both drug and alcohol use.

Information highlighting the association between violence and substance use can also be found in this report. Also see Ward and Applin (1998).

Case study: Ray

The following case study highlights some of the risks associated with substance use and mental illness.

Ray is a 29-year-old British man with a diagnosis of paranoid schizophrenia. He also has a drink problem and takes drugs if they are available, mainly cannabis, ecstasy and cocaine, but in the past he has used heroin (someone else injected him), and amphetamine. Ray also has a gambling problem. Ray's schizophrenia makes him feel that people are plotting to kill him. He believes he is 'in the frame' for a crime which he did not commit and that people are out to get him because of this. Sometimes he thinks people are watching him. Ray believes he has some protection from his parents and that as long as they are alive, the people plotting to kill him will not act.

Ray lived in the family home until recently but the situation there was difficult. His mother also had a mental illness and his father an alcohol problem. Violence in the home was not uncommon and, eventually Ray moved on because of his violence to his father, always at times when he (Ray) was intoxicated. Ray has one brother and one sister, both married with families of their own. He has some contact with them but they will not see him when he is drinking. When drinking Ray frequently gets himself into difficult and dangerous situations, but because he experiences blackouts, he often cannot remember what has happened. On occasions he has had 'one-night stands' during which he has had unprotected sexual intercourse. He also has criminal convictions for aggravated burglary, being drunk and disorderly, criminal damage and shoplifting, all related to his drinking. When Ray receives his benefits he usually spends money on drinking and gambling before meeting other financial commitments (for example, paying off debts and buying food).

Ray's mother has had a heart problem. She recently experienced a serious heart attack and died. Ray was very close to his mother and believed that she was able to protect him from the people plotting to kill him. He had always said that if anything happened to his mother he would kill himself. Although Ray had made good progress in moderating his drinking, he began drinking heavily again (a two-litre bottle of strong cider and 4–6 pints of standard strength lager each day). He said that he was drinking so that he didn't have to feel anything – in particular, the sadness of his mother's death and the feeling that he has not got much of a life. He has never held down a paid job, he does not have a girlfriend, he lives in a large hostel, he has debts of over £2500 and although he has drinking 'friends' he recognizes that they do not have his best interests at heart. When he is drinking heavily Ray tends to forget to go to the depot clinic and on occasions he has been so intoxicated that staff have felt it would be unsafe to give his medication. Despite periods of heavy use Ray does not appear to become physically dependent and can stop drinking without adverse physical effects.

Client's perception of situation, reasons for use and motivation to change

To complement the more specific information that is obtained during assessment it is important to gain some insight into the client's perceptions of their situation, their reasons for using and readiness for change. This, in conjunction with other information obtained, will also inform care planning and treatment interventions.

Prochaska and DiClemente (1986) have developed a model of change, which is widely used in the substance misuse field (Figure 17.2). Information to identify which stage most closely represents the client's position is likely to emerge during the course of the assessment. For example, a client may report that he is fed up with his wife and GP nagging him about his drinking when all he does is go down to the pub with his mates a few nights each week, and his only reason for attending this appointment is to get them off his back. This man is probably at the precontemplation, or perhaps, contemplation stage (he has, at least, presented to the service). Someone else might tell you that as a consequence of his drinking he has lost his job, has significant debts, his marriage has broken down, and his GP has told him that he has liver damage, he has now had enough and yesterday went to an Alcoholics Anonymous meeting. This man has almost certainly reached the active change stage. Future work would proceed very differently with these two people.

Understanding the client's reasons for using and the perceived advantages and disadvantages of their use can also be important in

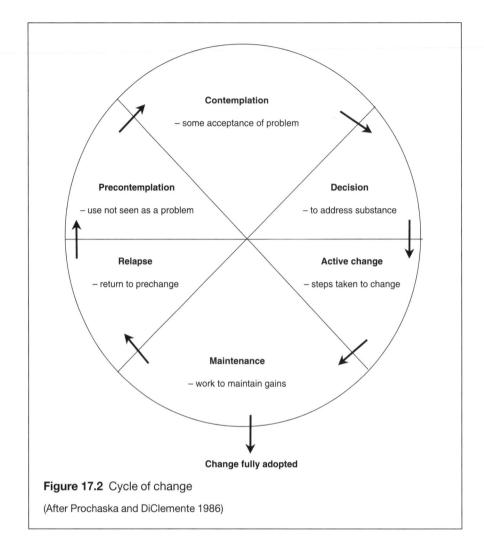

Figure 17.2 Cycle of change

(After Prochaska and DiClemente 1986)

highlighting areas for intervention. Reflecting on the disadvantages and problems associated with use can also serve to move someone on in the cycle of change.

Tools to aid assessment

Decision matrices

One way of enabling clients to explore their reasons for using substances, and identifying the disadvantages of use is through a decision matrix (see Figure 17.3). Clients who have sufficient literacy skills might complete a decision matrix between sessions. For those that do not the decision matrix might be used within sessions or as a framework which the nurse has in mind to guide interaction with the client.

Continuing to drink/use drugs	
Advantages	*Disadvantages*
Helps me to relax	Detrimental to health; e.g. liver damage, abscesses
Like the buzz	
	Electricity cut off
Relieves boredom	
	Have to be involved in crime to get money; risk of prison
Relieves stress	
Helps me to forget/block out feelings	Don't eat
Motivates to get things done	Row with partner
Gives me confidence, helps deal with social situations	Get into fights
	Makes me feel depressed

Stopping drinking/using drugs	
Advantages	*Disadvantages*
Health will improve	Lose drinking friends/social contacts
Can pay off debts	Have to deal with problems
Improve relationship with family	Have to cope with feelings
Feel less paranoid	Boredom
Feel less depressed	Lose identity
Keep out of trouble with the police	
Could get to college	

Figure 17.3 Decision matrix

Diaries

Diaries are further tools to aid assessment. Figure 17.4 is a drink diary. Information gained can provide baseline data about level of consumption, insights into motivations and triggers for drinking, and direct feedback to the client (from himself or herself) about their drinking. Diaries can be adapted to meet the needs of individual clients. For example, a person with depression might rate their mood alongside recording their alcohol intake.

In addition to use in initial-assessment decision, matrices and diaries can be used in ongoing work with clients. Diaries can enable clients to become aware of patterns and associations: for example, someone monitoring mood and alcohol intake may become aware that mood is lower when alcohol is being used. Such insights can enable clients to make informed choices about their use.

Day	How much and what type of alcohol	Times drinking started and ended	Who with	Where drinking took place	Number of units	Thoughts, feelings and consequences	Cost (£s)
Monday							
Tuesday							
Wednesday							
Thursday							
Friday							
Saturday							
Sunday							

Figure 17.4 Drink diary

Diaries are also a means of monitoring progress and, if gains have been made, looking back can provide encouragement to clients. The identification of triggers for substance use, whether this is through using decision matrices or diaries, highlights areas for work. For example, if someone uses as a means of dealing with boredom, work on structuring time would probably be helpful, whereas someone who uses to deal with feelings of tension may benefit from learning relaxation techniques.

Standardized instruments

Standardized instruments are sometimes used as part of the assessment process. Many tools exist, each with a specific purpose. Some are for initial screening; of these, some assess recent use: for example *AUDIT, The Alcohol Use Disorders Identification Test* (Babor *et al.* 1989), assesses use in the past 12 months), whereas others assess lifetime use: for example, MAST, Michigan Alcoholism Screening Test (Selzer 1971), CAGE (King 1986). Some are used to assess the severity of the problem: for example, SADQ, Severity of Alcohol Dependence Questionnaire (Stockwell *et al.* 1983), LDQ, Leeds Dependence Questionnaire (Raistrick *et al.* 1994), ASI, Addiction Severity Index (McLellan *et al.* 1992). Some are used to obtain baseline data so that change over time, or specific treatment outcomes, can be measured: for example, MAP, Maudsley Addiction Profile (Marsden *et al.* 1998).

The reliability and validity of many of these measures in people with mental health problems is unknown. Few tools have been designed specifically for people with a dual diagnosis and those that have, have been developed by researchers in the USA: for example, the DALI, the Dartmouth Assessment of Lifestyle Instrument (Rosenberg *et al.* 1998). It is uncertain how well measures developed in a different cultural context adapt to the British situation.

This section has described the key areas to be addressed in substance misuse assessment. Substance misuse cannot be seen in isolation; aspects of the person's life which have contributed to substance use, and the impact that use has on different aspects of the client's life must also be understood. While this may be desirable, in people with mental health problems disentangling symptomatology can be a challenge, even when a thorough assessment has been conducted.

The following section considers ways in which substance misuse can be addressed. As has been hinted, the separation between assessment and treatment is a rather artificial one. The nurse will continue to make an assessment of the client each time they meet. Moreover, aspects of the assessment process can themselves be interventions. For example, giving information and advice may stimulate behaviour change, and questioning the client may promote reflection on use and identification of areas to be addressed. If the nurse is alert to opportunities that arise he or she can respond in ways that enhance the client's motivation to change.

Approaches to treatment and care

A model for the treatment of people with a dual diagnosis

Treatment of people with a dual diagnosis requires an integration of principles from the mental health and substance misuse fields (Osher and Kofoed 1989). These authors propose a four-staged model: engagement, persuasion, active treatment and relapse prevention. These stages closely reflect Prochaska and DiClemente's (1986) stages of change and provide a framework for thinking about more specific interventions. Motivational interviewing (Miller and Rollnick 1991) and relapse prevention (Marlatt and Gordon 1985) have been linked to the persuasion and relapse prevention stages, respectively. Links with other substance misuse interventions can also be made. Figure 17.5 maps out these relationships. In practice, flexibility is required, movement between the stages can be fluid and aspects of the various interventions are likely to be utilized at each stage. The emphasis here is on substance misuse interventions but these should not be seen in isolation from mental health interventions (for example, medication management) which will also be crucial in working with people with a dual diagnosis. Relapse is usual rather than exceptional in people with substance misuse problems (Prochaska *et al.* 1992) and work with people with a dual diagnosis requires a long-term perspective, often lasting several years (Drake *et al.* 2001).

Stage of change (Prochaska and DiClemente 1986)	Treatment stage (Osher and Kofoed 1983)	Treatment approaches/interventions
Precontemplation	Engagement	Assertive outreach Harm minimization (e.g. needle exchange schemes, substitute prescribing) Brief interventions Information and advice Arrest referral schemes Drug treatment and testing orders
Contemplation decision	Persuasion	Motivational interviewing
Active change	Active treatment	Solution focused therapy Pharmacotherapy – detoxification Supportive counselling Complementary therapies
Maintenance	Relapse prevention	Relapse prevention Pharmacotherapy New skills development Lifestyle changes Structured day programmes Supportive accommodation Residential rehabilitation Individual counselling (substance misuse focused, other specialist focus or generic) Self-help groups, e.g. AA, NA, CARAT schemes

Figure 17.5 Relationships between stages of change, treatment stage and treatment approaches/interventions

Engagement

This stage concerns the development of a therapeutic alliance between client and professional. Persistence may be needed to engage the client and techniques associated with assertive outreach, such as visiting the client at home and helping sort out practical issues (for example, getting benefit payments, dealing with housing difficulties, providing clean injecting equipment) can serve to promote continued contact between client and nurse. Focusing on substance misuse is not the main aim at this stage. However, there may be scope for enhancing motivation and minimizing the harm associated with use.

Harm minimization is a specific approach to working with substance misusers which evolved in the 1980s, primarily in response to concerns about the transmission of HIV through the sharing of injecting equipment. Many substance misusers may not want, or may be unable to achieve abstinence, so the goal is to reduce associated harm – to the person themselves, their family and friends, and the wider society.

A key component of harm minimization is providing information and advice. This might include: safer injecting techniques, transmission routes of blood-borne infections, sexual health issues, recommended safe drinking limits, and the effects that various substances can have on physical and mental health. It is hoped that the client will respond by using substances in a safer way and take steps to live a more healthy lifestyle (for example, using condoms, having a hepatitis B vaccine). Needle exchange schemes have played an important part in this approach by giving out clean injecting equipment and providing for its safe disposal. Substitute prescribing on a maintenance basis (for example, methadone for heroin) has been another strategy. People can also be encouraged to use substances more safely by reducing the quantity and/or frequency of use, changing the route of administration (for example, from injecting to smoking), and reducing the intake of additional substances (for example, benzodiazepines and alcohol).

Although the goal for this stage is engagement, the nurse and client may only meet on one or two occasions. 'Minimal' or 'brief' interventions (Alcohol Concern 1997) in which verbal and/or written information and advice about substance misuse is given may be appropriate (there is some overlap between brief interventions and harm minimization). The acronym FRAMES has been used to summarize the elements of brief interventions.

F – *feedback* of current status and risk.
R – emphasis on the client having *responsibility* for change.
A – *advice* to change.
M – a *menu* of change options.
E – an *empathic* manner.
S – reinforcing the client's *self-efficacy*.

Brief interventions have been shown to be particularly effective for people with alcohol problems in the primary care setting but can be used more widely. Having received information, clients can make choices about their use, and their motivation to change may be influenced (Miller and Rollnick 1991).

In recent years there has been an increased emphasis on the criminal justice system encouraging drug users to engage with services. Arrest referral schemes aim to identify drug users when they have been arrested. They are assessed while in police custody and encouraged to access treatment from their local substance misuse service. A rather more coercive approach is a Drug Treatment and Testing Order (DTTO). This is a community sentence which can be issued by a court. Attendance at a treatment programme for 20 hours each week, regular drug testing and court reviews are required. Having this option, rather than, say, a custodial sentence, may push the person into thinking about change when they might not otherwise have done so (Turnbull *et al.* 2000).

Persuasion

In this stage the aim is to persuade the client that change would be desirable. Motivational interviewing (MI) is the key intervention (Miller and Rollnick 2002). The five principles of MI are to: express empathy, develop discrepancy, avoid argumentation, roll with resistance, and support self-efficacy. Specific techniques that might be used to develop discrepancy and nudge the person towards a decision to change include:

- education about substances and the potential problems which they may cause;
- re-framing past events and considering the role substance misuse may have had (for example, the possibility that a deterioration in mental state was triggered by substance misuse);
- feeding back objective test results (for example, liver function tests); and
- completing decision matrices.

Active treatment

In this stage the client and nurse identify and pursue goals. It is important that the goals are realistic. Achieving small goals can encourage the client and help to produce a sense of self-efficacy. Not achieving can create a sense of failure and trigger a return to precontemplation or contemplation stages. A solution-focused approach can be beneficial as it avoids emphasizing problems, seeks to enhance the client's sense of their own competence and ensures that he or she receives positive feedback (for example, Berg and Miller 1992; Berg and Reuss 1997).

Many people will decide to stop using substances altogether and some are able to gradually decrease use themselves. Others, however, will need pharmacological interventions to enable them to detoxify safely. Some people will detoxify in the community but others will require inpatient admission. Factors influencing this decision include: the number and quantity of substances being used, previous withdrawal experiences, physical and mental health, availability of support in the community, family responsibilities (for example, childcare), and personal preference. Maintaining the client's safety is essential. People who are using dangerous combinations of substances, have experienced withdrawal seizures, delirium tremens or whose physical health is very poor must be admitted to hospital. For people whose mental health tends to be unstable this may also be the best option, and once detoxified, time in an inpatient setting can allow a more thorough mental state assessment to be made.

Detoxification from opiates is usually undertaken by prescribing methadone linctus. An initial dose comparable to the quantity of illicit heroin (or other substance) being used is identified. The rate of reduction will vary from person to person. For community treatment it is recommended that methadone consumption is supervised by a professional for at least three months (DH 1999b). Continued supervision may be desirable for people whose mental health is unstable. Newer drugs which are being used in the detoxification of opiate users are buprenorphine (an opioid) and lofexidine (not an opioid but effective in the management of withdrawal symptoms).

Benzodiazepine detoxification is achieved by prescribing diazepam, a long-acting benzodiazepine, at an equivalent dose to the drug which was being taken and then reducing the dose. The reduction rate can be more rapid at the beginning, but clients are often extremely anxious about detoxification. A slow gradual reduction, which the client feels is achievable, is preferable to a more rapid one which makes the client overly anxious and may result in them obtaining illicit supplies.

Alcohol detoxification is achieved by prescribing a reducing regimen of a long-acting benzodiazepine (diazepam or chlordiazepoxide) over a period of about a week. Close monitoring of the client is required because of the risks if he or she drinks alcohol while taking benzodiazepines, and because of the severe complications that can be associated with withdrawal (for example, seizures).

People using stimulants, cannabis or ecstasy do not need pharmacological interventions to stop using. However, anti-depressants can be useful for people who have been using crack and cocaine, as low mood can persist for many weeks.

Clients may need high levels of support during detoxification, and those completing detoxification in inpatient settings are likely to feel well supported, with staff on hand and peer encouragement. For those detoxifying in the community the process may be more difficult. As well as making use of facilities accessible through substance misuse services (for example, supportive counselling and complementary therapies such as auricular acupuncture and shiatzu massage) enlisting the support of family and/or friends can be important.

Detoxification should not be seen in isolation. Coming off drugs is said to be the easy part, it is staying off that is more difficult. This will not be achieved unless the client has acquired new skills and made lifestyle changes. Work on these areas may run in parallel with the detoxification process and will certainly need to continue after.

Relapse prevention

In this stage it is assumed that change has been achieved and the aim is to ensure that gains which have been made are maintained. For people with mental health problems the notion of relapse is broader than a return to problematic substance misuse. They may also experience a relapse of their mental illness. For some people the two will be interrelated.

A specific approach for working with clients to prevent relapse has been developed by Marlatt and Gordon (1985). It uses cognitive behavioural strategies and the development of lifestyle change as its bases. The aim is to identify high-risk situations or triggers and develop strategies for coping with them without using substances. Effective coping enhances the person's sense of self-control. If substance use does occur this is seen as a lapse or slip-up which can be overcome, and from which learning can take place. In terms of Prochaska and DiClemente's (1986) model, the person returns to the active treatment stage rather than precontemplation, or contemplation. Such a perspective contrasts with the sense of failure and hopelessness which can be engendered if the client sees drinking or using drugs as a relapse which has put them 'back to square one'.

Situations/triggers for relapse are likely to be many and varied. These include: negative emotional states (for example, anger, anxiety, depression, boredom), positive emotional states (for example, celebrations), inter-personal conflicts (for example, with partner, family members, employer), social pressures (for example, at a party) and associations with particular places, people, times/dates or situations. Tools such as diaries and decision matrices can help clients identify their triggers. With the information gained strategies can be developed for dealing with these.

In conjunction with this approach to relapse prevention pharmaco-logical interventions may be beneficial. For people with opiate problems naltrexone can be helpful as it blocks the effects of opiates. Naltrexone has also been shown to reduce craving in drinkers. However, acamprosate is more commonly used for this purpose. Disulfiram (antabuse) acts as a deterrent to drinking as adverse consequences are experienced if alcohol is consumed (flushing, headache, palpitations, nausea and vomiting – in large amounts cardiac arrhythmias, hypotension and collapse may occur).

While preventing relapse is at the heart of a person's recovery or rehabilitation new skills and lifestyle changes will also be needed. A range of agencies may play a part in the person's rehabilitation and within them various methods might be used (for example, individual counselling, group work, skills training, recreational activities). Some people will choose community options, for example, a structured day programme or self-help group (such as Alcoholics Anonymous (AA) or Narcotics Anonymous (NA)). Others may decide that a residential project would better meet their needs. These range from supported hostel accommodation to more intensive therapeutic programmes. Within these there will be a variety of care philosophies – some have a religious basis, some are run on therapeutic community lines and some follow the '12 steps' of AA/NA. Alongside a focus on substance misuse, clients may engage in new activities (for example, going to a gym or attending an art class) and develop vocational skills (for example, computing). Clients may also benefit from services which address more specific problems (for example, childhood sexual abuse, bereavement issues). A social services community care assessor/care manager may work with the client to develop an ongoing treatment package. They have access to the finances required for some services.

With the increased emphasis on provision for drug users being made through the criminal justice system treatment can be accessed in prison through CARAT – counselling, assessment, referral, advice and throughcare – schemes. These provide interventions pertinent to each treatment stage.

Each client is different and a service which is helpful for one person may not be for the next. Some clients will attend several projects, others may not need further specialist input at all. At present, few projects are specifically set up for people with a dual diagnosis. While some mainstream substance misuse services are willing to work with this group their programme(s) may not be flexible enough to meet clients' needs. Some services, particularly residential projects, exclude people who have a severe mental health problem; and people with a history of self-harm, suicide attempts or violence are also likely to be excluded.

Throughout the treatment process clients may be involved with several different agencies. Services need to work together to find ways of sharing information so that clients can access help without having to negotiate unnecessary barriers. While there is an increasing recognition of this, the reality is often far from it, as Ken's experience illustrates.

Case study: Ken

Ken has an alcohol problem and a severe depressive disorder for which he has regular contact with his community mental health nurse (CMHN) and consultant psychiatrist. Ken decided that he wanted to stop drinking so was referred to the substance misuse team. The substance misuse nurse obtained detailed information about Ken's drinking from him but, with his permission, obtained other information from the mental health team. After a period working with the substance misuse team Ken became abstinent from alcohol and decided that he could benefit from a specialist dual-diagnosis day programme. Because this programme required social services community care funding Ken was referred to that team. He was assessed by them and funding was made available. He was then referred to the dual-diagnosis programme and assessed by the project staff there. Unfortunately, they felt unable to accept him. Although disappointed, Ken decided to approach another service that ran an alcohol day programme. They too wanted to assess him. This time Ken was accepted and he successfully completed the programme.

Ken is highly motivated and felt able to attend each of the assessment appointments. Many people with mental health problems would, or could, not have done so. Although services need to ensure that the people accessing them meet their criteria clients cannot be expected to attend repeated assessments in the way that Ken was. Unless protocols for sharing information, while maintaining client confidentiality, are developed the 'seamless service' advocated in the NHS Plan (DH 2000) will not be achieved.

Case study: Ray

To illustrate some of the treatment interventions, which can be used with people with a dual diagnosis, Ray's case is considered further.

Ray was referred to the substance misuse team from an inpatient psychiatric ward where he had been admitted following a deterioration in his mental state. This had stabilized and it was suggested that he might benefit from input for his substance misuse. The nurse visited him on the ward to begin the engagement process and gain some assessment information. Ray appeared open to looking at his use. Confidentiality was discussed and Ray was happy for information to be shared between the substance misuse and mental health teams, and his GP. He talked openly about his use.

He had recently been in trouble with the police and been in a fight in which he was badly assaulted. He said he had had enough of this sort of thing and wanted to cut down his drinking. From the outset the nurse sought to elicit such change talk to build his motivation. In order to maximize the chances of engaging Ray, initial sessions were held on the ward. Information to supplement that obtained by the substance misuse nurse was sought from Ray's CMHN and GP. An important early intervention was giving Ray information about units of alcohol and the possible effects that substance misuse could have on his physical and mental health as his knowledge base was low. Results of blood tests were obtained and showed abnormalities consistent with heavy drinking. These were explained to Ray and appeared to further motivate him. In the week following his hospital discharge Ray managed to remain abstinent from alcohol for four days. On each of those days he cooked himself a meal and began an exercise regimen. He was given positive feedback regarding this. Some discussion followed about what had been different on these days to those when he drank. Ray was unsure and it was suggested that he complete drink diaries which might provide some insights. Completing the diaries made Ray realize how much he was drinking and the amount of money he was spending on alcohol – he was surprised at this. They also enabled him to identify risk situations. These included: having money, one particular friend who often suggested they go to the pub, and boredom.

During one session Ray and the nurse together worked on completing a decision matrix. Among the potential advantages of stopping use were: the possibility of resuming a relationship with a past girlfriend (this ended because of his substance use), no longer ending up with cuts and bruises from falling or getting into fights when drunk, staying out of trouble with the police, getting some training to equip him for work, and having money to pay off his debts and eventually spend on things he wants, such as new clothes.

As time progressed, Ray started to attend appointments at the substance misuse team. He continued to complete drink diaries and these were discussed in sessions. Ray's drinking and drug use fluctuated. Some weeks he managed to remain completely abstinent and on others he would drink most days and use drugs if they were available. During the period after his mother's death he drank heavily for over two months. Ray came to recognize that when he was using more drugs he tended to be more paranoid. He also reported that when he was not drinking he felt much better, physically and emotionally.

Ray had often talked about attending a local alcohol agency which had a drop-in facility but he seemed unable to get there so the nurse went with him. After spasmodic attendance for a period he began attending regularly. Sometimes he would attend groups there too. This helped Ray to structure his time and his drinking reduced further. He increased contact with his brother and sister and enjoyed spending time with his nephews. The alcohol project ran a six-week structured day programme which required people to be abstinent during the course. Sessions were included on alcohol and health, assertiveness, dealing with emotions, problem solving and relapse prevention. Ray thought this would be helpful. It took him several months before he had minimized his drinking to a level where he realistically thought he could be abstinent for six weeks. However, he achieved this and is now attending the programme. He has also started looking for vocational courses which he might begin afterwards and has commenced acamprosate, a drug which helps to deal with craving. Ray is doing very well and there have been marked changes in his substance use and lifestyle over the past two years. However, (re)lapse is always a possibility. If/when he does lapse, it will be important to see this as a learning experience which can be overcome. In the meantime the professionals involved in his care continue to liaise and seek to provide a coordinated approach to his care.

Meeting the needs of families and carers

Despite the breakdown in relationships which can be associated with substance misuse many users do live with a partner, family or friends. This can often be a confusing and distressing experience for them. Some of these people will be actively involved in the care and treatment of the user and need specific knowledge for taking on this responsibility. Substance misuse services have not traditionally seen work with families as a core part of their remit, but even if clients do not want their family involved in their care and treatment, information can be provided (for example, about substances, their effects and complications, and the nature of care and treatment) without compromising the nurse–client relationship. Information should also be given about national organizations which are specifically set up to provide family and carer support. These organizations provide telephone helplines and some hold local meetings. Al-Anon and Al-Ateen (both on 020 7403 0888) work with people in contact with problem drinkers, the latter is targeted at teenagers, and Families Anonymous (020 7498 4680) focuses on people in contact with drug users. The *NSF for Mental Health* makes it clear that services involved with people with serious mental illness must attend to the needs of carers. If the person they are caring for has a substance misuse problem this includes meeting needs associated with this.

Older people

There is a tendency to think of substance misuse as an issue mainly concerned with younger people. Many people do stop using substances as they get older but some do not and others develop problems with substances in later life. There is no specific focus on substance misuse in the *NSF for Older People* (DH 2001a) but this group have been identified as a 'special population' in the Health Advisory Service dual diagnosis standards (Abdulrahim 2001). These note the need for older people's services to tackle misuse of alcohol, analgesics and tranquillizers and highlight the risk of falls in this population. Reducing falls is a *NSF for Older People* standard. Another area highlighted in the *NSF for Older People* is the effective and safe use of medication. Given that older people tend to be prescribed a range of medications, the possible interaction of alcohol and other illicit drugs with these needs to be considered.

Substance misuse, particularly alcohol, may be a factor in the presentation of several conditions which are common in elderly people, for example, memory problems, confusion and depression. Some disorders associated with old age such as brain disease or depressive illness might be factors which trigger drinking.

Case study: Joan

The following case study highlights some of the issues to consider when an older person has a drink problem.

Joan was a sprightly 74-year-old Scottish woman who had lived in London for many years. She approached the substance misuse service for help with her drinking, but found attending a daunting prospect. At the self-referral clinic the waiting area was crowded with an array of drug users and drinkers. Joan had to wait for some time before being seen and found the environment intimidating.

It appeared that there were several factors contributing to Joan's drinking. First, she was lonely. Her husband had died some years earlier and although the marriage had not been happy, Joan had spent several years being his carer as his health had been poor. Joan's sisters, with whom she had a good relationship, lived in Scotland. She had two daughters, one lived locally, the other about 60 miles away. The one living nearby had 'problems of her own'. Rather than being a support she was more of a burden. She would phone Joan late at night and spend an hour or more talking about her difficulties. Joan felt unable to terminate the conversations and was reluctant to involve her other daughter as she had a family to look after, 'a life of her own', and was preparing to move abroad. Joan's dog, who had been with her for many years, had recently died. She felt an intense sense of loss and not having the dog to take for a walk meant that her familiar routine was lost.

Moreover, Joan lived in a ground-floor flat and without the dog felt fearful for her safety, and was not sleeping well. Her flat was on an estate where many other older people were living. Joan was younger and less frail than the others so they looked to her for help and support. While Joan was willing to help people out, at times their demands seemed excessive and she found it difficult to refuse their requests.

Joan could go for several weeks and not drink at all but when her situation got on top of her she would buy a bottle of Scotch with the intention of having a glass or two, but once she started it was difficult to stop. It was not unusual for her to drink over half a litre of Scotch. The next morning she would feel physically unwell and guilty about her drinking. One way of dealing with this was to drink again, and in this way a binge would begin. When drinking heavily Joan would not eat. During one episode of heavy drinking Joan fell and was found on the floor by a relative who happened to be in the area and had called to see her. Fortunately, she was not badly hurt. On some occasions when Joan had been drinking heavily her GP would prescribe diazepam so that she could detoxify safely. Joan knew the dangers of taking diazepam and drinking so if she felt unable to maintain abstinence from alcohol she would not take the diazepam. This had resulted in her acquiring a store of diazepam. Sometimes when Joan had been drinking for a few days she would become depressed and feel suicidal. The daughter that lived nearby would usually become involved at these times. She contacted the mental health services and insisted that her mother be admitted to hospital. Joan was admitted to the elderly mental illness ward on a number of occasions. Once she had detoxified from alcohol her depression lifted and she returned home. As she did not have a formal psychiatric diagnosis she was not followed up by the mental health team but the substance misuse team nurse did keep in contact with her.

While Joan's circumstances are unique to her, many features of her situation are common to other people who develop drink problems in later life. Lack of routine or day-time structure, bereavement, loneliness, a sense that life is coming to an end and has little to offer can all be factors. Nurses need to be alert to the possibility of substance misuse being a factor in the presentation of older people and not think of it only as a younger person's problem. While substance misuse services may have a role to play, older people should be able to obtain help in a setting which is easily accessible and non-threatening to them. After her initial presentation Joan was seen at a clinic based at the local hospital and, on some occasions, she was seen at home.

Conclusion

This chapter has provided an overview of drug and alcohol use focusing on use by people with mental health problems. Concepts and terminology relating to substance misuse and dual diagnosis were explored. Information was provided about commonly misused substances, their mode of use, effects and complications as a basis for moving on to consider assessment. A staged model of treatment was described and interventions which might be used at each stage identified. Some attention has been paid to areas that relate to the NSFs for mental health and older people: the difficulties which people with a dual diagnosis may have in accessing service provision, the relationship between substance misuse and suicide, the needs of families and carers, and substance misuse in older people.

Although substance misuse was identified within the *NSF for Mental Health* some people thought that it was given insufficient attention. The Department of Health has now issued specific guidance on dual diagnosis (DH 2002a) and the extent to which local services are implementing it is being assessed through mechanisms, which monitor progress towards *NSF for Mental Health* and *NHS Plan* (DH 2000) standards. Dual diagnosis is also an area that is being recognized in other reports and policy developments, for example, the *National Suicide Prevention Strategy* (DH 2002c). Working with people who misuse substances can no longer be seen as a specialist area, it is a key aspect of mental health care and treatment and is the responsibility of all mental health professionals.

In summary, the main points of this chapter are:

- Substance misuse is common in people with mental health problems and all mental health professionals need knowledge and skills in this area.

- Dual diagnosis is a broad concept, which encompasses a wide range of people with varying levels of mental illness and substance use.

- The relationship between psychiatric illness and substance misuse is complex.

- A range of physical, psychiatric, interpersonal, social and legal complications can be associated with substance misuse.

- A variety of risks are associated with substance misuse, including suicide and violence.

- Assessment of substance misuse should be integral to mental health assessments.

- A client's readiness to change should guide treatment interventions.

- Working with people with a dual diagnosis requires flexibility and a long-term perspective.

- Attention should be given to the needs of families and carers.

- Substance misuse may occur at any age in a person's life.

- The various services in contact with people with a dual diagnosis need to develop partnership working so that, as far as possible, the client's experience is of seamless care provision.

Acknowledgement

Thanks to colleagues at South London and Maudsley Trust who commented on earlier drafts of the chapter.

Questions for reflection and discussion

1   List the substances you have used over the past few days and think about your reasons for using them.

2   Identify any ethical issues which might be encountered when working with people with a dual diagnosis.

3   Under what circumstances might you decide to break client confidentiality?

4   Look back at Ray's situation, identify the risks to Ray himself and the risks he may pose to others and consider strategies which might be put in place to manage these risks.

5   Look back at Joan's situation and identify possible interventions for her future care and treatment.

Annotated bibliography

- Banerjee, S., Clancy, C. and Crome, I. (eds) (2002) *Co-existing Problems of Mental Disorder and Substance Misuse (dual diagnosis): An Information Manual.* London: Royal College of Psychiatrists Research Unit. This information manual was written to accompany the DH Dual Diagnosis Good Practice Guide. It provides an overview of current thinking about dual diagnosis and is targeted at newcomers to the field as well as more experienced practitioners. It is organized into seven sections: conceptual and theoretical issues, problems in service provision, ethical issues and the Mental Health Act, assessment, interventions, organizational issues and information sources. The manual is available from the Royal College of Psychiatrists via their website www.rcpsych.ac.uk/cru

- Edwards, G., Marshall, E. J. and Cook, C.C. (2003) *The Treatment of Drinking Problems* (4th edn). Cambridge: Cambridge University Press. This is a comprehensive and detailed textbook on drinking problems which is targeted at clinicians.

- Department of Health (1999b) *Drug Misuse and Dependence – Guidelines on Clinical Management.* London: The Stationery Office. Although written with doctors in mind these guidelines are an easy read and provide information that will be valuable to anyone working with substance misusers. The guidelines are evidence based and identify current thinking on good clinical practice.

- Drugscope (2001) *Drug Abuse Briefing.* London: Drugscope. This briefing provides detailed information about the range of substances which can be misused. It covers their legal status, production and supply, prevalence, licit and illicit use, price and the effect of short- and long-term use.

• Other useful sources of information are 'Frank', formerly the National Drugs Helpline 0800 776600 and the Drugscope and Alcohol Concern websites (www.drugscope.org.uk and www.alcoholconcern.org.uk). Both provide up-to-date information for professionals and the public.

References

Abdulrahim, D. (2001) *Substance Misuse and Mental Health Co-Morbidity (Dual Diagnosis): Standards for Mental Health Services.* London: The Health Advisory Service.

Alcohol Concern (1997) *Brief Intervention Guidelines.* London: Alcohol Concern.

Alcohol Concern (2000) *Britain's Ruin?* London: Alcohol Concern.

American Psychiatric Association (1994) *Diagnostic and Statistical Manual of Mental Disorders.* Washington, DC: American Psychiatric Association.

Arseneault, L., Cannon, M., Poulton, R. *et al.* (2002) Cannabis use in adolescence and risk for adult psychosis: longitudinal prospective study, *British Medical Journal* **325**: 1212–13.

Babor, T., de la Fuente, J., Saunders, J. and Grant, M. (1989) *AUDIT, The Alcohol Use Disorders Identification Test: Guidelines for Use in Primary Care.* Geneva: World Health Organization.

Banerjee, S., Clancy, C. and Crome, I. (eds) (2002) *Co-existing Problems of Mental Disorder and Substance Misuse (dual diagnosis): An information manual.* London: Royal College of Psychiatrists Research Unit.

Bear, Z., Griffiths, R. and Pearson, B. (2000) *Childhood Sexual Abuse and Substance Use.* London: The Centre for Research on Drugs and Health Behaviour.

Berg, I.K. and Miller, S. (1992) *Working with the Problem Drinker: A Solution Focused Approach.* New York: Norton.

Berg, I.K. and Reuss, N. (1997) *Solutions Step by Step: A Substance Abuse Treatment Manual.* New York: Norton & Wylie.

Crome, I. (1999) Substance misuse and psychiatric co-morbidity: towards improved service provision, *Drugs: Education, Prevention and Policy* **6**: 151–74.

Department of Health (1995) *Sensible Drinking.* London: Department of Health.

Department of Health (1999a) *National Service Framework for Mental Health.* London: Department of Health.

Department of Health (1999b) *Drug Misuse and Dependence – Guidelines on Clinical Management.* London: The Stationery Office.

Department of Health (2000) *The NHS Plan.* London: The Stationery Office.

Department of Health (2001a) *National Service Framework for Older People.* London: Department of Health.

Department of Health (2001b) *Safety First: Five-Year Report of the National Confidential Inquiry into Suicide and Homicide by People With Mental Illness.* London: Department of Health.

Department of Health (2002a) *Mental Health Policy Implementation Guide: Dual Diagnosis Good Practice Guide.* London: Department of Health.

Department of Health (2002b) *Models of Care for Substance Misuse Treatment.* London: Department of Health.

Department of Health (2002c) *National Suicide Prevention Strategy for England.* London: Department of Health.

Drake, R.E., Bartels, S.J., Teague, G.B., Noordsky, D.L. and Clark, R.E. (1993) Treatment of substance abuse in severely mentally ill patients, *Journal of Nervous and Mental Disease* **18**: 606–11.

Drake, R.E., Noorsdy, D.L. and Ackerson, T. (1995) Integrating mental health and substance abuse treatments for persons with chronic mental disorders: a model, in A. Lehman and L. Dixon (eds) *Double Jeopardy.* Chur: Switzerland: Harwood Academic Press.

Drake, R., Essock, S., Shaner, A. *et al.* (2001) Implementing dual diagnosis services for clients with severe mental illness, *Psychiatric Services* **52**: 469–76.

Gossop, M., Marsden, J. and Stewart, D. (2001) *NTORS After Five Years: The National Treatment Outcome Research Study.* London: National Addiction Centre.

Gournay, K., Sandford, T., Johnson, G. and Thornicroft, G. (1997) Dual diagnosis of severe mental health problems and substance abuse/dependence: a major priority for mental health nursing, *Journal of Psychiatric and Mental Health Nursing* **4**: 89–95.

Johns, A. (2001) Psychiatric effects of cannabis, *British Journal of Psychiatry* **178**: 116–22.

King, M. (1986) At risk drinking among general practice attenders: validation of the CAGE questionnaire, *Psychological Medicine* **16**: 213–17.

Kipping, C. (1999) Dual diagnosis: meeting clients' needs, *Mental Health Practice* **3**: 10–15.

Krauz, M. (1996) Old problems – new perspectives, *European Addiction Research* **2**: 1–2.

Ley, A., Jeffery, D.P., McLaren, S. and Siegfried, N. (2002) Treatment programmes for people with severe mental illness and substance misuse, in *The Cochrane Library* (Issue 2) Oxford: Update Software.

Marlatt, G.A. and Gordon, J.R. (1985) *Relapse Prevention: Maintenance Strategies in the Treatment of Addictive Behaviours.* New York: Guilford Press.

Marsden, J., Gossop, M., Stewart, D. *et al.* (1998) The Maudsley Addiction Profile (MAP): A brief instrument for assessing treatment outcome, *Addiction* **93**, 1857–67.

McLellan, T., Luborsky, L., Cacciola, J. and Fureman, I. (1992) The fifth edition of the Addiction Severity Index: cautions, additions and normative data, *Journal of Substance Abuse Treatment* **9**: 461–80.

Meltzer, H., Lader, D., Corbin, T. *et al.* (2002) *Non-Fatal Suicidal Behaviour Among Adults Aged 16–74 in Great Britain.* London: The Stationery Office.

Miller, W. and Rollnick, S. (2002) *Motivational Interviewing: Preparing People to Change Addictive Behaviour* (2nd edn). New York: Guilford Press.

Osher, F.C. and Drake, R.E. (1996) Reversing a history of unmet needs: approaches to care for persons with co-occurring addictive and mental disorders, *American Journal of Orthopsychiatry* **66**: 4–11.

Osher, F. and Kofoed, L. (1989) Treatment of patients with psychiatric and psychoactive substance abuse disorders, *Hospital and Community Psychiatry* **40**: 1025–30.

Phillips, P. and Johnson, S. (2001) How does drug and alcohol misuse develop among people with psychotic illness? A literature review, *Social Psychiatry and Psychiatric Epidemiology* **36**: 269–76.

Prochaska, J. and DiClemente, C. (1986) Towards a comprehensive model of change, in W. Miller and N. Heather (eds) *Treating Addictive Behaviours: Processes of Change*. New York: Plenum.

Prochaska, J., DiClemente, C. and Nocross, J. (1992) In search of how people change: applications to addictive behaviours, *American Psychologist* **47**: 1102–12.

Raistrick, D., Bradshaw, J., Tober, G. *et al.* (1994) Development of the Leeds Dependency Questionnaire (LDQ): a questionnaire to measure alcohol and opiate dependence in the context of a treatment evaluation package, *Addiction* **89**: 563–72.

Rorstad, P. and Checkinski, K. (1996) *Dual Diagnosis: Facing the Challenge*. Kenley: Wynne Howard.

Rosenberg, S., Drake, R., Wolford, G. *et al.* (1998) Dartmouth Assessment of Lifestyle Instrument (DALI): A substance use disorder screen for people with severe mental illness, *American Journal of Psychiatry* **155**: 232–8.

Ryrie, I. (2000) Co-existant substance use and psychiatric disorders, in C. Gamble and G. Brennan (eds) *Working with Serious Mental Illness: A Manual for Clinical Practice*. London: Bailliere Tindall.

Selzer, M. (1971) The Michigan alcoholism screening test, *American Journal of Psychiatry* **127**: 1653–8.

Siney, C. (1999) *Pregnancy and Drug Misuse*. Hale: Books for Midwives Press.

Stockwell, T., Murphy, D. and Hodgson, R. (1983) The severity of alcohol dependence questionnaire: its use, reliability and validity, *British Journal of Addiction* **78**: 145–55.

Turnbull, P.J., McSweeney, T., Webster, R., Edmunds, M. and Hough, M. (2000) *Drug Treatment and Testing Orders: Final Evaluation Report*. London: Home Office.

Ward, M. and Applin, C. (1998) *The Unlearned Lesson*. London: Wynne Howard.

Webster, R. (1999) *Working with Black Crack Users in a Crisis Setting: The City Roads Experience*. London: City Roads.

World Health Organization (1992) *ICD-10 Classification of Mental and Behavioural Disorders*. Geneva: World Health Organization.

Zammit, S., Allebeck, P., Andreasson, S., Lundberg, I. and Lewis, G. (2002) Self reported cannabis use as a risk factor for schizophrenia in Swedish conscripts of 1969: historical cohort study, *British Medical Journal* **325**: 1199–203.

18

Mental health problems in childhood and adolescence

Robin Basu

Chapter overview

Child and adolescent psychiatry is concerned with the assessment and treatment of children's behavioural and emotional problems. In childhood, in the majority of disorders the symptoms shown by a child only become significant if these are of unusual intensity or duration, but are otherwise seen in most children at some point of their development.

In pre-school children, 7 per cent of children show moderate to severe problems and double that figure show milder problems. One of the most significant epidemiological studies was carried out in the 1960s by Rutter *et al.* (1970). The design and finding of this study have withstood the test of time. Rutter studied the 10- and 11-year-old population of the Isle of Wight. The estimated prevalence of psychiatric disorder in this group was 6.8 of which, 4 per cent were conduct and mixed disorders and 2.5 per cent emotional disorders. A survey of 1000 13-and 14-year-olds in Blackborough showed that disorders of a severity needing referrals to a clinic occurred in 21 per cent of boys and 14 per cent of girls. Studies in Oslo by Lavik (1977) and Boyle *et al.* 1987 show similar prevalence rates in adolescents.

The bulk of this chapter is devoted to describing the manifestations of mental distress and disorder in childhood and adolescence that nurses may encounter in the course of their work in a variety of practice settings. The chapter begins, however, with a discussion of those aspects of assessment that are particularly relevant when working with children and adolescents, since a full and comprehensive assessment is a prerequisite to successful treatment; readers are referred also to Chapters 7 and 8 of this book for a detailed consideration of the process of assessment.

Later sections of the chapter discuss principles of treatment, prevention of childhood psychiatric disorders and the views of users of child and adolescent psychiatric services. The importance of detection and skilled management of childhood and adolescent psychiatric disorders in the primary care setting is emphasized, since general practitioners (GPs) and other primary health care professionals are well placed to implement preventive interventions and manage less severe psychological problems in a non-stigmatizing care environment. To conclude, the chapter considers the nurses' role in the child and adolescent mental health field in the UK and how this may develop in the light of the *National Service Framework for Mental Health* (DH 1999).

In summary this chapter covers:

- Assessment.
- Manifestations of mental health problems in childhood, specifically:
    - pre-school problems;
    - hyperactivity;
    - autistic disordes;
    - conduct disorders;
    - emotional disorders of childhood;
    - disorders of social functioning;
    - elimination disorders;
    - child maltreatment;
    - Tourette's syndrome.
- Psychiatric disorders in adolescence, specifically:
    - obsessive compulsive disorder;
    - suicide and deliberate self-harm.
- Psychiatric disorders in childhood:
    - major affective disorders;
    - adolescent schizophrenia;
    - substance misuse in adolescence;
    - eating disorders.
- Somatizing in children and adolescence.
- Treatment of child and adolescent psychiatry.
- Prevention of child psychiatric disorders.
- Child and adolescent mental health problems in primary care.
- The nurses' role in child and adolescent services.

Classification of child and adolescent psychiatric disorders

The present system of classification for child and adolescent psychiatric disorders has focused primarily on symptomatology rather than aetiology. In child psychiatry, organic disorders in which psychiatric disorders arise secondary to physical causes are rare. Multi-axial classification takes into account different aspects of a patient's disorder and classifies the disorder along different axes giving a composite picture of the condition. The commonly used axes are:

- clinical psychiatric condition;
- intellectual level;
- specific delays in development;
- any medical conditions;
- abnormal psychosocial situation.

Classification should not be an end in itself and to be effective should be clinically relevant and aid communication on possible aetiology, treatment and prognosis classification.

The two main systems in use are the International Classification of Diseases (ICD) of the World Health Organization and the Statistical Manual (DSM) of the American Psychiatric Association. The DSM-IV and the ICD-10 provide clear descriptive criteria that must be met before a diagnosis can be made. The ICD-10 classification of Behavioural and Emotional Disorders with onset usually occurring in childhood and adolescents is coded separately (F90–F98) (see Table 18.1).

Assessment

It is essential to undertake a full and comprehensive assessment before embarking on treatment of the problems. It may take more than one meeting before an assessment is completed. Assessments should be carefully planned and time allowed to explore with the child and family their attitude to the referral. Most clinicians recommend a semi-structured approach as long as the relevant details of the history are completed.

The assessment process is complex and can be bewildering to patients with no previous experience of the process. At the onset, the nature, purpose and the length of the interview need to be clarified. Children and families need to be informed about their rights to confidentiality and any conditions under which you would have to disclose information obtained during the interview. There is no set format for interviewing families and assessment may involve interviewing the whole family, individual members or the parents and child separately.

The nature of the interview with the child will depend on the child's developmental age and maturity. With young children, this may involve free play, observation and drawing. Older adolescents often express a wish to be seen on their own. There are statutory obligations to report disclosure of abuse in line with national and local child protection procedures. It is important to keep the child's needs foremost in the mind.

The initial assessment may indicate a need for the collection of further information from other agencies who have contact with the family or child, and consent needs to be sought before such contact can be made. Decisions about psychometric testing, physical examination and laboratory tests need to be considered.

Table 18.1 F90–F98 Diagnostic Criteria for Research into Mental Disorders in Childhood and Adolescence

F90 *Hyperkinetic disorders*

Examples of these are:
F90.0 – Disturbance of activity and attention
F90.1 – Hyperkinetic conduct disorder

F91 *Conduct disorder*

Examples of these are:
F91.0 – Conduct disorder confined to the family context
F91.1 – Unsocialized conduct disorder
F91.2 – Socialized conduct disorder
F91.3 – Oppositional defiant disorder

F92 *Mixed disorders of conduct and emotions*

An example of this is:
F92.0 – Depressive conduct disorder

F93 *Emotional disorders with onset specific to childhood*

Examples of these are:
F93.0 – Separation anxiety disorder of childhood
F93.1 – Phobic anxiety disorder of childhood
F93.2 – Social anxiety disorder of childhood
F93.3 – Sibling rivalry disorder

F94 *Disorders of social functioning with onset specific to childhood and adolescence*

F94.0 – Elective mutism
F94.1 – Reactive attachment disorder of childhood
F94.2 – Disinhibited attachment disorder of childhood

F95 *Tic disorders*

F95.0 – Transient tic disorder
F95.1 – Chronic motor or vocal tic disorder
F95.2 – Combined vocal and multiple motor tic disorder (Gilles de la Tourette's syndrome)

F98 *Other behavioural and emotional disorders with onset usually occurring in childhood and adolescence.*

(After ICD-10, WHO 1993)

Issues to be addressed in a comprehensive assessment interview are listed in Figure 18.1.

Mental health problems in childhood

Pre-school problems

Pre-school problems such as sleep problems, tantrums and feeding problems are relatively common. Moderate to severe behavioural problems have been

History of presenting complaint

Nature of the problem, onset, frequency, duration
Beliefs of causation
What remedies have been tried
Who is affected by the problem
Why has help been sought now

The child's general functioning

Home
Family relationships, parents, siblings
Peer relationships in and out of school
Academic ability and performance
Emotions
Behaviour

Personal history

Pregnancy, problems during labour and delivery
Developmental milestones (physical, social, emotional)
Any disruptions to attachment/separation
Any anxiety relating to child's well-being or health
Reaction to starting school

Family history

Personal history of parents
Early upbringing
Schooling, peer relationships
Employment
Physical and mental history in the family
Family composition
History of pregnancy
Family strengths/weaknesses (problem solving)
Major life events, bereavement, stresses

Information from observation of family

Interaction between family members
Structure
Communication patterns
Family assessment of problems and ability to work with professional
Approach to parenting – consistency

Information from observation of the child

Appearance, build, attitude to referral
Motor, agitation, restlessness
Speech, communication, language
Attitude to other members

Mental state examination

Usually older children and adolescents where there is concern of abnormal mental functioning

Physical examination

Care plan

Figure 18.1 Issues to be addressed in a comprehensive assessment interview

found in 7 per cent with mild problems in a further 15 per cent, with a slight male excess (Richman *et al.* 1982; Lavigne *et al.* 1996). Disorders starting in pre-school years can persist into later life. Children with difficult temperaments are more likely to react to adverse family factors and present psychological difficulties beyond their pre-school years. Similarly, shy children are more likely to present with anxiety related problems later (Kagan *et al.* 1988).

Hyperactivity

The essential features of this disorder are developmentally inappropriate degrees of inattention, impulsiveness and hyperactivity. The British have used more stringent criteria in the diagnosis of 'hyperkinesis' with a point prevalence of 1.7 per cent (Taylor *et al.* 1996) with the condition being more frequent in boys. North Americans use a wider criteria for 'Attention Deficit Disorder' (ADHD) affecting around 10 per cent of children.

Aetiology

There is consensus that some genetic predisposition exists. Although family factors have also been implicated, their role in severe cases is unclear. Birth complications and diet play a part in a minority of cases.

Assessment is usually preceded by collecting information using the Conners' Teacher's and Parent's Questionnaires (Conners 1969, 1973). These questionnaires are used to screen children referred to the clinic prior to an appointment. The scores on the questionnaires are not diagnostic and cannot be used as a substitute for clinical assessment.

At the clinic, a full psychiatric history needs to be taken with particular emphasis on attention, activity levels and impulsiveness. The history should include details on parenting style, attachment patterns and social relationships. School reports from teachers are a valuable source of information as the problems may present themselves mainly in the school setting. Details of classroom behaviour, organizational skills and peer relationships can often confirm parents' concerns about hyperactivity.

Characteristic features

Marked restlessness, inattention and impulsiveness. Hyperactive children wriggle and squirm in their seats, find it hard to sit still in one place or experience difficulty persisting with any activity. In situations requiring attention and concentration, the child is easily distracted and seems not to listen when spoken to directly. Socially, such children find it hard awaiting their turn in activities or conversation, often blurting out answers before questions have been completed. For a diagnosis of hyperkinesis, the hyperactivity must be pervasive across different settings, for example, at home and at school. Both the British and North American criteria for diagnosis require a chronicity of at least six months of symptoms and onset before the age of 7.

Treatment

The long-lasting biological basis for the problems needs to be emphasized to teachers and parents. Support for the family is crucial regarding management of the child. Parents need to adopt a consistent attitude to parenting with clear guidelines for acceptable behaviour. Simple time-out procedures can be used for unacceptable behaviour. Encouraging the child's sustained attention on jigsaws and Lego can increase the child's attention span. More formal behaviour management techniques can be helpful with children who show milder versions of the problem or are too young for medication. Advice to teachers on the nature of the problem and the management of children with ADHD is crucial. Most children with hyper-active disorder require high levels of supervision and encouragement to remain on task.

Medication is by far the most effective treatment for hyperactivity. Psychostimulants, such as methylphenidate, have a beneficial effect on rest-lessness, inattentiveness and impulsiveness. Improvement in concentration and attention can increase academic performance leading to improved self-esteem and confidence. Common side effects of psychostimulant drugs include reduced appetite, weight loss and difficulty in falling asleep. Most children will need to continue medication at least until their early teens. Outcome can be determined by the presence of other concurrent disorders such as Asperger's syndrome, autism and conduct disorders.

Autistic disorders

Autistic disorders are also known as pervasive developmental disorders. Most professionals agree that three features are essential to the diagnosis. A general and profound failure to develop social relationships; language retardation and ritualistic and compulsive behaviour. Additionally, these abnormalities should manifest themselves before 30 months.

Prevalence

Community surveys have found prevalence rates of two per 10,000 increas-ing to 20 per 10,000 depending on how narrowly or broadly the disorder is defined. Boys are affected three times as much as girls.

Social impairment

The impairment of social development often reveals itself in infancy as the child appears aloof, fails to seek comfort from adults and generally shows a lack of interest in people. In half of the children with autism, some social interest and competence develops, although problems with empathy and social reciprocity remain.

Roughly 50 per cent of children fail to acquire useful speech. Acquisition of language is delayed and, when present, language abnormalities are common, including poor comprehension, intonation and pronominal reversal (for example using 'you' for 'I').

Ritualistic compulsive behaviours and interests

Common abnormalities include resistance to change, stereotyped, narrow and repetitive patterns of play (for example, lining up toys). Some children show intensive attachment to unusual objects or preoccupation and interests (train timetables, cricket scores). Early signs of a lack of social interest may be missed but, by the second or third year of life, their social deficits become more noticeable. Some children go through a stage when they lose previously acquired skills. Fifty per cent of children with autism have an IQ less than 50.

Asperger's syndrome

This condition is regarded by some as a milder version of autism. These children are often aloof, distant and lacking in empathy. There is usually no delay in the development of vocabulary and grammar, though other aspects of language are abnormal as in autism.

Management

Management includes appropriate assessment and school placement, and provision of advice and support for parents. Children with autism do well in a structured educational setting with behavioural programmes to reduce ritualistic behaviour, tantrums and aggressive behaviour while encouraging the child in task-orientated work. The use of neuroleptic medication, such as risperidone, chlorpromazine and haloperidol does not improve the core symptoms but does improve symptoms such as behavioural disturbance and aggression. Stimulants may reduce hyperactivity. The prognosis is better in children with higher intelligence and for children who acquire useful speech by the age of 5 years.

Conduct disorders

Conduct disorders consist of repetitive and persistent patterns of behaviour, which are age-inappropriate and violate accepted social norms. Children with conduct disorder often bully, intimidate or threaten others. Physical fights and cruelty to animals and people are not uncommon. Serious violation of rules, such as truanting, staying away from home and damage to property, often lead to forensic involvement. A category of family-based conduct disorders may be present where there is no significant disturbance or abnormality of social relationships outside the family. In older adolescents lack of punctuality and non-compliance with the requirements of employers leads to periods of unemployment.

Research has shown that many children with conduct disorders have poor academic achievement and a third of children have specific reading disorders (Rutter *et al.* 1970, 1975). Disruptive behaviour in the classroom is common leading to poor interpersonal relationships.

Oppositional defiant disorder

This is a sub-type of conduct disorder in younger children. Usually there is an absence of behaviour that violates the law or seriously interferes with the rights of others.

Juvenile delinquency

This is a socio-legal concept defined as a person who has attained the age of criminal responsibility and has been found guilty of a crime. Most offences are against property rather than persons. Personal violence accounts for less than 10 per cent. Factors associated with juvenile delinquency include large family size, low socio-economic status and income, and a family history of criminality in parents and siblings. There is a strong association with broken homes with high levels of disorder and poor parental supervision.

Good care planning demands a full history of functioning at school and at home. Due to the wide spectrum of problems, a number of agencies (social services, health, education) may be involved with the family. Behaviour management approaches, parent training and problem-solving approaches have been advocated as effective. In juvenile delinquency multi-systemic therapy involving close multi-agency work with family therapy, assertiveness training and problem-solving training has been shown to be effective in reducing re-offending (Sheldrick 1994).

School refusal

Children who present with problems of school attendance represent 5 per cent of clinic referrals. The problem can present in a variety of ways including abdominal pain and headaches in the mornings before setting out for school. Onset may be abrupt in which case a precipitating factor can be found, or gradual with the child increasingly reluctant to attend school. The child is often fearful of separating from the parent and leaving home. There is often a lack of authority on the part of the parents to enforce attendance. Emotional over-involvement by the parents can also play a part. In contrast to the school-phobic child, truants stay away from school to engage in other activities without the knowledge of their parents. Truancy is linked to conduct disorder, male sex, large families, parental criminality and poor supervision at home.

Treatment and management involves dealing with the underlying condition particularly separation anxiety. Family therapy to help parents enforce school attendance may be necessary. Effective liaison with the school is essential to deal with issues such as bullying and to harness teachers' support. Change of schools rarely helps unless there are particular problems, for example, distance from school, academic ability, necessitating change. Medication is not helpful in most cases.

Emotional disorders of childhood

The Isle of Wight studies (Rutter 1976) diagnosed anxiety disorders in 2 per cent of 10- and 11-year-olds. The most common anxiety disorders are separation anxiety, disorders of childhood, generalized anxiety disorder, specific phobias and social anxiety disorders of childhood.

Separation anxiety disorders

Anxiety arises in response to separation from parents and other attachment figures. It is most prominent during the pre-school years. When the intensity of anxiety is developmentally inappropriate and handicapping, separation anxiety disorder is diagnosed. Children with this condition are reluctant to let their parents out of their sight and complain of physical symptoms, for example, headaches, stomach ache and nausea when separation is enforced (in the mornings before setting out for school). Behaviour management techniques, reward systems using star charts to motivate change and graded exposure to increasing separation have been found to be helpful.

Generalized anxiety disorders

This is present in roughly 3 per cent of children who experience persistent anxieties and worries which are not related to a particular event or situation. Somatic complaints are common. Relaxation and cognitive therapy have been shown to be helpful.

Phobic anxiety disorders

Specific phobias are common in early childhood. Animal phobias are common before the age of 2–4. Anxiety leads to avoidance and distress. It is more common in girls. Desensitization, support and cognitive techniques have been found to be helpful.

Disorders of social functioning

This category includes selective mutism, reactive attachment disorders of childhood and disinhibited attachment disorders of infancy.

Selective mutism

The main problem in this condition is the child's refusal to talk in certain situations while conversing normally in others. Generally, normal speech is present while in a minority there are problems of articulation and speech production. Milder forms present themselves at the start of school life and are usually transitory. Behavioural and family therapy result in a good prognosis for 50 per cent of cases.

Attachment disorders

The motion of attachment in infants was strongly influenced by the writings of John Bowlby (1980). According to these theories, a child needs to be attached to a protective figure as biologically adaptive. Children develop attachments to a relatively small number of figures. This relationship offers a secure base from which the child explores the world around them. Although all children develop attachments, the quality of the attachments vary greatly and can be measured by how distressed the child becomes when separated and by the child's response to reunions. Based on the quality of these attachments, securely attached children do much better than insecurely attached children although not all of those do badly.

Elimination disorders

Enuresis

Many would argue whether enuresis should be seen as a mental health problem. Enuresis may be primary when bladder control has never been achieved or secondary when bladder control is lost after a child has acquired bladder control for at least six months. Boys are more prone to nocturnal enuresis (bed wetting at night) while girls are more prone to diurnal enuresis. Once continence is achieved relapse occurs most commonly around the age of 5 or 6. The male:female sex ratio for nocturnal enuresis rises from 1:1 at the age of 5 to nearly 2:1 in adolescence (Shaffer 1994).

Aetiology

Seventy per cent of enuretic children have a first-degree relative with a history of wetting. Enuretic children are more likely to show other developmental delay; language and motor delays being twice as common as among controls. Delay beyond 20 months in starting toilet training is associated with a higher incidence of enuresis. Girls with enuresis are more likely to suffer from urinary tract infections (5 per cent of 5-year-old enuretics). Enuresis is associated with stressful life events at the age of 3–4 years and these include early separations, birth of siblings, accidents and admissions to hospital. Enuresis is associated with social disadvantage and institutional care (Douglas 1973).

Management

A detailed assessment should include a full psychiatric assessment. Physical causes need to be excluded and urinary microscopy and culture carried out in all cases. Treatment is unlikely to be successful unless the child and family are motivated. Behavioural interventions as well as pharmacological treatments have proven to be effective. Using a simple star chart to record dry nights can be effective. If enuresis persists the use of an enuresis alarm is recommended. Originally the device consisted of a buzzer and a pad which was placed under the bedsheet at night. Current models are portable and the pad can be attached to the child's pyjamas. In both devices when the child wets, the buzzer is set off and the child is expected to go to the toilet. Cure rates of 50+ per cent are reported although a third of children relapse. For resistant cases an intensive form of therapy called the dry-bed training is recommended. This works better with older and motivated children. This technique involves hourly waking during the first night and practice of proper toileting habits. The medication of choice is desmopressin which is effective in 70 per cent of children. Relapse rates are, however, high. Low dosage tricylic anti-depressants, for example, imipramine have been shown to be effective.

Encopresis

Encopresis or faecal soiling is the voiding of faeces in inappropriate places and usually involves the soiling of the child's clothes. At the age of 7, the prevalence in boys is 2.3 per cent and 0.7 per cent in girls with a male:female ratio of almost 3.5:1. By the age of 11, less than 1 per cent of children soil themselves once a month (Hersov 1994).

Faecal soiling can occur for a variety of reasons. Some children fail to achieve continence as they have never learned bowel control and this is termed primary faecal soiling. This is usually found in the context of inconsistent or coercive toilet training practice. Treatment involves educating parents in proper toilet training methods on realistic targets and reinforcement of achievement by the child. Star charts can be used to record success. Fear of using the toilet can lead to some children soiling their clothes. General reassurance and rewards for appropriate use of the toilet can help resolve the problem.

In some children encopresis may occur as a result of long-standing faecal retention. The original cause may be emotional or physical but, in time, leads to constipation. Chronic constipation can lead to hard faeces acting as a plug. Liquid and semi-solid stools eventually leak past the plug causing soiling. This form of soiling arises as a result of constipation with overflow leading to soiling.

Appropriate measures need to be adopted to unblock the bowel by using a laxative such as senna in combination with a stool softener such as Lactulose, although enemas may be needed in resistant cases. Family counselling and training in appropriate toilet training methods is essential. Close monitoring and support to families helps motivate parents in keeping to an agreed programme.

Soiling can occur in children who have achieved continence when they experience stressful situations such as physical or sexual abuse. The main aim of treatment is to reduce stress.

The provocative or aggressive soiler deliberately defecates onto furniture or smears walls with faeces. There is an association with dysfunctional family systems based on social disorganization and coercive and abusive child-rearing practices. Management and treatment usually needs the co-ordinated input of several agencies including social services and education.

Child maltreatment

There are wide variations in the reported incidence of child abuse and neglect based on variation in definition and methods used to estimate prevalence. Types of abuse include:

- physical abuse – non-accidental injury, burns, fractures, bruises;
- emotional abuse – threats, hostility, failure to protect;
- sexual abuse – penetrative, non-penetrative; and
- neglect – lack of appropriate care and nurture, stimulation and supervision.

Causes of child abuse

The causative factors are complex and multi-factional. Parents who abuse children have often been victims of abuse themselves. Perpetrators often have problems in a number of areas including vocational and social skills, substance abuse, poor education and low income. Abuse is often seen as a part of dysfunction formerly with poor parent–child bonding and attachment. Abuse may also take place in institutional care, schools and children's homes.

Management

The first aim is to prevent further abuse and to involve child protection services in assessment and investigation of the case to ensure the safety and protection of the child. Removal from home to hospital may be necessary. The second aim is to provide inter-agency help to meet the child's social, emotional and psychological needs while providing support to the family.

Psychiatric disorders in adolescence

Although adolescence is often associated with a period of stress and turmoil, most adolescents manage the transition between childhood and adulthood without major problems. It is a period, however, during which there are major changes in body image, self-esteem, relationships with parents and mood. Awareness about sexual orientation and identity are also heightened.

The rate at which children mature differs with early maturing boys showing some social advantage over boys who mature later. Early maturing girls, on the other hand tend to experience some depression and anxiety compared with late maturers. Discomfort and embarrassment about body shape and size are comparatively greater in this group. Conflicts with parents and emotional and behavioural problems are also more commonly experienced.

The term 'identity crisis' was used originally by Erikson (1968), to describe the process of development during adolescence, leading to a well-developed notion of self. Experimentation with different roles and beliefs is not uncommon. There are large differences in the rate and pace of change in the development of personal identity. This period of change before identity crisis is resolved was termed 'identity confusion' by Erikson (1968).

Adolescence is a period of transition between childhood and adulthood and, in most cultures, is heralded by the onset of puberty while termination is often socially and culturally determined. The interplay of social and biological influences play an important part in the disorders of adolescence. Prevalence rates for disorder range from 8–20 per cent (Rutter *et al.* 1970; Boyle *et al.* 1987; Lavik 1977).

Emotional conduct disorders are the most commonly diagnosed and, in a proportion of adolescents, are the continuation of unresolved disorders in earlier childhood. Conduct problems become more pronounced with the onset of adolescence and may result in forensic involvement. Substance misuse is likely to play a part in disturbed and offending behaviour.

Anxiety disorders related to school attendance, phobias and agoraphobia may have its onset in adolescence. Obsessive-compulsive disorders presenting with obsessional ideas, ruminations and ritual and can be associated with anxiety, depression or Tourette's syndrome.

Depressive disorders, mania and bipolar disorders are more common during adolescent than in childhood. Self-harm and suicide rates also show an increase. A proportion of children with pervasive developmental disorders develop epilepsy during adolescence. Behavioural disturbance can increase and children may show difficulties in understanding and expressing sexual behaviour.

Although schizophrenia can occur in younger children, its onset before puberty is rare. Males are more vulnerable and it is usually preceded by a stage of behavioural and social difficulties and this may make early diagnosis difficult.

Eating disorders, such as anorexia nervosa and bulimia nervosa have their onset during adolescence. In anorexia nervosa onset before puberty is uncommon. The prevalence rises from 0.1 per cent in 11- to 15-year-olds to 1 per cent in 16- to 18-year-olds; the male/female ratio being 1:10. Bulimia peaks a few years later (Steinhausen 1994).

Obsessive-compulsive disorder

While there are striking similarities between the phenomenology of obsessive-compulsive disorder (OCD) in children and adults, significant differences exist in terms of gender distribution, co-morbidity, familial contribution and developmental issues.

Epidemiology

Roughly a third of adults have their first symptoms before the age of 15. Earlier estimates of OCD from child psychiatric clinics range from 0.2 per cent to 1.2 per cent but more recent studies suggest prevalence rates ranging between 1 and 4 per cent (Rapoport *et al.* 1994).

Characteristic features

Obsessions are recurrent, intrusive thoughts, ideas or images or impulses that the person experiences as ego-dystonic and intensely distressing. One of the core characteristics of obsession in adults is that they are resisted. Resistance to obsessions and compulsions in children is, however, not always present. Common obsessions in childhood focus on contamination, harm or death, and symmetry. Compulsions are repetitive physical or mental acts that the person feels driven to perform in response to that obsession. The purpose of the compulsion is usually to reduce anxiety or magically prevent a dreaded event. Compulsive behaviour can become so extreme that it interferes with normal social functioning. Common examples are checking, touching, washing and repeating acts.

The average age of onset is 7½ to 12½ years and is earlier in boys than in girls, and peaks firstly in adolescent and then in early adulthood. The male/female ratio in childhood OCD is 3:2 (Rapoport *et al.* 1994).

Differential diagnosis

Normal childhood ritual such as bedtime routine and collecting are not uncommon in early childhood. Symptoms of OCD can present secondary to primary depressive disorders. Children with the autistic spectrum group of disorders may present with repetitive behaviour and sometimes develop full-blown symptoms of OCD. Symptoms of OCD can be associated with schizophrenia and anorexia. Obsessive compulsive symptoms occur in up to two thirds of patients with Tourette's syndrome.

Treatment and management

OCD is a chronic condition and needs long-term commitment to its management. Cognitive behavioural therapy, advice on management, involving carers and parents and medication have all shown to be effective. Exposure and response prevention has been shown to be effective in reducing symptoms. Advice to parents about how to respond to their child's demands that they take part in ritualized behaviour helps reduce anxiety and tensions in the family.

Clomipramine, a tricyclic drug has shown to be effective in symptom reduction, although side effects such as weight gain and sedation can affect compliance. Other drugs which have been found to be effective include fluvoxamine, fluoxetine, sertraline and paroxetine.

Suicide and deliberate self-harm

Completed suicide is rare before puberty but its incidence increases during older adolescence. It is estimated that the figures for Britain are roughly five suicides per million children aged 10–14 years. The suicide rate in North America has been increasing during the last several decades and there is an excess of males who commit suicide at all ages (Shaffer 1974; Shaffer *et al.* 1996).

Factors seen in the background of adolescents who commit suicide include disruptive home circumstances, higher rates of psychiatric disorder in family members and previous suicidal threats in roughly half of all cases during the 24 hours prior to the suicide. High rates of psychiatric disorder are common in older adolescents who commit suicide.

While hanging and carbon monoxide poisoning are common methods used by males, girls are more likely to overdose themselves. The risk of suicide is greater in adolescence. A careful assessment of risk should be undertaken in every case, taking into account family history of mood disturbance and past attempts at self-harm.

Deliberate self-harm (DSH)

Deliberate self-harm peaks at adolescence and is generally low in childhood. Suicidal ideation is relatively common in adolescence with 10–20 per cent experiencing such thoughts over the past year. DSH is generally uncommon in early childhood and is more common in boys. After the age of 12, DSH is five times more common in girls than boys. Self-poisoning is the common form among girls (Shaffer *et al.* 1996).

Common features found in the background of children attempting DSH include broken homes, discordant family life with psychosocial conflict. Parental psychiatric disorder and substance abuse/alcohol abuse are more common. A history of sexual abuse or physical abuse may be present. Roughly one fifth of the children will have made a previous attempt at DSH (Shaffer 1974).

Assessment

All children who self-harm should have a full psychiatric assessment. Children who commit DSH may be seen in Accident and Emergency departments or be admitted to an inpatient ward where they can be seen once the toxic effects of an overdose have been dealt with. As DSH commonly involves adolescents, clear protocols need to be in place to meet the needs of these children so that they do not fall into the gaps between the medical and mental health services for children and those for adults. Factors indicating the suicide risk of children following an incident of DSH are shown in Table 18.2. Most children who self-harm should be offered follow-up after assessment.

Table 18.2 Suicide risk assessment in children following deliberate self-harm (DHS)

	Low risk	*High risk*
Location of overdose	In public, for example, on school bus	Isolated in the woods, locked room
Timing	Intervention likely	Intervention unlikely
Precipitants	Impulsive – following argument with girl/boyfriend	Extensive premeditation
Preparations in anticipation of death	No suicide note	Suicide notes stating arrangements for funeral, etc.
Attitude following overdose	Relieved about safe outcome	Still expressing suicidal intent
Revaluation of problems precipitating DSH	Positive, for example, school taking problems more seriously	Negative – outlook pessimistic

Management

Where family factors are prominent, involvement of the family is beneficial. They should be encouraged to see DSH as serious and play a role in minimizing further risk of DSH. Individual therapy aimed at helping the children to refrain from the problem and adopt a problem-solving approach has shown to be beneficial.

Tourette's syndrome

This condition has been recognized for over 150 years. Tourette's syndrome affects 3–5 per 10,000 children. Prevalence is ten times greater in children than it is in adults and occurs four times more commonly in males than in females (Robertson 1989).

Clinical characteristics

The mean age of onset of symptoms is 7 years and the essential features of the illness are the existence of multiple motor tics and at least one vocal tic. The most common symptoms involve eye-blinking, and tics affecting the face, neck or head. The onset of vocalization usually occurs later than the motor tics. Coprolalia, the inappropriate and involuntary uttering of obscenities, is seen in about a third of patients seen at the clinic. The manifestation of the tics varies in response to different conditions. Anxiety, stress and fatigue can aggravate tics. Concentration on controlling the symptoms can lead to temporary disappearance of symptoms. Children with Tourette's syndrome are disproportionately likely to be obsessional. Attention deficit hyperactivity disorder occurs in roughly 25–50 per cent. An association with exhibitionism, anti-social behaviour, aggression and self-infurious behaviour has been suggested.

Treatment

For the milder versions, explanation and reassurance to teacher, parents and the child has been shown to be sufficient. Parents benefit from contact with self-help groups. The mainstay of treatment is medication; the most commonly used ones being haloperidol, pimozid and sulpiride. Clonidine has also shown to be beneficial, particularly when Tourette's syndrome is present with comorbid features of ADHD (Robertson 1989).

Progressive Tourette's syndrome runs a lifelong course with symptoms waxing and waning over time. In up to a third, the tics symptoms remit by late adolescents while an additional third show significant improvement in symptoms.

Major affective disorders

Affective disorders are discussed in Chapter 14 of this book. This section considers those aspects that are particularly relevant in children and adolescents.

Depression

As a symptom depression is relatively common, with 10 per cent of 10-year-olds being described as depressed by their parents in the Isle of Wight study (Rutter *et al.* 1970). This figure rose to 40 per cent in cases of 14-year-olds who reported feeling miserable.

There is now general acceptance that children can suffer from adult-type depression. Studies have demonstrated depressive symptomology starting before puberty, continuing into adolescence and adulthood. There are, however, some important differences with children being relatively more reactive to their environment than adults. The presence of behavioural problems is common in depressed children and may mask an underlying depression.

Prevalence

Up to 1–2 per cent of pre-pubertal children and 2–5 per cent of adolescents are thought to suffer with major depressive disorders. The sex ratio changes with age with there being more pre-pubertal boys than girls with depression while, after puberty, there is a female preponderance.

Causes

Depressed children are more likely to have parents with depression. Parents with depression are also more likely to have children who are depressed. Studies suggest a strong genetic loading while environmental factors clearly play an important role. Family dysfunction, alcoholism and anti-social behaviour are associated with pre-pubertal depression.

As with adult depressive disorder, depressed mood, hopelessness, misery and tearfulness are common. Changes in the young person's experience of school and social life may often herald the onset of depression. Low self-esteem, feelings of worthlessness and self-blame are not uncommon. Changes in appetite and weight loss are less common than in adults. Suicidal thoughts and behaviour may lead to referral by worried parents or teachers.

The onset of depression in adolescence may be acute or insidious. While brief periods of low moods are not uncommon in children, evidence of sustained low mood needs to be elicited for a diagnosis of depressive disorder. It is not uncommon for parents to be unaware of depression in their children: there is often a precipitant for the episode of depression and some children may have been victims of physical or sexual abuse.

Treatment

The major aims of treatment are to reduce depression, to promote social and emotional functioning and help the family in understanding and dealing with the adolescent's illness.

In severe cases of depression where there is a high risk of self-harm the child may need admission to an inpatient unit. Milder cases are seen as outpatients. Individual therapy, particularly cognitive behavioural psychotherapy (CBT) has been shown to be effective. CBT helps develop cognitive strategies for dealing with negative thoughts and helps in developing problem-solving techniques. CBT is covered in Chapters 10 and 15 of this book, and the practical application of behavioural and cognitive techniques in Chapters 24 and 25.

While early trials showed promising results with tricylic anti-depressants, subsequent trials failed to show significant benefits over placebo (Harrington 1992; Hazell 1995). The selective serotonin reuptake inhibitors (SSRI) have been shown to be more effective than placebos. It is now the first line treatment of choice where medication is indicated. Resistant depression presenting with severe suicidal risk may need to be treated with ECT in specialist units (Edwards 1994).

Mania

Manic disorders are rare before puberty. In pre-pubertal children, symptoms of mania may be confused with attention deficit hyperactive disorder. Manic patients present with irritability, euphoria or elated mood and insomnia. They tend to be hyperactive and may engage in reckless and impulsive behaviour.

Manic episodes may be part of a bipolar affective disorder with episodes of depression and mania. Onset is usually during adolescence or early adulthood. Neuroleptic drugs or lithium are commonly used to control acute episodes.

Adolescent schizophrenia

As discussed in Chapter 13 schizophrenia first presents typically in early adult life and is relatively rare in childhood. The majority of cases seen in children tend to have an onset in adolescence. Making a firm diagnosis is often difficult because of the limited verbal skills of the children and the confusion between vivid normal fantasy life and psychotic thinking.

Children with schizophrenia often present with earlier developmental delays and poor premorbid functioning. Developmental delays are particularly common in the areas of language development, reading and bladder control. A third of children also show difficulties in forming socio-emotional relationships. The onset of schizophrenia is usually insidious. The recognition of symptoms during the early phase may be common to other childhood psychiatric disorders before merging with the prodromal symptoms preceding the onset of psychotic symptoms. There is usually a strong family history of psychosis/schizophrenia.

The main features of the clinical picture are delusional beliefs, thought disorder, hallucinations and disorders of affect. Delusions in schizophrenia include paranoid delusions and beliefs that thoughts are being withdrawn or broadcast from one's head or externally controlled. Associations between thoughts may be loosened and move between topics in an unrelated way. In extreme cases the patient may be incoherent. Hallucinations are most often auditory and may consist of voices discussing the patient or repeating their thoughts out loud. Emotionally, the patient often presents as flattened, inappropriate or blunted. Adolescent schizophrenia is generally characterized by prominent negative features (inappropriate affect and avolition) rather than prominent delusions or hallucinations when compared with adult schizophrenia.

Before starting treatment it is important to seek consent from the patient and adults holding parental responsibility. Assessment of competence to give consent needs to be tailored to the young person's age and understanding of the purpose, nature and likely effects and risks. Inpatient admission should be considered where there is serious risk to the safety of the young person or others. Lack of insight and poor compliance with treatment are other factors which need to be considered. Alternatively, the patient may be treated as a day patient or an outpatient.

Many of the antipsychotic drugs used in adults are not licensed for younger patients. The newer atypical antipsychotic drugs are increasingly the first line treatment of choice. Olanzapine and risperidone have been used with good effect. During the acute phase, benzodiazepine may be used to relieve distress or reduce behavioural disturbances.

Psychoeducation of parents and the patient about the illness, treatment and prognosis, helps their understanding of an illness which can be frightening and stigmatizing. Cognitive behavioural strategies and supportive counselling may be beneficial.

Substance misuse in adolescence

There is increasing evidence of a rise in substance abuse among British adolescents. A survey of British 15- to 16-year-olds found that almost half had tried illicit drugs at some time (Fergusson and Horwood 2000). While most children who experiment with illicit drugs do not go on to habitual abuse of drugs, the earlier the onset, the more persistent the habit becomes and some will become substance dependent as adults.

While a proportion of illicit drug-abusing children go on to adult dependence, there are significant differences in the pattern of abuse among adolescents and adults. Children with conduct disorders are more likely to misuse drugs. The risk is increased in children with conduct disorder and hyperactivity. Adult role models and peer group drug use have a strong influence on adolescent drug abuse. Inhaling organic solvents is particularly associated with adolescent abuse and social adversity.

There is some evidence to suggest that multiple drug use is more common among adolescents than adults with an irregular pattern of abuse rather than chronic use. As a result, dependence among adolescents in relatively uncommon.

While substance misuse is more likely to respond to early treatment in adolescence, motivation in accepting treatment can be poor. It is often the concern of others which leads to referral. There is an increased risk of suicidal ideation and attempted suicide with children, not uncommonly first presenting following an episode of deliberate self-harm. Drug use is a major risk in completed suicide.

Among adolescent females involved in drug misuse, affective symptoms are likely to be more common while, in males, conduct disorders predominate. As adolescent drug abusers do not readily present themselves for treatment, an assertive approach needs to be adopted usually involving other agencies such as probation, social services and education. Although alcohol dependence is uncommon, in cases where dependence has developed, detoxification is required. Detoxification for dependence on other illicit drugs follows the same programme as in adults. Individual counselling in primary care settings using the brief intervention techniques have shown significant reduction in alcohol misuse (Swadi 2000).

Family influences play a significant role in the onset and progression of drug misuse; and family therapy approaches using techniques such as the multi-dimensional family therapy have been shown to be beneficial. Group therapy involving peers based on the Alcoholics Anonymous model helps in providing support and relapse prevention.

Adolescents need considerable support to abstain from drug use. Inter-agency support and help with education, accommodation and training is important. Drug and alcohol use is discussed in detail in Chapter 17.

Eating disorders in children and adolescents

Eating disorders are conditions in which there is excessive preoccupation and concern with control of body weight and shape, with grossly restricted food intake. The term 'eating disorder' in children and adolescents covers a range of early onset conditions where one or all of the psychological, social and physical areas of functioning is involved. The spectrum of eating disorders in childhood and early adolescence covers the following: early onset anorexia nervosa, bulimia nervosa, food avoidance emotional disorder (FAED), selective eating, and pervasive refusal syndrome. It is important to note that eating disorders can arise secondary to other disorders such as depression, and obsessive-compulsive disorders. Eating disorders are covered also in Chapter 16 of this volume.

Childhood onset anorexia nervosa

The co-ordinal features of childhood onset anorexia nervosa are:

- failure to maintain weight gain or actual weight loss in relation to age;
- determined food avoidance;
- abnormal concerns/preoccupation with weight and shape; and
- amenorrhoea in post-menarcheal adolescents or delayed or arrested puberty.

Incidence and prevalence

In adolescent populations the prevalence of anorexia is estimated to be 0.1 to 0.2 per cent, and is lower in younger children. Most clinics report an increase in the number of referrals to specialist services and there is some evidence of an increase in incidence. Among adolescents, 5–10 per cent of cases occur in males while in younger male children the numbers may be up to a third.

The aetiology of eating disorders is complex and needs to be viewed from a bio-psychosocial perspective. A number of biological factors may play a part, including endocrine dysfunction affecting the hypothalmic pituitary gonadal axis and genetic factors although its exact effects remain uncertain.

Although a number of psychological and familial factors have been implicated as playing a role in the pathogenesis of anorexia nervosa, there is insufficient empirical evaluation for these hypotheses. Cultural and social factors are also important. Earlier studies suggested a preponderance of higher social class, although this is not marked in adolescence (Fossen *et al.* 1987). Generally, eating disorders are reported more frequently in societies where food is plentiful and thinness is valued. The risk of anorexia is high in occupations such as modelling and ballet dancing where there is an emphasis on slimness.

Clinical description

The onset is usually within a few years of menarche but cases can be as young as 8 years. The onset is usually insidious and the first indication in post-menarcheal females is the cessation of menstruation. The most significant feature is food avoidance leading to severe weight loss. Patients are often secretive and adolescents are likely to avoid unsupervised meals such as school lunches. Distortions of body image are common, with denial of weight loss even when grossly underweight. Other associated symptoms include excessive physical activity in an attempt to lose weight and burn off calories. Preoccupation with preparing food and feeding others is not uncommon. With decreasing weight the physical effects of starvation become evident. Patients complain of tiredness, lethargy, constipation and cold extremities. It is important to bear in mind that in severe cases death may occur.

Due to the poor motivation of adolescents with anorexia, engagement of the patient and the family into therapy is crucial. Teenagers who live with their parents are usually managed on an outpatient basis. Care plans should set out clear goals for weight restoration and involve parents and teachers with the consent of the patient. With younger patients the parents are encouraged to take charge and supervise meal times.

Family therapy, individual counselling and cognitive behavioural psychotherapy have all been shown to be beneficial. Individual psychotherapy is helpful in addressing interpersonal issues which may have precipitated the illness and encouraging problem-solving strategies to deal with them. In recent onset cases, intensive family therapy is more useful than hospitalization and individual counselling. However, in severe cases hospitalization may need to be considered.

Bulimia nervosa

This is an eating disorder characterized by episodes of binge eating. During these episodes large amounts of food are consumed over short periods. The condition should not be diagnosed in patients with a diagnosis of anorexia nervosa up to 50 per cent of whom also binge eat.

Periods of binge eating are usually preceded by intense craving or preoccupation with food and intractable urges to overeat. The fattening effects of the food are countered in a number of ways, including periods of starvation following binges or by self-induced vomiting and purging. Although fear of becoming fat and concerns about body weight are common, usually body weight is close to normal.

The majority of patients are female and clinical presentation is usually several years later than patients with anorexia nervosa, patients most commonly presenting between 20 and 25 years of age. Patients usually describe loss of control over eating as the most significant problem. Up to 50 per cent vomit and binge eat or both on a daily basis. As this behaviour is associated with shame and guilt, self-induced vomiting is usually secretive. Disorders of mood with depression guilt and suicidal thought may be present. Impulsiveness in the form of promiscuousness and shoplifting of food is present in some cases.

Management

Most adolescents can be treated on an outpatient basis. Cognitive behaviour therapy addressing maladaptive thought processes leading to the problems has shown to be effective.

Somatizing in children and adolescents

Most professionals accept the need to take a holistic approach bringing together the physical and psychological dimensions in the assessment and treatment of children and adolescents. Complaints of somatic symptoms are common in children presenting with psychological problems. This chapter deals more specifically with conditions in which the main complaints are of somatic symptoms and where there is inadequate explanation in terms of a physical cause.

Developmental factors play an important role in the presentation of these disorders. Parental attitudes to 'illness behaviour' in children include the extent to which concessions are made for responsibility for alterations and lifestyle and medical consultation. Very young children are less able to convey psychological distress based on their verbal competence and cognitive development.

The categories of somatic disorder differ based on the nature, chronicity and impact of unexplained somatic symptoms. There are certain factors associated with an increased reporting of physical symptoms; girls consistently report more symptoms, the gender difference becoming more marked during adolescence. This may, in part, be related to the increase in symptom reporting associated with the onset of menarche. Other factors, including temperament and conditions such as anxiety and depression, family discord, major life events, poor parental care and experience of abuse are also significant factors.

Dissociative disorders

The most common symptom in young people is loss of motor function but loss of function in any modality may be reported. Complaints of sensory loss involving sight, hearing or consciousness are not uncommon. The symptoms present as an 'epidemic' particularly involving girls where large numbers of children in a class report the same symptoms. True prevalence is difficult to estimate as transient disorders are not brought to medical attention. Unlike the individual form, the disorder may arise in a number of individuals within a closed community, such as a school or children's home. This variety of disorder is often described as 'epidemic hysteria'.

Diagnosis of the condition is fraught with difficulties as a proportion of children diagnosed on follow-up have been shown to be suffering from an organic condition. Children who are referred usually have had extensive physical investigations. It is important to engage the family in exploring the psychological stressor without stigmatizing the patient as malingering. Individual and family work has been shown to be helpful.

Chronic fatigue syndrome

This is a condition in which severe disabling fatigue persists for over six months (three months in children) and is associated with a variety of other associated symptoms unexplained by primary physical or psychiatric causes. The most significant complaint on presentation is one of fatigue often preceded by a flu-like illness from which complete recovery has not been made. Associated low mood, mental fatigue and inability to concentrate are not uncommon. Girls are more affected than boys.

The aetiological model is complex and physical and psychological factors have been suggested. The presence of persistent viral infection, muscular dysfunction, immune dysfunction and electrolyte imbalance have all been implicated. Low mood, anxiety and depression are not uncommon and, in up to a third of cases, depression may be present. While most cases remain ambulant, in very severe forms, children may be confined to a wheelchair and remain disabled from taking part in normal activity over a period of years. These children often present in paediatric clinics and may be resistant to transfer to child and adolescent mental health services as they see the principle cause of the problems as organic. It is best to adopt a supportive role while remaining open to discussion about the relative contribution of physical and psychological factors involved. Individual work with the child in using behavioural and cognitive strategies in goal-setting and encouraging graded rehabilitation has been found to be beneficial. It is important to involve the family in examining attitudes to illness and in encouraging compliance with treatment plans.

Factitious disorders

These present from middle childhood and are seen more commonly in girls. Existing minor physical problems are often exaggerated through interference to make the condition look more dramatic. There is often a need for medical attention with repeated presentation at Accident and Emergency departments. There is an overlap with other somatizing disorders.

In the severe and chronic forms, difficulties in attachment and bonding, temperamental traits and abusive experience have been found. Low self-esteem and poor social skills and peer relationships may be present. Individual work addressing these difficulties has shown to be of help.

Principles of treatment in child and adolescent psychiatry

Once a comprehensive assessment has been completed, the child and parents need to be involved in drawing up a treatment plan. The successful rate of treatment will depend on the extent to which they feel their wishes, fears and anxieties have been addressed during the initial meetings. It is useful for the therapists and the family/child to set out some targets for what will be seen as a successful outcome of treatment.

Diagnostic labels are helpful if parents and the child have an understanding of the criteria used for making a diagnosis and its potential for treatment. Caution needs to be exercised, however, as diagnostic labels can be seen as stigmatizing and parents often withdraw from treatment for fear of being 'labelled'. Diagnosis has potential benefits as it is a concise way in which information, regarding the nature, origin and prognosis for a particular child, can be conveyed. It also allows for special provisions to be made to meet the child's needs (special school, statementing).

Clinical governance, the framework through which NHS organizations are held accountable for the quality of services, has emphasized the need for evidence-based practice. The National Institute for Clinical Effectiveness has produced guidelines for the diagnosis and management of ADHD with particular reference to the use of stimulants (Techology Appraisal Guidance No. 13 National Institute for Clinical Excellence).

There is fairly strong evidence of efficacy for the use of medication in hyperkinesis, parent training in conduct disorders and family therapy in the treatment of anorexia in adolescents. Behaviour treatments for soiling and enuresis have also been found to be effective. On the other hand, there is very little evidence that the use of tricylics in adolescent depression and social skills' therapy in clinic settings for peer relationship problems are effective.

Prevention of child psychiatric disorders

The Department of Health publication *Saving Lives* (1999), emphasized disease prevention and health promotion as one of its objectives. Specific mention was made of the reduction of suicide as a mental health target. The paper also acknowledged the importance of the mental health of children and adolescents and their vulnerability to physical, intellectual and emotional behaviour disorders which, if untreated, could have serious implications for adult life.

Three types of prevention are recognized. The aim of primary prevention is to reduce the possible incidence of a disorder in a population before its onset. Secondary prevention is aimed at early diagnosis and intervention to minimize the impact on the patient and carers. Tertiary prevention has the goal of limiting the physical social effects of the disorder (Caplan 1964). In undertaking primary preventative intervention, several factors need to be considered and these include risk factor, protective factors and the vulnerability of the individual to a particular disorder. Risk factors may arise from the genetic background, problems during pregnancy and maternal infection or malnutrition. Good antenatal care can help to minimize these risks. Primary preventative work can also protect the child from the adverse effects of birth trauma, accidents, exposure to infection, deprivation and abuse through timely intervention.

Protective factors include adaptable temperament, a good relationship with a significant adult caretaker and experience of areas in which the child has a good experience such as sports or school. Several studies (Masten *et al.* 1988; Rutter 1990) have shown that a proportion of children exposed to gross deprivation and severe stress are resilient to developing psychiatric disorder, although the precise reasons why some children are resilient is not understood. The formation of secure attachments and the ability to be self-reflective are seen as protective factors. The need for secondary and tertiary preventative work in early identification and intervention is discussed further below.

Child and adolescent mental health problems in primary care

Although childhood psychiatric disorders are relatively common, only 1 in 10 of cases is seen in specialist mental health services for children. Two to 5 per cent of children attending primary care during any one year present with emotional or behavioural disorders. Pre-school children present predominantly with oppositional deficient disorder, while school-age children present with emotional and conduct disorders. Primary care recognition of disturbance is an important factor in referral to specialist mental health services. Children are less likely to be referred unless they present with overt psychological problems.

GPs are often the first point of contact in the referral system. They are in a unique position to implement preventative intervention and deal with less severe psychological problems. They have knowledge of the family's circumstances and can offer a service which is less stigmatizing. There is an increasing emphasis on collaborative support from specialist mental health services and paediatric services focusing on primary care intervention targeting high risk populations.

Many primary care practices employ counsellors, community psychiatric nurses and psychologists offering consultation and assessment in primary care settings. The appointment of primary care liaison workers offering consultation-liaison has helped reduce referrals to increasingly long waiting lists for specialist child mental health services. They also have an input in enhancing GP skills in managing milder cases and making more appropriate referrals to specialist services. The future of consultation and collaborative working will need modification as primary care trusts move from being commissioners to providers of specialist child mental health services.

The role of nurses in child and adolescent services

The Audit Commission document *Children in Mind* (1999) described a four-tier model for the delivery of child and adolescent services. Tier 1 services are provided by primary care and other front-line services offering advice for mild to moderate problems and promoting mental health.

Tier 2 services are generally provided by specialist professionals working on their own with links to primary care (Tier 1 services) and the specialist multi-disciplinary CAMHS services (Tier 3). Tier 4 services deal with complex severe cases with links to inpatient child and adolescent beds.

As with all nursing posts, commitment to ongoing continuing professional development and lifelong learning is essential. There are a range of courses and developmental opportunities for registered nurses working within child and adolescent mental health services. A number of these were approved by the former English National Board and include child and adolescent mental health nursing for nurses.

Nurses with specialist training in child and adolescent psychiatry are uniquely placed to work in all four tiers of the service. At Tier 1, nurses are able to take on the role of primary care mental health workers (PMHWs). Besides providing first line intervention they have a role to support other professionals working in primary care and provide links between Tier 1 and specialist services. PMHWs also play an important role as gatekeepers to specialist services.

Nurses with specialist training in a range of therapies, including cognitive behavioural therapy, family therapy and counselling, work independently at Tier 2 level on their own or as members of the Tier 3 multi-disciplinary service. At Tiers 3 and 4, community psychiatric nurses will increasingly play a central role in the services for adolescents with first onset psychosis. Services for this group are currently being developed in line with recommendations in the *National Service Framework for Mental Health.*

While there is an emphasis on multi-disciplinary working in inpatient adolescent units, nurses provide care and therapeutic input as the core group of specialists who outnumber other professionals. Children admitted to such units often need medication for serious psychotic problems, and careful assessment of risk and monitoring of the effects of medication is an important role for nurses.

Health visitors and school nurses with training in child development and assessment of children are uniquely placed to provide a service at Tier 2 level with support from specialist CAMHS services and are seen as less stigmatizing services for mild to moderate cases. There is evidence that community treatment of mothers with postnatal depression by child health nurses can lead to greater levels of improvement than a control group (Holden *et al.* 1989).

Opportunities exist for the appointment of nurse consultants to Tier 4 services although such posts are relatively new within child and adolescent services.

Users' views

Users of child and adolescent mental health services represent a large group of stakeholders including children, their families, schools, social services and others. Primary Care Trusts are important stakeholders with GPs often acting as gatekeepers to the service. User organizations, focus groups and meetings of stakeholders are increasingly involved in decisions about service planning and delivery. Views from such meetings indicate a need for greater clarity about the range of services offered by child and adolescent mental health services and the roles of professionals working within the service. Problems with access to the service and waiting times for first appointments are also concerns. Parents have indicated a need for greater support in their role of parenting.

In response to user views, services are being developed to provide out-of-hours support through the provision of respite, day and crisis response services. User concerns over the lack of collaborative inter-agency work in the provision and delivery of services has been reflected in a number of documents published by the Department of Health. In response to these concerns, children's services are increasingly jointly commissioned by Health Education and Social Services. Common protocols for assessment of children's needs have been developed.

The appointment of primary care mental health workers based in primary care has made it possible for the mild and moderate cases to be seen within the primary care setting. Trained health visitors and school nurses are able to provide a less stigmatizing service with the support of specialist services offering consultation and liaison. Schools are increasingly offering

Tier 2 services. There is still a need however to involve stakeholders and users more widely in the planning, delivery and evaluation of services provided by children's services. The Government Paper on Improving Quality and Accountability through Clinical Governance Initiatives offers further opportunities for user involvement in monitoring and evaluation of child and adolescent services.

Conclusion

In summary, the main points of this chapter are:

- Nurses may encounter mental distress and mental illness in children and adolescents in a wide variety of clinical practice settings. This chapter describes the manifestations of the more common mental health problems that children may experience and treatment approaches.

- Compared with the high profile of adult mental health, the significance of the mental health needs of children has only recently been recognized. A National Service Framework for Children is to be published soon. One of the key objectives will be to set national standards and break down barriers between agencies providing services to children.

- There are substantial areas of overlap between childhood mental health and physical health particularly during the pre-school and early school years. A tiered service offers nurses a variety of roles in primary care and in specialist teams.

- Service users' views are important in guiding the future development of child and adolescent mental health services (CAMHS). They have highlighted concerns with access to the service and waiting times, and the need for greater support to people in their parenting role.

- There are strong links also between childhood psychiatric disorders and growing areas of public concern such as adult community drug and alcohol misuse.

- Increasingly there is an emphasis on preventive work and pressure to allocate an increasing proportion of resources to primary prevention, that is to measures taken to reduce the incidence of specific disorders in a population not currently suffering from those disorders (Caplan 1964).

Questions for reflection and discussion

1   Consider what more might be done to improve services for children and adolescents presenting with mental health problems in a primary care setting with which you are familiar.

2 Should children's services be provided under one umbrella? What are the potential benefits? What are your feelings about children's services being provided by a Children's NHS Trust?

3 Should child psychiatry align itself with community paediatrics or adult mental health?

4 What specialist roles could nurses play in bridging the gap between services for adolescents and adult mental health?

5 What services could be nurse led? Is there scope for generic workers to be trained to undertake most of the functions within child and adolescent mental health services (CAMHS)?

Annotated bibliography

- Barker, P. (1992) *Basic Child Psychiatry*. Oxford: Blackwell Science Publishers. I recommend this book to trainees in child psychiatry. It is extremely well written and is a useful reference book for clinical situations experienced in everyday practice.
- Rutter, M. and Taylor, E. (eds) (2002) *Child and Adolescent Psychiatry* (4th edn). Blackwell Publications. The fourth edition is one of the most comprehensive textbooks in child and adolescent psychiatry and is highly recommended for readers wishing to research topics in depth. It outlines recent research findings and current thinking in the field.

References

American Psychiatric Association (1994) *Diagnostic and Statistical Manual of Mental Disorders, DSM-IV* (4th edn). Washington, DC: American Psychiatric Association.

Audit Commission (1999) *Children in Mind: Child and Adolescent Mental Health Services*. Portsmouth: Holbrooks Printers.

Barker, P. (1992) *Basic Family Therapy* (3rd edn). Oxford: Blackwell.

Bowlby, J. (1980) *Attachment and Loss: III. Loss, Sadness and Depression*. London: Hogarth and New York: Basic Books.

Boyle, M.H., Offord, D.R., Hofman, H.G. *et al.* (1987) 'Ontario child health study: methodology', *Archives of General Psychiatry* **44**: 826–31.

Caplan, G. (1964) *Principles of Preventative Psychiatry*. New York: Basic Books.

Conners, C.K. (1969) A teacher rating scale for use in drug studies with children. *American Journal of Psychiatry* **127**: 884–8.

Conners, C.K. (1973) Rating scales for use in drug studies with children. *Psychopharmacology Bulletin: Special issue on Pharmacotherapy with children* **9**: 24–84.

Department of Health (1999) *Saving Lives: Our Healthier Nation*. White Paper, July. DOH Public Health Division.

Douglas, J.W.B. (1973) Early disturbing events and later enuresis, in I. Kolvin,

R. Mackeith and S.R. Meadow (eds) *Bladder Control and Enuresis, Clinics in Developmental Medicine*, Nos 48/49, 109–17. London: Heinemann/Spasibics International Medical Publications.

Edwards, J.G. (1994) Drugs in focus: 14. The selective serotonin reuptake inhibitors in the treatment of depression. *Prescribers' Journal* **35**: 197–204.

Erikson, E. ([1960] 1965) *Childhood and Society*. London: Penguin.

Erikson, E.H. (1968) *Identity: Youth and Crisis*. New York: Norton.

Fergusson, D.M., and Horwood, L.J. (2000) Does cannabis use encourage other forms of illicit drug use? *Addiction* **95**: 505–20.

Fossen, A., Knibbs, J., Bryant-Waugh, R. and Lask, B. (1987) Early onset anorexia nervosa, *Archives of Disease in Childhood* **62**: 114–18.

Harrington, R.C. (1992) Annotation: the natural history and treatment of child and adolescent affective disorders. *Journal of Child Psychology and Psychiatry* **33**: 1287–302.

Hazell, P., O'Connell, D., Heathcote, D., Robertson, J. and Henry, D. (1995) Efficacy of tricyclic drugs in treating child and adolescent depression: a meta-analysis. *British Medical Journal* **310**: 897–901.

Hersov, L. (1994) Faecal soiling, in M. Rutter, E. Taylor and L. Hersov (eds) *Child and Adolescent Psychiatry: Modern Approaches* (3rd edn). Oxford: Blackwell Science, pp. 520–8.

Holden, J.M., Sagoysky, R. and Cox, J.L. (1989) Counselling in a general practice setting: controlled study of health visitor intervention in treatment of postnatal depression. *British Medical Journal* **298**: 223–6.

Kagan, J., Reznick, J.S. and Snidman, N. (1988) Biological basis of childhood shyness. *Science*, **240**: 167–71.

Lavik, N.J. (1977) Urban-rural differences in rates of disorder. A comparative psychiatric population study of Norwegian adolescents, in P.J. Graham (ed.) *Epidemiological Approaches in Child Psychiatry*. London: Academic Press, pp. 223–51.

Lavigne, J.V., Gibbons, R.D., Christoffel, K.K. *et al.* (1996) Prevalence rates and correlates of psychiatric disorders among pre-school children, *Journal of the American Academy of Child and Adolescent Psychiatry* **35**(2): 204–14.

Masten, A.S., Garmezy, N., Tellegan, A. *et al.* (1988) Competence and stress in school children. The moderating effects of individual and family qualities, *Journal of Child Psychology and Psychiatry* **29**: 745–64.

Rapoport, J.L. *et al.* (1994) Obsessive-compulsive disorder, in M. Rutter, E. Taylor and L. Hersov (eds) *Child and Adolescent Psychiatry: Modern Approaches* (3rd edn). Oxford: Blackwell Science, pp. 441–54.

Richman, N., Stevenson, J. and Graham, P.J. (1982) *Pre-school to School: A Behavioural Study*. Behavioural Development: A Series of Monographs. 228. London: Academic Press.

Robertson, M.M. (1989) The Gilles de la Tourette syndrome: the current status. *British Jounral of Psychiatry* **154**: 147–69.

Rutter, M. (1976) Isle of Wight studies, 1964–1974, *Psychological Medicine* **6**: 313–32.

Rutter, M. (1990) Psychosocial resilience and protective mechanisms, in J. Rolf, A.A. Masten, D. Cicchetti, K.H. Neuchterlein and S. Weintraub (eds) *Risk and Protective Factors in the Development of Psychopathology* New York: Cambridge University Press, pp. 79–101.

Rutter, M. and Taylor, E. (eds) (2002) *Child and Adolescent Psychiatry* (4th edn). Blackwell Publication.

Rutter, M., Tizard, J. and Whitmore, K. (eds) (1970) *Education, Health and Behaviour* (this is the original description of the first Isle of Wight study). London: Longman.

Rutter, M., Shaffer, D. and Sturge, C. (1975) *A Guide to a Multi-Axial Classification Scheme for Psychiatric Disorders in Childhood and Adolescence*. London: Department of Child and Adolescent Psychiatry, Institute of Psychiatry.

Shaffer, D. (1974) Suicide in childhood and early adolescence. *Journal of Child Psychology and Psychiatry*, **15**: 275–291. (This is an excellent descriptive study of completed suicide in 12–14 year olds; most other studies focus on older teenagers.)

Shaffer, D. (1994) Enuresis, in M. Rutter and L. Hersov (eds) *Child and Adolescent Psychiatry: Modern Approaches* (3rd edn). Oxford: Blackwell Science, pp. 505–19.

Shaffer, D., Gould, M.S., Fisher, P. *et al.* (1996) Psychiatric diagnosis in child and adolescent suicide. *Archives of General Psychiatry* **53**: 339–48.

Sheldrick, C. (1994) Treatment of delinquents, in M. Rutter, E. Taylor and L. Hersov (eds) *Child and Adolescent Psychiatry: Modern Approaches* (3rd edn). Oxford: Blackwell Science, pp. 968–82.

Steinhausen, H.-C. (1994) Anorexia and bulimia nervosa, in M. Rutter, E. Taylor and L. Hersov (eds) *Child and Adolescent Psychiatry: Modern Approaches* (3rd edn). Oxford: Blackwell Science, pp. 425–40.

Swadi, H. (2000) Substance misuse in adolescents, *Advances in Psychiatry Treatment*, Vol. 6, pp. 201–10.

Taylor, E., Chadwick, O., Heptinstall, E. and Danckaerts, M. (1996) Hyperactivity and conduct problems as risk factors for adolescents development, *Journal of the American Academy of Child and Adolescent Psychiatry* **35**: 1213–26.

World Health Organization (1993) *The ICD-10 Classification of Mental and Behavioral Disorders: Diagnostic Criteria for Research*. World Health Organization, Geneva.

19

The older person with dementia or other mental health problems

John Keady and Peter Ashton

Chapter overview

In this chapter we consider dementia and other mental health problems in older people with reference to the *NSF for Older People* (Department of Health (DH) 2001), which is described as a 'key vehicle' (p. 5) for ensuring that the needs of older people are at the heart of the UK government's reform programme for health and social services. We pay particular attention to Standard 7 of this policy document entitled 'mental health in older people'. While Standard 7 alludes to the broad range of diagnostic categories that affect older people, the conditions of depression, suicide and dementia are specifically, and repeatedly, referred to as the priority areas for support, intervention and service attention. Taking this focus as the lead, therefore, these three conditions form the main thrust and direction of this chapter.

If a more rounded account of the range of mental health conditions experienced by older people is required, we would suggest access to more substantial texts such as those by Norman and Redfern (1997) and Smyer and Qualls (1999). Further details about these two texts are in the annotated bibliography of recommended reading at the end of this chapter. Echoing the specific focus of Standard 7, the chapter will also emphasize the 'community orientation' (DH 2001: 91) of mental health services for older people thereby supporting the policy imperative of identifying the hallmarks of quality service provision.

In order to place each of these issues within an appropriate context, the chapter starts by briefly examining the growth of mental health policy for older people in the UK, with a primary focus on dementia. The central discourses of Standard 7 of the *NSF for Older People* (DH 2001) will then be addressed and applied to each of the three diagnostic conditions given above. We use a case study in each of the areas of depression and dementia to help illustrate some of the key ethical and clinical challenges that are present for mental health nurses involved with the client group. Finally, the chapter pulls together some of the major challenges that are present for mental health nurses and identifies areas from Standard 7 where further attention and research activity would prove helpful in moving the agenda forward.

This chapter covers:

- Background to the NSF for older people.
- What does the NSF for older people cover?
- Depression in older people: an overview.
- Suicide in later life.
- Depression: risk assessment, treatment and intervention.
- Depression in later life: a case study.
- Dementia: a human condition.
- Family care: exploring the meaning of need.
- Evidence-based care: outcome studies in dementia.
- Sharing the diagnosis of dementia: a case study.

Background to the *NSF for Older People*

Prior to the launch of the *NSF for Older People* (DH 2001), policy formation for mental health and older people in the UK had been, at best, fragmented and poorly developed. An early illustration of this fragmentation can be found in a report conducted by Thomson *et al.* (1951) on behalf of the Birmingham Regional Hospital Board. This study was focused on the care of the 'ageing and chronically sick' and was primarily funded to explore the potential for this group to 'choke' (bed-block) hospital infirmary wards; the study also addressed an alternative care paradigm of older people (and the chronically sick) remaining at home supported by their families. At the time it was thought that 'grave hardship and public scandal' would result if no action was taken to remedy the situation and thereby recommendations were required to ameliorate inadequate service provision.

Reading through the detailed and sensitively constructed report, it would appear that few lessons have been learnt over the years. For instance, the report suggested that it would be both 'unfortunate' and 'inefficient' if the care of the aged were to be 'divided between self-contained departments of different authorities' (Thomson *et al.* 1951: 5). Similarly, and with admirable foresight, the report's authors also urged reform to be directed towards the 'prevention of complete disability in the senile' (p. 47). Indeed, this was further developed in the report by the need for infirmaries to build extensions to their accommodation in order to meet the distinct needs of those with 'mild senile dementia' (p. 128). Arguably, this recommendation has, over the years, developed into the provision of memory clinics, although their availability remains patchy across the UK (Wilcock *et al.* 1999). More-over, to this day, studies continue to reveal that older people with dementia (and other mental health conditions) in acute hospital settings are mis-understood and have inadequate access to specialist nursing care (see Shah *et al.* 1998).

During the 1980s attempts at providing a strategic vision for mental health services for older people were usually provided by the representative bodies of the medical and nursing professions who were concerned about its 'Cinderella' status as compared to other areas of the (mental) health service (see, for illustration, The Royal College of Physicians' report *Organic Mental Impairment in the Elderly* (1981) and the joint report by the Royal College of Physicians and the Royal College of Psychiatrists, *Care of Elderly People with Mental Illness: Specialist Service and Medical Training* (1989)). It is fair to suggest that these reports were also concerned with upholding the 'distinctiveness' of mental health work with older people, a debate that con-tinues to the present with the separation, for good or bad, of older people from the *NSF for Mental Health* (DH 1999a).

A cursory review of later policy documents that have a direct bearing on the lives of older people with mental health needs (see Alzheimer's Disease Society 1995, DH 1995, 1996, 1997; NHS Confederation and the Sainsbury Centre for Mental Health 1997), while varying in their depth and sophistica-tion, are unified by a common absence – that of a meaningful evaluative strategy that sets targets on service improvement and limits on how far such service shortfalls should be tolerated. The need to start setting, and measuring, standards of good practice was brought home by the launch of the report *Forget Me Not: Mental Health Services for Older People* at the start of this century (Audit Commission 2000).

Conducted in 12 areas of England and Wales this influential study used a range of instruments to measure current practice in primary, secondary and tertiary care settings, including surveys of general practitioners (GPs), carers' individual case information and case file analysis. Interestingly, for older people with functional mental health problems, it was found that this group were well able to articulate their own needs and that – unsurprisingly perhaps – their self-reported priorities were 'similar to those of younger people with mental health problems' (Audit Commission 2000: 14). These priorities were listed as:

- information about services and treatments;
- respect, dignity and confidentiality;
- a choice of appropriate services at times when they are needed;
- education and training for participation in service planning;
- involvement in decisions about their care and services in general.

(Audit Commission 2000: 14–15)

The report also identified the importance of practising cognitive behavioural therapy (CBT) and that older people with depression would benefit from having a regular visitor to their home, even though it was recognized that such visits might not cure the depression. Furthermore, three key aims of a mental health service for older people were listed (Audit Commission 2000: 15) and these were stated as being able:

1 to maintain the mental health of older people and to help preserve their independence;

2 to support family carers as well as older people themselves;

3 to provide intermittent or permanent residential care for those who are so disabled that it is the most practical and humane way of looking after them.

In the area of dementia care, particularly in its early identification, the report (Audit Commission 2000) presented some worrying findings. For example, of the total number of GPs surveyed (n = 1000+ (representing 55 per cent of the study sample)) only around one half of respondents believed that it was important to look actively for early signs of dementia and to make an early diagnosis. As the report went on to explain, many of the GPs saw no point in looking for an incurable condition with a typical GP response being listed as: '*Dementia is untreatable, so why diagnose it?*' (2000: 21). In contrast, almost 9 out of 10 GPs in the survey believed it was important to look for early signs of depression and to make a diagnosis.

Arguably, of even more concern than the expressed nihilistic attitudes towards those with (suspected) dementia, less than one half of the GPs questioned said that they used any specific tests or protocols to help them diagnose the condition. Moreover, only one third said that they used specific tests or protocols to detect the signs of depression. Clearly, much work needs to be done if the situation is to improve, and similar to the situation faced by nursing (Nolan *et al.* 2001), it is recommended that GPs (and the wider primary health care team (PHCT)) receive better training and education on mental health and older people.

In their follow-up report published in February 2002, the Audit Commission (2002a) synthesized the results of a series of local audits conducted on mental health services for older people. These local audits were all conducted in England and were commissioned after the publication of the first Audit Commission report in January 2000. The 2002(a) report also drew attention to the main elements of Standard 7 of the *NSF for Older People* (DH 2001), as will be shortly addressed, and integrated these targets into the report's findings. However, before moving on to this aspect of the chapter, it is important to mention that the 2002(a) Audit Commission report continued to highlight the problems experienced by GPs in identifying mental health problems early in their course, particularly dementia. Similarly, health and social care agencies were encouraged to develop joint plans for commissioning and delivering integrated services based on good information and involving key partners. In this latter recommendation there is more than a passing resemblance to that made by Thomson *et al.* in 1951. It is, therefore, important to not only digest the recommendations that such reports present, but, more importantly to actively seek, and evaluate, their integration into mainstream service practice and management. Arguably, it is the enactment of this notion, coupled with the philosophies of 'value for money' and 'consumer empowerment', that the UK Labour government have grasped so firmly and which has emerged to inspire the entire development of the NSFs. It is to a consideration of the main constituents of *NSF for Older People* (DH 2001) that we now turn.

What does the *NSF for Older People* cover?

The need to start benchmarking national service standards for the mental health care of older people was reflected, in England, in the publication and dissemination of the *NSF for Older People* (DH 2001).[1] This contains eight standards, as follows:

1   rooting out age discrimination;
2   person-centred care;
3   intermediate care;
4   general hospital care;
5   stroke;
6   falls;
7   mental health in older people;
8   the promotion of health and active life in older age.

Within the *NSF for Older People* the eight standards are supported by advice on local delivery, monitoring mechanisms and national support available to assist in their implementation. As the policy document makes clear, the *NSF for Older People* is 'the key vehicle' (DH 2001: 5) for ensuring that the needs of older people are at the heart of the reform programme for health and social services. While each of these standards has an impact upon the life of an older person, Standard 7 specifically addresses 'mental health in older people' with the overarching aim: 'To promote good mental health in older people and to treat and support those older people with dementia and depression' (DH 2001: 90).

Accordingly, Standard 7 is built squarely on the foundations of depression and dementia and, later on, also aligns its recommendations to the cause of younger people with dementia. Moreover, Standard 7 provides a salient reminder that under-detection of mental illness in older people is 'widespread' and complicated by the fact that many older people live alone without a close support network (see also Tuokko *et al.* 1999; Gilmour 2002). Standard 7 also emphasizes the need to 'treat and support' older people with mental health needs around a community-orientated model that is underpinned by three key interventions, namely:

1   promoting good mental health;
2   early recognition and management of mental health problems; and
3   access to specialist care (DH 2001: 91).

As also highlighted in the Audit Commission reports from 2000 and 2002(a), a focus on early recognition and management is particularly important as it is here where the person with the (undiagnosed) condition will first come into contact with a member of the PHCT, usually their GP. As Standard 7 makes clear, early recognition and prompt treatment of depression can reduce distressing symptoms and prevent more serious consequences such as 'physical illness, adverse effects upon social relationships, self neglect or self-harm/suicide' (DH 2001: 94). It is recommended that the assessment of psychiatric, psychological and social factors in depression include: history taking and examination of mental state, the use of assessment scales to aid diagnosis, and the carrying out of a physical examination and investigations. Furthermore, within the *NSF for Older People*, advice on the treatment of depression is provided in Standard 7 in the following way (2001: 95):

The treatment of depression involves:

- Making the diagnosis and giving the person an explanation of their symptoms.

- Assessment of risk. Especially suicidal intent, and looking for coexisting physical problems, especially possible dementia or physical illness.

- Giving information about the likely prognosis and options for packages of care.

- Making appropriate referrals to help with the fears and worries, distress, practical and financial issues that will affect the person and the carer.

- Prescribing anti-depressant medicines, taking into account the use of therapeutic dosages, anticipated side effects, known contra-indications of anti-depressants, and being sure that older people are able to take their medicines.

- Offering psychological therapies alongside anti-depressant drug treatment. The evidence suggests that the most effective treatments for depression are cognitive behaviour therapy, interpersonal therapy or brief, focused analytic therapy, offered by a trained person. Counselling in primary care may also be effective for depression at the less severe end of the spectrum.

In the area of dementia care, Standard 7 identifies the role of the National Institute of Clinical Excellence (NICE) in recommending that the drugs donepezil, rivastigmine and galantamine should be available through the NHS as a treatment component for people with mild to moderate Alzheimer's disease (for a useful review on the most recent drug treatments for Alzheimer's disease see Jones 2002). Conditions are attached to the availability of these drugs and these are: a mini-mental state examination

(MMSE) (Folstein *et al.* 1975) score of 12 or above; a diagnosis of Alzheimer's disease made in a specialist clinic; and treatment to follow specialist assessment, including tests of cognitive, global and behavioural functioning.

Within Standard 7 advice is also given on the treatment of dementia (DH 2001: 98), and this is repeated below as it provides a baseline for establishing good practice in community and residential settings.

Treatment of dementia always involves:

- Explaining the diagnosis to the older person and any carers, and where possible giving relevant information about sources of help and support.

- Giving information about the likely prognosis and options for packages of care.

- Making appropriate referrals to help with fears and worries, distress, practical and financial issues that affect the person and their carer.

- At all stages, emphasizing the unique qualities of the individual with dementia and recognizing their personal and social needs.

- Using non-pharmacological management strategies such a mental exercise, physical therapy, dietary treatment alongside drug therapy.

- Prescribing anti-psychotic drugs for more serious problems, such as delusions, and hallucinations, serious distress or danger from behaviour disturbance.

To support these objectives, Standard 7 also suggests that there should be a specialist mental health service for people with dementia if, for instance, their diagnosis is uncertain, there are safety concerns or a risk assessment is necessary. Again, such advice becomes highly relevant for nurses in this area of work as it provides a framework for assessment, intervention and practice evaluation.

In this connection, we will now provide a further elaboration of these guidelines and suggest how mental health nurses can better understand some of the key concepts that underpin Standard 7 and the *NSF for Older People* (DH 2001) more generally. This begins in the areas of depression and suicide.

Depression in older people

Depression is a complex and multi-faceted mental experience that reflects changes in a person's emotions, cognitions, physical state and behaviours. Generally, the diagnosis of clinical depression is based on either the International Statistical Classification of Diseases and Related Health Problems (ICD-10) (World Health Organization (WHO) 1993) or the Diagnostic and Statistical Manual of Mental Disorders (DSM-IV) (American Psychiatric Association 1994). As Table 19.1 reveals, people who experience depression frequently report having most, if not all, of the experiences described.

Table 19.1 Main characteristics of depression

Emotions

The emotional aspect of depression often presents with the person reporting (or being observed having), depressed mood most of the day, nearly every day. This is often characterized by expressions of sadness, despair and tearfulness.

Cognitions

Associated with the above emotions, depressed people will often experience and describe thoughts of a negative nature. People often report having negative thoughts about themselves that frequently refer to a sense of guilt, unworthiness, disappointment, hopelessness and helplessness. For example, '*There is no point to life any more, I am no longer needed*.' These thoughts can be so extreme that they can be accompanied by further thoughts relating to suicide, '*My family would be better off without me*.' Many people also report lower levels of concentration and attention that can lead to impaired judgement.

Behaviour

Coexisting with the above thoughts, people frequently describe changes in their everyday behaviour. People will often report having a loss of interest and pleasure in everyday and social activities. People frequently start to spend more time on their own, withdraw from social activity and can have diminished interest in sexual activity. People often state that these changes are due to a lack of interest, energy or ability to concentrate. However, in some cases where there is coexisting agitation, there may be increased activity in the form of restlessness, pacing and an inability to relax.

Physical experiences

From a physical perspective, people often report having disturbed sleep which can include waking in the night, difficulty getting off to sleep or early morning rising. As a consequence, people frequently experience irritability and excessive fatigue. Many people also report having a diminished appetite stating that they are not hungry or can no longer make the effort to prepare meals. Prolonged disturbance of eating can result in weight loss and loss of energy.

Source: ICD-10 (WHO 1993) and DSM-IV (APA 1994)

Types of depression

The characteristics outlined in Table 19.1 can manifest themselves in different ways and there are considerable variations in how older people experience depression. This can range from a low level of dysphoria (i.e. unhappiness) to major clinical depression resulting in serious and comprehensive changes to the person's well-being. Furthermore, the depression may have been in existence for varying lengths of time. For some people, the depression is of an episodic nature, perhaps resulting from a significant life event. For others, there may be a history of long-term misery and unhappiness. Depression therefore needs to be viewed from the perspective of symptom intensity and duration. The picture for depression is further complicated by the debate around the existence of sub-types of depression such as reactive-endogenous, neurotic-psychotic, primary-secondary, and the existence of the following different ways of classifying depression:

- bipolar affective disorder;
- depressive episode;
- recurrent depressive disorder;
- persistent mood (affective) disorders (including dysthymia);
- reaction to severe stress, and adjustment disorder.

(ICD-10 classification: WHO 1993)

and

- major depression (single episode or recurrent);
- bipolar disorders;
- dysthymia;
- minor depressive disorder;
- mixed anxiety-depressive disorder.

(DSM-IV classification: American Psychiatric Association 1994)

While the utilization of the above classifications may be useful for clinical diagnosis and research purposes, from a nursing perspective it is how the older person experiences and interprets these features that are the crucial issues. Without such an understanding, nursing care will, we suggest, fail to be person-centred.

Epidemiology of depression

Although there have been many attempts to examine the existence of depression in older people, accurate estimates of the prevalence of depression can be problematic due to the use of different instruments and the focus on different types of depression. Beekman *et al.* (1999) review of studies into the prevalence of depression in older people within the general population reports rates within the range of 2.9–15.9 per cent, with the lower rates for major depression and the higher rates for minor depression. Moreover, in a UK-based community survey by Lindesay *et al.* (1989) of approximately 1000 older people in an urban area, 4.3 per cent were identified as suffering from severe depression, with a further 13.5 per cent experiencing depression to a mild to moderate degree. While there appears to be differences in the prevalence of different types of depression, there is an agreement that depression is the most common mental health problem experienced by older people (Banerjee *et al.* 1996). Furthermore, depression in older people presents itself in a variety of different settings:

- Banerjee (1993) found evidence of depression in 26 per cent of people receiving home care services from a local authority social services department.
- Pitt (1991) reported a prevalence rate of depression of 5–40 per cent in 'geriatric' inpatient populations.

- Ames (1991) identified a figure of 40 per cent in a UK study of older people living in residential homes.
- Koenig *et al.* (1988) report rates up to 45 per cent for older people in medical settings.
- MacDonald (1986) identified the existence of depression in 31 per cent of all older people attending their GP.

Within these and other studies, other important information about depression in later life has been identified. For instance, both Wragg and Jeste (1989) and Teri and Wagner (1991) have suggested that as many as 30 per cent of people with Alzheimer's disease have a coexisting major depressive disorder. There also seems to be a strong association with loss events, poverty and social isolation (Katona 1994), the coexistence of physical disease and recent bereavement (Murphy 1982) and depression being more common in women (Copeland *et al.* 1987). Also, depression appears to have a poorer prognosis than in younger people with higher mortality rates (Murphy 1983), and high rates of persistence and recurrence (Cole 1990). For example, Musetti *et al.* (1989) found that previous episodes of depression in older people were as high as 67 per cent. However, these findings may well have been influenced by inappropriate, or even non-existent, treatment and management regimens (see also Benbow 1992). Unfortunately, many older people with depression, both severe and less severe, are often not diagnosed (Blanchard and Mann 1994) or not identified (Iliffe *et al.* 1993; Audit Commission 2000, 2002a,b). This is of particular concern given the high risk of suicide that is found within the older population (Diekstra 1989), an issue that we now consider in a little more detail.

Suicide in later life

As stated earlier, one of the significant cognitive aspects of depression is the tendency for people to have strong negative thoughts that can relate to a sense of hopelessness, helplessness, guilt and unworthiness. The intensity, duration and content of these beliefs can have serious consequences in terms of suicidal ideation, with people experiencing a strong sense of helplessness and hopelessness, being more at risk of self-harm and suicide (Ashton and Keady 1999).

While there has been an ongoing reduction in the number of older people committing suicide within the general population of England and Wales (Hoxey and Shah 2000), older people still experience the highest rates for suicide, particularly males over the age of 75 years (Murphy 1988; Diekstra 1989; Clarke and Fawcett 1992) – an issue that appears to be a multinational phenomenon (Pearson *et al.* 1997; Snowdon 1997). Furthermore, McIntosh (1992) has indicated that there is a ratio of 4:1 of attempted suicide to successful suicide in older people, compared with between 8:1 and 20:1 in the general population. Based on these figures, suicidal behaviour in older people is more likely to have a fatal outcome. While not all older people who commit suicide are clinically depressed, results from studies have identified a strong correlation between depression, suicide and attempted suicide (Draper 1996). Indeed, Barraclough *et al.* (1974) found that there was a diagnosis of depressive illness in 87 per cent of suicides they examined. In a more recent study, Cattell and Jolley (1995) reviewed 100 cases of suicide in Manchester, and they found that in 61 per cent of the successful attempts the person had a clinically recognizable depressive illness.

Of further significance, in Hepple and Quinton's (1997) study of 100 people over 65 who had attempted suicide, a significant number went on to make further attempts or achieve fatal outcomes. From their cohort, all five of the male repeat attempts resulted in death. They also state that those at risk of further self-harm are most likely to be suffering from persistent depression and to be in contact with mental health services. It is, therefore, important to specifically address this issue in nursing assessment of older people with depression who come into contact with mental health services. Furthermore, a focus on this issue will help service providers and policy makers continue to make progress towards an overall 15 per cent target reduction in suicide outlined in *The Health of the Nation* (DH 1992) report, and the proposed further reduction of one sixth of the 1996 baseline by the year 2010 outlined in the document *Saving Lives: Our Healthier Nation* (DH 1999b).

To work towards the achievement of these reductions there is a need to be aware of possible contributory factors that apply to people who attempt or achieve suicide. The review of attempted suicide by Draper (1996), and reviews of suicide by Barraclough *et al.* (1974), Cattell and Jolley (1995) and Lindesay (1997), draws attention to the following range of risk factors:

- the presence of depressive symptoms or disorder;
- social isolation and living alone;
- chronic physical illness and pain;
- males more than females commit suicide;
- females more likely to engage in parasuicide;
- more evidence in people from lower social class;
- the person is single, divorced or widowed;
- there is a history of incapacity for forming close relationships, dependency and difficulty coping with change;
- previous episode of attempted suicide;
- recent significant aversive life event;
- alcohol abuse.

Given that the critical periods of risk for those already undergoing treatment for depression is within the first few hours after admission to an inpatient psychiatric unit, and the first few weeks after discharge (Baldwin 1993), mental health nurses working either in the hospital or community settings have a pivotal role in risk assessment, treatment and intervention. It is to each of these areas that the chapter will now turn.

Depression: risk assessment, treatment and intervention

Risk assessment

As stated earlier, and coupled to the advice outlined in Standard 7 of the *NSF for Older People* (DH 2001), depression is a complex and multi-faceted condition that impacts upon the physical, psychological and social aspects of a person's life, including their spouse/significant other, relatives and friends. Therefore, to establish the person's needs and goals, it is recommended that a comprehensive assessment be conducted that examines the existence of physical, psychological and social factors. Whether the assessment is carried out in hospital or in the community, it is necessary for the assessment to be thorough, detailed, comprehensive and continuous.

It is also important to recognize that depression is a very personal experience that can be very painful for the individual. Sharing their experience may be very difficult, challenging and emotional for some people. It is, therefore, important for the mental health nurse to draw on and use their interpersonal skills in a sensitive and supportive manner. From the outset it is also crucial that the person recognizes that they can be helped, and this is especially important with patients who express some suicidal ideation.

During the initial assessment, the therapeutic relationship also needs to be developed. The nurse should demonstrate a warm, attentive, concerned manner and be non-judgemental in response to what the older person may disclose. The use of empathic responses will help the person feel listened to and understood. When conducting the assessment it is important to identify the way in which the person is experiencing the(ir) depression, and the manner in which they have attempted to cope with their difficulties. From the outset, the nurse needs to encourage the patient to share their thoughts, feelings and actions and help them to understand their depression. This can be achieved through explanation or by giving the patient a handout on depression. Many patients find this information reassuring in that it helps them to realize that they are not 'going mad' or that they are not the only ones to have experienced the condition.

In the initial stages of the assessment it is important to explore and get an insight into the following aspects of the person's life:

- the subjective experience of depression in terms of symptoms, their intensity and duration;
- any precipitating events;
- current and possible previous coping strategies;
- consequences of the depression for both the older person and any significant others;
- suicidal ideation;
- current medication;
- previous history of depression;
- current health state.

Examination of these issues will help to build up an understanding of the older person's depression, its meaning for them, and form the basis for future nursing interventions. Interviews with relatives or friends can provide an additional source of information that can both clarify and provide a clearer picture of the existing situation. Observational information should also be used as it makes a vital contribution to the initial and ongoing assessment process. The assessment process can also be assisted through the use of formal rating scales and assessment tools. However, as Burns *et al.* state:

> ... determining which scale should be selected must always follow an analysis of the underlying purpose ... is the scale to be used to screen a population, assess severity of symptoms, or to help with diagnosis or to monitor change?
>
> (2002: 161)

From a nursing perspective, tools for assessing symptoms, monitoring change and screening in the community would be the most relevant and one, or a combination of tools, from the following list could be helpful:

- Beck Depression Inventory-II (Steer *et al.* 2000). This is a validated 21-item self-report scale of depressive symptoms in which the patient indicates the existence and severity of symptoms. The scale is not designed to diagnose depression but to assess and monitor changes to symptoms.
- Hamilton Rating Scale for Depression (Hamilton 1960). This scale would be completed by the nurse and used to assess the severity of depression, rather than as a diagnostic tool.
- Hospital Anxiety and Depression Scale (Zigmond and Snaith 1983). Again, this is a self-report instrument that measures anxiety and depression. Flint and Rifat (2002) have recently subjected it to a validation study with older patients with encouraging results.
- Geriatric Depression Scale (Yesavage *et al.* 1983; Shiekh and Yesavage 1986). This is a self-report assessment tool for depression. The 1986 tool is a shorter (15-item version) of the original instrument.
- Schwab-Gilleard Depression Scale (Schwab and Holzer 1973). This is a short self-report instrument for the assessment of depression and is particularly useful in its ability to discriminate depression from dementia. The Schwab-Gilleard Depression Scale has been subjected to a validation study, assessing depression in residential homes with positive outcomes (Richardson and Hammond 1996).

Treatment and intervention

The nursing contribution to the treatment of depression should consider psychological, physical, pharmacological and social interventions. While the treatment of depression in older people has traditionally focused on the use of pharmacotherapy (Shepherd *et al.* 1981; Larson *et al.* 1991), the use of medication has produced mixed results. As an illustration, Georgotas *et al.*

(1986) reported that between 30 and 40 per cent of individuals with major depressive disorder did not achieve a satisfactory improvement from initial treatment with anti-depressants. In a follow-up study of depressed older people in local authority homes, Ames (1990) experienced 'disappointing results' with a poor response to psychotropic medication. Furthermore, it has also been suggested that the sole use of drug therapy may produce a poor outcome for some patients (Murphy 1983; Gerson *et al.* 1988). Flint (1995) suggests that a number of factors could be contributing to these outcomes such as an incorrect diagnosis, inadequate dose and duration of medication, poor compliance, presence of physical illness, concurrent medications contributing to depression and ongoing psychosocial factors.

Richter *et al.* (1983) also suggest that many older people who receive anti-depressants are prescribed sub-therapeutic doses, possibly because of the increased risk of side effects. Even when the correct dose is prescribed, non-compliance can be a problem. For example, in Kendrick and Bayne's (1982) study of older people receiving care in their own homes, only 57 per cent were compliant with the prescribed medication. Conversely, older people who do comply with prescription regimens are more likely to experience side effects because of increased susceptibility to adverse drug reactions (Epstein 1978). Indeed, older people are vulnerable to almost all side effects of drugs because of changes in absorption, metabolism and excretion leading to elevated drug levels in the body and prolonged half-life of the drugs (Whitlock and Evans 1978; Wood *et al.* 1988; Harper *et al.* 1989). This increased susceptibility to adverse drug reactions and side effects may also contribute to non-compliance or premature discontinuation of treatment. However, with careful medical management and the following nursing support, medication can make a positive contribution to the treatment of depression:

- Encourage compliance through explanation, education, the possible use of medication dispensers, and the involvement of significant others.

- Closely monitor the effects of medication, both in terms of symptom relief and side effects.

- Ensure the person prescribing the medication is regularly informed of all aspects of its impact on the person.

In addition to medication, electro-convulsive therapy (ECT) may be prescribed for the treatment of depression. Benbow's (1989) review of the use of ECT in the treatment of depression in older people concluded that older people respond to ECT just as well as younger people do. Furthermore, Kendell (1981) has suggested that older people are able to tolerate ECT very well, and it seems to have a positive impact in cases of endogenous depression (Fraser and Glass 1980; Benbow 1987).

For some time now, there has been a growing body of evidence to support the use of psychological therapies with older people (Woods 1992). In a study of behavioural, cognitive and brief psychodynamic therapy, Thompson *et al.* (1987) reported that all three therapies achieved positive outcomes in the treatment of depression. Furthermore, these psychological therapies have been reported to be effective with reactive and endogenous forms of depression (Gallagher and Thompson 1983). However, as stated in Standard 7 of the *NSF for Older People* (DH 2001), CBT seems to be emerging with the strongest evidence base for practice efficacy (see also Charlesworth *et al.* 2000). In support of this assertion, Thompson *et al.* (1986) examined the evidence for the use of cognitive therapy and came to the conclusion that 'cognitive therapy, engaged on a one to one basis, is efficacious in the treatment of clinically depressed older adults'. In a later study by Leung and Orrell (1993), which centred on the efficacy of brief focused cognitive therapy, results described a positive outcome with 92 per cent of the patients diagnosed on the DSM III-R (American Psychiatric Association 1987) as major depression were functioning well at discharge at the time of the one-year follow-up.

However, other studies have suggested that CBT can also be effective when provided in a group format. In Beutler *et al.*'s (1987) study an attempt was made to compare the effectiveness of alprazolam and group cognitive therapy with older adults experiencing depression. Their results showed that patients receiving group cognitive therapy showed consistent improvement in self-reported symptoms, compared to non-group patients, and were less likely to prematurely terminate treatment. Furthermore, the researchers concluded that positive benefits observed during therapy were continued through the follow-up phase, suggesting that patients had learnt something of benefit.

Given the positive outcomes achieved from the use of CBT, nurses should consider its use as part of their psychological component of care. In addition to psychological therapy, many older people may benefit from social support. Encouraging the patient to re-establish previous social activity and contacts can help reverse the social isolation that may have emerged. It is also important for the nurse not to underestimate the physical aspect of the older person's needs. Some depressed older people may have ongoing physical problems that cause discomfort or reduce mobility. The nurse should pay particular attention to these needs and respond where appropriate. There may also be a need to ensure that the patient has an adequate diet and to provide encouragement with self-care. In conclusion, the achievement of Standard 7 of the *NSF for Older People* (DH 2001) will be progressed if nurses provide high quality evidence-based practice. Given that depression in later life usually affects different aspects of the person's life, effective care and treatment is more likely to be achieved through the use of multi-disciplinary assessment, treatment and liaison. It is this focus that the following case study attempts to reveal.

Depression in later life: the case of Mrs Jones

This case study provides a clinical illustration of the characteristics of depression and risk of suicide, and the nurse's role in the assessment, treatment and support of an older person experiencing a reactive type of clinical depression. The case study is built from the clinical experience of one of the chapter authors (PA), although certain details in the case study have been changed to maintain confidentiality.

Background

Mrs Jones is a 69-year-old retired nurse who had been referred by her GP to the older person community mental health team in North Wales, with an initial diagnosis of depression. The letter from the GP indicated that Mrs Jones has been suffering from depression for the 'last four months' and that it was 'probably a reaction to the death of her husband, who had died six months ago after living with dementia for five years'. Mrs Jones had been offered some anti-depressant medication but has been reluctant to take it.

Mrs Jones has two grown-up children who live in other parts of the country. While she is in contact with her children, it is mainly via the telephone as they both live some distance away.

Initial nursing assessment

Following this referral, arrangements were made for her to be seen at home by PA. On commencing the first visit, PA endeavoured to establish a good rapport with Mrs Jones through the careful use of non-verbal and verbal responses. These included shaking Mrs Jones's hand when introducing himself, maintaining good eye contact, active listening and the use of empathic, reflective and summarizing responses to communicate a sense of understanding and interest in what Mrs Jones had to say.

PA then suggested that it might be helpful if Mrs Jones could share with him a little about how she was feeling and proceeded to use mainly open-ended questions to encourage Mrs Jones to talk about how she felt. Questions were used to explore the meaning and nature of Mrs Jones's depression. This involved a careful exploration of the emotional, cognitive, behavioural and physical aspects of her depression, and its duration and intensity. To assist with the recording of this information, PA used the Beck Depression Inventory-II (Steer *et al.* 2000) which, as highlighted earlier, is a scale consisting of 21 questions relating to the common characteristics of depression. While this would normally be completed by the older person him/herself, PA introduced and used this form to help demonstrate its use, and provide a baseline level of symptoms and their severity.

From a cognitive perspective, Mrs Jones stated that her depression started to emerge shortly after the death of her husband, whom she had cared for during his illness. She described this time as being 'very difficult' but felt it was 'the least she should do' given their close relationship. However, some three weeks before her husband's death, Mrs Jones finally, and reluctantly, agreed to his admission into the local mental health unit for respite care. It was during this time that Mr Jones died. Mrs Jones expressed thoughts relating to guilt, being a failure and of 'letting her husband down'. She also expressed thoughts relating to wanting to be with her husband and there being 'no future or point to life any more'. At an emotional level, Mrs Jones expressed sadness and was tearful throughout the first meeting.

Given the potential for suicide in depressed older people and the existence of the following risk factors in the case study: negative thoughts, a recent aversive life event, reduced social contacts, living alone, and being widowed; it was necessary to ascertain whether there was any significant risk of self-harm or suicide. While many of the risk factors were present and Mrs Jones expressed negative thoughts about her future, when asked to respond to the question on suicide in the BDI-II, she scored 1 (the lowest score) by answering 'I have had thoughts about killing myself, but I would not carry them out.' Mrs Jones also stated that she hadn't actually thought about how to end her life, and didn't think she would have the courage to do this as it would upset her son and daughter. These responses seemed to suggest a low risk of self-harm.

From a physical perspective, Mrs Jones stated that she wasn't sleeping very well and was always feeling very tired. She said her appetite had gone and she was unable to muster any enthusiasm for cooking. Behaviourally, Mrs Jones stated that she did not go out of the house for long periods of time, and even when she did, she tried to avoid contact with people she previously knew. Before this event Mrs Jones had had a very active social life and also worked a few hours a week for a local voluntary agency. However, Mrs Jones stated that this had stopped when she had to focus on meeting her husband's needs. Mrs Jones also stated that she could no longer be bothered to do the household chores as 'nobody called anyway'. Mrs Jones also stated that she previously took pride in her own appearance but was now 'disinterested' in herself.

After exploring the different aspects of Mrs Jones depression, and completing the BDI-II form, the score was calculated and shared with Mrs Jones. The initial score was 21 and this reflected a 'moderate level' of depression. Mrs Jones was then helped to clarify her problems and how life might be if positive changes could be made to improve her situation. Mrs Jones felt her main problems were a lack of energy, a sense of loss, guilt about being a failure, and having no purpose or pleasure in life any more. Mrs Jones said she would like life to be better and agreed to work with PA to try and improve the way she was experiencing her life. PA then completed the care plan with Mrs Jones and provided her with a copy.

Interventions

As previously stated, interventions need to be chosen for their relevance and potential to bring about positive changes within the problematic aspects of life. However, the option of medication was ruled out because Mrs Jones did not think it would help and she was reluctant to become dependent on it. Given that Mrs Jones's depression appeared to be of the reactive type, it was felt that social support and interpersonal therapy, based on the principles of CBT, would be a suitable treatment option. This was provided by PA, who, over the next few sessions, worked to the following three-point plan:

1   To engage on a sessional treatment plan of CBT in order to work on negative thoughts relating to guilt, being a failure and having a purpose in life. This involved Mrs Jones keeping a 'thought diary' in order to provide a focus for work on her negative thoughts. Within the psychotherapy aspect of interventions, Mrs Jones was encouraged to reflect on the validity and helpfulness of her current thoughts and to consider the development of more helpful alternative thoughts. Between sessions, Mrs Jones was encouraged to progressively engage in more activities to accumulate further evidence of alternative, more helpful, beliefs.

2   To re-establish activities previously enjoyed, using activity scheduling and mastery and pleasure rating. This included contacting some old friends and colleagues from her voluntary group, going out more for walks to the local shops and going to the hairdresser to counter social isolation and raise self-esteem.

3   The ongoing weekly use of the Beck Depression Inventory-II (Steer *et al.* 2000) to monitor depressive symptoms and evaluate improvement.

Outcome

After five weekly, and a further five fortnightly, one-hour visits, Mrs Jones demonstrated considerable improvement. The scores on the BDI-II forms moved from an initial score of 21 (moderately depressed) to 6 (a low level of unhappiness). While Mrs Jones still has some reservations about allowing her husband to go into hospital, she no longer strongly believes that she had failed her husband. From a social perspective, she has now re-established contact with several of her old friends and is considering helping out at the voluntary agency.

This case study amply illustrates how a mental health nurse, using their knowledge of depression and suicide, and interpersonal and psychotherapy skills, helped to bring about a positive change in an older person's life. It also reflects the degree of training that is necessary if the objectives raised in Standard 7 of the *NSF for Older People* (DH 2001) are to be fully met. This need for further information and development is now taken into the area of dementia care with an emphasis on its early recognition and subjective adjustment to its onset.

Dementia: a human condition

To coincide with World Alzheimer's Day, on 21 September 2000 the Alzheimer's Disease International (ADI) produced a bold and colourful pamphlet to outline their 'Charter of Principles' (ADI 2000) for the care of people with dementia and their carers. These principles are illustrated in Table 19.2.

Table 19.2 ADI Charter of Principles

1   Alzheimer's disease and related dementias are progressive, incapacitating diseases of the brain that have a profound impact on persons with dementia and members of their families.
2   A person with dementia continues to be a person of worth and dignity, and deserving the same respect as any other human being.
3   People with dementia need a physically safe living environment and protection from exploitation and abuse of person and property.
4   People with dementia require information and access to coordinated medical and welfare services. Anyone who is thought to have the disease needs medical assessment and those with the disease require ongoing care and treatment.
5   People with dementia should as far as possible participate in decisions affecting their daily lives and future care.
6   The family carers of a person with dementia should have their needs relating to the care assessed and provided for and should be enabled to take an active role in this process.
7   Adequate resources should be available and promoted to support people with dementia and their carers throughout the course of the disease.
8   Information, education and training on the disease, its effects and how to provide care must be available to all those involved in the assistance of people with dementia.

Source: ADI (2000)

Alongside these principles, and included in the same publication, the ADI (2000) also produced an overview of the worldwide projections of dementia dividing the figures between the developed and developing world. Within these pages it was revealed that in the year 2000 18 million people across the world lived with a dementia (11 million in the developing world, 7 million in the developed world), with the overall figure projected to rise to 34 million by the year 2025 (24 million in the developing world, 10 million in the developed world). The ADI also suggested that around half this total will have Alzheimer's disease and that age is the most significant risk factor for developing dementia, a finding that is consistent with other studies in the field (see, for example, Dillmann 2000).

In the UK the Alzheimer's Society (formerly known as the Alzheimer's Disease Society) revealed that, at present, some 500 people per day develop a dementia and that, in the UK, around 800,000 people currently have a dementia (Alzheimer's Society 2000). As our society has an ageing population, by the year 2021 it is estimated there will be nearly one million people with a dementia living in the UK (Alzheimer's Society 2000), a figure that is expected to rise to 1.2 million in 2050 (DH 2001). Significantly, a high percentage (around 20 per cent) will live alone with the condition and face the additional risk of self-neglect, abuse (financial and physical) and (unreported) self-injury (see also Alzheimer's Disease Society 1994; Tuokko *et al.* 1999). As importantly, behind each figure is a human being with a support system (however tenuous this may at first appear) who will also be touched by its onset and progression, a network that stretches from neighbours to family members and on to local communities. Indeed, studies have consistently demonstrated that the stressors faced by family carers of people with dementia are among the most burdensome of all chronic illnesses, with carers prone to an increased risk of depression, stress, loneliness and self-injury (for a comprehensive review, see Briggs and Askham 1999). For example, in a 1-year longitudinal study of family care giving for a person with dementia conducted by Baumgarten *et al.* (1992), the authors found a direct correlation between worsening caregiver depression and an inability to cope with increased 'challenging behaviour' from the person with dementia. Such a correlation, it was suggested, led the carer to consider 'giving up' the care-giving role and seek institutional care for the person with dementia. However, as this, and other studies have found, such a decision does not automatically lead to a lessening of caregiver stress and is often accompanied by raised feelings of guilt (see Woods 1997), feelings that may remain unresolved for many after the formal aspect of care giving has ceased.

In recent years, and as indicated in Standard 7 of the *NSF for Older People* (DH 2001), the advent of the recent drugs for Alzheimer's disease has also provided a challenge to primary care to diagnose the condition earlier, an outcome that has not always figured highly in GP consultations (Rait *et al.* 1999; Audit Commission 2000; Iliffe and Drennan 2001). However, an earlier diagnosis and communication of this to the person concerned is essential if those living with a dementia are to benefit from a range of positive outcomes, such as access to memory rehabilitation (Clare 1999) and early-stage support groups (Yale 1995). Such a paradigm shift has recently led nurses in dementia care to begin to explore their role within memory clinic environments (see for example: Rogers and Dupuis 1999; Royal College of Nursing Institute 1999; Adams and Page 2000) and in leading therapeutic programmes for people at the beginnings of their dementia (LaBarge and Trtanj 1995; Hawkins and Eagger 1999, 2002).

The recognition that the *NSF for Older People* (DH 2001), particularly Standards 2 and 7, was influenced by the experiences and voices of people with an early diagnosis of dementia should not be underestimated. In particular, a short book written by the Reverend Robert Davis at the end of the 1980s (Davis 1989) about his descent into Alzheimer's disease, proved highly influential in articulating the early adjustment process and a welcome (and necessary) addition to the literature. Others who also wanted to communicate their experience later joined this lone voice and have their experiences validated. Such texts included: McGowin (1993) *Living in the Labyrinth: A Personal Journey Through the Maze of Alzheimer's*; Henderson (1998) *Partial View: An Alzheimer's Journal*; and Boden (1998) *Who Will I Be When I Die?* Coupled with the person-centred movement outlined earlier in the chapter, the need for self-expression has recently culminated in people with dementia putting forward their needs for self-advocacy on an international platform (Friedell and Bryden 2002). This expression is also represented through internet-based activities such as the Dementia Advocacy and Support Network International (www.dasninternational.org) (see also Bryden 2002).

While Standard 7 of the *NSF for Older People* (DH 2001) correctly highlights the importance of early detection of dementia in primary care, it is equally necessary to consider the next phase of personal (and familial) adjustment to the diagnosis. Arguably, it is in this transition where mental health nurses can have the greatest impact in helping people to articulate and cope with their new-found situation. Accordingly, for those nurses who work in the field, it is important to recognize that people with dementia maintain an insight (awareness) into their condition and can utilize positive coping behaviours. Keady and Nolan (1995a,b) were among the first researchers to look at this adaptation and developed the Index for Managing Memory Loss (IMMEL) as an instrument to assess specific positive coping behaviours used by people with dementia. Included in the 42-item IMMEL scale were such coping behaviours as: routines, accepting memory loss and finding ways of overcoming it, writing in a personal diary, using lists and other memory aids, staying in familiar surroundings, exhibiting humour, information seeking, constant repetition to self to help remember, and practising relaxation techniques. The data, from which the IMMEL scale was developed, was based on qualitative interviews with 10 individuals with dementia and their caregivers (Keady and Nolan 1995a).

The study by Harris and Durkin (2002) built upon the emerging area of research that examines the coping and adaptation behaviours of people in early stage Alzheimer's disease. This study was based on qualitative interviews conducted with 22 people in early stage Alzheimer's disease and their carers. The analytic framework from which these narratives were examined was organized around common themes of successful coping and adaptation to early stage Alzheimer's disease that emerged from the data. From the analysis of these narratives, it was noted that the people who adapted successfully used multiple coping strategies from a range, and these, together with a brief summary of its meaning, are listed below:

- *Acceptance and ownership:* People in early stage Alzheimer's who were coping positively were able to face the reality of their diagnoses and sought no blame for it.

- *Disclosure:* Telling friends, family members, neighbours, and when appropriate, acquaintances that they were diagnosed with probable Alzheimer's disease was a powerful release and coping strategy for many of the people interviewed.

- *Positive attitude and self-acceptance:* Individuals who were coping successfully were able to face Alzheimer's disease from a positive perspective and accept themselves.

- *Role relinquishment and replacement:* Individuals who relinquished the necessary social roles because of dementia, but replaced them with new roles or adapted previous roles, were seen to fair the best.

- *Innovative techniques/use of technology:* Individuals were very creative in finding coping techniques to deal with their dementia. Harris and Durkin (2002) gave an example of one man in their sample using travellers' cheques instead of 'normal bank cheques' in his daily transactions as he could no longer write a cheque. With travellers' cheques the person with early Alzheimer's disease just had to sign his name and if he lost the cheque, it could be replaced.

- *Fluidity:* Being able to go with the flow of the disease allowed individuals to manage the daily stresses of dementia.

- *Utilizing pro-active skills:* This action-oriented approach occurred in a number of different ways. The researchers found some people with dementia utilize 'energy efficiency' in their management of their lives; for instance, one person in the study reported doing chores in the morning rather than the afternoon when he was more fatigued.

- *Connection with past activities:* Using skills that one developed before the diagnosis and finding meaningful uses for them in the 'here and now' was a common theme discussed in a number of narratives.

- *Anticipatory adaptation:* Anticipating needs in the future allows people with Alzheimer's disease to not only become familiar with their next challenge, but also to begin to integrate new behaviours. This anticipation assists the person to adapt to a realistic view of their disease giving them a chance to plan and thus exercise and maintain control.

- *Altruism:* The ability to still be a productive member of society and give back to their communities was seen as a meaningful coping behaviour for those interviewed.

- *Holistic practices:* Some people with Alzheimer's disease reported enjoying learning new relaxation techniques, such as reiki, tai' chi, meditation, yoga and guided imagery.

- *Spirituality:* For a number of the individuals interviewed by the researchers, their spiritual beliefs were a source of comfort and support, especially on their bad days.

As Harris and Durkin (2002) go on to explain, this range of positive coping behaviours assists individuals with early stage Alzheimer's disease to adapt to the challenges of living with dementia by increasing their resilience to the stressors. Moreover, the range of coping behaviours also provided people with some feelings of control over their condition and helps to instil a sense of hope. Living with the impact of Alzheimer's disease, and other dementias, is not a passive activity and, we would suggest, a primary role for the mental health nurse is to identify and support such positive coping techniques while working to minimize more negative patterns of coping.

Family care: exploring the meaning of need

The impact that exhibited behaviours of people with dementia had on carers provided the initial, and overwhelming, focus for social research enquiry. Such findings had their roots in an early, and seminal, study by Grad and

Sainsbury (1965). These authors measured the burden placed on carers when elderly psychiatric patients were discharged home from an institutional setting. In so doing, they distinguished between objective burden, that is, the 'behavioural dysfunctions' and practical problems that were encountered by the carer, and subjective burden, the carer's emotional adjustment in terms of increased stress, lowered morale and so on. In dementia care this conceptualization of 'burden' can also be seen in a UK study by Sanford (1975), which was one of the first to explore stress and the experience of caring at home for a person with dementia.

In this study the author interviewed 50 family carers whose relative was attending a geriatric unit in one of three district general hospitals in London. The focus of the study was on carers whose dependant had experienced dementia for some time and the interviews explored the subjective and objective circumstances of care. His findings were that behavioural disturbances, such as sleep disturbance (including night wandering and shouting) and communication difficulties were poorly tolerated by carers and caused the greatest feelings of stress. On the other hand, attending to their dependant's activities of daily living caused comparatively little upset to the carer, particularly those tasks relating to the person's basic human needs such as feeding and washing.

Sanford (1975) also commented that services, in the guise of district nurses, intervened in areas of the carer's life where they felt best able to cope, but tended to overlook the more debilitating aspects of care as perceived by the carer. To improve this situation Panzarine (1985) later suggested that community practitioners might best intervene during the caregiver's period of anticipatory coping, i.e. at the time when the carer is deciding what future action to take, thus helping to ameliorate the further build-up of stressors. This relationship between stress and coping informed the majority of caregiving studies in dementia (see Rabins *et al.* 1982; Quayhagen and Quayhagen 1988; Pearlin *et al.* 1990), and it is, therefore, important to have a more complete understanding of this area of the literature.

Early studies on coping tended to focus on the relationship between coping, the stressors of life and their effect on health status (see, for instance, Janoff-Bolman and Marshall 1982). In order to better understand this process, Morrissey *et al.* (1990) suggested that the context of stress is an important factor in determining coping and advocated that the transactional model of stress best characterizes this relationship. The transactional model builds on the work of Lazarus (1966) and, as the name suggests, views stress as resulting from a transaction between an individual and his or her environment. It is based upon a process of assessment, or appraisal, in which, initially, an individual considers the nature of an event and decides whether it poses a threat, harm or challenge. This period of consideration is known as the primary appraisal. If as a result of this appraisal a response is perceived as necessary, the potential response is compared to the individual's available coping resources (secondary appraisal). A coping response is selected and its effect on the original demand is then assessed (reappraisal).

Stress is only said to result when there is a perceived mismatch between the nature of the demand and the individual's ability to respond effectively, by reducing the degree of perceived threat, harm or challenge. Using this approach the crucial determinant is not the objective nature of the demand (stressor) itself, but its appraised impact. Hence, carers in Sanford's (1975) study were able to tolerate the seemingly stressful event of their dependant's incontinence, but were less well able to manage the social embarrassment that such behaviours evoked. In other words, events only become stressors when the mind identifies them as such (see Spaniol and Jung 1987). This distinction is important as it allows for the possibility of the same event being differentially stressful for different people, or even for the same person at different points in time.

A study conducted in the USA by Hirschfield (1981, 1983) made a significant contribution to advancing understanding on the meaning of care from the experiences of carers of people with dementia. The author interviewed 30 caregivers of people with dementia (the sample also including unstructured interviews with seven people with mild cognitive impairment), and developed the concept of 'mutuality' as 'the most important variable' (1983: 26) to explain the social relationship between families and the person with dementia. In outlining the properties of 'mutuality', Hirschfield suggested that: 'it grew out of the caregiver's ability to find gratification in the relationship with the impaired person and meaning from the caregiving situation. Another important component to mutuality was the caregiver's ability to perceive the impaired person as reciprocating by virtue of his/her existence' (1983: 26).

Thus mutuality grew out of the carer's ability to find meaning, gratification and reciprocity in their care giving role (see also Horowitz and Shindelman 1983). According to Hirschfield (1981, 1983) mutuality was seen as existing within four parameters:

1   high mutuality from within the relationship (internally reinforced mutuality);
2   high mutuality due to circumstances (externally reinforced mutuality);
3   low mutuality;
4   no mutuality survived.

Feelings of low mutuality were synonymous with poor adjustment within the family and negative feelings towards the person with dementia. This negative adjustment was as likely to be present in those caring for a person with mild dementia as those caring in later stages. Hirschfield (1983) outlined three other variables that influenced the planned continuation of home care, these being: management ability, morale and tension. Interestingly, the operational definition of tension included the feeling of 'being tied down', and this was conceptualized as the carer's restricted opportunity for free time and lack of individual privacy. Indeed, it was the combination of low/no mutuality coupled with 'severe tension' that Hirschfield (1983) believed to be the driving force for carers considering admission into care of the person with dementia, and thus predicting the breakdown of home care (for a validation of this hypothesis see later studies: Gilhooly 1986; Lieberman and Kramer 1991; Cohen *et al.* 1993; Aneshensel *et al.* 1995; Cahill 1997; Steeman *et al.* 1997; Hope *et al.* 1998). Hirschfield illustrated the existence of this phenomenon via the following case example of 'no mutuality existing':

> I used to love my father; I used to love to see him come through the door. Now when he comes I hate it. It is like my emotions have changed. I hate to think that I hate my father now, but I just hate the disease he has. It's like I consider him dead three or four years ago . . . some people say 'that's your father' but when you hear a door banging all night long you can't sleep.
>
> (Hirschfield 1983: 28)

It's uncertain if it is the person with dementia or the disease that is being blamed in this case example, but it highlights the importance of establishing the nature and quality of the relationship during professional assessment of need.

In a large-scale longitudinal study covering all stages of what they describe as the 'care-giving career', Aneshensel *et al.* (1995) have identified 'role captivity', i.e. the caregiver's perception of being trapped by care-giving responsibilities, as being particularly relevant to the breakdown of care. Indeed, caring at home for someone with dementia is a stressful and, at times, self-injurious process. In a survey of 1303 carers in the UK conducted by the Alzheimer's Disease Society it was found that 97 per cent were experiencing some form of emotional health problem, such as stress, tiredness or depression. In addition, 36 per cent had a physical complaint (for example, back pain) as a direct result of being a carer (Alzheimer's Disease Society 1993). In the same report, the Alzheimer's Disease Society found that 34 per cent of carers had not been offered a full assessment and 59 per cent complained that the person they cared for did not receive regular check-ups by a doctor or nurse. Depressive symptoms and behavioural problems in people with dementia have been reported to be the most stressful for carers, with the most powerful predictors of psychological distress in carers being depression and mood-related signs of depression in the person with dementia (Donaldson *et al.* 1998).

Evidence-based care: outcome studies in dementia

Arguably, most outcome studies in dementia care practice have focused upon carers and, in particular, on measuring the effectiveness of carer interventions in structured group-work (for a review, see Miller and Morris 1993). To date there remain relatively few published accounts of outcome studies on clinical effectiveness in dementia care practice. Indeed, identifying appropriate outcome measures is difficult in relation to the person with dementia, with a progressive decline in function, and the validity of self-report quality of life measures is open to question. For the family caregiver outcome measures such as the level of strain, burden or depression is readily available (for a review, see Briggs and Askham 1999). However, as intimated earlier, the needs of the carer and those of the person with dementia may at times conflict, especially in relation to respite and continuing care admissions (Cohen *et al.* 1993). Remaining in the community is at times regarded as an index of outcome for older people with dementia, with the implicit, but unsupported, assumption that their quality of life is inevitably worse in a residential home.

Knight *et al.*'s (1993) meta-analysis indicates that psycho-educational programmes and respite care services have more positive effects on caregiver stress than service coordination alone. Studies from Australia and the USA on family-based interventions have shown reduced rates of institutionalization of people with dementia (see Woods 1995). However, a British study by O'Connor *et al.* (1991), that involved the input of a multi-disciplinary team (but not a specific psycho-educational approach), failed to make an impact; indeed, people with dementia living alone entered continuing care more rapidly than those not receiving the intervention.

A further study involved the controlled evaluation of four Admiral Nurse Service teams in the North Thames Region (Woods *et al.* 1999). Admiral Nurses provide a specific community nursing service where the focus of attention is on the carer of the person with dementia. In this study it was found that carers referred both to the Admiral Nurse Services and a comparison mental health service for older people showed a reduction in the general level of distress over the length of the study (8 months). However, carers receiving an Admiral Nurse Service were seen to exhibit a significantly greater decline in anxiety over the follow-up period. Moreover, Woods and his colleagues suggested that this carer-oriented focus did not detract from the overall quality of life/care for the person with dementia. However, in the conclusion to their report, the authors emphasized the importance of considering the interaction between the carer and person with dementia as a future research agenda. We highlight some of these dilemmas in the following short case study.

Sharing the diagnosis of dementia

The following case study is taken directly from a 15-month intervention project that was funded by the Department of Health and undertaken in Gwynedd, North Wales (Wenger *et al.* 2000). The focus of the experimental research was on early intervention in dementia care and was conducted in primary care. The project employed two clinical specialists to pilot a psycho-social intervention at this early stage of the diagnosis of dementia to see whether or not such a package improved adjustment and coping patterns, both for the family and the person with the dementia. Of the two clinical dementia-care specialists, one was an experienced social worker and the other a community psychiatric nurse (CPN) with a long history of service development and clinical care for people with dementia and their families. Professor Bob Woods, a well-known clinical psychologist in the field of mental health and older people and one of the authors of this chapter (JK) undertook the clinical supervision over the length of the project. Forming part of the caseload of the dementia-care specialists, the following (anonymous) case study illustrates some of the complexities and dilemmas that were faced by the workers (and their supervisors) at this point in the diagnostic and intervention cycle.

Case study: Mr and Mrs Thomas

This case concerns a couple in their late 80s. Mr Thomas retired from running his own shop about 15 years ago. Mrs Thomas used to help out in the business and attended to all the bookkeeping, form filling and administrative tasks of the business. Mr Thomas, a wartime refugee from eastern Europe, feels that his English is not up to the task of explaining his needs and wants. He has been treated and diagnosed for throat cancer, which is in remission but which the GP expects will return and eventually result in Mr Thomas's death.

Mrs Thomas has significant memory impairment and finds it increasingly difficult to cope. She still retains responsibility for all the paperwork and finances of the household but regularly loses pension and bank books, bills and invoices and everything else that she takes responsibility for. Mrs Thomas is not willing to give up responsibility for these tasks.

Mrs Thomas was assessed at the local hospital and it was confirmed that she probably has Alzheimer's. The GP shared the diagnosis with Mrs Thomas but Mrs Thomas asked the GP not to tell her husband about it. Mr Thomas is extremely concerned about his wife but she refuses to allow the diagnosis to be shared with him; indeed, she sometimes forgets what it is the GP has told her although she is aware of her failing memory and powers to concentrate.

Some questions and dilemmas

Standard 7 of the *NSF for Older People* (DH 2001) indicates that 'treatment in dementia . . . always involves explaining the diagnosis to the older person and any carers and where possible giving relevant information about sources of help and support' (p 104). After reflecting on this statement and the information provided in the case study, do you think that:

- Mr Thomas has a right to know of his wife's diagnosis?
- The GP is acting reasonably in not telling Mr Thomas of his wife's diagnosis?
- The GP should persuade Mrs Thomas to let Mr Thomas know the diagnosis?
- The GP has other reasons/motivations for not intervening more effectively in this case?

Read through the case study once again and ask yourself the following questions:

- What role would I play if I were the worker assigned to this couple?
- Whom would I involve to help provide ongoing support to the couple?
- What sort of support would I need if I were the primary worker in this case?

It is always tempting to think that there is a correct solution to these questions and those raised in the case study. In trying to find a path through this ethical maze, we (i.e. the dementia-care specialists and their supervisors) had to weigh up the complex issues raised by this case and support the right of Mrs Thomas not to inform her husband of her diagnosis. However, the non-disclosure was raising severe tensions between the couple and the denial of information (from Mrs Thomas to her husband) was leading to a negative cycle of blame and recrimination, events that were undoubtedly affecting the couple's quality of life.

To help the workers during their period of intervention, at the end of each visit the dementia-care specialists were prompted, with the assistance of Mrs Thomas, to draw an ecomap (a pictorial representation of relationships using representative symbols: for further explanation see Dobson 1989) to chart the family dynamics and perceived closeness of the couple. Over time, this built up a picture of relationship change. Moreover, the ecomaps were then used (with permission) as a primary source of case material during clinical supervision. By using this approach it became easy to see that the couple were pushing one another further and further away, and a root cause of this conflict was anxiety over disclosure. To try and overcome this situation, a strategy was then formulated with Mrs Thomas that allowed her to rehearse her fears and concerns about the impact of informing her husband of the diagnosis with one of the dementia-care specialists. This approach allowed Mrs Thomas to confront and voice her fears within a safe environment. Indeed, in the course of this procedure, Mrs Thomas initially disclosed that she did not want her husband informed of her diagnosis as she did not want to 'burden him even more with my troubles' prior to his death. After allowing Mrs Thomas time to work through these emotions, and the prospect of her husband's death, she came to the conclusion that her husband had a 'right to know what was wrong' and that it was 'no good keeping secrets'. Mrs Thomas then decided that she wanted to share her diagnosis of Alzheimer's disease with her husband in the presence of the dementia-care specialist. This 'opening up' of the diagnosis from wife to husband was achieved some five months after it was first given to Mrs Thomas. After its sharing, Mr Thomas was able to put a name to his wife's condition and a meaning to her actions, something he attached great importance to during the remaining months of his life.

The case study highlights some important human emotions and conflicts that can be raised during the push for an earlier diagnosis of dementia. It must be remembered who 'owns' the diagnosis and as professionals we must be prepared for all possible outcomes for the use of this information. By turning the tables from the empowerment of carers to that of the person with dementia brings with it a series of challenges to professionals and their ability to feel 'in control' of a situation. To help cope with such emotions and practice dilemmas, it is vital that dementia-care practitioners, and those who work with all older people with mental health needs, have regular and supportive clinical supervision. There is little doubt that the involvement of people with dementia in all aspects of care and service provision will increase in the years ahead. However, as the *NSF for Older People* (DH 2001) makes explicit, it is also important that the needs of carers remain a service priority.

Finally, in this section, we think it important to briefly review the influence of Tom Kitwood at the Bradford Dementia Group to the development of dementia care and to the person-centred movement that sits at the heart of the *NSF for Older People* (DH 2001). Briefly, the principle source of person-centred care emanated from a stream of social research from the Bradford Dementia Group that began in the mid-1980s under the leadership of Tom Kitwood and his colleagues (see Kitwood 1988, 1989, 1990, 1993, 1997; Kitwood and Bredin 1992a,b; Kitwood and Benson 1995). In particular, Kitwood applied the concept of personhood to the field of dementia care and defined its characteristics in the following way: 'It [personhood] is a standing or status that is bestowed upon one human being, by others, in the context of relationship and social being. It implies recognition, respect and trust. Both the according of personhood, and the failure to do so, has consequences that are empirically testable' (Kitwood 1997: 8).

Thus in this paradigm the experience of dementia is not simply seen as the sum total of a diagnostic label, but as an evolving dynamic that embraces the whole person and covers ethical, social-psychological and neurological significance. In this framework the dialectic tension that exists between 'us' (professional carers) and 'them' (person with dementia) is withdrawn and the onus placed firmly on the 'us' to remove barriers to understanding and build bridges towards meaningful dialogue and communication (see also Killick and Allan 2001).

In keeping with the underpinning philosophy of the *NSF for Older People* (DH 2001), the last sentence of the above extract also reveals an important facet of Kitwood's approach to dementia care, that of measurement and testability. Prior to such a stance, an approach of therapeutic nihilism pervaded the field of dementia care whereby the provision of 'safety and security' were key nursing interventions for the person with dementia (Keady and Adams 2001a,b). In developing the tools of measurement, Kitwood (1990, 1997) observed care practices in continuing care settings and compiled a list of 'depersonalizing tendencies' (Kitwood 1997: 46) that were grouped together to form a 'malignant social psychology' that impacted upon the life of the person with dementia. Originally comprising of 10 elements (Kitwood 1990), Kitwood later extended these to 17 as shown in Table 19.3.

From the components of such a list it was possible to then measure their relevance for the person by recording examples of their duration, frequency, level of observed upset and so on. This process of documentation became known as Dementia Care Mapping (Kitwood and Bredin 1992b),

Table 19.3 Main features of a 'malignant social psychology'

Treachery:	the use of dishonest representation or deception in order to obtain compliance;
Disempowerment:	doing for a dementia sufferer what he or she can still do, albeit clumsily or slowly;
Infantilization:	implying that a dementia sufferer has the mentality or capability of a baby or young child;
Condemnation:	blaming; the attribution of malicious or seditious motives, especially when the dementia sufferer is distressed;
Intimidation:	the use of threats, commands or physical assault; the abuse of power;
Stigmatization:	turning a dementia sufferer into an alien, a diseased object, an outcast, especially through verbal labels;
Outpacing:	the delivery of information or instruction at a rate far beyond what can be processed;
Invalidation:	the ignoring or discounting of a dementia sufferer's subjective states; especially feelings of distress or bewilderment;
Banishment:	the removal of a dementia sufferer from the human milieu, either physically or psychologically;
Objectification:	treating a person like a lump of dead matter; to be measured, pushed around, drained, filled and so on;
Ignoring:	carrying on (in conversation or action) in the presence of a person as if they were not there;
Imposition:	forcing a person to do something, overriding desire or denying the possibility of choice on their part;
Withholding:	refusing to give asked-for attention, or to meet an evident need;
Accusation:	blaming a person for actions or failures that arise from their lack of ability, or their misunderstanding of the situation;
Disruption:	intruding suddenly or disturbingly upon a person's action or reflection; crudely breaking their frame of reference;
Mockery:	making fun of a person's 'strange' actions or remarks; teasing, humiliating, making jokes at their expense; and
Disparagement:	telling a person that they are incompetent, useless, worthless and so on, giving them messages that are damaging to their self-esteem.

Source: Kitwood (1997: 46–7)

a technique that has proved invaluable in helping to define the quality of life (and quality of care) received by people with dementia in continuing care environments (Brooker *et al.* 1998; Younger and Martin 2000). As a specific programme of training, Dementia Care Mapping continues to be offered by the Bradford Dementia Group in the UK and it is anticipated that its usefulness will, in future, be applied to domestic (community-based) settings (Brooker and Rogers 2001).

Conclusion

In this chapter we have focused on the stated aim of Standard 7 of the *NSF for Older People* (DH 2001), which is to 'treat and support those older people with dementia and depression' and articulate some of the underlying tensions and approaches that currently exist in both the literature and practice. While there are many positives in the development of Standard 7, one area that is absent in the strategy is on professional preparation for practice with older people with mental health needs. The policy documents and literature we have reviewed in preparing this chapter has, time and time again, spelled out the inadequacy of practitioner training and knowledge in the field (see, for example, Audit Commission 2000, 2002a,b). However, it would be unwise to place this criticism solely at the door of GPs. Recently, in the dementia care field, some commentators have begun to question the value of CPNs in terms of both carer support (Pickard and Glendinning 2001) and in the models used to guide their day-to-day work with family carers (Carradice *et al.* 2002). Indeed, the study by Pickard and Glendinning suggests that carers value help with personal care tasks, but that the CPNs in their sample (n=12) failed to provide such a service and generally constructed their usefulness through 'advice and moral support' (2001: 8). There was little evidence of skills sharing with carers in this study, and still less of an evaluation strategy to gauge the efficacy of the intervention. In our opinion it is essential that the mental health nursing profession grasps the importance of this finding and begins to mobilize a response to such criticism.

In summary, the main messages of this chapter are:

- To date work with older people has not always been promoted with vigour on training programmes, or viewed as a worthwhile career option (Skog *et al.* 1999; Courtney *et al.* 2000); this needs to change.

  For example, on this former point, a recent extensive survey on student nurses' preparation for gerontological practice has revealed a paucity of attention to the mental health care of older people within the 'Project 2000' foundation programme (Nolan *et al.* 2001). Arguably, of even more concern, this finding extended to student nurses on specialist mental health branch programmes. Similarly, qualified mental health nurses involved in the care of older people require access to high quality specialist courses that are available locally and provide a skills-orientated focus, such as a foundation in psychotherapy with older adults (Orbach 1996).

- In addition to promoting such positive values and the acquisition of psychotherapuetic skills, it is important that mental health nurses working with older people actively engage in strategies of mental health promotion (cf. Chapter 2). This is a significant challenge for the profession as the literature reveals a virtual absence of specific studies that cover this topic. However, we would suggest that mental health nurses are in a prime position to develop, undertake and evaluate such programmes. For instance, one arm of a health promotion programme could include a role for the mental health nurse in primary care undertaking the screening of blood pressure in addition to other assessments based around the area of cognitive functioning. Such an activity may help to identify those older people who may be at an increased risk of developing a vascular dementia (DH 1992; McIntosh and Woodall 1995).

- Finally, for clinical work to be effective, it is important that interventions are paced to the understanding and belief structures of those older people who are experiencing the condition. We concur with Whitehouse (2000) who suggests that, in dementia care, a key challenge for the future is to develop programmes of support that improve the quality of life of both the person with dementia and the carer. This approach, Whitehouse (2000) argues, should be undertaken through the assessment of: cognition; behaviour function; and social, economic and spiritual factors.

    With a little imagination, and the additional element of ethnic minority perspectives (Dilworth-Anderson and Gibson 1999), such a programme of assessment is transferable to all older people who experience a mental health need in old age and provides a platform for interpreting the statements of 'treatment' that are expressed in Standard 7 of the *NSF for Older People* (DH 2001) and repeated earlier in this chapter.

    We would hope that mental health nurses are at the forefront of such assessments and take a lead in translating these factors into effective and meaningful programmes of intervention. Older people deserve nothing less than our highest standards of care practice.

Questions for reflection and discussion

1   Is my current nursing assessment of depressed older people person-centred and holistic in nature?

2   What should I be considering in my nursing assessment to ensure effective need and risk assessment?

3   How could I improve the likely success of any medication prescribed?

4   For each patient/family that I encounter, what psychosocial interventions should be used?

5   How will we know if our interventions are working and are effective?

Note

1   As at April 2004, an NSF for Older People Implementation Planning Group has been established to develop a similar framework for Wales with the final version due in June 2005 (see National Assembly for Wales, 2002: 63. website: http://www.wales.nhs.uk/sites/home.cfm (accessed 25 March 2004).

Annotated bibliography

- Norman, I.J. and Redfern, S.J. (eds) (1997) *Mental Health Care for Elderly People*. Edinburgh: Churchill Livingstone. This is a comprehensive and accessible introduction to mental health and older people edited by two respected nurse academics. Contributors to the book are drawn from the UK and the text is divided into four sections, the third of which has eight chapters on therapeutic interventions. Essential reading for all mental health nurses with an interest in the topic.
- Smyer, M.A. and Qualls, S.H. (1999) *Aging and Mental Health*. London: Blackwell. Written by two American psychologists, this book provides an introduction to ageing and mental health and is an excellent resource for those working in the field. The book provides a succinct summary of the psychodynamic, behavioural and family systems models of ageing that would be of particular value to student nurses.
- Woods, R.T. (ed.) (1999) *Psychological Problems of Ageing: Assessment, Treatment and Care*. Chichester: Wiley. This book comprises 12 chapters that initially formed part of the more substantial textbook *Handbook of the Clinical Psychology of Ageing* (John Wiley and Sons, 1996, also edited by R.T. Woods). As stated in its Preface, the book is a 'day-to-day resource for clinical psychologists' although there is much in the text that is applicable to the work of mental health nurses involved in the care of older people. For example, the chapters on 'Cognitive behaviour therapy' (by Leah Dick and her colleagues) and 'Psychodynamic therapy and scientific gerontology' (by Bob Knight) provide an evidence-base for intervention and should be required reading for all mental health nurses.
- Sabat, S.R. (2001) *The Experience of Alzheimer's Disease: Life Through a Tangled Veil*. Oxford: Blackwell. Written by a respected clinical psychologist in the USA, this book presents new challenges to the dementia-care profession by confronting underlying assumptions about what it is to live with dementia. Specifically, Steven Sabat constructs a new way of thinking about 'the self' and its assumed loss in people with dementia. The book is peppered throughout by case study material and extends the boundaries on the efficacy of therapeutic work with people with dementia.
- Cantley, C. (ed.) (2001) *A Handbook of Dementia Care*. Buckingham: Open University Press. Written by 22 UK-based contributors (including

the editor) this comprehensive publication provides readers with an authoritative overview of the latest advances in dementia care. The book has a person-centred philosophy to its structure, and the contents address a range of topic areas, for example, biomedical perspectives, UK policy initiatives, therapeutic advances and service development. The latter topic includes advice on how to include people with dementia and families in developing and evaluating new services. A thoroughly recommended book for students at either undergraduate or postgraduate levels; existing practitioners will also gain much from a familiarity with the text.

References

Adams, T. and Page, S. (2000) New pharmacological treatments for Alzheimer's disease: implications for dementia care nursing, *Journal of Advanced Nursing*, **31**(5): 1183–8.

Alzheimer's Disease International (2000) *World Alzheimer's Day Bulletin*. London: Alzheimer's Disease International.

Alzheimer's Disease Society (1993) *Deprivation and Dementia*. London: Alzheimer's Society.

Alzheimer's Disease Society (1994) *Home Alone with Dementia*. London: Alzheimer's Society.

Alzheimer's Disease Society (1995) *Dementia in the Community: Management Strategies for General Practice*. London: Alzheimer's Society.

Alzheimer's Society (2000) *Introduction to Dementia*. London: Alzheimer's Society.

American Psychiatric Association (1987) *Diagnostic and Statistical Manual of Mental Disorders* (3rd edn, revd) (*DSM-III-R*) Washington, DC: American Psychiatric Association.

American Psychiatric Association (1994) *DSM-IV: Diagnostic and Statistical Manual of Mental Disorders* (4th edn). Washington, DC: American Psychiatric Association.

Ames, D. (1990) Depression among elderly residents of local authority residential homes: Its nature and efficacy of intervention, *British Journal of Psychiatry* **156**: 667–75.

Ames, D. (1991) Epidemiological studies of depression among the elderly in residential and nursing homes, *International Journal of Geriatric Psychiatry* **6**: 347–54.

Aneshensel, C.S., Pearlin, L.I., Mullan, J.T., Zarit, S.H. and Whitlatch, C.J. (1995) *Profiles in Caregiving: The Unexpected Career*. San Diego, CA: Academic Press.

Ashton, P. and Keady, J. (1999) Mental disorders of older people, in R. Newell and K. Gournay (eds) *Mental Health Nursing: An Evidence-based Approach*. London: Churchill Livingstone.

Audit Commission (2000) *Forget Me Not: Mental Health Services for Older People*. London: Audit Commission.

Audit Commission (2002a) *Forget Me Not 2002: Developing Mental Health Services for Older People in England*. London: Audit Commission.

Audit Commission (2002b) *Losing Time: Developing Mental Health Services for Older People in Wales*. London: Audit Commission.

Baldwin, R. C. (1993) Depressive Illness, in R. Jacoby and C. Oppenheimer (eds) *Psychiatry in the Elderly*. Oxford: Oxford University Press, pp. 676–719.

Banerjee, S. (1993) Prevalence and recognition rates of psychiatric disorder in the elderly clients of a community care service, *International Journal of Geriatric Psychiatry* **8**: 125–31.

Banerjee, S., Sharmash, K., and Macdonald, A.J.D. (1996) Randomised controlled trial of effect of intervention by psychogeriatric team on depression in frail elderly people at home, *British Medical Journal* **313**: 1058–61.

Barraclough, B.M., Bunch, J. and Nelson, B. (1974) A hundred cases of suicide: clinical aspects, *British Journal of Psychiatry* **125**: 355–73.

Baumgarten, M., Battista, R.N., Infante-Rivard, C. *et al.* (1992) The psychological and physical health of family members caring for an elderly person with dementia, *Journal of Clinical Epidemiology* **45**(1): 61–70.

Beekman, A.T.F., Copland, J.R.M. and Prince, M.J. (1999) Review of community prevalence of depression in later life, *British Journal of Psychiatry* **174**: 307–11.

Benbow, S.M. (1987) The use of electroconvulsive therapy in old age psychiatry, *International Journal of Geriatric Psychiatry* **2**: 25–30.

Benbow, S.M. (1989) The role of electroconvulsive therapy in the treatment of depressive illness in old age, *British Journal of Psychiatry* **155**: 147–52.

Benbow, S.M. (1992) Management of depression in the elderly, *British Journal of Hospital Medicine* **48**(11): 726–31.

Beutler, L.E., Scogin, F., Kirkish, P. *et al.* (1987) Group cognitive therapy and Alprazolam in the treatment of depression in older adults, *Journal of Consulting and Clinical Psychology* **55**: 550–6.

Blanchard, M. and Mann, A. (1994) Depression in primary care settings, in E. Chiu and D. Ames (eds) *Functional Psychiatric Disorders of the Elderly*. Cambridge: Cambridge University Press.

Boden, C. (1998) *Who Will I Be When I Die?* East Melbourne, Australia: Harper Collins Religious.

Briggs, K. and Askham, J. (1999) *The Needs of People with Dementia and Those who Care for Them*. London: Alzheimer's Society.

Brooker, D. and Rogers, L. (eds) (2001) *Dementia Care Mapping: Think Tank Transcripts*. University of Bradford, UK: Bradford Dementia Group.

Brooker, D., Foster, N., Banner, A., Payne, M. and Jackson, L. (1998) The efficacy of dementia care mapping as an audit tool: report of a 3-year British NHS evaluation, *Aging & Mental Health* **2**(1): 60–70.

Bryden, C. (2002) A person-centred approach to counselling, psychotherapy and rehabilitation of people diagnosed with dementia in the early stages, *Dementia: The International Journal of Social Research and Practice* **1**(2): 141–56.

Burns, A., Lawlor, B. and Craig, S. (2002) Rating scales in old age psychiatry, *British Journal of Psychiatry* **180**: 161–7.

Cahill, S.M. (1997) 'I often think I wish he were here': Why do primary carers institutionalise family members with dementia? *Australian Social Work* **50**(3): 13–19.

Cantley, C. (ed.) (2001) *A Handbook of Dementia Care*. Buckingham: Open University Press.

Carradice, A., Shankland, M. and Beail, N. (2002) A qualitative study of the theoretical models used by UK mental health nurses to guide their assessments with family caregivers of people with dementia, *International Journal of Nursing Studies* **39**(1): 17–26.

Cattell, H. and Jolley, D.J. (1995) One hundred cases of suicide of elderly people, *British Journal of Psychiatry* **166**: 451–7.

Charlesworth, G., Riordan, J. and Shepstone, L. (2000) Cognitive behaviour therapy (CBT) for depressed carers of people with Alzheimer's disease and related disorders (Protocol for a Cochrane review), in *The Cochrane Library* **4**, 2000. Oxford: Update Software.

Clare, L. (1999) Memory rehabilitation in early dementia, *Journal of Dementia Care – Research Focus* **17**(6): 33–8.

Clarke, D.C. and Fawcett, J. (1992) Review of empirical risk factors for evaluation of the suicidal patient, in B. Bongar (ed.) *Suicide: Guidelines for Assessment, Management and Treatment*. New York: Oxford University Press.

Cohen, C.A., Gold, D.P., Shulman, K.L. *et al.* (1993) Factors determining the decision to institutionalise dementing individuals: a prospective study, *Gerontologist* **33**(6): 714–20.

Cole, M.G. (1990) The prognosis of depression in the elderly, *Canadian Medical Association Journal* **142**: 633–9.

Copeland, J.R.M., Dewey, M.E., Wood, N. *et al.* (1987) Range of mental illness among the elderly in the community, *British Journal of Psychiatry* **150**: 815–23.

Courtney, M., Tong, S. and Walsh, A. (2000) Acute-care nurses' attitudes towards older patients: A literature review, *International Journal of Nursing Practice* **6**(2): 62–9.

Davis, R. (1989) *My Journey into Alzheimer's Disease*. Amersham-on-the-Hill, Buckinghamshire: Scripture Press.

Department of Health (1992) *The Health of the Nation: A Strategy for Health in England*. London: HMSO.

Department of Health (1995) *Building Bridges: A Guide to Arrangements for Inter-agency Working for the Care and Protection of Severely Mentally Ill People*. London: HMSO.

Department of Health (1996) *Assessing Older People with Dementia in the Community: Practice Issues for Social and Health Services*. Wetherby: HMSO.

Department of Health (1997) *At Home With Dementia: Inspection of Services for Older People with Dementia in the Community*. London: HMSO.

Department of Health (1999a) *National Service Framework for Mental Health: Modern Standards and Service Models*. London: Department of Health.

Department of Health (1999b) *Saving Lives: Our Healthier Nation* (Cm 4386). London: Department of Health.

Department of Health (2001) *National Service Framework for Older People: Modern Standards and Service Models*. London: Department of Health.

Diekstra, R.F.W. (1989) Suicide and attempted suicide: An international perspective, *Acta Psychiatrica Scandinavica* **80**: 1–24.

Dillmann, R.J.M. (2000) Alzheimer disease: epistemological lessons from history?, in P.J. Whitehouse, K. Maurer and J.F. Ballenger (eds) *Concepts of Alzheimer Disease: Biological, Clinical and Cultural Perspectives*. Baltimore, MD: The Johns Hopkins University Press.

Dilworth-Anderson, P. and Gibson, B.E. (1999) Ethnic minority perspectives on dementia, family caregiving and interventions. *Generations* **XXIII**(3): 40–5.

Dobson, S. (1989) Genograms and ecomaps, *Nursing Times* **85**(51): 54–6.

Donaldson, C., Tarrier, N. and Burns, A. (1998) Determinants of carer stress in Alzheimer's disease, *International Journal of Geriatric Psychiatry* **13**: 248–56.

Draper, B. (1996) Attempted suicide in old age, *International Journal of Geriatric Psychiatry* **11**: 577–87.

Epstein, L.J. (1978) Anxiolytics, antidepressants and neuroleptics in the treatment of geriatric patients, in M. Lipton, A.D. Mascio and K. Killman (eds) *Psychopharmacology: A Generation of Progress*. New York: Raven Press.

Flint, A.J. (1995) Augmentation strategies in geriatric depression, *International Journal of Geriatric Psychiatry* **10**: 137–46.

Flint, A.J. and Rifat, S.L. (2002) Factor structure of the hospital anxiety and depression scale in older patients with major depression, *International Journal of Geriatric Psychiatry* **17**: 117–23.

Folstein, M.F., Folstein, S.E. and McHugh, P.R. (1975) Mini-mental state: a practical guide for grading the cognitive state of patients for the clinician, *Journal of Psychiatric Research* **12**: 189–98.

Fraser, R.M. and Glass, I.B. (1980) Unilateral and bilateral ECT in elderly patients: A comparative study, *Acta Psychiatrica Scandinavica* **62**: 13–31.

Friedell, M. and Bryden, C. (2002) A word from two turtles: A guest editorial. *Dementia: The International Journal of Social Research and Practice* **1**(2): 131–3.

Gallagher, D. and Thompson, L.W. (1983) Effectiveness of psychotherapy for both endogenous and non-endogenous depression in older adults, *Journal of Gerontology* **38**: 307–12.

Georgotas, A., McCue, R.E., Hapworth, W. *et al.* (1986) Comparative efficacy and safety of MAOIs versus TCAs in treating depression in the elderly, *Biological Psychiatry* **21**: 1155–66.

Gerson, S., Plotkin, D. and Jarvik, L. (1988) Antidepressant drug studies 1964–1986, Empirical evidence for ageing patients, *Journal of Clinical Psychopharmacology* **8**: 311–32.

Gilhooly, M.L.M. (1986) Senile dementia: factors associated with caregiver's preference for institutional care, *British Journal of Medical Psychology* **57**: 34–44.

Gilmour, H. (2002) *Dementia in Fermanagh Northern Ireland*. Stirling: Dementia Services Development Centre, University of Stirling.

Grad, J. and Sainsbury, P. (eds) (1965) An evaluation of the effects of caring for the aged at home, in *Psychiatric Disorders in the Aged*. WPA Symposium, Manchester: Geigy.

Hamilton, M. (1960) A rating scale for depression, *Journal of Neurology, Neurosurgery and Psychiatry* **23**: 56–62.

Harper, C.M., Newton, P.A. and Walsh, J.R. (1989) Drug induced illness in the elderly, *Postgraduate Medicine* **86**(2): 245–56.

Harris, P. and Durkin, C. (2002) Building resilience through coping and adapting, in P. Harris (ed.) *The Person with Alzheimer's Disease: Pathways to Understanding the Experience*. Baltimore, MD: The Johns Hopkins University Press.

Hawkins, D. and Eagger, S. (1999) Group therapy: sharing the pain of diagnosis, *Journal of Dementia Care* **7**(5): 12–14, 38.

Hawkins, D. and Eagger, S. (2002) Group therapy: sharing the pain of diagnosis, in S. Benson (ed.) *Dementia Topics for the Millennium and Beyond*. London: Hawker Publications.

Henderson, C. (1998) *Partial View: An Alzheimer's Journal*. Dallas, TX: Southern Methodist University Press.

Hepple, J. and Quinton, C. (1997) One hundred cases of attempted suicide in the elderly, *British Journal of Psychiatry* **171**: 42–6.

Hirschfield, M.J. (1981) Families living and coping with the cognitively impaired, in L.A. Copp (ed.) *Care of the Ageing: Recent Advances in Nursing*. Edinburgh: Churchill Livingstone.

Hirschfield, M.J. (1983) Home care versus institutionalization: family caregiving and senile brain disease, *International Journal of Nursing Studies* **20**(1): 23–32.

Hope, T., Keene, J., Gedling, K., Fairburn, C.G. and Jacoby, R. (1998) Predictors of Institutionalizing for People with Dementia Living at Home with a Carer, *International Journal of Geriatric Psychiatry* **13**(10): 682–90.

Horowitz, A. and Shindelman, L.W. (1983) Reciprocity and Affection: Past Influences on Current Caregiving, *Journal of Gerontological Social Work* **5**(3): 5–20.

Hoxey, K. and Shah, A. (2000) Recent trends in elderly suicide rates in England and Wales, *International Journal of Geriatric Psychiatry* **15**: 274–9.

Iliffe, S. and Drennan, V. (2001) *Primary Care and Dementia*. London: Jessica Kingsley.

Iliffe, S., Tai, S.S, Haines, A. *et al.* (1993) Assessment of elderly people in general practice: depression, functional ability and contact with services, *British Journal of General Practice* **43**: 371–4.

Janoff-Bolman, R. and Marshall, G. (1982) Mortability, well-being and control: a study of population of institutionalized aged, *Personality and Social Psychology Bulletin* **8**: 691–8.

Jones, R.W. (2002) Drug treatment of Alzheimer's disease, *Reviews in Clinical Gerontology* **12**: 165–73.

Katona, C.L.E. (1994) *Depression in Old Age*. Chichester: John Wiley.

Keady, J. and Adams, T. (2001a) Community mental health nursing and dementia care, *Journal of Dementia Care – Research Focus* **9**(1): 35–8.

Keady, J. and Adams, T. (2001b) Community mental health nursing in dementia care: their role and future, *Journal of Dementia Care – Research Focus* **9**(2): 33–7.

Keady, J. and Nolan, M. (1995a) IMMEL: assessing coping responses in the early stages of dementia, *British Journal of Nursing* **4**(6): 309–14.

Keady, J. and Nolan, M. (1995b) IMMEL 2: working to augment coping responses in early dementia, *British Journal of Nursing* **4**(7): 377–80.

Kendell, R.E. (1981) The present status of electroconvulsive therapy, *British Journal of Psychiatry* **139**: 265–83.

Kendrick, R. and Bayne, R. (1982) Compliance with prescribed medication by elderly patients, *Canadian Medical Association Journal* **11**: 961–2.

Killick, J. and Allan, K. (2001) *Communication and the Care of People with Dementia*. Buckingham: Open University Press.

Kitwood, T. (1988) The technical, the personal and the framing of dementia, *Social Behaviour* **3**: 161–80.

Kitwood, T. (1989) Brain, mind and dementia: with particular reference to Alzheimer's disease, *Ageing and Society* **9**(1): 1–15.

Kitwood, T. (1990) The dialectics of dementia: with particular reference to Alzheimer's disease, *Ageing and Society* **10**(2): 177–96.

Kitwood, T. (1993) Person and process in dementia, *International Journal of Geriatric Psychiatry* **8**: 541–5.

Kitwood, T. (1997) *Dementia Reconsidered: The Person Comes First*. Buckingham: Open University Press.

Kitwood, T. and Benson, S. (eds) (1995) *The New Culture of Dementia Care*. London: Hawker Publications.

Kitwood, T. and Bredin, K. (1992a) Towards a theory of dementia care: personhood and well-being, *Ageing and Society* **12**: 269–87.

Kitwood, T. and Bredin, K. (1992b) A new approach to the evaluation of dementia care, *Journal of Advances in Health and Nursing Care* **1**(5): 41–60.

Knight, R.G., Lutzky, S.M., Macofsky-Urban, F. (1993) A meta-analytic review of interventions for care-giver distress: recommendations for future research. *Gerontologist* **33**: 240–8.

Koenig, H.G., Meador, K.D. and Cohen, H.J. (1988) Detection and treatment of major depression in older medically ill hospitalised patients, *International Journal of Psychiatric Medicine* **18**(1): 17–31.

LaBarge, E. and Trtanj, F. (1995) A Support Group for People in the Early Stages of Dementia of the Alzheimer Type, *Journal of Applied Gerontology* **14**(3): 289–301.

Larson, D.B., Lyons, J.S., Hohmann, A.A., Beardsley, R.S. and Hidalgo, J. (1991) Psychotropics prescribed to the US elderly in early to mid 1980's: Prescribing patterns of primary care practitioners, psychiatrists and other physicians, *International Journal of Geriatric Psychiatry* **6**: 63–70.

Lazarus, R.S. (1966) *Psychological Stress and the Coping Process*. New York: McGraw-Hill.

Leung, M.N.S. and Orrell, M.W. (1993) A brief CBT group for the elderly: who benefits? *International Journal of Geriatric Psychiatry* **8**: 593–8.

Lieberman, M.A. and Kramer, J.H. (1991) Factors affecting decisions to institutionalize demented elderly, *Gerontologist* **31**(3): 371–4.

Lindesay, J. (1997) Suicide in later life, in I.J. Norman and S.J. Redfern (eds) *Mental Health Care for Elderly People*. Edinburgh: Churchill Livingstone.

Lindesay, J., Briggs, K. and Murphy, E. (1989) The Guys/Age Concern survey prevalence rates of cognitive impairment, depression and anxiety in an urban elderly community, *British Journal of Psychiatry* **155**: 317–29.

MacDonald, A.J.D. (1986) Do GPs miss depression in elderly patients? *British Medical Journal* **292**: 1365–8.

McGowin, D.F. (1993) *Living in the Labyrinth: A Personal Journey Through the Maze of Alzheimer's Disease*. Cambridge: Mainsail Press.

McIntosh, I.B. and Woodall, K. (1995) *Dementia: Management for Nurses and Community Care Workers*. Dinton: Mark Allen Publishing.

McIntosh, J.L. (1992) Suicide in the Elderly, in B. Bongar (ed.) *Suicide: Guidelines for Assessment, Management and Treatment*. New York: Oxford University Press.

Miller, E. and Morris, R. (1993) *The Psychology of Dementia*. Chichester: John Wiley and Sons.

Morrissey, E., Becker, J. and Rupert, M.P. (1990) Coping resources and depression in the caregiving spouses of Alzheimer patients, *British Journal of Medical Psychology* **63**: 161–71.

Murphy, E. (1982) Social origins of depression in old age, *British Journal of Psychiatry* **141**: 135–42.

Murphy, E. (1983) The prognosis of depression in old age, *British Journal of Psychiatry* **142**: 111–19.

Murphy, E. (1988) Prevention of depression and suicide, in B. Gearing. M. Johnson and T. Heller (eds) *Mental Health Problems in Old Age*. Chichester: John Wiley and Sons.

Musetti, L., Perugi, G., Soriani, A. *et al.* (1989) Depression before and after age 65: a re-examination, *British Journal of Psychiatry* **155**: 330–6.

National Assembly for Wales (2002) *When I'm 64 . . . and More: The Report from the*

Advisory Group on a Strategy for Older People in Wales. Cardiff: National Assembly for Wales.

Nolan, M., Davies, S., Brown, J., Keady, J. and Nolan, J. (2001) *Longitudinal Study of the Effectiveness of Educational Preparation to Meet the Needs of Older People and Carers: The AGEIN (Advancing Gerontological Education in Nursing) Project.* London: English National Board for Nursing, Midwifery and Health Visiting.

Norman, I.J. and Redfern, S.J. (eds) (1997) *Mental Health Care for Elderly People.* Churchill Livingstone: London.

NHS Confederation and the Sainsbury Centre for Mental Health (1997) *The Way Forward for Mental Health Services.* London: HMSO.

O'Connor, D.W., Pollitt, P.A., Brook, C.P.D., Reiss, B.B. and Roth, M. (1991) Does early intervention reduce the number of elderly people with dementia admitted to institutions for long-term care? *British Medical Journal* **302**: 871–5.

Orbach, A. (1996) *Not Too Late: Psychotherapy and Ageing.* London: Jessica Kingsley.

Panzarine, S. (1985) Coping: conceptual and methodological issues, *Advances in Nursing Science* **7**(4): 49–57.

Pearlin, L.I., Mullan, J.T., Semple, S.J. and Scaff, M.M. (1990) Caregiving and the stress process: an overview of concepts and their measures, *Gerontologist* **30**(5): 583–94.

Pearson, J.L., Conwell, Y., Lindesay, J., Takahashi, Y. and Caine, E.D. (1997) Elderly suicide: a multi-national view, *Aging & Mental Health* **1**(2): 107–11.

Pickard, S. and Glendinning, C. (2001) Caring for a relative with dementia: the perceptions of carers and CPNs, *Quality in Ageing-Policy, Practice and Research* **2**(4): 3–11.

Pitt, B. (1991) Depression in the general hospital setting, *International Journal of Geriatric Psychiatry* **6**: 363–70.

Quayhagen, M.P. and Quayhagen, M. (1988) Alzheimer's stress: coping with the caregiving role. *Gerontologist* **28**(3): 391–6.

Rabins, P.V., Mace, N.L. and Lucas, M.J. (1982) The impact of dementia on the family, *Journal of the American Medical Association* **248**: 333–5.

Rait, G., Walters, K. and Iliffe, S. (1999) The diagnosis and management of dementia in primary care, *Generations* **XXIII**(3): 17–23.

Richardson, C.A. and Hammond, S.M. (1996) A psychometric analysis of a short device for assessing depression in elderly people, *British Journal of Clinical Psychology* **35**: 543–51.

Richter, J., Barsky, A.J. and Hupp, J.A. (1983) The treatment of depression in elderly patients, *Journal of Family Practice* **17**: 43–7.

Rogers, A.C. and Dupuis, M.E. (1999) The role of a CNS in a memory clinic, *Clinical Nurse Specialist* **13**(1): 24–7.

Royal College of Nursing Institute (1999) *Nursing in memory clinics: resource pack.* Oxford: Royal College of Nursing Institute.

Royal College of Physicians (1981) Organic mental impairment in the elderly: implications for research, education and the provision of services. A report of the Royal College of Physicians by the College Committee on Geriatrics, *Journal of the Royal College of Physicians of London* **15**(3): 141–67.

Royal College of Physicians and the Royal College of Psychiatrists (1989) *Care of Elderly People with Mental Illness: Specialist Service and Medical Training.* London: Royal College of Physicians.

Sabat, S.R. (2001) *The Experience of Alzheimer's Disease: Life Through a Tangled Veil*. Oxford: Blackwell.

Sanford, J.R.A. (1975) Tolerance of debility in elderly dependents by supporters at home: its significance for hospital practice, *British Medical Journal* **3**: 375–6.

Schwab, J.J. and Holzer, C.E. (1973) Depressive symptomatology and age. *Psychosomatics* **14**: 135–41.

Shah, A., Karasu, M. and De, T. (1998) Nursing staff and screening for depression among acutely ill geriatric patients: a pilot study, *Aging & Mental Health* **2**(1): 71–4.

Shepherd, M., Cooper, B., Brown, A. and Kalton, G. (1981) *Psychiatric Illness in General Practice*. Oxford: Oxford University Press.

Shiekh, J. and Yesavage, J. (1986) Geriatric Depression Scale: recent findings in development of a shorter version, in J. Brink (ed.) *Clinical Gerontology: A Guide to Assessment and Intervention*. New York: Howarth Press.

Skog, M., Grafström, M., Negussie, B. and Winblad, B. (1999) Change of outlook on elderly persons with dementia: a study of trainees during a year of special education, *Nurse Education Today* **19**: 472–9.

Smyer, M.A. and Qualls, S.H. (1999) *Aging and Mental Health*. London: Blackwell.

Snowdon, J. (1997) Suicide rates and methods in different age groups: Australian data and perceptions, *International Journal of Geriatric Psychiatry* **12**(2): 253–8.

Spaniol, L. and Jung, H. (1987) Effective coping: a conceptual model, in A.P. Hatfield and H.P. Lefley (eds), *Families of the Mentally Ill: Coping and Adaptation*. London: Cassell.

Steeman, E., Abraham, I.L. and Godderis, J. (1997) Risk profiles for institutionalization in a cohort of elderly people with dementia or depression, *Archives of Psychiatric Nursing* **XI**(6): 295–303.

Steer, R.A., Rissmiller, D.J. and Beck, A.T. (2000) Use of the Beck Depression Inventory-II with depressed geriatric inpatients, *Behaviour Research and Therapy* **38**: 311–18.

Teri, L. and Wagner, A. (1991) Assessment of depression in patients with Alzheimer's disease: concordance between informants, *Psychology and Aging* **6**: 280–5.

Thompson, L.W., Davies, R., Gallagher, D. and Krantz, S. (1986) Cognitive therapy with older adults, *Clinical Gerontologist* **3**(4): 245–79.

Thompson, L.W., Gallagher, D. and Breckenridge, J.S. (1987) Comparative effectiveness of psychotherapies for depressed elders, *Journal Consulting Clinical Psychology* **53**: 385–90.

Thomson, A.P., Lowe, C.R. and McKeown, T. (1951) *The Care of the Ageing and Chronic Sick*. Published for the Birmingham Regional Hospital Board. London: E. & S. Livingstone.

Tuokko, H., MacCourt, P. and Heath, Y. (1999) Home alone with dementia, *Aging & Mental Health* **3**(1): 21–7.

Wenger, G.C., Woods, B., Keady, J., Scott, A. and White, N. (2000) *Dementia Action Research and Education*. Final Report to the Department of Health December 2000. University of Wales, Bangor: Institute of Medical and Social Care Research.

Whitehouse, P.J. (2000) History and the future of Alzheimer's disease, in P.J. Whitehouse, K. Maurer and J.F. Ballenger (eds) *Concepts of Alzheimer's Disease:*

Biomedical, Clinical and Cultural Perspectives. Baltimore, MD: The Johns Hopkins University Press.

Whitlock, F.A. and Evans, L.E.J. (1978) Drugs and depression, *Drugs* **15**: 53–71.

Wilcock, G.K., Bucks, R.S. and Rockwood, K. (eds) (1999) *Diagnosis and Management of Dementia: A Manual for Memory Disorders Teams.* Oxford: Oxford University Press.

Wood, K.A., Harris, M.J., Morreale, A. and Rizos, A.L. (1988) Drug induced psychosis and depression in the elderly, *Psychiatric Clinics of North America* **11**(1): 167–93.

Woods, B., Wills, W., Higginson, I., Whitby, M. and Hobbins, J. (1999) *An Evaluation of the Admiral Nurse Service: An Innovative Service for the Carers of People with Dementia.* London: NHS Executive North Thames R & D Directorate.

Woods, R.T. (1992) Psychological therapies and their efficacy, *Reviews in Clinical Gerontology* **2**(2): 171–83.

Woods, R.T. (1995) Dementia care: progress and prospects, *Journal of Mental Health* **4**(2): 115–24.

Woods, R.T. (1997) Why should family caregivers feel guilty? in M. Marshall (ed.) *State of the Art in Dementia Care.* London: Centre for Policy on Ageing.

Woods, R.T. (ed.) (1999) *Psychological Problems of Ageing: Assessment, Treatment and Care.* Chichester: Wiley.

World Health Organization (1993) *The ICD-10 Classification of Mental and Behavioural Disorders: Diagnostic Criteria for Research.* Geneva: World Health Organization.

Wragg, R.E. and Jeste, D.V. (1989) Overview of depression and psychosis in Alzheimer's disease, *American Journal of Psychiatry* **146**: 577–87.

Yale, R. (1995) *Developing Support Groups for Individuals with Early-Stage Alzheimer's Disease: Planning, Implementation and Evaluation.* London: Health Professions Press.

Yesavage, J., Brink, T., Rose, T. *et al.* (1983) Development and validation of a geriatric depression screening scale, *Journal of Psychiatric Research* **17**: 37–49.

Younger, D. and Martin, G.W. (2000) Dementia care mapping: an approach to quality audit of services for people with dementia, *Journal of Advanced Nursing* **32**(5): 1206–12.

Zigmond, A.S. and Snaith, R.P. (1983) The hospital anxiety and depression scale, *Acta Psychiatrica Scandinavica* **67**: 361–70.

20

The person who uses forensic mental health services

Phil Woods

Chapter overview

Users of forensic mental health services are usually referred to as mentally disordered offenders, a term which covers mentally disordered persons who have broken or who are alleged to have broken the law (DH and Home Office 1992). The National Association for the Care and Rehabilitation of Offenders (NACRO) defines this patient group as:

> Those offenders who may be acutely or chronically mentally ill; those with neuroses, behavioural and/or personality disorders; those with learning difficulties; some who, as a function of alcohol and/or substance misuse, have a mental health problem; and any who are suspected of falling into one or other of these groups. It also includes those offenders where a degree of mental disturbance is recognised even though that may not be severe enough to bring it within the criteria laid down by the Mental Health Act 1983. It also applies to those offenders who, even though they do not fall easily within this definition – for example, some sex offenders and some abnormally aggressive offenders – may benefit from psychological treatments.
>
> (NACRO 1993: 4)

Forensic mental health nurses are responsible for the day-to-day management and care of this population in a variety of assessment and treatment settings, which include prisons, high security hospitals, medium secure units, low secure units, acute mental health wards, specialized private hospitals, psychiatric intensive care units, court diversion schemes, and outpatient, community and rehabilitation services.

This chapter addresses problems faced by people with mental health problems in forensic care and the challenges facing their professional carers. The chapter considers:

- the speciality of forensic mental health nursing;
- prevalence and incidence of mental disorder among those in forensic care;
- the relationship between mental health problems and mental disorder, including psychopathology of offences;
- policy developments in forensic mental health care;
- challenges for practice including: taking account of service users' views, risk assessment and its management, forging therapeutic relationships, and providing gender sensitive services;
- the research and development agenda.

What is forensic mental health nursing?

The historical development of forensic mental health nursing has been intrinsically linked with that of generic mental health nursing. Care has been provided by nurses in controlled environments since bedlam (Tarbuck 1994). Its history can be traced as a unique thread through the development of Broadmoor, Rampton and Ashworth special hospitals, and the foundation of regional secure units in the 1980s (Topping-Morris 1992).

According to Topping-Morris (1992) and McCourt (1999) forensic mental health nursing dates back only as far as this period, coinciding with the introduction of the regional secure unit programme. However, Dale *et al.* (2001) suggests that there are three phases of development: an initial inert stage, when the work largely took place within large high security hospitals that were shrouded in secrecy (1863–1985), a stage of awakening that commenced with new services being developed and nurses being eager to describe their experiences (1985–95), and, from about 1996 to the present, a more empirical stage, when evidence is beginning to emerge from funded research, from doctoral degrees and scrutiny of services to assess their adherence to evidence-based practice and clinical governance.

Mullen (2000) defines forensic mental health as:

An area of specialisation that, in the criminal sphere, involves the assessment and treatment of those who are both mentally disordered and whose behaviour has led, or could lead, to offending. In the civil sphere forensic mental health has a more complex remit, not only being involved in the assessment and treatment of those who have potentially compensatable injuries but also providing advice to courts and tribunals on competency and capacity.

(2000: 307)

In some parts of the world forensic nursing represents a very specific specialism such as in the USA where sexual assault nurse examiners (SANE), forensic nurse examiners and forensic nurse investigators can be found. In the UK, however, the role is somewhat different. The International Association of Forensic Nurses defines forensic nursing as:

> ... the application of the forensic aspects of health care combined with the bio-psychosocial education of the registered nurse in the scientific investigation and treatment of trauma, and/or death of victims and perpetrators of violence, criminal activity, and traumatic accidents. The forensic nurse provides direct services to individual clients, consultation services to nursing, medical, and law-related agencies, as well as providing expert testimony in areas dealing with questioned death investigative processes, adequacy of service delivery, and specialised diagnoses of specific conditions as related to nursing.
>
> (1999: 2)

A study of nursing in secure environments by the United Kingdom Central Council for Nursing Midwifery and Health Visiting (UKCC) and the University of Central Lancashire (UCLancs) (1999) used a variety of methods to identify a number of key skills for staff that were relevant primarily to: relationships, boundaries, communication and counselling and more specifically to:

- safety and security;
- assessment and observation, including risk assessment and management;
- management of violence and aggression, control and restraint, de-escalation techniques;
- therapies and treatments, including cognitive-behavioural therapy and psychosocial interventions;
- knowledge of offending behaviour and appropriate legislation;
- report writing;
- jail craft (a term used to describe the prison context and culture); and
- practical skills, including primary health care, first aid and practice nursing.

(UKCC and UCLancs 1999: 58)

Peternelj-Taylor's (2000) requirements of the forensic mental health nurse listed in Box 20.1 show that these are similar to those of requirements of mental health nurses generally, although maintaining a non-judgemental attitude is probably more difficult in forensic than in other mental health settings.

This is demonstrated by case studies in Boxes 20.2 to 20.4, which illustrate the very damaged lives of patients with whom forensic mental health nurses work and the problems facing these patients and their professional carers.

These case studies illustrate that forensic services are called upon to provide assessment and treatment for some of the most damaged people in the country, many of whom have been in receipt of forensic services for many years and for whom, once ready to leave secure care, future placements are hard to find.

Box 20.1 Requirements of the forensic mental health nurse

- having respect for and maintaining the dignity for another human being, no matter how horrific the crime they have committed;
- role modelling by teaching pro-social values;
- having excellent listening and assessment skills;
- being flexible and able to adapt therapy to the individual;
- believing people can change;
- being self-aware of their values and belief systems;
- having confidence in their own abilities;
- having an enriched understanding of sub-cultures;
- having excellent report writing skills;
- being able to recognize one's limitations;
- being able to motivate change;
- demonstrating assertiveness;
- having a non-judgemental attitude;
- having a mature attitude and approach;
- drawing on life experiences.

(After Peternelj-Taylor 2000)

Box 20.2 Case study: Jack

Jack was admitted to a high-security hospital following conviction for the rape of his neighbour. He had a long history of mental disorder and had many previous admissions for this. Jack had been diagnosed previously with a functional psychosis. But more recently a psychiatrist felt he had an underlying anti-social personality disorder. Jack stated that at the time of the offence he felt well. His outpatient records did not confirm this as he was becoming increasingly difficult to engage in his treatment plan. When the police arrested Jack he told them that he had been raping women for years and had also attempted to rape others without success. The police could not confirm any of Jack's claims into unsolved crimes but took his admissions seriously. Jack had been detained in the high-security hospital for seven years now and, although some episodes of psychosis had been noted, he had been well settled generally and did not present any management problems. Jack refused to undertake any treatment to reduce the chance of him raping again. He had previously indicated to a member of staff that if he did it again he would probably kill the woman so she could not tell on him this time. Jack was due for a Mental Health Review Tribunal soon and his care workers were concerned about the outcome.

Box 20.3 Case study: Philip

Philip is a man in his late 20s who was transferred to a medium secure unit from prison. He has a long history of arson and violence towards those in authority and was given a 10-year prison sentence for setting his bail hostel room on fire and causing grievous bodily harm to the hostel staff when they intervened. He has a primary diagnosis of personality disorder but he was considered suitable for treatment in the unit's personality disorder ward. Since being admitted to this ward Philip has refused to be cooperative with assessment processes or to engage actively in treatment with 'screws' (nursing staff), and has harmed himself several times. He assaulted a member of nursing staff seriously and continues to verbally threaten staff and other patients. He has been nursed in an observation area of the ward for the last two months and attempts to return him to the main part of the ward precipitates threatening behaviour and attempted assault, which results in staff restraining him and returning him to the observation area.

Box 20.4 Case study: James

James is a man in his late 40s with mental illness and mild cognitive impairment. His illness is long-standing, with the first signs appearing in his late teens. Since the onset of his illness James has been institutionalized in one setting or another. He is detained currently in high-secure psychiatric care, where he has remained for over 20 years. James's case notes describe him in the past as 'a schizophrenic of the paranoid and violent type'. Over the years his clinical presentation has been little changed. He has a fixed and rigid personality, complex delusional system, lack of coping skills, refuses to accept ownership for his own actions, lacks insight, and generally is not accepted by other patients as a member of any ward community. He has a long history of violent and impulsive behaviour, which eventually resulted in the death of another person and consequently his contact with the high-secure psychiatric services via the courts. He was admitted under Section 37 of the Mental Health Act (DHSS 1983) with Section 41 restrictions for discharge. During his prolonged stay in the forensic services he has been troublesome and disruptive and one attempt to rehabilitate him through medium-secure services ended in failure. James is once again being considered for discharge to a medium-secure unit.

Mentally disordered offenders who are sentenced to prison for their crimes will serve their time and be released; there may be conditions attached to their release but they still do have to be released. However, if mentally disordered offenders are detained under a Restriction Order they cannot be released until deemed to be at low risk of re-offending. This places a large responsibility on forensic practitioners who must gaze into their crystal balls and make a judgement about their patients' future behaviour. Of course, they cannot know for certain what these people will do in future; but one thing is certain, if a patient who is released re-offends the public and media outcry will mean that the forensic service will be shouldered with at least some responsibility for their crime. This is a hard but simple fact of forensic mental health practice.

Prevalence and incidence of mental health problems in care

Forensic mental health services provide assessment and treatment for people suffering from the full spectrum of mental disorders who have committed a variety of crimes. Most service users suffer from a mental illness. Some have a psychopathic or other personality disorder, and a small and diminishing number suffer from mental impairment.

According to statistics on mentally disordered offenders in England and Wales for the year 2001 (Johnson and Taylor 2002) there were 3002 patients within the mental health system subject to a restriction order of the Mental Health Act (1983). During 2001 there were 980 admissions and 314 discharges to the community of these restriction orders. Furthermore, there was a fall in the number detained in high-security hospitals and a rise in those detained in other hospitals. Forty-two per cent of people admitted to forensic services during 2001 had been charged with or convicted of violence against the person. Seventy-three per cent of those detained suffered from a mental illness and 14 per cent from psychopathic disorder as defined by the Act. Eighty-four per cent of people admitted during 2000 were diagnosed as mentally ill and 3 per cent as suffering from psychopathic disorder.

Coid *et al.* (1999) retrospectively recorded, from a representative sample, all admissions to secure forensic psychiatry services over a seven-year period. They found that 84 per cent suffered from mental illness and 16 per cent from personality disorder. Furthermore, they found that proportionally more personality disordered patients were admitted to high-security than medium-secure care (28 per cent and 14 per cent, respectively).

Jamieson *et al.* (2000) reported on referral and admission trends in high-security hospitals over the 10-year period 1986–95. Overall they found no decrease in referrals but admissions fell by 16 per cent with some regional variation. Admission under the Mental Health Act (1983) classifications of psychopathic disorder and mental impairment had significantly decreased whereas under mental illness they had remained relatively stable. There was a decrease in admissions directly from court but an increase in the number of men from prison particularly pre-trial. Overall, there was an upward trend in the admissions of restricted patients. They concluded that there was a continuing demand for high security beds and that, although there was a drop in the number of admissions, these include individuals with pressing needs who made substantial demands on the service.

Butwell *et al.* (2000) examined residency and discharge within the high-security hospitals. They found an 8 per cent fall in the annual number of patients during the 10-year period, particularly within the Mental Health Act (1983) classification of mental impairment categories. However, the number of resident male patients classified as mentally ill was sustained over time. This was in spite of increased numbers of patients discharged to other institutions, fewer admissions and the introduction of new treatments for schizophrenia.

Women service users

The most comprehensive review to date of the literature on women and secure psychiatric services by Lart *et al.* (1998) reported that women, although making up less than 20 per cent of the population of forensic mental health settings, were a heterogeneous group. They covered a wide age range, and had diverse personal, psychiatric and forensic histories. This review reported two types of service provision: one in which women were an afterthought (wards are segregated, several male but only one female ward) and the other which offered gender-blind provision (mixed gender-wards).

According to *Women in Special Hospitals* (1997) women are less likely to have restriction orders imposed under the Mental Health Act (1983), less likely to have index offences of a violent or sexual nature, but more likely to have an index offence of arson. A higher proportion of women than men in high-security care in England and Wales are admitted from NHS mental health services; most such admissions are of people regarded as difficult to manage within lower levels of security (Lart *et al.* 1998). Coid *et al.* (1999) reported that proportionately more women admitted to forensic mental health services over a seven-year period suffered from personality disorder (32 per cent) rather than mental illness (12 per cent), and that those with personality disorder were on average younger on admission. Johnson and Taylor (2002) report that the number of women detained in forensic mental health services under restriction orders has been relatively stable over a 10-year period (11–12 per cent).

A relatively high proportion of those on the caseload of any forensic mental health service, whether in the health, social care sector or criminal justice system, suffer from one or more personality disorders. Moreover, many patients diagnosed with a mental illness have co-morbid personality disorder. Personality disorder within the UK is clouded by the legal classification of psychopathic disorder with the result that different studies use different terms. Some studies use a legal classification when defining a case, some refer to personality disorder and others to both.

A significant proportion of mentally disordered offenders find themselves at some time within the prison system. Some will be diverted to forensic mental health services shortly after remand, others will be diverted at sentencing and others will be diverted following the passing of a custodial sentence. Singleton *et al.*'s (1998) survey of psychiatric morbidity among prisoners reports a high prevalence of personality disorder in all populations: 78 per cent of male prisoners on remand, 64 per cent of male prisoners serving their sentence, and 50 per cent of the total population of women prisoners in both groups. Further, they report anti-social personality disorder as having the highest prevalence rate: 63 per cent, 49 per cent and 31 per cent, respectively. In relation to functional psychosis (i.e. schizophrenia, manic depression), they found rates of 7 per cent for sentenced male prisoners, 10 per cent for males on remand and 14 per cent for female prisoners. Further, they report that schizophrenic or delusional disorders were more common than affective disorders.

The Department of Health (2000c) reports that two thirds of the high-security hospital population in England and Wales have committed serious crimes: homicide, 26 per cent; wounding, 37 per cent; and various types of sexual offence, 9 per cent. Coid *et al.* (1999) report that there was an increase in admissions of mentally-ill people to forensic services following non-criminal behaviours, mainly because of violence or threatened violence. In contrast, the principal reason for admitting people suffering from personality disorder following a non-criminal offence was deliberate self-harm (mainly self-mutilation). For those admitted following a criminal offence, mentally-ill people were admitted mainly for minor crimes of violence, and those suffering from personality disorder for serious sexual offences and arson.

Buchanan's (1998) follow-up study of patients discharged from high-security hospitals between 1982 and 1983 found that within 5½ years following discharge 24 per cent had been convicted of a criminal offence (9 per cent for a serious offence, 8 per cent for a violent offence, 5 per cent for a sexual offence) and that within 10½ years a criminal conviction had been recorded against 31 per cent (14 per cent for a serious offence, 14 per cent for a violent offence, 7 per cent for a sexual offence). Men were more likely to have been convicted than women, as were those who were younger on discharge and those with more extensive criminal records. Moreover, those classified as psychopathic disorder were significantly more likely than those classified as mentally ill to be reconvicted within 10½ years following discharge.

In summary, these trends show that young men are predominant users of forensic mental health services in the UK. The majority is diagnosed as having a mental illness, and those suffering from personality disorders also constitute a substantial group. Among current admissions the largest single group are those with histories of violence against the person.

The relationship between mental health problems and criminality

The relationship between mental health problems and criminality is at best tenuous, and is traditionally viewed as the potential for violent offending. According to Blumenthal and Lavender:

> the question of whether individuals suffering from a mental disorder have a greater propensity for violence than the general population has been controversial. Early research found that psychiatric patients were

no more likely to be violent than the rest of the population, but recent studies have established a consistent, albeit modest, relationship.

(2000: 1)

There is a widespread view that mental disorder is linked to violent offending, perhaps fuelled by the media frenzy that is seen when a particularly horrific or extraordinary crime takes place. 'He must be mad to undertake such a bad act' and similar phrases are often heard, indicating the belief that some acts could not possibly be carried out by a mentally stable person. In some sense lay reasoning and indeed professional opinion at times suggests madness and badness to be explicitly linked. A consequence of this is that public opinion tends to drive the political agenda. Thus, controversial policies such as the UK government's draft Mental Health Bill (DH 2002) which arises from a political agenda which conflicts with professional views of mental health problems.

According to Mason and Mercer (1999) the relationship between mental disorder and criminality has much to do with how mental disorder and criminal behaviour are socially defined and constructed. Furthermore, research studies, which have investigated this relationship, have been criticized for their methodological limitations. Among these are the failure of studies to take sufficient account of the criminalization of the mentally ill, the medicalization of deviance, and confounding differences between comparison groups (Blumenthal and Lavender 2000). Criminalization of the mentally ill is a particular problem for such studies because it means that mentally ill people are more likely to be arrested for the same offence than non-mentally ill people. In contrast the medicalization of deviance means that more deviant behaviours, including violent acts, are becoming the province of psychiatry and therefore more violent people are becoming psychiatric patients. A further limitation of many research studies is that subjects tend to be those in high-risk groups making comparison with the general population questionable.

Case linkage studies using conviction rates have, however, shed some light on the relationship between mental disorder and criminality. In a large Swedish birth cohort study, men who had been treated for a major mental disorder such as major affective disorder, schizophrenia, paranoid states and psychoses, were 2.56 times more likely to be convicted of an offence and 4.2 times more likely to be convicted of a violent offence by the age of 30 than men without a history of major mental disorder. For women, the relative risks were 5.02 and 27.5 respectively (Hodgins 1992). Wessely *et al.*'s (1994) UK case linkage study of people diagnosed with schizophrenia over a 20-year period, matched for age and sex with other psychiatric diagnoses, found that the risk of conviction was increased 3.3 times for schizophrenic women, but there was no difference for men. However, men with schizophrenia had a 3.8, and women suffering from schizophrenia a 5.3, times greater risk of conviction for assault or serious violence. Hodgins *et al.* (1996) in a later cohort study that sought to address some methodological weaknesses of the previous studies found that, compared with the general population, women with a major mental disorder had a relative risk of 8.66 and men 4.48 of committing a single violent crime.

Much of the research into the relationship between criminality and mental disorder has examined major mental disorder or personality/ psychopathic disorders. The link between the latter has been frequently demonstrated. However, the learning disabled offender has only been considered by relatively few studies. An exception is Alexander *et al.* (2002) who report on referrals to a forensic learning disability service. These researchers found that those referred were mainly men (81 per cent) who had a mild/borderline learning disability (82 per cent); many had prior service contact (92 per cent), in addition a high proportion abused alcohol or drugs (57 per cent) and many suffered from co-morbid schizophrenia (33 per cent) or personality disorder (58 per cent). Index offences included violence to others (30 per cent), sexual offences (22 per cent), and arson (10 per cent). A high proportion (76 per cent) had at least one previous conviction. Learning disabled people who offend may have limited skills in communicating and forming relationships with others, and limited strategies for coping with frustration and anger. Interestingly, Lyall *et al.* (1995) report that many staff who care for this patient group would tolerate offending behaviour and be reluctant to report offences to the police, even when the offence was serious, such as sexual or physical assault which results in the victim requiring hospital treatment.

The associations between personality disorder and criminality have been dealt with earlier in this chapter. Patients with personality disorders are some of the most difficult to manage in forensic mental health settings. Personality disorder manifests itself in many different behavioural repertoires, many of these starkly anti-social. Melia and Moran describe succinctly challenges faced by nurses caring for these patients within a personality disorder unit in a high-security hospital:

> ... there is a psychosocial pattern demonstrable through the manner in which individuals perceive, interpret and relate to their environment and to others. In acknowledging this and trying to provide a treatment service for this challenging group of individuals it is crucial that 'relationship' is recognized as a key pathway towards providing appropriate clinical treatment.

(2000: 468)

The balance to be struck between treatment and care of these patients and simply managing their behaviour is a matter for political and professional debate. A crucial question, for planners, providers and commissioners of services, however, is what interventions and regimes have been demonstrated to work.

The author's recent systematic review of the literature in relation to the effectiveness of nursing interventions with personality disorders (Woods and Richards 2002) found that there was a flimsy evidence base for nursing interventions, whether delivered in isolation or as part of a multi-professional treatment programme. The review highlighted the importance of further research into the day-to-day nursing care of these patients.

Psychopathology of offending

Violence and homicide

Violence is a more common phenomenon than homicide. Moreover aggression is often linked to violence yet can occur without violence. Aggression can be covert or overt, yet violence is considered as more destructive than aggression and is often associated with dangerousness. Violence will always have a victim, although the motive may not always be clear.

Indictable violent offences include:

- murder offences (murder, attempted murder, threat or conspiracy to murder);

- manslaughter offences (manslaughter – section 2 Homicide Act 1957 [diminished responsibility], other manslaughter – child destruction, causing death by dangerous driving, infanticide); and

- assault and robbery offences (wounding, grievous bodily harm, other act endangering life, assault, actual bodily harm, robbery, assault with intent to rob).

Although sexual offences could be included here they are considered in a separate section. Some common non-indictable violent offences include: aggravated assault, assault on a constable, common assault, possession of an offensive weapon, and drunkenness.

The psychopathology of violent mentally-ill offenders is complex yet certain risk factors are identified in the literature. These include: youth, male gender, previous violence, relationship instability, positive symptoms of mental illness, alcohol or drug misuse, lack of insight, poor coping skills, prior supervision failure, negative attitudes, impulsivity, and unresponsiveness to treatment.

Fire raising or arson

Fire raising or arson has immense destructive power and as such evokes fear in many professionals and the public alike. Relatively speaking, it accounts for only a small proportion of all crimes. However, the number of arson offences recorded by the police rose by 14 per cent between 2000/01 and 2001/02, and levels have risen by over 70 per cent since the mid-1990s (Crime in England and Wales 2001/2002 – Jon Simmons and colleagues: personal communication).

As with other crimes the motives and circumstances surrounding arson are complex, yet some have tried to classify them. Faulk (1988) suggested two categories: Group I where fire is a means to an end; and Group II where the fire itself is the phenomenon of interest. Later Rix (1994) suggested 15 motive categories following his study of 153 arsonists: revenge, excitement, vandalism, cry for help/attention, rehousing, attempted suicide, carelessness, psychotic, financial, cover-up, other manipulative, heroism, proxy, anti-depressant, and political.

According to Prins (1994) there are some general characteristics of arsonists. They are mostly young males who have considerable relationship difficulties. Many have alcohol problems, many are not very intelligent and many have had unstable childhoods and suffer from serious psychological disturbance. A direct sexual motive is rare, but many have difficulty in forming sexual relationships and many have problems in dealing with feelings of anger or frustration at real or imagined wrongs.

As these characteristics demonstrate arsonists are often individuals with complex problems and needs. The additional problems of mental disorder exacerbate the challenges of treatment and rehabilitation.

Sexual offences

A useful starting point is Prins's (1994: 199) definition of non-criminal sexual behaviour as 'those forms of sexual activity between two adults which is acceptable to both parties, do not involve coercion, exploitation or degradation, and do not affront the notion of decency prevailing at the time'. Therefore, the assumption must be that any behaviour outside of this can be considered sexually inappropriate or an offence.

Indictable sexual offences include: buggery or attempt, indecent assault on a male, rape or attempted rape, indecent assault on a female, unlawful sexual intercourse, and gross indecency with a child. Perkins (1991) classifies sex offenders as either compensatory, displaced aggression, sadistic or impulsive/opportunistic. Sexual offending constitutes a small proportion of all crime, about 5 per cent according to Crime in England and Wales 2001/2002 (Simmons and colleagues: personal communication). However, this crime is very underreported.

Not surprising, most sexual offences are committed by men. Some result in more serious crime such as murder. It is not possible to generalize about the psychopathology of sexual offending because reasons are complex, offences varied and sexual offenders are not a homogenous group. Treatment tends to focus on reducing the offender's denial and minimization of the offence, changing the cognitive distortions relevant to the aberrant behaviour, increasing victim empathy, modifying deviant sexual preferences, improving problem-solving and coping skills, improving social and communication skills, and constructing a relapse-prevention plan.

▌Policy developments in forensic mental health care

Recent policy documents identify forensic mental health care as a priority area for development. *Modernising Mental Health Services* (DH 1998) and the *National Service Framework for Mental Health* (DH 1999) priorities include addressing gaps in services for people with severe and enduring mental illness who require secure accommodation, closer integration of services and strengthening assessment criteria and outcome measures. *The NHS Plan* (DH 2000a) further emphasizes these priorities particularly with regard to inappropriate levels of detention and long-term provision. It makes a financial commitment to provide extra resources and staffing, specifically in relation to high-security services and the management of people with severe personality disorder.

The UK government plans integration of high-security and medium-secure services within the overall mental health care system, the aim being to provide a seamless service for patients. Much of this integration has already been accomplished. New services are trying to operate within a whole-systems approach to ensure that the service as a whole has adequate facilities to provide care pathways for patients that facilitate their smooth progression through appropriate levels of security.

Additional secure places are being provided, with high priority being given to the regional development of long-term medium- and low-secure facilities. This development aims to alleviate system pressures within medium-secure services currently. In these services beds are 'blocked' by those patients who require long-term care, with the result that people with mental health problems continue to be placed inappropriately within prisons.

The government White Paper, *Reforming the Mental Health Act in England and Wales* (DH 2000b) set out proposals that will have a significant impact on the care of mentally disordered offenders. Chapter 4 of the White Paper discusses the compulsory care and treatment of mentally disordered offenders. Although many of its proposals support existing provisions within the current Mental Health Act (1983), it does make some important suggestions for improvement. When an offender comes before the court it will have a wider range of disposal options than currently, which can take account of the nature of the offence, the risk to others from possible repeat offending and assessment of the offender's treatment needs. There is also a new single power of remand for assessment and treatment.

The most controversial component of *Reforming the Mental Health Act* is Part II, which deals with mental disorder and public protection. Included here are proposals for managing dangerous people with severe personality disorder; these are discussed later in this chapter. The White Paper proposes, also, new statutory powers for the assessment and treatment of high-risk patients in civil proceedings, and for the assessment and treatment of high-risk mentally disordered offenders. Integral to this part of the Act is information sharing and risk management and service development for managing these high-risk individuals. The draft Mental Health Bill is, at the time of writing, out for consultation, and it seems likely that many of these proposals will be incorporated within the future legislative framework for mental health care.

The Journey to Recovery: The Government's Vision for Mental Health Care (DH 2001) sets targets and sets out spending plans for forensic mental health services. According to this report:

- An additional 200 long-term secure beds will be provided, so enabling 400 patients now in high-secure accommodation to move to more appropriate less secure facilities.

- Detection and treatment of the 5000 prisoners at any one time who could have a serious mental illness will be improved.

- New partnerships between the NHS and local prisons will ensure that all those detected will receive treatment, and none will leave prison without a care plan and a care coordinator.

- More suitable services, in secure as well as community settings, will be developed for those with severe personality disorder, who pose a risk to other patients, staff, the public and to themselves. Many of these are the most needy and disadvantaged people in our society; the aim is to help them accept responsibility for their problems and, by changing their behaviour, work towards their successful reintegration into the community.

Court liaison

A government circular (Home Office 1990) and a review of services for mentally disordered offenders (DH and Home Office 1992) advocated that wherever possible a mentally disordered offender (or alleged offender) should receive care and treatment from services other than those provided by the criminal justice system. This policy continues, as a result of which numerous court liaison schemes have evolved with the aim of identifying the mentally disordered offender in need of mental health care rather than custodial care either prior to the court, from the court, or from remand and prison.

The point at which diversion occurs depends largely on whether the Crown Prosecution Service is prepared to discontinue criminal proceedings. Its decision must take account of several factors, including: the severity of the offence, circumstances surrounding the offence, the likely penalty, the age of the offender (youth or old age and infirmity), the complainant's attitude and presence of mental illness or stress (Prins 1992).

In the case of the more serious, violent mentally disordered offender, it is almost inevitable that they will spend a period in custody either awaiting a psychiatric report, or transfer for further assessment or treatment (Joseph 1990; Robertson *et al.* 1994). Due to legislation within the Bail Act (1976) the mentally disordered offender is more likely than the non-mentally disordered offender to be remanded into custody, even when charged with a non-custodial offence; the main reason for this is the 'protection of the defendant' (Joseph 1990) and a general tendency to regard the mentally disordered as dangerous (Robertson 1988).

Diversion from the criminal justice system to the mental health system has been criticized for being somewhat arbitrary (Davis 1994), dependent on such factors as: the enthusiasm and motivations of individuals concerned with the defendant (i.e. defence or prosecution lawyer, or judge) (Cooke

1991); and dominant perceptions of available resources (Exworthy and Parrott 1993).

Diversion as a concept is also not without its critics, who argue that diversion schemes fail to preserve public interest. Others argue that such schemes violate the rights of the accused because they erode their right to a custodial sentence and they place undue pressure on them to participate in treatment (McKittrick and Eysenck 1984). The current Review of the Mental Health Act is likely to erode these rights further where the mentally disordered offender is considered a particular danger to society.

To what extent should mentally disordered offenders be held responsible for their actions? And how much consideration should be given to the views of the victim? (Prins 1992). These are important questions. One might argue that the formal legal process can be a valuable way of testing a mentally disordered offender's concept of reality (Smith and Donovan 1990).

Challenges for nursing practice

Patients who find themselves in forensic mental health services have the most complex problems and needs, and have often found themselves in trouble with the courts, in many cases for extreme acts of violence. Some have not actually been charged or convicted of an offence but their behaviour has brought them to the attention of the police. Those with the most complex needs are likely to be placed in high-security hospitals for, on average, seven or eight years (Department of Health 2000c). With rehabilitation through the medium-secure services being two years or more, this extends an average length of stay to 10 years or more. However, some patients may find themselves within the services for a much longer period – some in excess of 20 years. Moreover, a high proportion of patients remain in contact with either forensic mental health or mental health services for most of the rest of their lives. Consequently, detaining and caring for mentally disordered offenders is an expensive demand on today's mental health services.

Nursing these patients is not easy. They require complex treatment plans that focus fundamentally on reducing risk of harm to others. But some patients simply cannot engage in treatment, while others will refuse to do so. So treatment plans need to be developed in the context of risk assessment and consequent management of the risks identified, that will not only reduce risk while in care but also the risk of future offending when the patient returns to live in the community.

According to McCann (1999) the internal tensions and conflicts within forensic mental health care raises questions about the kinds of treatment and care that should be provided, and about the balance to be struck between care and punishment, custody and containment, and empowerment and control.

Nurses are charged with managing the day-to-day care and treatment of forensic patients and are faced with complex and challenging behaviour, sometimes with only limited experience and additional training. Many patients are: unwelcome receivers of care, treatment resistive, 'act-out' an extreme spectrum of behaviours; and display a high level of violence and aggression. Rask and Rahm Hallberg's (2000) study of forensic psychiatric nursing care in Sweden reports that the nurse's role consists mainly of actions related to activities of daily living, medical psychiatric actions, informing and educating patients and families, and assessing patients.

In a later paper Rask and Levander (2001) highlight interventions used by nurses in the context of the nurse–patient relationship. They report the most commonly used interventions as social interaction, regular communication and social skills training. The most common focus in the verbal nurse–patient interaction in this study involved nurses explaining consequences of patients' behaviour to them, confronting and encouraging patients to talk about their crime or behaviours, interpretative communications, and communication about functions of daily life. These findings, although useful, provide only a very narrow view of the process of forensic mental health nursing practice.

This section focuses on challenges to nursing practice that are particularly relevant to the forensic setting. These are:

- taking account of service users' views;
- risk assessment and its management;
- forging therapeutic relationships; and
- providing gender sensitive services.

For information on other aspects of forensic nursing, readers are referred to the annotated reading list at the end of this chapter.

Taking account of service users' views

In many cases users of forensic mental health services are unwilling partners in care. In most cases patients are detained against their will, the majority having been committed to the care of forensic services by the court following conviction for an offence. User perceptions of care processes must be taken into account but how and when to do so are issues of continual debate. This is in part because forensic services must pursue joint goals of care and custody, which may suggest divergent interventions and approaches; striking the right balance between the duty of care and of custody is difficult to achieve. Indeed some forensic services are explicitly led security measures and directions, which cannot be influenced by the views of service users because they exist for the protection of staff, patients and the public.

Given the limitations of patient empowerment within forensic services, it is not uncommon, however, for patients to be represented at ward or unit management team meetings. Patients' views are relevant to the way that forensic services function and they should be invited to suggest what developments should occur. However, the extent to which these can be acted upon may be limited.

In view of the particular difficulties involved in patients expressing their views directly, patient advocates are particularly important in forensic settings. Advocacy services are developing quickly with the aim of ensuring that the views of all groups of service users from the full range of ethnic backgrounds are heard.

Risk assessment and management

The assessment and management of risk (the focus of Chapter 8) is the core business for forensic mental health professionals. This is not surprising since mentally disordered offenders are in receipt of care and treatment because they present a risk to themselves or others. Entangled in the process of risk assessment and management is the concept of dangerousness. This term was once considered outdated, but is once again current owing to recent government documents which describe mentally disordered offenders in terms of their dangerousness. Dangerousness is the potential to cause serious physical and psychological harm to others. It incorporates also fear-inducing, impulsive and destructive behaviours that are displayed or have been displayed by a person in the past.

For the forensic mental health nurse risk assessment is concerned mainly with three highly interrelated components: the risk posed in the past, now, and in the future. It is concerned also with two key questions: will reoffending occur?; and what is the potential for change? The main problem which forensic mental health nurses face in their approaches to risk assessment, and its management, is that it is affected to a large degree by who defines the risk and how it is defined (McClelland 1995). Pollock and Webster (1990) and Monahan and Steadman (1994) point out that assessments need to be: systematic and based on the population undergoing assessment; require identified risk factors being broken down into manageable components; for these to be further assessed through effective treatment planning; and for outcomes to be evaluated through monitoring recovery status.

Forensic mental health professionals are expected to be able to assess risk adequately (Bingley 1997), but, this key skill relies heavily on clinical judgement since 'no other measurement device is available' (Chiswick 1995). Thus, the difficult question arises as to how mental health nurses might be best prepared for this task. Borum (1996) makes three recommendations to improve clinical practice in risk assessment: improve assessment technology; develop clinical practice guidelines; and develop training programmes and curricula. Although these recommendations appear straightforward, forensic mental health nurses need to bear in mind that even the most careful risk assessment is complicated by the assessor's inability to control for future physical and social circumstances. For example, the patient may do something completely out of the blue, something which could never have been predicted.

Many forensic mental health professionals rely upon the *actuarial* or *statistical* approach to risk assessment, which involves the use of predictive factors (often historical variables) known to be associated to risk in the population being risk assessed. Although this approach can act as an anchor for risk assessment processes, a clinical approach is required to provide sufficient evidence for the reduction of risk. This approach looks for professional opinion and evidence concerning a patient's self-presentation and considers also situational and clinical variables. The clinical risk assessment approach looks for explanations of specific violent behaviour and is concerned with: how individuals behave, how they react in various situations, how they have been known to behave, how willingly they accept treatment, and how much insight they have into their condition.

However, as Webster *et al.* (1995) rightly point out, in their endeavour to produce 'safe' conclusions, clinicians tend to vastly overrate the likelihood of future violence. This results in 'false positive' errors, whereby an individual is predicted to be violent but, in fact, does not turn out to be so. It has been suggested that these errors should not be viewed entirely as poor clinical practice but as part of the risk itself, arising from the social pressure for false positive errors rather than false negative ones (Shah 1978). This is not surprising, since what is being asked is, will an individual be violent in the future? This is rather like crystal-ball gazing, as violent behaviours stem from a complex array of causal factors including personality, developmental influences and environmental effects.

Risk assessment should be followed by a risk management plan which focuses on the likelihood of the probability or outcome occurring. Vinestock (1996) describes this as a method of balancing probable consequences of decisions, which assists in formalizing the decision-making process in relation to the risk of harm to self or others.

The risk management plan should state the nature or level of the risk specifically. The situational context of the risk should be stated as should the relationships between the risky behaviours presented. Next, for the plan to be effectively evaluated, it is important for it to be reviewed continuously. These reviews need to be time-bound and, above all, the plan and evaluations need to be communicated to all relevant people involved in the care process.

Doyle (1999: 49) identifies seven key questions, which can assist the forensic mental health nurse in estimating the level of risk:

- What is the likelihood of harm occurring?
- How often is this likely to occur?
- What possible outcomes may there be?
- Who is at risk?
- What is the immediacy of the risk?
- What is the timescale for assessment?
- What are the circumstances which are likely to increase or decrease the risk?

However, for risk management to be effective clear statements of anticipated risk and how these can be avoided need to be made, so minimizing the possible impact of any risk. In effect, therefore, if the nurse has a detailed knowledge of an individual's personal, mental health, forensic history, then the early warning signs of any risk can be anticipated. In turn, the risk management plan can focus specifically on the responses required to deal with these potential or anticipated risks, and monitor their effects on risk reduction through implementation of the plan. This is, in essence, dynamic risk assessment.

Good practice dictates which responses are appropriate in response to risks that occur. This may involve physical restraint or isolation from others on the unit to allow the individual to talk about (ventilate) their feelings on a one-to-one basis. It is crucial that the individual is informed of the risk(s) that have been identified, what will happen if they occur, and why. In practice, this may involve the patient being given the opportunity to select from a range of alternative management strategies. For example, some very powerful men are petrified of being injected with a major tranquillizer and, therefore, other forms of medication in crisis may be more beneficial; and women who have been sexually abused may be terrified of being physically restrained on their back, if this position was used when they were abused. Therefore, they should be restrained only with their front to the floor.

Successful risk management requires nurses as individuals and as members of a multi-disciplinary clinical team to ask rhetorical questions that include:

- Do we have the personal and professional experience and resources to manage the risk?
- Is our working environment amenable to manage the risk (for example, physical layout, potential weapons)? and (particularly within the community),
- Are the carers, friends or neighbours likely to hinder the risk management plan?

Forging therapeutic relationships

The struggle to find the balance between care and custody is a continual burden for forensic mental health professionals – even more so for forensic mental health nurses. Nurses provide most of the security on the wards where they are also expected to therapeutically engage with the person who they may have to search before going on a rehabilitation trip, or handcuff before a visit to court. How can therapeutic relationships develop among the day-to-day management tasks which nurses are expected to undertake within forensic mental health care? There are no easy answers, but much depends on the ability of the nurse to forge relationships as a medium for delivering care.

An important consideration here is the role of professional values.

Values

As health care professionals, forensic nurses are expected to leave their personal values at home and provide care for individuals whose very existence may be in conflict with these personal values and belief. Somehow forensic mental health nurses are expected to step outside their role as, for example, a parent, and provide care and treatment for those people who have abused children who may be the same age as their own.

According to Williams and Dale (2001), six professional values are important when caring for mentally disordered offenders:

- respect for the patient as a human being, regardless of behaviour, offending history or diagnosis;
- acceptance and application of current concepts of ill health and needs for care and treatment operated by the medical and psychiatric professions;
- not judging patients;
- applying an equally high quality of care to every patient;
- treating all patients with equality and fairness;
- maintaining confidentiality.

Set against this somewhat idealist view of applying values to forensic mental health practice are realistic descriptions of the challenges facing forensic nurses that show just how real the struggle is for forensic mental health nurses. Swinton points out that:

> Forensic nurses are called upon to care for people who have committed acts that are often horrific, frightening, repulsive and extremely difficult for most people to understand or identify with. They are frequently called upon to offer care to patients whose aggressive and unpredictable behaviour means that the primary therapeutic goal may be to develop and maintain some kind of workable equilibrium.
> (Swinton 2000: 113)

Furthermore, Swinton and Boyd indicate that forensic mental health nurses are caught in a dilemma:

> on the one hand, they are faced with the difficult reality of having to respect the personhood of individuals who show little respect for themselves or for others; who are frequently aggressive and violent, sometimes dishonest, often deceitful; and who may appear to have little or no remorse for the antisocial acts they may have perpetrated. On the other hand, their professional role means that it is not possible for them to offer any kind of meaningful nursing care if they do not or cannot respect the personhood of the other.
> (Swinton and Boyd 2000: 136)

These are the real issues that forensic mental health nurses have to deal with before they are ever able to fully accomplish the professional values that

Williams and Dale provide. Many nurses will be able to find their own answers, others will simply leave the specialty. However, ignoring the value base of forensic nursing is not an option for nurses; the conflicts that may arise between personal and professional values must be faced.

Aiyegbusi (1998) informs us that forensic mental health nursing, as in other branches of mental health nursing, is concerned predominately with the effective use of interpersonal relationships with patients. The ability to establish a therapeutic relationship is one of the most important competencies, as the nurse–patient relationship affects every aspect of the nursing process and the quality of care given. According to Aiyegbusi (1998) a coherent theoretical framework necessarily needs definition, in the light of psychically complex and disturbing situations that nurses may encounter when attempting to work therapeutically with patients whose internal working models for relationships may be grossly disturbed by their formative developmental experiences.

Killian and Clark (1996) highlight the challenges associated with applying humanistic interventions, instead of more mechanistic ones, in forensic mental health nursing. They point out that the exchange of physical boundaries for the security provided by relationships that patients develop with nurses, places a large demand upon nursing staff. 'They (the staff) have to provide both emotional and practical (physical) containment, whilst allowing at the same time for optimum conditions of therapeutic interaction' (1996: 102). Further, they observe that mostly nurses have to work out the right balance between their custodial and more clinical role for themselves.

In summary, the therapeutic relationship is central to forensic mental health nursing practice established by the nurse with his or her patients. Through the effective use of this relationship, nurses make a major contribution to accurate assessment and effective management of risk and so strike a balance between their duties of care and custody.

Providing gender sensitive services

As Ifill (1998) points out '. . . female patients in a predominately male setting do not always receive services that are geared to their needs' and '. . . most provision is set up for the majority, in this case men' (1998: 14–15). Neglect of the special needs of women in forensic care is being addressed. Standards have been developed for women's services by the Working Group for Women Service Users in Forensic Psychiatry and these are being implemented and monitored currently in many secure units and hospitals (MacKenzie and Morgan-Clark 2000).

According to Byrt *et al.* (2001) forensic service developments for women have focused on the following areas:

- privacy and dignity and freedom from sexual harassment;
- women's needs related to culture, religion, sexual orientation and disability;

- appropriate levels of physical and relational security;
- increasing opportunities for participation and choice;
- access to appropriate advocacy;
- access to children, partners and family members;
- provision of care and treatment, which both values women and meets their psychological, physical, and other health needs;
- gender sensitive training for staff.

Scott and Parry-Crooke (2001) surveyed 154 members of professional teams working with women in a high-security hospital, in three medium-secure units (an adolescent secure unit for young women, a prison health care unit and a community forensic team) to assess their training needs. The response rate to the survey is not reported directly but appears to be only 39 per cent. Nevertheless, the survey was valuable in identifying issues in relation to working with women offenders which professional staff wanted to understand more.

Organizational and institutional issues included:

- gender-based issues with male colleagues who work with women;
- ward crises and why they are constant;
- development and adaptation of treatment protocols to the particular needs of women;
- dynamics of women living together in secure settings;
- effects of racism and cultural differences;
- women's social roles and their interaction with mental health;
- managing fragile relationships; and
- why some women are in prison and not hospital.

In relation to personal and individual issues respondents identified their need for greater understanding of:

- self-harm;
- manipulative behaviour among women;
- engaging women who are unwilling to look at what's involved in problematic behaviour;
- empowering individual women;
- boundaries around staff/women relationships;
- encouraging women's independence; and
- responding to disclosures.

These lists are extensive, although perhaps not exhaustive. What is clear, however, is that many care and treatment issues exist for women and that the development of gender-sensitive services is unlikely to be achieved overnight. However, increased awareness by forensic health care professionals of the special needs of women is a good starting point.

Parry-Crooke *et al.*'s (2000) study of women in forensic mental health services identified several sources of dissatisfaction in their relationships with staff. These included: inaccessibility of staff, staff not believing what they were saying or thinking that they were making things up, being inattentive or not making an effort to understand them; and being infantilized.

Forensic mental health research and development

Significant improvements in practice can be achieved only if concerted research and development takes place focused on key areas which have a bearing on clinical practice. Currently within England and Wales there is a dedicated research programme for forensic mental health care. This programme has established research priorities and has commissioned a series of expert papers, on topics that are likely to be priorities for research and development in the years ahead. The topics covered by these papers are:

- *Antisocial Personality Disorder: Children and Adolescents* (Bailey 2002);
- *Dual Diagnosis of Mental Disorder and Substance Misuse* (McMurran 2002a);
- *Prison Health care* (Shaw 2002).
- *Social Division and Difference: Black and Ethnic Minorities* (Ndegwa 2002);
- *Sex Offender Research* (Grubin 2002);
- *Social Division and Difference: Women* (Bartlett 2002);
- *Mental Illness and Serious Harm to Others* (Taylor 2002).
- *Personality Disorder* (McMurran 2002b);
- *Neurobiological Approaches to Disorders of Personality* (Dolan 2002).

Conclusion

Forensic mental health care is a very challenging area of nursing work, but it can be rewarding too. Central are issues of risk assessment and management. Forensic nurses need to have excellent interpersonal skills and be able to critically question their own values and judgements if they are to work effectively with this challenging patient group. Forensic services are a priority for future development, which should result in improved security and standards of treatment and care of mentally disordered offenders. Future investment will also open up further professional and career opportunities for forensic nurses and provide them with opportunities to establish the specialty clearly within the mental health nursing field.

In summary, the main points of this chapter are:

- Forensic mental health nurses are called upon to provide assessment and treatment to some of the most damaged people in the country, many of whom have been in receipt of forensic services for many years. Clients tend to be young males who suffer from mental illness or a personality disorder. Those with histories of violence against the person constitute the largest single group.

- The psychopathology of violent mentally-ill offenders is complex, but risk factors identified in the literature include: youth, male gender, history of previous violence, relationship instability, positive symptoms of mental illness, alcohol or drug misuse, lack of insight, poor coping skills, prior supervision failure, negative attitudes, impulsivity and unresponsiveness to treatment.

- Key skills for nursing staff working in secure environments are concerned with: relationship, boundaries, communication and counselling, and more specifically with:
    - safety and security;
    - assessment and observation, including risk assessment and management;
    - management of violence and aggression;
    - therapies and treatments;
    - knowledge of offending behaviour and relevant legislation;
    - report writing;
    - jail craft; and
    - practical skills, such as first aid.

- Many users of forensic mental health services require complex treatment plans that focus fundamentally on reducing the risk of harm to others. These plans need to be developed in the context of risk assessment and consequent management of the risks identified, the aim being not only reduction of risk while an inpatient, but also reduction of the risk of future offending following discharge.

- Striking the right balance between their duty of care and of custody is a constant challenge for forensic mental health nurses.

Questions for reflection and discussion

1 Taking an example of a forensic service you know or have visited, and consider the practical implications for nurses and patients of attempts by the service to strike a balance between care and custody.

2 How far is it possible for forensic mental health nurses to establish helping relationships with patients who resent their presence?

3 You are allocated to nurse a patient who is detained in a special hospital for having committed sexual and violent offences against children. What

emotions might this evoke in you? How might you manage these in the context of your professional relationship with the patient?

4   What risks need to be taken into consideration when discharging a mentally disordered offender from hospital to live in the community?

Annotated bibliography

- Chaloner, C. and Coffey, M. (eds) (2000) *Forensic Mental Health Nursing: Current Approaches*. Oxford: Blackwell Science. This is an informative text, underpinned by a sound evidence base, which emphasizes the practical application of theory and research findings in clinical practice. A key emphasis throughout the text is the role of forensic mental health nursing within multi-disciplinary and multi-agency teams and services.
- Dale, C., Thompson, T. and Woods, P. (eds) (2001) *Forensic Mental Health: Issues in Practice*. London: Harcourt Publishers Ltd. This is a multi-professional, relevant, practical and comprehensive text which addresses the context and development of effective practice in forensic mental health care.
- Fernando, S., Ndegwa, D. and Wilson, M. (1998) *Forensic Psychiatry, Race and Culture*. London: Routledge. Probably the best resource for research and practice issues in relation to race and culture to date.
- Kettles, A., Woods, P. and Collins, M. (eds) (2002) *Therapeutic Interventions for Forensic Mental Health Nurses*. London: Jessica Kingsley. Written by experts in the growing field of forensic mental health care, this book explores current and emerging interventions in forensic nursing and the care of the mentally disordered offender, with an emphasis on clinical practice and competence.
- Mason, T. and Mercer, D. (1999) *A Sociology of the Mentally Disordered Offender*. London: Longman. Provides a refreshing and certainly welcome look at the concept of the mentally disordered offender from a sociological perspective. The main theme is the analysis of crime and mental disorder, and the complex and often grey areas that lie between these two concepts.
- Mercer, D., Mason, T., McKeown, M. and McCann, G. (eds) (2000) *Forensic Mental Health Care: A Case Study Approach*. Edinburgh: Churchill Livingstone. An excellent text which provides immense insight into working with mentally disordered offenders. It brings together a range of disciplines and expertise in the field and is a valuable resource for anyone working in forensic care.
- Robinson, D. and Kettles, A. (eds) (2000) *Forensic Nursing and Multidisciplinary Care Of The Mentally Disordered Offender*. London: Jessica Kingsley. This text provides a valuable insight into caring for the

mentally disordered offender from an international perspective. It tries to draw out exactly what is special about the forensic nurse.

- Taylor, P.J. and Swan, T. (eds) (1999) *Couples in Care and Custody*. Oxford: Butterworth-Heinemann. This text provides a valuable resource and insight into couples' relationships in forensic care. The text is well edited and underpinned by a research and practice base.

References

Aiyegbusi, A. (1998) *Personality Disorder and Nursing at Ashworth Hospital: A Position Paper*. Evidence to the inquiry into the personality disorder unit at Ashworth Hospital Authority. Unpublished.

Alexander, R.T., Piachaud, J., Odebiyi, L. and Gangadharan, S.K. (2002) Referrals to a forensic service in the psychiatry of learning disability, *British Journal of Forensic Practice* **4**(2): 29–33.

Bailey, S. (2002) *Antisocial Personality Disorder: Children and Adolescents*. Liverpool: NHS National Programme on Forensic Mental Health Research and Development.

Bartlett, A. (2002) *Social Division and Difference: Women*. Liverpool: NHS National Programme on Forensic Mental Health Research and Development.

Bingley, W. (1997) Assessing dangerousness: protecting the interests of patients, *British Journal of Psychiatry* **170**(32): 28–9.

Borum, R. (1996) Improving the clinical practice of violence risk assessment, *American Psychologist* **51**(9): 945–56.

Blumenthal, S. and Lavender, T. (2000) *Violence and Mental Disorder: A Critical Aid to the Assessment and Management of Risk*. London: Jessica Kingsley.

Buchanan, A. (1998) Criminal conviction after discharge from special (high security) hospital: incidence in the first 10 years, *British Journal of Psychiatry* **172**: 472–6.

Butwell, M., Jamieson, E., Leese, M. and Taylor, P. (2000) Trends in special (high security) hospitals 2: residency and discharge periods, 1986–1995, *British Journal of Psychiatry* **176**: 260–5.

Byrt, R., Lomas, C., Gardiner, G. and Lewis, D. (2001) Working with women in secure environments, *Journal of Psychosocial Nursing* **39**(9): 42–50.

Chiswick, D. (1995) Dangerousness, in D. Chiswick and R. Cope (eds) *Seminars in Practical Forensic Psychiatry*. London: Gaskell.

Coid, J., Kahtan, N., Gault, S. and Jarman, B. (1999) Patients with personality disorder admitted to secure forensic psychiatry services, *British Journal of Psychiatry* **175**: 528–36.

Cooke, D.J. (1991) Treatment as an alternative to prosecution: offenders diverted for treatment, *British Journal of Psychiatry* **158**: 785–91.

Dale, C., Woods, P. and Thompson, T. (2001) Nursing, in C. Dale, T. Thompson and P. Woods (eds) *Forensic Mental Health: Issues in Practice*. London: Harcourt Publishers Ltd.

Davis, S. (1994) Factors associated with the diversion of mentally disordered offenders, *Bulletin of the American Academy of Psychiatry and Law* **22**(3): 389–97.

Department of Health and Home Office (1992) *Review of Health and Social Services for Mentally Disordered Offenders and Others Requiring Similar Services, Final Summary Report Cm 2088*. London: HMSO.

Department of Health (1998) *Modernising Mental Health Services: Safe, Sound and Supportive*. London: HMSO.

Department of Health (1999) *Mental Health National Service Framework: Modern Standards and Service Models*. London: HMSO.

Department of Health (2000a) *The NHS Plan: A Plan for Investment: A Plan for Reform*. London: HMSO.

Department of Health (2000b) *Reforming the Mental Health Act in England and Wales*. London: HMSO.

Department of Health (2000c) *Report of the Review of Security at the High Secure Hospitals*. London: HMSO.

Department of Health (2001) *The Journey to Recovery: The Government's Vision for Mental Health Care*. London: HMSO.

Department of Health (2002) *Draft Mental Health Bill*. London: The Stationery Office.

Dolan, M. (2002) *Neurobiological Approaches to Disorders of Personality*. Liverpool: NHS National Programme on Forensic Mental Health Research and Development.

Doyle, M. (1999) Organizational responses to crisis and risk: issues and implications for mental health nurses, in T. Ryan (ed.) *Managing Crisis and Risk in Mental Health Nursing*. Cheltenham: Stanley Thornes.

Exworthy, T. and Parrott, J. (1993) Evaluation of a diversion from custody scheme at magistrates' courts, *Journal of Forensic Psychiatry* **4**(3): 497–505.

Faulk, M. (1988) *Basic Forensic Psychiatry*. Oxford: Blackwell Science.

Grubin, D. (2002) *Sex Offender Research*. Liverpool: NHS National Programme on Forensic Mental Health Research and Development.

Hodgins, S. (1992) Mental disorder, intellectual deficiency, and crime: evidence from a birth cohort, *Archives of General Psychiatry* **49**: 476–83.

Hodgins, S., Mednick, S.A., Brennan, P.A., Schulsinger, F. and Engberg, M. (1996) Mental disorder and crime: evidence from a Danish birth cohort, *Archives of General Psychiatry* **53**: 489–96.

Home Office (1990) Provision for mentally disordered offenders, *Circular 66/90*. London: Home Office.

Ifill, C. (1998) One of a kind, *Nursing Times* **94**(27): 14–15.

International Association of Forensic Nurses (1999) *Scope and Standards of Forensic Nursing Practice*. Washington, DC: American Nurses Association.

Jamieson, E., Butwell, M., Taylor, P. and Leese, M. (2000) Trends in special (high security) hospitals 1: referrals and admissions, *British Journal of Psychiatry* **176**: 253–9.

Johnson, S. and Taylor, R. (2002) *Statistics of Mentally Disordered Offenders 2001: England and Wales*. London: Home Office.

Joseph, P. (1990) Mentally disordered offenders: diversion from the criminal justice system. *Journal of Forensic Psychiatry* **1**(2): 133–8.

Killian, M. and Clark, N. (1996) The multi-disciplinary team – the nurse, in C. Cordess and M. Cox (eds) *Forensic Psychotherapy: Crime, Psychodynamics and the Offender Patient: part II mainly practice*. London: Jessica Kingsley, ch. II-8-ii, pp. 101–6.

Lart, R., Payne, S., Beaumont, B., MacDonald, G. and Mistry, T. (1998) *Women and Secure Psychiatric Services: A Literature Review*. York: NHS Centre for Reviews and Dissemination.

Lyall, I., Holland, A.J. and Collins, S. (1995) Offending by adults with learning disabilities and the attitudes of staff to offending behaviour: implications for service development, *Journal of Intellectual Disability Research* **39**(6): 501–8.

MacKenzie, J. and Morgan-Clark, C. (2000) Measuring progress and improving quality, in C. Kaye and T. Lingial (eds) *Race, Culture and Ethnicity in Secure Psychiatric Practice: Working with Difference*. London: Jessica Kingsley, pp. 94–203.

McCann, G. (1999) Care of mentally disordered offenders, *Mental Health and Learning Disabilities Care* **3**(2): 65–7.

McClelland, N. (1995) The assessment of dangerousness: a procedure for predicting potentially dangerous behaviour, *Psychiatric Care* **2**: 17–19.

McCourt, M. (1999) Five concepts for the expanded role of the forensic mental health nurse, in P. Tarbuck, B. Topping-Morris and P. Burnard (eds) *Forensic Mental Health Nursing: Strategy and Implementation*. London: Whurr.

McKittrick, N. and Eysenck, S. (1984) Diversion: a big fix?, *Justice of the Peace*, 16 June, pp. 377–9, 393–4.

McMurran, M. (2002a) *Dual Diagnosis of Mental Disorder and Substance Misuse*. Liverpool: NHS National Programme on Forensic Mental Health Research and Development.

McMurran, M. (2002b) *Personality Disorder*. Liverpool: NHS National Programme on Forensic Mental Health Research and Development.

Mason, D. and Mercer, D. (1999) *A Sociology of the Mentally Disordered Offender*. London: Longman.

Melia, P. and Moran, T. (2000) Triumvirate nursing – a secure system for the delivery of nursing care, in T. Thompson and P. Mathias (eds) *Lyttle's Mental Health and Disorder* (3rd edn) chapter 22. Edinburgh: Bailliere Tindall.

Monahan, J. and Steadman, H.J. (eds) (1994) *Violence and Mental Disorder: Developments in Risk Assessment*. Chicago, IL: University of Chicago Press.

Mullen, P.E. (2000) Forensic mental health, *British Journal of Psychiatry* **176**: 307–11.

NACRO (1993) Community Care and Mentally Disturbed Offenders: Policy paper 1. London: NACRO.

Ndegwa, D. (2002) *Social Division and Difference: Black and Ethnic Minorities*. Liverpool: NHS National Programme on Forensic Mental Health Research and Development.

Parry-Cooke, G., Oliver, C. and Newton, J. (2000) *Good Girls: Surviving the Secure System*. London: University of North London/WISH.

Perkins, D. (1991) Clinical work with sex offenders in secure settings, in C.R. Hollin and K. Howells (eds) *Clinical Approaches to Sex Offenders and Their Victims*. Chichester: Wiley.

Peternelj-Taylor, C. (2000) The role of the forensic nurse in Canada, in D. Robinson and A. Kettles (eds) *Forensic Nursing and Multi-disciplinary Care of the Mentally Disordered Offender*. London: Jessica Kingsley.

Prins, H. (1992) The diversion of the mentally disordered: some problems for criminal justice, penology and health care, *Journal of Forensic Psychiatry* **3**(3): 431–43.

Prins, H. (1994) *Offenders, Deviants or Patients?* London: Routledge.

Pollock, N. and Webster, C. (1990) The clinical assessment of dangerousness, in R. Bluglass and P. Bowden (eds) *Principles and Practice of Forensic Psychiatry*. Edinburgh: Churchill Livingstone.

Rask, M. and Levander, S. (2001) Interventions in the nurse–patient relationship in forensic psychiatric nursing care: a Swedish survey, *Journal of Psychiatric and Mental Health Nursing* **8**: 323–33.

Rask, M. and Rahm Hallberg, I. (2000) Forensic psychiatric nursing care – nurses' apprehension of their responsibility and work content: a Swedish survey, *Journal of Psychiatric and Mental Health Nursing* 7: 163–77.

Rix, K.B. (1994) A psychiatric study of adult arsonists. *Medicine, Science and the Law* **34**: 21–34.

Robertson, G. (1988) Arrest patterns among mentally disordered offenders, *British Journal of Psychiatry* **153**: 313–16.

Robertson, G., Dell, S., James, K. and Grounds, A. (1994) Psychotic men remanded in custody to Brixton Prison, *British Journal of Psychiatry* **164**: 55–61.

Scott, S. and Parry-Crooke, G. (2001) Gender difference matters. *Mental Health Today*, October: 18–21.

Shah, S. (1978) Dangerousness: a paradigm for exploring some issues in law and psychology, *American Psychologist* **33**: 224–38.

Shaw, J. (2002) *Prison Healthcare*. Liverpool: NHS National Programme on Forensic Mental Health Research and Development.

Singleton, N., Meltzer, H., Gatward, R., Coid, J. and Deasy, D. (1998) *Psychiatric Morbidity Among Prisoners in England and Wales*. London: The Stationery Office.

Smith, J. and Donovan, N. (1990) The prosecution of psychiatric inpatients, *Journal of Forensic Psychiatry* **1**: 379–83.

Swinton, J. (2000) Reclaiming the soul: a spiritual perspective on forensic nursing, in D. Robinson and A. Kettles (eds) *Forensic Nursing and Multi-disciplinary Care of the Mentally Disordered Offender*. London: Jessica Kingsley.

Swinton, J. and Boyd, J. (2000) Autonomy and personhood: the forensic nurse as moral agent, in D. Robinson and A. Kettles (eds) *Forensic Nursing and Multi-disciplinary Care of the Mentally Disordered Offender*. London: Jessica Kingsley.

Tarbuck, P. (1994) The therapeutic use of security: a model for forensic nursing, in T. Thompson and P. Mathias (eds) *Lyttle's Mental Health and Mental Disorder* (2nd edn). London: Churchill Livingstone.

Taylor, P. (2002) *Mental Illness and Serious Harm to Others*. Liverpool: NHS National Programme on Forensic Mental Health Research and Development.

Topping-Morris, B. (1992) A historical and personal view of forensic nursing services, in P. Morrison and P. Burnard (eds) *Aspects of Forensic Psychiatric Nursing*. Aldershot: Avesbury.

United Kingdom Central Council for Nursing Midwifery and Health Visiting and University of Central Lancashire (1999) *Nursing in Secure Environments*. London: UKCC.

Vinestock, M. (1996) Risk assessment: 'a word to the wise'?, *Advances in Psychiatric Treatment* **2**: 3–10.

Webster, C.D., Eaves, D., Douglas, K. and Wintrup, A. (1995) *The HCR-20 Scheme: The Assessment of Dangerousness and Risk, Version 1*. Simon Fraser University and Forensic Psychiatric Services Commission of British Columbia.

Wessely, S.C., Castle, D. and Douglas, A.J. (1994) The criminal careers of incident cases of schizophrenia, *Psychological Medicine* **24**: 483–502.

Williams, P. and Dale, C. (2001) The application of values in working with patients in forensic mental health settings, in C. Dale, T. Thompson and P. Woods (eds) *Forensic Mental Health: Issues in Practice*. London: Harcourt Publishers Ltd, chapter 13.

Women in Special Hospitals (1997) *Annual Report 1996–1997*. London: Wish.

Woods, P. and Richards, D. (2002) *The Effectiveness of Nursing Interventions with Personality Disorders: A Systematic Review of the Literature*. Available from http://www.fnrh.freeserve.co.uk/pdsysreview.html.

21

The person with a personality disorder

Simon Houghton and Leah Ousley

Chapter overview

The concept of personality disorder is both complex and controversial. There is no consensus regarding their mere existence let alone the diagnosis of specific types and subsequent treatment approaches. There continues to be an ongoing debate regarding the amenability of personality disorders to both psychological and pharmacological interventions that is reflected in the ambiguity of the legal status of such a diagnosis. What little is agreed in the field of personality disorders is the difficulty in engaging this group of people within mainstream mental health services and the complexity of delivering meaningful care. Such service delivery is complicated further by the lay understanding of the notion of the 'psychopath'. This chapter will disentangle many of these concepts and provide the reader with a clearer understanding of the issues involved in nursing the person with a personality disorder.

This chapter covers:

- the concept of personality disorder;
- the legal status of personality disorder;
- the diagnosis and classification of specific personality disorders;
- the epidemiology of personality disorders;
- assessment models and methods;
- treatment approaches and their relative effectiveness;
- principles of nursing care;
- an outline of the concept of psychopathy.

Introduction

Personality disorders are common and invariably disabling conditions. However, many people with personality disorder function very well with little distress. Unfortunately, there are others who, because of the severity of the disorder, suffer significant levels of distress, and can place a heavy burden on those who provide care for them. As is the case for all mental disorders, the vast majority of care for the person with a personality disorder is delivered in primary care. For those individuals with the most significant levels of distress or difficulty there may be a need for specialist secondary or tertiary services. At present there are very few specific services for people with a personality disorder. As such their care will often be delivered through general adult mental health services. This may lead to particular difficulties that will be explored more fully within this chapter.

The concept of personality disorder

The concept of the personality goes directly to essence of what we are as human beings. Questions such as, Who we are? How well we know ourselves? or, How well do others know us? are commonly asked but prove difficult to answer. Personality then is what makes us who we are, and makes us different from other people. In the clinical world of abnormal psychology it is common to meet people who have become depressed, are experiencing unusual sensory phenomena, or have experienced great trauma at some time. Despite these difficulties all these people have a personality.

What then forms a disordered personality? In order to answer this we must first agree on what constitutes a personality. Millon and Davis (2000) describe it as 'a complex pattern of deeply embedded characteristics that are expressed automatically in almost every area of psychological functioning'. Although there is no universally accepted view of the personality, a common approach to the study of personality and personality disorder is the trait approach. This approach attempts to explain the whole sphere of human behaviour and subjective experience in terms of a small number of constructs. Among trait theorists the current leading model is known as the 'Five Factor Model' (Millon and Davis 2000). The five factors described being openness, conscientiousness, extroversion, agreeableness and neuroticism. It is proposed within this model that these five dimensions alone can describe all human personalities. However, descriptions of abnormal personality in terms of these factors may have limited clinical relevance and as such so-called lower-order traits, sub-divisions of the five factors, have been identified that may be more representative of the scope of human personality (see Box 21.1, Livesley 1998).

Box 21.1 Sixteen lower-order traits

Affective lability	Anxiousness	Callousness
Cognitive dysregulation	Compulsivity	Conduct problems
Insecure attachment	Intimacy avoidance	Narcissism
Oppositionality	Rejection	Restricted expression
Social avoidance	Stimulus-seeking	Submissiveness
Suspiciousness		

(After Livesley 1998)

Definitions of personality disorder

Personality disorder is a clinical construct used to describe various clusters of human behaviour and experience that are generally regarded as functionally impaired or psychologically distressing, and that arise from inflexible and maladaptive personality traits. It should be noted that personality disorders are descriptions of a narrow section of generally recognizable personalities that are of interest to clinicians. As such they do not describe personality in general.

Psychopathy

As will be highlighted the concept of 'psychopathy' is currently confused. In England and Wales psychopathic disorder is a legal classification of mental disorder within the Mental Health Act (1983). Currently, however, psychopathy, or psychopathic (personality) disorder is not classified within either major diagnostic system, DSM-IV or ICD-10, as a mental disorder. The legal position of psychopathic disorder, its assessment, identification and treatment is discussed later in this chapter.

Legal status of personality disorder

Within England and Wales there has been a legal classification of 'psychopathic disorder' since the Mental Health Act (1959) was passed into law (Jones 2003) (cf. Chapter 6). This included the concept of the compulsory admission of people deemed to have 'persistent disorders of mind which resulted in abnormally aggressive or seriously irresponsible conduct on the part of the patient, and require or are susceptible to treatment'. This legal definition was simplified although made no less ambiguous with the introduction of the Mental Health Act (1983). This defines psychopathic disorder as 'a persistent disorder or disability, which results in abnormally aggressive or seriously irresponsible conduct on the part of the person concerned'.

This new legal definition appears to remove the caveat that the disorder require or be susceptible to treatment. However, the definition of psychopathic disorder is only applicable to detention under sections 3, 37 and 47. Each of these sections of the Mental Health Act (1983) deem that a patient be detained due to them suffering with a psychopathic disorder, cannot be compulsorily admitted unless it can be shown that their treatment 'is likely to alleviate or prevent a deterioration in their condition' (Jones 2003). However, the legal meaning of psychopathic disorder is not universally agreed. It was concluded by the Report of the Department of Health and Home Office Working Group on Psychopathic Disorder (1994) that, 'It is generally accepted that the term psychopathic disorder does not represent a single clinical disorder but is a legal category describing a number of severe personality disorders, which contribute to the person committing anti-social acts, usually of a recurrent or episodic type.' There is no legal classification of psychopathic disorder (or personality disorder) in Scotland (Mental Health (Scotland) Act 1984) or Northern Ireland (Mental Health (Northern Ireland) Order 1986).

Dangerous and severe personality disorder

Proposed new legislation for England and Wales has identified a category of personality disorder described as dangerous and severe personality disorder (DSPD). Issues surrounding the development and implementation of this legislation are discussed further in Chapter 20.

Diagnosis and classification of personality disorders

Currently personality disorders are diagnosed by the recognition of a set of diagnostic criteria. Within both DSM-IV (APA 2000) and ICD-10 (WHO 1992) personality disorders are described as a mixture of both psychological traits and overt behaviours. Each diagnostic system describes the concept of personality disorder upon which subsequent specific diagnoses should be based. DSM-IV describes a personality disorder as 'an enduring pattern of inner experience and behaviour that deviates markedly from the expectations of the individual's culture, is pervasive and inflexible, has an onset in adolescence or early adulthood, is stable over time, and leads to distress or impairment'.

The specific personality disorders are then grouped into three clusters based on descriptive similarities. Cluster A disorders are described as 'odd or eccentric', Cluster B as 'dramatic, emotional, or erratic', and Cluster C as 'anxious or fearful'. However, this clustering system has been found to have limited validity, although has been useful in some research and educational situations (Tyrer 2000).

As can be seen in Table 21.1, ICD-10 and DSM-IV differ in their classification and description of specific personality disorders. Psychological

Table 21.1 DSM-IV and ICD-10 personality disorders

	DSM-IV	ICD-10
Cluster A	**Paranoid** Distrustful; suspicious	**Paranoid** Excessive sensitivity; suspicious
	Schizoid Indifferent to social relationships; emotionally detached	**Schizoid** Emotionally cold and detached
	Schizotypal Interpersonal and social deficits; odd beliefs and thinking	No equivalent
Cluster B	**Antisocial** Disregard for violation of rights of others	**Dissocial** Callous unconcern for others; aggression; irresponsibility; irritability
	Borderline Instability of relationships, self-image and mood; impulsivity	**Emotionally unstable** **(a) Borderline** Unclear self-image; intense, unstable relationships; impulsivity; self-harm **(b) Impulsive** Inability to control anger; quarrelsome; unpredictable mood
	Histrionic Excessive emotionality; attention-seeking; suggestibility; superficiality	**Histrionic** Self-dramatization; egocentric; manipulative behaviour
	Narcissistic Grandiose; lack of empathy; arrogance; need for admiration	No equivalent
Cluster C	**Avoidant** Fear of negative evaluation; socially inhibited; feelings of inadequacy; hypersensitivity	**Anxious** Tension; self-consciousness; hypersensitive; restricted lifestyle
	Dependent Persistent dependence; submissive	**Dependent** Subordinated personal needs; needs constant reassurance; fails to take responsibility for actions
	Obsessive-compulsive Perfectionist; inflexible	**Anankastic** Indecisiveness; doubt; cautious; pedantic; rigid

(After Tyrer 2000)

traits such as sensitivity and impulsivity mixed with descriptions of behaviour such as violence and self-harm, have led to discussions as to whether these diagnoses reflect true personality disorders or are actually descriptions of social deviance (Arntz 1999).

Each diagnostic system agrees that a diagnosis of personality disorder can only be made where the psychological traits and/or behaviours have been present since adolescence or early adulthood. Clearly then, a marked change in behaviour or personal characteristics, in response to a specific situational stressor cannot be included as evidence of the presence of a personality disorder. Similarly the behaviours and/or traits should permeate the whole of the person's experience; in other words, personality disorders cannot be active or inactive dependent on circumstances. Importantly, only when the identified traits and/or behaviours cause significant functional impairment or subjective distress can a diagnosis of personality disorder be made. The traits and behaviours displayed by a person with a diagnosis of personality disorder will commonly lead to difficulties in developing and maintaining close relationships or holding down regular employment.

For a firm diagnosis of personality disorder within ICD-10, the patient must fulfil a set of specified criteria. However, within the DSM-IV classification system a set of criteria are provided of which the person must meet a number, but not all, for a positive diagnosis to be made. As such the system of diagnosis as set out by DSM-IV can lead to a number different combinations of traits and behaviours resulting in the same diagnosis. For example, it has been calculated that there are 848 different combinations of criteria that can construct a diagnosis of anti-social personality disorder, and 247 combinations to meet criteria for borderline personality disorder (Arntz 1999).

Epidemiology

Epidemiology has been defined as 'the study of the health of human populations', the functions of which are to discover the factors affecting health, to determine the causes of ill health, to identify populations at risk of ill health, and to evaluate the effectiveness of health programmes (Terris 1992).

Prevalence of personality disorders

Measuring the prevalence of personality disorders is difficult. There is no consensus on the definition, diagnosis or classification of the specific disorders. There is also much debate on operational definitions of psychological traits inherent in personality disorder, but little agreement. As such varied estimates of the prevalence are published due to the variation in definition applied, and measurement tool implemented. Coid (2003) collated much of the most recent data obtained in community surveys (see Table 21.2). The figures cited represent the results of surveys using interviews with participants.

There is broad agreement that the prevalence of personality disorders increases dramatically among psychiatric hospital populations, with estimates ranging between 36 per cent and 67 per cent of inpatients suffering a personality disorder (NIMHE 2003). Similarly, personality disorders are more common in offender populations. Estimates for remanded male

Table 21.2 Prevalence of personality disorder in community surveys

Personality disorder	% of population
Anti-social	0.6–3.0
Borderline	0.7–2.0
Narcissistic	0.4–0.8
Histrionic	2.1
Paranoid	0.7–2.4
Schizoid	0.4–1.7
Schizotypal	0.1–5.6
Avoidant	0.8–5.0
Dependent	1.0–1.7
Compulsive	1.7–2.2
Any	4.4–13.0

(After Coid 2003)

prisoners are around 78 per cent, for sentenced male prisoners that falls to 64 per cent; and 50 per cent of all female prisoners are thought to have a recognizable personality disorder (Singleton *et al.* 1998).

Course of personality disorders

By definition a personality disorder is stable over time (APA 2000). As such once the features of a personality disorder have become recognized during adolescence or early adulthood it can be expected that the observed pattern of thinking, behaving and feeling will be relatively stable and unchanging. However, it has been found that particularly anti-social and borderline personality disorders can become less recognizable with age (Coid 2003). Typically the traits and behaviours associated with anti-social personality disorder reduce in severity by middle age, with only 20 per cent still diagnosable by 45 years of age (Coid 2003). Similarly patients with borderline personality disorders have been found to exhibit the most severe symptoms in their mid-20s followed by improvement in their late-30s. Indeed, Paris (1988) reported that 15 years post-diagnosis most patients no longer meet criteria for borderline personality disorder. However, other personality disorders may become more rigid over the patient's lifetime, such as obsessive-compulsive and schizotypal (APA 2000).

Co-morbidity of personality disorders

The co-morbidity of mental illness with personality disorder is a controversial topic, made difficult by disagreement over diagnosis and the fundamentals of personality structure. However, there would appear to be four possible points of view:

1   Personality disorder and mental illness cannot exist simultaneously. This position perhaps provides the weakest argument, with little empirical

evidence. However, the process of medical diagnosis perhaps implies that each is mutually exclusive.

2   All mentally ill people have a personality disorder. This may have some validity, as there is increasing evidence that those people with a mental illness may have a biological vulnerability, which may include some personal characteristics. However, the evidence for this position seems to suggest that those personality differences are not of a severity to enable a diagnosis of personality disorder.

3   Some personality disordered people will develop mental illness but that each can occur separately. This view is the one implied by the DSM classification system whereby both clinical mental disorder and personality disorder can be diagnosed on different axes. Current research evidence would suggest that there is significant co-morbidity between personality disorder and mental illness but that there is not an absolute or predictable link (Dowson and Grounds 1995).

4   Personality disorder is a chronic neurotic disorder. This view observes that many features of personality disorders are similar to those observed in non-psychotic mental illness such as anxiety and mood disorders. It is argued that they are merely present for the person's life from an earlier onset than those other neurotic disorders seen later in life (Murray *et al.* 1997).

Assessment of personality disorders

Chapter 7 of this book discusses client assessment in detail. Below we comment on specific aspects of assessment that are most relevant to the person with suspected personality disorder.

The methods with which health care professionals assess an individual for personality traits and disorders encompass a wide range of techniques, which invariably reflect professional background and agenda. Ideally, the assessment would bring together evidence from all disciplines, using interview, structured assessment tools, observation and third-party information to corroborate facts and findings. There are pitfalls associated with an over-reliance on mentally thumbing through the criteria of diagnostic tools such as DSM-IV (APA 2000) or ICD-10 (WHO 1992) following a non-specific interview or basic assessment, similarly through a reliance on self report.

Self-report measures

Self-report measures that look to measure personality correlate with mood state and irrelevant things, which leads to questions as to how reliable or valid self-report measures are. Self report as a stand-alone assessment can miss subtleties, particularly in measuring criminality (see Table 21.3). Such tests may be further affected by a general lack of insight and deceit.

Table 21.3 Types of assessment and predictive reliability by assessment method

	Diagnostic (PCL-R, PCL-SV)	Self report (MCMI-III, MMPI-2)
Content	+++	–/+
Stability	++	+
Lying	+++	–/+
Crime	++	+

(After Hart 2001)

Despite many self-report measures being developed only three have an adequate body of psychometric data (Lilienfield *et al.* 1997). One such tool is the MCMI-III (Millon 1994). Fortified and refined to align itself with the framework of the DSM-IV, the MCMI-III is a 175-item clinical assessment tool with profiles based on 24 clinical scales, designed only for the purpose of diagnostic screening and clinical assessment for adults who have eighth-grade reading abilities. Despite the well reported validity and reliability of self-report measures such as the MCMI-III in diagnosing traits and disorders of personality (Lilienfield *et al.* 1997), the differences in the constructs of psychopathy and anti-social personality disorder as defined within DSM-IV results in their use not being recommended in the assessment of psychopathy.

Observation

Observation is an under-utilized assessment method that can be highly effective in identifying both personality traits and coping styles. It may be controlled or uncontrolled depending largely on whether they are pre-arranged or unplanned observations of ongoing behaviours. Similarly, these may be recorded freehand or through using a structured response sheet to monitor what is seen and heard.

Self observation, that is the maintaining of thought or behaviour diaries, can offer a useful insight into the individual's perception of themselves. As with self-report measures of any kind, important cognitions can be shrouded in what the individual may think we want to hear. This is in itself an important tool and can give the assessor a valuable insight in to how the person views themselves, others and the world around them. Aiken (1996) suggests that in order to be truly valid, observations should be objective and unobtrusive, which may be difficult to achieve when working within the psychiatric setting where patients are aware that they are being observed. There are further difficulties in attempting to be objective while the majority of the professional's time is taken up in getting to know the individual. It is questionable how objective the nurse can be with regard to observation while he or she is within a therapeutic relationship with the individual. Observation is not merely a tool for watching but a valuable tool for engagement.

Whether the observations are formal or informal they offer the clinician a way in, and the individual a chance to understand and participate fully in their care.

Interview

Personality assessment via interview is perhaps the most popular method of choice by clinicians. It may provide the interviewer with a rich source of information, such as,

- the nature of the individual's problems (including duration, severity and manifestation);
- the coping ability of the individual, triggers, and protective factors;
- what has worked in the past, and what strategies may be useful for the future (Aiken 1996).

The assessor must guard against using the assessment interview as an 'easy way out'. That is, a quick interview in the comfort of an office is no substitute for a comprehensive assessment covering all fields in order to back up, quantify and indeed qualify information gathered and received.

The interviewer should be friendly but neutral, avoid prying yet show interest. The interview should demonstrate that its sole purpose is to understand not only the difficulties experienced but also the individual themselves. It should, therefore, reflect their perspective, countered against observations, written reports and self-report tests. The style of interview should be somewhat directive, using a high proportion of open questions and reflection. The extract from an assessment interview in Box 21.2 illustrates these points.

Box 21.2 Extract from an assessment interview

Nurse: Would you tell me about your relationship with your girlfriend?

Patient: What for?

Nurse: At the moment I am carrying out an assessment. It is important for me to get a picture of the whole of you and your circumstances in order to know how we might help you with the difficulties you spoke about earlier.

Patient: But my girlfriend hasn't got anything to do with my problems.

Nurse: That may be so, but it may be that at some point she could help with some of the therapy we might move onto.

Patient: How do you mean?

Nurse: Well it may be that the difficulties with your temper that you talked about occur mainly in certain situations and it may be useful to practise different behaviours in some of those situations. Your girlfriend might be able to support you in doing that, making it a little less daunting.

Misuse and unauthorized use of tests

The use of tools such as the MCMI-III (Millon 1994) or the PCL-R (Hare 1991) should not be taken lightly. Those who use or supervise the use of the MCMI-III should have a sufficient background in test logic, theory of clinical practice and psychometric methods (Skinner and Pakula 1986).

According to Hare, 'the potential for harm is considerable if the PCL-R is used incorrectly or if the user is not familiar with the clinical and empirical literature pertaining to psychopathy' (1991: 5).

Principles of assessment

It is important that the assessor look at interpersonal style, affect and behavioural facets using a multitude of assessment methods, and over time. No diagnostic procedure, regardless of type should be measured against a standard of absolute accuracy (Millon and Davis 2000) due to the errors within all.

Absolute labels of personality disorder, including psychopathy, are not always entirely useful. They can act as a barrier for therapeutic approaches under a banner of 'nothing works'. It is, however, clinically relevant and beneficial to identify particular traits and personality difficulties that may hinder treatment approaches. This in turn will enable both the individual patient and professional to navigate an effective route for functioning to an optimum degree within society.

Treatment of personality disorders

This section outlines the main treatment approaches adopted when working with people with personality disorders and discusses their relative efficacy.

Behavioural and cognitive approaches

There is evidence that behavioural and cognitive approaches (discussed also in Chapters 24 and 25) can be effective in the treatment of people with personality disorders. The main approaches evaluated include schema-focused therapy (Young 1994), dialectical behaviour therapy (Linehan *et al.* 1991; Verheul *et al.* 2003) and long-term cognitive behavioural therapy (Bateman and Fonagy 2000).

Schema-focused therapy

Schema-focused therapy is an approach developed as a result of observations of the difficulties encountered when applying a traditional cognitive therapy model to patients with personality disorder. These difficulties included the diffuse presentation of patients with personality disorders, the high prevalence of interpersonal problems, an overly rigid style of thinking and behaviour, and a resulting avoidant pattern of coping with new situations. Young (1994) hypothesized that a wider conceptual approach was needed to engage these people that makes sense of the whole of the personality disordered patients difficulties. As such he developed a therapy that incorporates traditional cognitive therapy techniques but marries these with interpersonal and experiential interventions, using the concept of schema as the unifying element. Schema have been described as 'the basic rules that people live by' (Freeman and Leaf 1989), and are thought to develop out of early life experience. Young (1994) proposed a subset of schema that he termed Early Maladaptive Schema, and that these serve as templates for processing and defining later behaviour. The aim of schema-focused therapy, then, is to help the patient challenge these early maladaptive schemas through a range of behavioural experiments, cognitive restructuring and interpersonal techniques within the therapeutic relationship. As yet there is only weak evidence of the validity of Young's (1994) concept of early maladaptive schema and no strong evidence of the effectiveness of the schema-focused approach (Leichsenring and Leibing 2003).

Dialectical behaviour therapy

Dialectical behaviour therapy is a long-term, cognitive behavioural therapy package of interventions evaluated as having some effectiveness in the treatment of patients with a borderline personality disorder (Linehan *et al.* 1991). This form of therapy derives from the hypothesis that the core difficulty encountered by patients with a borderline personality disorder is an inability to self-regulate emotional arousal. This, it is suggested, is the factor that leads to the cluster of behaviours that have collectively become recognized as borderline personality disorder. This treatment approach generally lasts a minimum of 12 months and would contain individual cognitive behavioural psychotherapy focusing mainly on motivational issues, including the motivation to stay alive and remain in treatment. This therapy is conducted alongside skills training groups with the goal of teaching self-regulation of emotional states through the practising of new skills. The therapists delivering this treatment package are recommended to receive intensive clinical supervision and frequent consultation with each other.

Until recently the evidence for the effectiveness of dialectical behaviour therapy was seen as promising but largely weak due to small sample sizes, and the fact that the majority of trials had been conducted by the therapy's originator. However, a Dutch study has recently published the results of a large randomized controlled trial comparing dialectical behaviour therapy and treatment as usual for patients with borderline personality disorders (Verheul *et al.* 2003). The results of this study demonstrated that dialectical behaviour therapy led to statistically and clinically significant reductions in self-mutilating behaviours and self-damaging impulsive acts. These differences could not be attributed to any differences between the treatment groups.

Cognitive-behaviour therapy

Cognitive-behavioural therapy protocols for people with personality disorder have generally agreed on the need to modify standard therapy approaches with an emphasis on a greater degree of individualized case formulation to guide and inform subsequent intervention design. To this end it is recommended that the therapist be more active than may be traditionally expected, and that the therapist should expect to tolerate a greater degree of negative transference. It is generally recommended that the therapy be longer term, with 12–20 months (or more) of treatment not uncommonly recommended (Freeman and Jackson 1998). This long-term traditional approach to the treatment of personality disorder has yielded some promising early results in studies of effectiveness (Bateman and Tyrer 2003), but as yet these studies are statistically underpowered and as such have limited generalizability.

Psychodynamic approaches

The psychodynamic view of personality disorders is based on a developmental model of personality with the aim of helping the patient understand how the past influences the present with the use of interpretation. Treatment will generally be long term focusing on the therapeutic relationship between the patient and therapist, emotional experience and defence mechanisms. The therapist will use the relationship developed between therapist and patient, known as transference, as the means of understanding how the patient relates to other people.

The evidence for the effectiveness of psychodynamic approaches to personality disorder is scarce. The few randomized studies that exist suggest that this approach may be helpful to patients with borderline personality disorder (Bateman and Fonagy 2001), and that a brief psychodynamic therapy may be more effective than a waiting list control (Winston *et al.* 1994).

Pharmacological approaches

Anti-psychotic, anti-depressant and mood stabilizing drugs have all been used in the treatment of personality disorders. It appears that some atypical anti-psychotic drugs can reduce symptoms such as depression, interpersonal sensitivity, anger and paranoia in patients with borderline personality disorder (Zanarini and Frankenberg 2001). However, this study was relatively small (n = 28) and so should be regarded as preliminary evidence only.

Anti-depressants have also been recommended in the treatment of borderline personality disorder, being found to reduce impulsiveness, anger and depression (Coccaro and Kavoussi 1997). Mood stabilizers such as lithium and carbamazepine have been used in the treatment of mood disturbance for patients with personality disorder. However, there is little evidence that they offer any further benefits to these patients (Bateman and Tyrer 2003).

Principles of nursing care

There are a number of practical principles that should be considered when nursing patients with personality disorders. Issues such as the development of an appropriate therapeutic relationship, team working, supervision and support, are perhaps even more important when working with personality disordered patients, than with other patient groups.

Therapeutic relationships and engagement

The development of a therapeutic relationship is of crucial importance in the delivery of effective health care interventions to mentally disordered people. This is perhaps even more crucial when that person has a personality disorder. The centrality of an appropriate therapeutic relationship is emphasized by all three major psychological approaches to therapy. The humanistic school would propose that a therapeutic relationship is necessary and indeed sufficient in the delivery of a therapy that enables personality change (Rogers 1957). The psychodynamic therapist would encourage the development of a therapeutic relationship as a vehicle by which the patient can explore their past and current relationships with others. This knowledge, derived from the workings of the therapeutic relationship, would in turn generate insights that allow the person to change. Finally, the learning theorists have more recently come to understand that cognitive and behavioural therapies can be made more effective when delivered in the context of a strong therapeutic relationship (Schaap *et al.* 1993).

Rogers (1957) emphasized what he termed core conditions in the development of a therapeutic relationship, those being warmth, empathy and genuineness. The application of these skills led to the therapist having unconditional positive regard for the patient and so enabling the exploration of internal issues that would lead to a realization and change. While not all schools of psychological therapy agree with the mechanism of change proposed by Rogers (1957), it has become widely accepted that he identified the key ingredients to developing therapeutic relationships with people.

There are particular issues when developing therapeutic relationships with personality disordered patients. These are largely dependent on the observed behaviours within that individual that have attracted the diagnosis of personality disorder. Specific examples are shown in Table 21.4.

As such it is important that these deficits within the personality-disordered patient are recognized and do not prevent the development of a potentially otherwise helpful relationship. The nurse charged with engaging a personality-disordered patient in their care and treatment (cf. Chapter 22 of this book) may need to accept certain behaviours within that relationship that might cause concern or be considered unusual in relationships with non-personality disordered patients. For example, a patient with a borderline personality disorder may split the nursing team into those staff that are definitely OK and those that are definitely not, resulting in behaviours such as over-dependence or overt hostility. In normal circumstances the

Table 21.4 Behaviours inherent in specific personality disorders that may inhibit the development of therapeutic relationships

Personality disorder	Associated behaviours
Paranoid	Suspiciousness
Schizoid	Indifference
Schizotypal	Poor social skills
Anti-social	Disregard for others
Borderline	Unstable relationship building
Histrionic	Attention seeking
Narcissistic	Lack of empathy
Avoidant	Socially inhibited
Dependent	Reassurance seeking
Obsessive compulsive	Indecisiveness

Box 21.3 Development of a therapeutic relationship with a patient with a borderline personality disorder

Background Tina is a 26-year-old woman with a diagnosis of borderline personality disorder. She was admitted to a regional secure unit six months ago under Section 37 of the Mental Health Act (1983), following a conviction for arson with intent to cause harm. Tina has a history of self-harming behaviours since the age of 12 when she took an overdose of her mother's anti-depressants. On that occasion her next-door neighbour took her to hospital, after Tina told her what had happened. Since this time Tina has taken many further overdoses, cut her arms, stomach and legs repeatedly, and has burned her arms with cigarettes and lighters. Tina has had many short-term sexual relationships but relates that she felt a great deal for each of her previous partners. She is in regular contact with her mother who continues to have mental health problems. Tina was first in trouble with the police when she was 11-years-old following her stealing from local shops. Since this time she has had many convictions for minor offences but has never been previously incarcerated.

   In hospital Tina was allocated Sheila as her named nurse. Sheila is a charge nurse on the admissions ward with many years' experience of nursing acutely mentally ill people. Tina quickly warmed to Sheila stating that she found talking with her 'comforting'. During the first three months of Tina's admission she found it increasingly difficult to maintain control over her impulses to self-harm and in fact was burning herself on an almost daily basis. During this time Sheila found she was spending increasing amounts of time with Tina offering support, reassurance and distraction from thoughts of self-harm. Gradually, it was observed that Tina reduced the frequency of self-harming behaviour, particularly when Sheila was on duty. Tina felt less able to control her impulsive behaviour at other times, reporting that she did not feel she could approach other staff as she could Sheila.

team may wish to try to modify these behaviours but in this case it may be helpful to tolerate these extremes in order to maintain some engagement with at least a part of the nursing team.

Box 21.3 provides describes briefly the formation of a therapeutic relationship by a nurse with a patient with a borderline personality disorder.

Team working

While the nurse builds a therapeutic relationship with the patient it is crucial that the other members of the care team behave in a manner likely to help foster this relationship while maintaining the integrity of the individual nurse. As has previously been highlighted, the personality-disordered patient will typically find it difficult to build relationships, particularly more than one close rapport. The role of the team then becomes to reinforce and maintain the boundaries set by the nurse. Clinical experience suggests that this boundary setting is a therapeutic task that many teams find difficult to institute. However, such a consistent approach is crucial if the personality-disordered patient is to receive consistent reinforcement of appropriate behaviours. Where these boundaries are not maintained consistently the patient is unlikely to learn the desired socially acceptable behaviours that the team aim to encourage.

Supervision and support

It is recommended that nurses working with people with personality disorder have frequent individual clinical supervision. The development of therapeutic relationships with such patients will be difficult and cause the nurse much anxiety. Supervision allows the nurse to explore and problem-solve these aspects of the care they are delivering. In order that the supervision is helpful to the nurse it should focus on monitoring the maturity of the therapeutic relationship. The supervisor should seek information from other members of the team on their observations of the relationship and this should be fed back to the nurse. An over-reliance on the nurse's own account of the relationship could allow them to ignore difficulties that are emerging but are not yet clear to the nurse. Changing the terms of such a relationship can then be achieved in small increments with a minimum of distress to the patient. If these difficulties go unnoticed then it is likely that changes in the relationship will be more difficult for the patient to assimilate.

The whole care team should meet regularly to discuss the wider approach to the person with a personality disorder. Again this will limit the distress to the patient and allow the maintenance of relationships through periods of change. Issues that the team should particularly attend to include boundaries and the implementation of consistent treatment approaches.

Psychopathy: a special case

The much bandied-around, indeed, maligned label of psychopathy has little to do with real individuals with such a complex disorder of personality. It is usually that which accompanies individuals with challenging behaviours and reflects not a state of psychopathy but a felt sense of professional inadequacy in caring for those who refute help offered and take far more than they give.

The emergence of psychopathy as a clinical construct over the last century belies its early existence. Indeed, individuals through the ages have demonstrated evidence of this devastating disorder (McCord and McCord 1964; Cleckley 1976; Millon 1981), defined by Pinel (1801) as insanity without delirium, a status which he regarded as morally neutral. Prichard (1837) on the other hand defined the construct as moral insanity, 'a madness consisting of morbid perversion of natural feeling, affection, inclinations, temper, habits, moral dispositions and natural impulses . . . without insane illusion or hallucination'. The debate as to whether the psychopath is mad or bad, or simply diabolical has continued across the generations. Indeed there are those that simply deny its existence, which is at best unhelpful.

Within modern mental health care we have the benefit of the research by those such as Hare (1998, 1999) not only in shedding light on the existence of the clinical construct of psychopathy but allowing the operationalization of the construct using psychometric procedures with established validity and reliability. He describes psychopathy as socially devastating, encompassed by a complex plethora of interpersonal, behavioural and affective characteristics. These are underpinned by a callousness and lack of empathy, together with a repetitive and all pervasive violation of expectations and social norms. Hare (1991) uses a factor model to distinguish between these aspects of psychopathy (see Table 21.5).

Research demonstrates that the key elements of psychopathy, including the broad content of personality style and criminal versatility, are stable over time and are associated with deceitfulness and criminality. Despite the correlation of crime and psychopathy, some psychopaths invariably manage to remain outside the criminal justice system, though those that deviate from society's rules run the gamut of possible offending (Hart and Hare 1997). However, it is the ease with which the psychopath engages in dispassionate violence that makes society reel.

The flippant use of the term psychopathy that trips off the tongues of not only the day's society but clinicians diagnosing the disorder treads a difficult path. The ease with which clinicians use DSM-IV criteria for anti-social personality disorder to apply a diagnosis of psychopathy is alarming and can only lead to unfortunate consequences. Psychopathy is not synonymous with, yet is often confused with the diagnostic category of anti-social personality disorder. This distinction is often lost on clinicians. The majority of individuals with anti-social personality disorder are not psychopaths. Those individuals diagnosed as psychopathic may well demonstrate

Table 21.5 Construct of psychopathy within its factor structure

Factor 1 – Interpersonal style	*Factor 2 – Behavioural style*	*Items which do not load to either factor*
Glibness/superficial charm	Need for stimulation/proneness to boredom	Promiscuous sexual behaviour
Grandiose sense of self-worth	Parasitic lifestyle	Many short-term marital relationships
Pathological lying	Poor behavioural controls	Criminal versatility
Conning/manipulative	Early behavioural problems	
Lack of remorse or guilt	Lack of realistic long-term goals	
Shallow affect	Impulsivity	
Callous/lack of empathy	Irresponsibility	
Failure to accept responsibility for ones own actions	Juvenile delinquency	
	Revocation on conditional elease	

(After Hare 1991)

all or some of the features of the anti-social, but are also likely to show evidence of criteria for narcissistic and/or histrionic personality disorder, earning their place as a special case (see Figure 21.1).

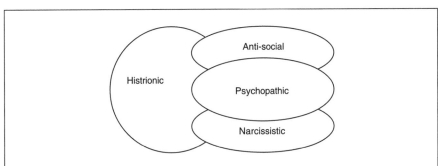

Figure 21.1 The relationship between psychopathy and other diagnosable personality disorders (after Hare 2002)

Conclusion

Working with people with a personality disorder is complex, challenging and anxiety provoking. The range of behaviours that the personality-disordered person demonstrates can in turn anger, frustrate and threaten those charged with caring for them. However, there is cause for optimism. Evidence suggests that the traits of personality disorders can change over time. The nurse can be central to this change process, engaging the patient in a therapeutic relationship that can be the conduit for further behavioural and interpersonal change. Through consistent reinforcement of behaviours, and ongoing assessment of outcome the nurse will be the change agent for the person with a personality disorder.

In summary the main points of this chapter are:

- The concept of personality disorder describes a complex variety of human behaviour and experience. These behaviours are regarded as functionally impaired or psychologically distressing.

- There is a legal classification of 'psychopathic disorder' describing a number of severe personality disorders that result in anti-social acts. This legal definition of psychopathy does not relate to what is clinically understood as psychopathy.

- There are two broadly similar classifications of personality disorders that identify specific types of disorders.

- Personality disorders are prevalent in society. They are generally recognized in adolescence or early adulthood, and the behaviours, thinking styles and feelings reported will be relatively stable over time.

- The use of a wide range of assessment methods is recommended. Interview, questionnaires, previous assessments, reports of friends and family are all vital in obtaining a clear and whole picture of the person with a personality disorder.

- There is evidence that the person with a personality disorder can change behaviours and thinking styles as a result of psychological interventions, most notably forms of cognitive and behavioural therapies.

- Principles of nursing people with personality disorders include the development of helpful therapeutic relationships, maintenance of agreed boundaries, and a consistent team approach. The nurse should receive frequent individual clinical supervision and the team should meet regularly to maintain its approach to the care.

- Psychopathy is a description of a complex and severe personality disorder not classified within the main index systems. It is highly correlated with criminality and as such more prevalent in secure settings. The care of the psychopath is extremely challenging and likely to be undertaken over a long period of time.

Questions for reflection and discussion

1. What is the legal status of personality disorders?
2. From Table 21.1, identify which characteristics of a personality disorder are psychological traits and which are behaviours.
3. How may the nurse referred to in Box 21.2 enhance the assessment of this patient's difficulties?
4. Discuss the potential benefits and pitfalls in the relationship between Tina and Sheila as described in Box 21.3.
5. Consider the treatment approaches you have witnessed being implemented with patients that have a personality disorder. Were they evidence based? Were they ethical? Were they effective?
6. Describe the core features of psychopathy, and distinguish these from the features of other types of personality disorder.

Annotated bibliography

- Tyrer, P. (2000) *Personality Disorders: Diagnosis, Management and Course* (2nd edn). Oxford: Butterworth Heinemann. A well-researched and thorough book that covers all aspects of personality disorder in great depth.
- Arntz, A. (1999) Do personality disorders exist? On the validity of the concept and its cognitive-behavioural formulation and treatment, *Behaviour Research and Therapy* **37**: S97–S134. An interesting and readable paper that challenges the reader to review his or her own thoughts on personality disorders. Theory and practice are well linked, particularly in relation to psychological approaches.
- Freeman, A. and Jackson, J.T. (1998) Cognitive behavioural treatment of personality disorders, in N. Tarrier, A. Wells and G. Haddock (eds) *Treating Complex Cases: The Cognitive Behavioural Approach*. Chichester: Wiley. Description of adaptations thought to enhance the therapeutic experience for people with personality disorders. Although written with therapy in mind, many of the recommendations apply equally well to the general philosophy of care required.
- Hare, R. (1993) *Without Conscience: The Disturbing World of the Psychopath Among Us*. London: Guilford Press. An engaging and illuminating book written for the interested lay reader.

References

Aiken L.R. (1996) *Rating Scales and Checklists: Evaluating Behaviour, Personality, and Attitudes*. Chichester: Wiley.

American Psychiatric Association (APA) (2000) *Diagnostic and Statistical Manual of Mental Disorders – Text Revision*, 4th edn (DSM-IV). Washington, DC: APA.

Arntz, A. (1999) Do personality disorders exist? On the validity of the concept and its cognitive-behavioural formulation and treatment, *Behaviour Research and Therapy* **37**: S97–S134.

Bateman, A.W. and Fonagy, P. (2000) Effectiveness of psychotherapeutic treatment of personality disorder, *British Journal of Psychiatry* **177**: 13–143.

Bateman, A. and Fonagy, P. (2001) Treatment of borderline personality disorder with psychoanalytically oriented partial hospitalisation: an 18-month follow-up, *American Journal of Psychiatry* **158**: 36–42.

Bateman, A.W. and Tyrer, P. (2003) *Effective Management of Personality Disorder*. London: Department of Health.

Cleckley, H. (1976) *The Mask of Sanity* (5th edn). St Louis, MD: Mosby.

Coccaro, E.F. and Kavoussi, R.J. (1997) Fluoxetine and impulsive aggressive behaviour in personality disordered patients, *Archives of General Psychiatry* **54**: 1081–8.

Coid, J. (2003) Epidemiology, public health and the problem of personality disorders. *British Journal of Psychiatry* **182** (suppl.44): s3–s10.

Department of Health and the Home Office (1994) *Report of the Department of Health and Home Office Working Group on Psychopathic Disorder*. London: HMSO.

Dowson, J.H. and Grounds, A.T. (1995) *Personality Disorders: Recognition and Clinical Management*. Cambridge: Cambridge University Press.

Freeman, A. and Jackson, J.T. (1998) Cognitive behavioural treatment of personality disorders, in N. Tarrier, A. Wells and G. Haddock (eds) *Treating Complex Cases: The Cognitive Behavioural Approach*. Chichester: Wiley.

Freeman, A. and Leaf, R.C. (1989) Cognitive therapy applied to personality disorders, in A. Freeman, K.M. Simon, L.E. Beutler and H. Arkowitz (eds) *Comprehensive Handbook of Cognitive Therapy*. New York: Plenum Press.

Hare, R.D. (1991) *Psychopathy Checklist – Revised (PCL-R) Manual*. New York: Multi-Health Systems.

Hare, R.D. (1998) Psychopaths and their nature. Implications for the mental health and criminal justice systems, in T. Millon, E. Simonsen, M. Birket-Smith and R.D. Davis (eds) *Psychopathy: Antisocial, Criminal and Violent Behaviour*. New York: Guilford Press.

Hare, R.D. (1999) Psychopathy as a risk factor for violence, *Psychiatric Quarterly* **70**: 181–97.

Hare, R.D. (2002) Psychopathy Checklist – Revised. Presentation at Lakeside Hotel, Cumbria, UK. September.

Hart, S. (2001) Psychopathy Checklist – Revised. Presentation at Rampton Hospital, Nottinghamshire, UK. 26–27 February.

Hart, S. and Hare, R.D. (1997) Psychopathy: Assessment and association with criminal conduct, in D.M. Stoff, J. Breiling and S.D. Maser (eds) *Handbook of Antisocial Behaviour*. Chichester: Wiley.

Jones, R. (2003) *Mental Health Act Manual* (8th edn). London: Sweet & Maxwell.

Leichsenring, F. and Leibing, E. (2003) The effectiveness of psychodynamic therapy and cognitive behaviour therapy in the treatment of personality disorders: a meta-analysis, *American Journal of Psychiatry* **160**: 1223–32.

Lilienfield, S.O., Purcell, C. and Jones-Alexander, J. (1997) Assessment and anti-social behaviour, in D.M. Stoff, J. Breiling and S.D. Maser (eds) *Handbook of Antisocial Behaviour*. Chichester: Wiley.

Linehan, M.M., Armstrong, H.E., Suarez, A., Allmon, D. and Heard, H. (1991) Cognitive behavioural treatment of chronically parasuicidal borderline patients, *Archives of General Psychiatry* **48**: 1060–4.

Livesley, W.J. (1998) Suggestions for a framework for an empirically based classification of personality disorder, *Canadian Journal of Psychiatry* **43**: 137–47.

McCord, W. and McCord, J. (1964) *The Psychopath: An Essay on the Criminal Mind.* New York: D. Van Nostrand.

Mental Health Act (1983) London: HMSO.

Mental Health (Scotland) Act (1984) London: HMSO.

Mental Health (Northern Ireland) Order (1986) London: HMSO.

Millon, T. (1981) *Disorders of Personality: DSM-III, Axis II.* New York: Wiley.

Millon, T. (1994) *MCMI-III Manual.* Minneapolis, MN: National Computer Systems.

Millon, T. and Davis, R. (2000) *Personality Disorders in Modern Life.* New York: Wiley.

Murray, R., Hill, P. and McGuffins P. (1997) *The Essentials of Postgraduate Psychiatry* (3rd edn). Cambridge: Cambridge University Press.

National Institute for Mental Health in England (NIMHE) (2003) *Personality Disorder: No Longer a Diagnosis of Exclusion.* London: NIMHE.

Paris, J. (1988) Follow-up studies of borderline personality disorder: a critical review, *Journal of Personality Disorders* **2**: 189–97.

Pinel, P. (1801), cited in R.D. Hare (1993) *Without Conscience: The Disturbing World of the Psychopath Among Us.* London: Guilford Press.

Pritchard, J.C. (1837) *A Treatise on Insanity and Other Diseases.* Philadelphia, PA: Harwell, Barrington & Harwell.

Rogers, C.R. (1957) The necessary and sufficient conditions of therapeutic personality change, *Journal of Consulting Psychology* **21**: 95–103.

Schaap, C.A.S., Bennun, I., Schindler, L. and Hoogduin, K. (1993) *The Therapeutic Relationship in Behavioural Psychotherapy.* Chichester: Wiley.

Singleton, N., Meltzer, H., Gatward, R., Coid, J. and Deasy, D. (1998) *Psychiatric Morbidity Among Prisoners.* London: Office of National Statistics.

Skinner, H.A. and Pakula, A. (1986) Challenge of computers in psychological assessment, *Professional Psychology: Research & Practice* **17**: 44–50.

Terris, M. (1992) The Society for Epidemiologic Research (SER) and the Future of Epidemiology, *American Journal of Epidemiology* **136**: 909–15.

Tyrer, P. (2000) *Personality Disorders: Diagnosis, Management and Course* (2nd edn). Oxford: Butterworth Heinemann.

Verheul, R., Van Den Bosch, L.M.C., Koeter, M.W.J. *et al.* (2003) Dialectical behaviour therapy for women with borderline personality disorder: 12-month, randomised clinical trial in The Netherlands, *British Journal of Psychiatry* **182**: 135–40.

Winston, A., Laikin, M., Pollack, J. *et al.* (1994) Short-term dynamic psychotherapy of personality disorders, *American Journal of Psychiatry* **15**: 190–4.

World Health Organization (WHO) (1992) *The ICD-10 Classification of Mental and Behavioural Disorders: Clinical Descriptions and Diagnostic Guidelines.* Geneva: WHO.

Young, J.E. (1994) *Cognitive Therapy for Personality Disorders: A Schema Focused Approach*. Sarasota, FL: Professional Resource Press.

Zanarini, M.C. and Frankenberg, F.R. (2001) Olanzapine treatment of female borderline personality disorder patients: a double blind, placebo-controlled pilot study, *Journal of Clinical Psychiatry* **62**(11): 849–54.

PART 4

Core procedures

22

Engaging clients in their care and treatment

Marc Thurgood

Chapter overview

This chapter defines engagement, outlines its importance for mental health - care and identifies the key principles of individual practice and service delivery that best promote it. Criticisms of mental health services that draw upon the experience of service users are described and argued to be the starting point from which services need to change. Barriers and solutions to engagement are expanded upon with reference to key marginalized groups and recommendations for practice illustrated by case-study examples. The issues raised here echo those raised in other chapters of this volume, in particular Chapters 5, 10 and 29.

Introduction

Over the past decade there has been an increasing policy emphasis upon mental health care for people with severe and enduring mental illness and promoting their 'engagement' with mental health services (DH 1999). This reflects a recognition that many people in this group have often been excluded from effective help and that their negative experience of the mental health system has left them feeling mistrustful and alienated, with some living in conditions of extreme poverty and neglect (Muijen 1996; SCMH 1998; Dean and Craig 1999; Craig and Timms 2000). The challenge facing mental health services as a whole, and nurses in particular, is to find ways to engage this hard-to-engage group of people.

This chapter focuses on this problem and how nurses might best work to engage their clients. It draws primarily upon literature on the assertive outreach model of community care, which has been defined as an approach that engages high-risk severe mentally ill clients with complex needs who are resistant to contacting services; proactively reaches out to clients in their own territory in the community; assesses need comprehensively, develops individually tailored care packages and effectively coordinates care across agencies; and optimises the rehabilitative potential of clients by delivering clinical interventions that enhance client functioning.

(Ryan 1999: 2)

The assertive outreach model highlights issues that are relevant to engaging service users in all treatment and care settings.

What is 'engagement'?

Engagement can be defined broadly as providing a service that is experienced by service users (including carers) as acceptable, accessible, positive and empowering. If clients perceive a mental health service in this way they are more likely to use it. Creating such a service has implications for both the quality of the relationships that service users have with their individual workers and also for the nature of the services of which these workers are a part.

At a personal level, each client has their own opinion of mental health services that are influenced by factors such as their past experience, ethnicity and culture, needs, difficulties, strengths and aspirations, and the sense that they make of their own experience of mental ill-health, and what helps. Establishing and maintaining relationships with clients that are experienced as helpful is fundamental to engagement. To do this requires nurses to learn about their clients' unique perspectives and to respect them as valid and meaningful. Respect for the client's viewpoint provides the basis for collaborative working and open negotiation around informed choices for care and treatment.

Service users value mental health nurses as a professional group (Rogers *et al.* 1993; Rogers and Pilgrim 1994) and nurses are well placed to improve mental health care practice by virtue of their relatively high contact with clients through their care coordination role and their traditional emphasis on forming long-term therapeutic relationships with clients (cf. Chapter 3). As 'natural allies' (Repper 2000: 585), nurses are able to develop a good understanding of their clients' wider lives and aspirations, and to gain insights into their problematic experiences of services and social deprivation (Campbell and Lindow 1997). These insights are the starting point for engagement.

At an organizational level the engagement agenda has contributed to the implementation of new approaches to service delivery that have taken into account service users' criticisms of traditional mental health services. Examples of these approaches include assertive outreach, home treatment and crisis services in the community, separate community services for black and ethnic minority service users and psychosocial interventions for psychosis (DH 1999, 2001). Service users have also created their own 'self-help' services (for example, Clubhouse, the Hearing Voices Network) and are increasingly involved in the design, delivery and appraisal of services. Mental health professionals are now required to share their power with users. Joint-working between statutory mental health, voluntary and social services sectors, particularly with regard to meeting social needs (such as supported housing), is also now recognized as being crucial for effective engagement. The notion of 'recovery' (that people with severe mental illness have the right to and are capable of leading rewarding lives through employment, education and leisure/social opportunities when given access, choice and support) (cf. Chapter 5) supports the development of partnerships between service users and mainstream organizations to promote greater social inclusion (see, for example, NIACE/NIMHE 2003).

If engagement is to be achieved, nurses need to demonstrate their commitment to these organizational and ideological changes. Critical appraisal of one's own work with clients and of the wider service within which individual nurses operate (for example, team and locality service) is essential. Challenging and changing practice in response to the needs and criticisms of service users and involving them in this process needs to be seen as a fundamental part of a service that engages effectively with its clients.

Why some clients don't engage with their care and treatment

Some clients do not engage with their care and treatment because:

- Clients vary in their willingness and ability to engage. Much depends on their previous experience, both of life and of services, and the extent to which their mental ill-health affects their capacity to cooperate with the help offered.
- Services themselves have created significant barriers to engagement in the way that they have been organized and delivered.
- Service users are not always given what they most want.

Service user related factors

Past experience

Many people with mental health problems mistrust statutory services and feel ambivalent or openly hostile towards them, for good reasons. The Sainsbury Centre's review of care for people with severe mental illness who are hard to engage with services (SCMH 1998) points out that many clients' contacts with mental health services may have been characterized by long periods of neglect while in the community and by traumatic experiences of hospitalization at times of crisis (often by detention under the Mental Health Act 1983) with subsequent poor continuity of community support on discharge. An overemphasis on physical treatments (often with bad side effects from medication) at the expense of psychosocial interventions and social support may be experienced by service users as dehumanizing and punitive. Discrimination and insensitivity from mental health service staff (on the grounds of gender, race, culture, sexuality and lifestyle – such as substance use and homelessness) has been a common complaint. Black and ethnic minority clients have been particularly alienated by discriminatory negative experiences, including being subject to more severe and coercive treatments, poorer access to 'talking treatments' and cultural and language barriers in assessments (see also SCMH 2000; DH 2003).

The social disadvantage often associated with mental illness may have also contributed to the traumatic histories of our clients and their experiences of other statutory services could have been as negative as their experience of mental health services. Childhood abuse, local authority care as a child or having their own child taken into care by social services, contact with the criminal justice system in their youth or during a mental health crisis, and difficult dealings with housing and benefits departments are commonplace findings of psychosocial assessments (SCMH 1998). Unstable or inadequate housing is also a common problem and many clients with a history of homelessness relate stories of losing their accommodation through eviction as a consequence of having received insufficient help for their mental health problems (Dean and Craig 1999).

The effects of mental illness

The difficulties associated with serious mental ill-health may also play a major part in an individual's capacity to engage with services. People who have psychotic experiences or significant psychological and emotional instability may find it extremely hard to form trusting and lasting relationships with others. For example, persecutory thinking and the hearing of threatening or derogatory voices can often lead to social withdrawal as a coping strategy and the refusal of even the most basic of survival needs, such as taking up state benefits. Delusional explanations for one's situation, particularly if these relate to services, can be a considerable barrier. Defensive aggression or other anti-social behaviours (for example, begging and petty crime as a survival strategy) can similarly serve to distance someone from help. Cognitive impairments such as difficulties with generating and ordering thoughts, concentration, memory and abstract problem solving will often impede someone's ability to effectively seek out assistance. The use of illicit substances and alcohol as a form of 'self-medication' for chronic distress (or 'symptoms') can serve to exacerbate these problems. Less obvious, but equally disabling, are the 'negative symptoms' of schizophrenia. Loss of volition, motivation and interest ('get-up-and-go') can result in the most extreme self-neglect, whereby the daily tasks of self-care that most of us take for granted can seem insurmountable.

Added to this, the long-term effects of social isolation and loneliness through the progressive loss of meaningful occupation, relationships and income, coupled with the stigmatizing status of being labelled as mentally ill can have a devastating effect on self-esteem and confidence. Many clients experience persecution, exploitation and rejection in their daily lives. This further compromises their ability to assertively communicate their needs and set goals for the future.

Service-related factors

The Sainsbury Centre (SCMH 1998) has identified the main service-related barriers to engagement as:

- difficulties around establishing lead responsibility for care coordination;
- fragmentation of services resulting in poor joint-working between agencies; and
- rigid, service-centred practice.

The complexity of need for many people with serious mental illness necessitates coordinated input from a range of agencies. The separation of physical health care, mental health care, substance misuse services, and housing and welfare support typify the traditional rigidity of service boundaries. This can lead to disputes about which agency should take lead responsibility for a client's care with the result that much needed help is denied. The tragic impact of this has been demonstrated by many inquiries into failures of community care (SCMH 1998).

Geographical catchment area boundaries across agencies can serve to exclude people from receiving services, particularly those with no permanent address. The 'no fixed abode' (NFA) hospital admission rota that often dictates which service will take on a homeless client in crisis is inherently discriminatory and commonly prevents continuity of contact with any one service (essential for long-term engagement). It has been argued that this 'lottery approach' to allocation of homeless people to services ignores the fact that many homeless people have a history of local connection to an area (Timms 1996).

Other service-centred approaches, such as formal appointment systems, do not always meet need and can be positively discouraging. It is unrealistic to always expect someone with a severe mental illness and overwhelming social problems to be sufficiently organized and motivated to attend appointments at a service base or to respond to letters. Non-attendance at appointments will often result in discharge particularly if demand on the service is high (Timms 1993). Some service users therefore tend to delay seeking help until a crisis occurs (via an A & E department, for example). The resulting interventions are too often brief and inadequate, which serves to further alienate the client (Craig and Timms 2000). It is important to note that excellent interventions with clients by individual professionals may often be rendered less effective, or ineffective, by the service framework within which they take place.

A diagnosis of 'personality disorder' (cf. Chapter 21) can lead people to be excluded from receiving help because the disorder is not perceived as a 'severe mental illness' or it may be seen as 'untreatable' and, therefore, beyond the remit of mental health services. Care is also often refused if this label is used in response to anti-social or criminal behaviours. At the same time, other services (such as social care agencies) can paradoxically also refuse help to this group of people on the grounds of a history of high contact with mental health services (SCMH 1998). Many people with a diagnosis of personality disorder are frequent users of mental health services, albeit on the margins, and may experience episodes of 'treatable' mental illness such as psychosis or depression. Mental health policy is now addressing these difficulties through recognition that adequate services need to be provided, some by mental health trusts, and by providing consultation guidelines for best practice and a commitment to funding specialist personality disorder services (NIMHE 2003) (cf. Chapter 4).

Division of responsibility between specialist substance misuse services and mental health teams has meant that clients have often fallen between services. Substance misuse can mean that engagement is even more difficult to achieve due to a worsening of symptoms, increased risk factors (aggression, violence, self-harm and self-neglect), loss of housing and chaotic use of crisis services. Conflicting approaches to the option of coercive treatment for mental illness and the need for motivated voluntary treatment for substance misuse makes this issue difficult to resolve – for example, how does one respond to the intoxicated person with psychosis (SCMH 1998)? Current mental health policy states that mental health services should expect substance misuse in clients with mental illness. The aim is for mental health services to deliver concurrent high quality care and treatment both for the underlying mental illness and the substance misuse via integration with specialists in substance misuse services and by the specialist training of workers within community mental health teams (DH 2002).

Services have often been required to provide managers with evidence of short-term outcomes via brief interventions and 'through-put' to demonstrate their effectiveness and thereby guarantee further funding. This emphasis on through-put data (for example, the numbers of referrals and discharges of clients travelling through a service on their way to a 'cure') has led to criticism of what has been argued to be an overly medical model (SCMH 1998) that is often inappropriate (Craig and Timms 2000). For people with disabling long-term mental illness, short-term improvement is often unrealistic and cure, in the medical sense, is unachievable. Emphasizing short-term outcomes may lead to mental health teams pushing for 'better' results by oppressively imposing interventions on their clients and denying them choice with resulting disengagement from the service. Sustained engagement needs to be an important criterion by which to judge the success of mental health services.

Services neglect what service users want

Repper's (2000) review of studies of service-user views alerts us to the fact that traditional mental health services have not delivered what service users want. In summary service users want:

- practical, socially-oriented support which encompasses help in claiming state benefits and paying bills and in ensuring an adequate income, adequate housing, education, employment, daily living skills, childcare, and satisfying relationships and social networks;
- to be listened to, respected, trusted and demonstrably cared about by friendly, tolerant and non-judgemental workers who are sensitive to and advocate for client preference;
- to be given good quality information and genuine choice around options for care and treatment and help to access appropriate specialist services, including both inpatient units and alternatives to hospital admission when in crisis;
- 'specialist' interventions including help to understand their diagnosis and its potential implications, information and support to achieve an acceptable level of medication, help to cope with symptoms such as worrying beliefs and voices, help to recognize signs of relapse and prevent crises and help in planning ways to cope with crises.

What can be done to engage clients?

Strategies for engaging people with mental health problems have been identified by a number of publications (for example, Morgan 1998; Perkins and Repper 1998; SCMH 1998; DH 1999, 2003; Craig and Timms 2000; Repper 2000; Williamson 2003). These are drawn on below, together with my current clinical experience as a worker in an assertive outreach team, to identify principles of engagement, which nurses may wish to consider in their practice. These principles of engagement cover two areas:

- the values and relationship-building interventions of workers;
- the values and organization of the service to support these interventions.

Values and relationship-building interventions of workers

A needs-led, client-centred approach

Allowing the client's priorities to set the agenda wherever possible quickly establishes a working alliance. Socially-orientated help, particularly with urgent practical issues (for example, the basic survival needs of housing, income, clothing, food) is often the most effective engagement strategy for people who are most unwilling to engage with mental health services.

Flexibility, responsiveness and creativity

Taking the service to the client on their terms as far as possible will make it more accessible and increase the likelihood of engagement. Negotiation around the timing, venue and what will be done together is needed, and may mean some inconvenience for the worker. The frequency, duration and nature of contact needs to be adapted in response to the client's preference and changing priority of need.

Optimism and hope – viewing clients positively

Instilling hope and building self-esteem are real incentives for clients to remain in contact. Focusing on strengths in the context of an acknowledgement of the disabling long-term effects of illness, discrimination and stigma is important as is recognizing that clients have considerable survival skills and have often coped with far greater difficulties than many other people. Demonstrating a commitment to the possibility of change by not dismissing clients' ambitions but instead seeking realistic ways for them to begin to work towards achieving them creates a positive working climate.

Perseverence, patience and realism

Nurses need to allow for setbacks and to accept a slow or non-existent pace of progress if pessimism is to be avoided. Viewing relapse as part of recovery and taking a long-term view with regard to sustained engagement as a marker of success is a more constructive approach.

Seeing the client as expert and being willing to compromise and negotiate

It is important to avoid a power struggle with clients by trying to impose your own model or explanation on clients. Learning from clients by respecting their perspective on their own experiences as valid and meaningful will inform the process of engagement. This requires an acceptance and tolerance by the nurse of the client's right to reject interventions or to disagree with advice (for example, regarding use of medication) and an openness to explore differences and find acceptable ways forward.

Advocacy and challenging oppressive practice

If they are to genuinely engage with services clients need to be heard and taken seriously. Helping clients to represent their views at care review meetings and including them in Care Programme Approach (CPA) care plans, involving independent advocates where necessary, and highlighting approaches that are overly coercive or paternalistic is essential. Adequate information on individual rights, including the complaints procedures, will also help to create a climate of cooperation.

Positive risk-taking

Allowing clients the freedom to learn and gain from experience where possible (taking into account assessment of risk), even if there is the possibility of failure, promotes engagement by avoiding overly controlling practice. This can be facilitated by a collaborative risk-management approach which involves an open exploration of risk history and honesty about the likely consequences of risk behaviours, coupled with reaching agreement on relapse prevention and coping with crises.

Choice and the sharing of good information

Many clients will have been progressively disempowered by their experiences and regaining a sense of control and self-direction is central to engagement. Active involvement through the promotion of informed choice by providing accessible information about the range of options for care and treatment, including facilitating access to appropriate self-help and non-statutory organizations, will help to restore this. Avoidance of psychiatric jargon is important, as it is a stigmatized and alienating barrier to understanding, but explanations of these terms need to be given as necessary. Finding a meaningful language that is acceptable to the client (for example, 'voice hearing' as opposed to 'auditory hallucinations') should be supported by the provision of educative user-friendly literature and time for discussion.

Cultural sensitivity and anti-discriminatory practice

It is important to recognize that clients' experience of services as discriminatory and oppressive has often been a reason for disengagement. There needs to be active enquiry about cultural beliefs and practices and the respectful consideration of them in care planning. Provision of access to trained interpreters in a preferred language, choice of gender and ethnicity of worker where possible, and the involvement of local religious and cultural organizations will all serve to break down cultural barriers and promote engagement.

Honesty, genuineness, trust and respect

Showing your human side to clients is very important. Non-defensive statements about one's limitations, such as 'I don't know but we could find out', is one way of showing this, as is use of humour and having ordinary, problem-free general conversation. Being seen to deliver and do what you say you will do, honesty if you can't or if there are difficulties or delays, communication of any unforeseen changes to your agreed plan and apologizing for any shortcomings on your part will build trust and respect. Clients can be very forgiving if these features of the relationship are in place.

Values and organization of the service

Some service models are inherently better placed to optimize engagement (for example, assertive outreach and early intervention teams), in that they have the advantage of an explicitly targeted client group with engagement as a stated central goal, and are able to 'gate-keep' referrals and limit workers' caseload size to allow sufficient time for more intensive and comprehensive interventions. The relatively recent integration of mental health and social services in many community teams has helped to address the problems of service fragmentation outlined earlier in this chapter. However, whatever the service model or setting, clinical experience suggests that there are key features of a service which will determine how well (or not) it engages with its clients.

Commitment to engagement

A stated commitment to engagement is needed to underpin all aspects of the team's work and should be central to its operational policy and service specification. Acceptability, accessibility, empowerment, choice and involvement are values that need to be formalized in this way.

Service user involvement

Commitment of a clinical team to engage clients is unlikely to be achieved in full unless there is an effective mechanism for involving clients in team development. Service user-led satisfaction surveys can be a useful way of canvassing opinion but will be perceived as tokenistic if their findings are not then drawn upon to inform changes in practice. The whole team, therefore, needs to be open to criticism and willing to act together positively in response. Service user participation in staff selection can help to ensure that positive attitudes prevail. Being interviewed by a service user prior to joining a team can be an effective way of conveying core service values to a new staff member and establishing their commitment to them.

Effective teamwork

The challenges of engaging a client group that often presents with high risk, complex needs and several concurrent mental health problems means that individual workers may experience a high degree of stress and will be unable to work effectively in isolation. A mutually supportive and respectful team climate is essential if effective teamwork is to be fostered. This can be promoted by good quality clinical debate and team problem solving and care planning that shares responsibility by drawing upon the expertise of all members of the multi-disciplinary team.

Staff support and development

If a team is to engage with its clients it also needs to effectively engage with its staff. Regular clinical supervision by competent and experienced practitioners is needed to facilitate good practice by providing a safe learning environment for workers to recognize achievements, effectively manage their caseload and to feel supported enough to acknowledge their own limitations and gaps in expertise and to ask for advice. This has to be complemented by a commitment to continuing staff training (both external and in-house) and the demonstrable encouragement, valuing, recognition and sharing of good practice and staff innovations within the team.

Leadership

Role-modelling positive and professional attitudes by team managers and senior practitioners is essential to maintain adherence of all workers to the core values and aims of the team. A management style that involves all members in an ongoing critical appraisal of the team's aims, objectives, work and direction is important as it facilitates ownership and commitment to the principles of good practice with regard to engagement.

Joint-working across agencies

Establishing effective working partnerships with relevant allied agencies is essential if the needs of clients are to be fully attended to and their engagement achieved. Central to this is recognition that no one team or service can provide everything, an appreciation of the complementary possibilities of joint-working, and a willingness to work together with other agencies for the best outcomes for clients. The Care Programme Approach (CPA) is the statutory framework intended to facilitate this, and good practice guidelines for its implementation need to be adhered to. Service-level agreements between agencies that commonly work together are an effective way of establishing agreed protocols for joint-working, and should include both statutory and voluntary sectors (for example, primary care, community and inpatient mental health services, voluntary sector housing providers and social services). Collating information on relevant wider community resources (for example, self-help groups, work-skills training and employment agencies, educational, social and leisure opportunities) and making creative use of them in care planning will go some way towards engaging with the priorities of clients.

Resources

Adequate resourcing of services is required if clients are to receive the help that they wish for, and this is an issue that is usually beyond the control of individual workers or their line managers. However, teams should make their views known and need to proactively use the existing mechanisms within their organization to constructively lobby for improvements. Alliances with service users in this respect can be very persuasive. Complementary crisis services with 24-hour access and adequate provision of supported housing projects are just two current areas of shortfall. At a team level, working to achieve a realistic caseload size for individual workers is important for retaining a motivated workforce.

Illustrative case studies

In this section two case studies are presented which illustrate some barriers to and strategies for promoting engagement of clients in their care and treatment.

Case study: Terry

Terry is 36 years old with a 10-year history of street homelessness and itinerancy. He often mutters to himself and is suspicious, isolative and aggressive towards others, particularly after binge drinking alcohol. He is often to be seen angrily shouting and gesticulating at passers-by and has been the victim of several assaults. He is extremely thin and wears heavily soiled clothing. He has been excluded from several day centres due to his threatening behaviour.

Barriers to engagement

- hostility towards mental health services due to his exclusion from effective help following a misdiagnosis of his schizophrenia in earlier life and labels of personality disorder and alcohol dependence;
- negative experiences of other services including evictions from hostels, exclusion from day centres and several charges for petty crime;
- persecution and harassment by members of the public;
- long-term isolation and social withdrawal;
- frightening psychotic experiences and threatening behaviour, complicated by alcohol use.

Strategies to promote engagement

- Compulsory hospital admission after limited success of non-coercive engagement strategies and in response to increased risk;
- close working between the inpatient team and community team care coordinator, including frequent visits to Terry to provide continuing contact, support, advocacy, and to build trust with an emphasis on engagement around his priorities of maintenance and collection of benefits and wish for clothing and housing;
- facilitation of a carefully planned discharge to voluntary sector high-support special-needs housing with involvement of the housing team in visiting him on the ward prior to the move;
- strengthening the working relationship with Terry by: negotiation and respect for Terry's preference to have relatively brief contacts with staff and his wish to continue to live a largely isolative lifestyle, optimizing benefits entitlement via the securing of disability living allowance, and mutual agreement on the goals of preventing further hospital admissions and a return to homelessness;

- long-term joint-working between the community mental health, housing and home treatment teams in developing acceptable ways to manage risk, build on daily living skills and maintain community tenure;
- gradual, strengths-focused exploration of Terry's past life experiences and illness, pattern of relapse, risk factors and relapse prevention strategies including medication use;
- assistance with working towards his aspirations of renewing contact with his family and returning to his home town.

Case study: Femi

Femi is a 25-year-old single Nigerian man who has experienced a gradual social decline following the death of his mother six years ago with whom he had lived. He now lives in a low-support flat after a period staying in emergency hostels. He has been unemployed for the past four years and has only infrequent contact with his extended family which he experiences as being rather critical of him. He is often distressed by the experience of commanding voices, unpleasant physical sensations and the belief that he is being controlled by persecutory spirits. He feels embarrassed by his involuntary laughter that often occurs when he is in company and, there-fore, tends to isolate himself, but has mentioned a wish to find paid employment and thereby regain a social network and a girlfriend. He is extremely sensitive to suggestions that he may be mentally ill and can become very irritable and dismissive of attempts to discuss treatment options, sometimes expressing the belief that services are in conspiracy with the spirits.

Barriers to engagement

- distressing psychotic experiences that impede Femi's ability to trust and feel confident with others;
- negative experience of several dismissals from work and long-term unemployment;
- estrangement from his family with consequent loss of status as the eldest son and disconnection from his own community;
- cultural differences around the explanatory model for his difficulties, complicated by the stigma attached to the mental illness model;
- reluctance to engage with discussion about 'symptoms' and to cooperate with advice regarding medication use.

Strategies to promote engagement

- Discussion at the multi-disciplinary clinical review meeting confirms that Femi's need to regain a sense of control over his life should inform all interventions.
- Femi's daily difficulties and aspirations are explored respectfully and empathically from his own cultural perspective and in a way that avoids

use of psychiatric jargon. A potential power struggle is avoided via an open acknowledgement and acceptance of differences of opinion and of the mistrust that he sometimes feels.

- Agreement is reached by the mutual identification of the goals of improving his sleep, reducing unpleasant experiences and eventually returning to work.

- There is an exploration of the approaches that Femi finds helpful and unhelpful with a view to modifying them through negotiation. For example: respecting Femi's wish to take control at the beginning of visits by deciding whether or not he wishes to discuss 'symptoms' and medication (this can be either 'helpful' or 'unhelpful' depending on how he is feeling); and a flexible approach to medication use whereby Femi is encouraged to try varying doses and assess advantages and disadvantages of this.

- There is a negotiated change of allocation to a Nigerian housing support worker with whom Femi has developed a good rapport. Consequent joint-working gradually involves key family members via formal and informal contacts to build understanding and restore relationships. Input from the family's church pastor to meet Femi's spiritual needs and provide advice.

- Appointments are facilitated with the local disability employment adviser and a referral is made to a supported work-skills training project.

Conclusion

Sustained engagement, often through 'low-level' relationship-building interventions allied to an emphasis on socially oriented practical help (housing, benefits, etc.), needs to be an important criterion by which to judge the success of mental health services. To engage their clients, nurses and other mental health professionals must be willing to relinquish the traditional power relationship of expert–recipient and to use the skills of sensitive compromise. This emphasis requires flexibility and a willingness by mental health workers to put aside their specialist skills in the initial stages of their relationships with clients. 'Psychiatric' interventions (medication and CBT, for example) may be best introduced later when trust and greater stability has been established (SCMH 1998).

In summary the main points of this chapter are:

- Engagement in treatment and care of people with serious mental illness is now a national policy and mental health nurses are in a key position to help facilitate this.

- Many service users have valid reasons to mistrust services, and this must be acknowledged.

- Engagement requires both individual workers and services to change their traditional practices by responding positively to criticisms by service users and directly involving them in the process of change.
- There are key principles of engagement that should underpin individual practice and service delivery, whatever the service setting.
- An individualized and socially oriented approach to care provides a foundation for effective engagement.

Questions for reflection and discussion

1   In what ways have services failed to engage effectively with clients?
2   What principles for practice can help individual workers to engage their clients effectively in care and treatment?
3   Using examples of client work from your own experience, identify possible barriers and solutions to engagement. What needs to change and how might you begin to address these changes?
4   How could your service or team optimize the engagement of its clients?

Annotated bibliography

- Brooker, C. and Repper, J. (eds) (1998) *Serious Mental Health Problems in the Community. Policy, Practice and Research*. London: Bailliere Tindall. Covers in detail many of the issues referred to in this chapter, and includes useful case examples.
- Perkins, R. and Repper, J. (1998) *Dilemmas in Community Mental Health Practice. Choice or Control*. Abingdon: Radcliffe Medical Press. Provides a thorough exploration of the challenges and complexities of practice with regard to empowering and engaging service users.
- Sainsbury Centre for Mental Health (1998) *Keys to Engagement. Review of Care for People with Severe Mental Illness who are Hard to Engage with Services*. London: SCMH. A key text that states the case for assertive outreach and the need for services to change.

References

Campbell, P. and Lindow, V. (1997) *Changing Practice: Mental Health Nursing and User Empowerment*. London: MIND/Royal College of Nursing.

Craig, T. and Timms, P. (2000) Facing up to social exclusion: services for homeless mentally ill people, *International Review of Psychiatry* **12**: 206–11.

Dean, R. and Craig, T. (1999) *Pressure Points: Why People with Mental Health Problems Become Homeless*. London: Crisis.

Department of Health (DH) (1999) *A National Service Framework for Mental Health. Our Healthier Nation*. London: HMSO.

Department of Health (DH) (2001) *The Mental Health Policy Implementation Guide*. London: Department of Health Publications.

Department of Health (DH) (2002) *Mental Health Policy Implementation Guide. Dual Diagnosis Good Practice Guide*. London: Department of Health Publications.

Department of Health (DH) (2003) *Delivering Race Equality: A Framework for Action. Mental Health Services Consultation Document*. London: Department of Health Publications.

Morgan, S. (1998) The assessment and management of risk, in C. Brooker and J. Repper (eds) *Serious Mental Health Problems in the Community: Policy, Practice and Research*. London: Bailliere Tindall.

Muijen, M. (1996) Scare in the community: Britain in moral panic, in T. Heller, J. Reynolds, R. Gomm, R. Muston and S. Pattison (eds) *Mental Health Matters: A Reader*. Basingstoke: Macmillan/Open University.

NIACE/NIMHE (2003) *Access to Adult Education for People Diagnosed with Mental Health Problems. Report of a National Postal Survey of Colleges of Further Education, Local Authority Adult Education Services and Workers' Educational Associations*. National Institute of Adult Continuing Education/National Institute for Mental Health (England) Partnership Project. www.nimhe.org.uk

NIMHE (2003) *Personality Disorder; No Longer a Diagnosis of Exclusion. Policy Implementation Guidance for the Development of Services for People with Personality Disorder*. England: National Institute for Mental Health. www.nimhe.org.uk

Perkins, R. and Repper, J. (1998) *Dilemmas in Community Mental Health Practice. Choice or Control*. Abingdon: Radcliffe Medical Press.

Repper, J. (2000) Adjusting the focus of mental health nursing: Incorporating service users' experiences of recovery, *Journal of Mental Health* **9**(6): 575–87.

Rogers, A., Pilgrim, D. and Lacey, R. (1993) *Experiencing Psychiatry; Users' Views of Services*. London: MIND.

Rogers, A. and Pilgrim, D. (1994) Service users' views of psychiatric nurses, *British Journal of Nursing* **3**: 16–18.

Ryan, P. (1999) *Assertive Outreach in Mental Health*, Nursing Times Clinical Monographs No. 35. London: NT Books/Emap Healthcare.

SCMH (1998) *Keys to Engagement. Review of Care for People with Severe Mental Illness who are Hard to Engage with Services*. London: Sainsbury Centre for Mental Health.

SCMH (2000) *Breaking the Circles of Fear. A Review of the Relationship Between Mental Health Services and African and Caribbean Communities*. London: Sainsbury Centre for Mental Health.

Timms, P. (1993) Mental health and homelessness, in K. Fisher and J. Collins (eds) *Homelessness, Health Care and Welfare Provision*. London: Routledge.

Timms, P. (1996) Management aspects of care for the homeless mentally ill. *Advances in Psychiatric Treatment* **2**: 158–65.

Williamson, T. (2003) Enough is Good Enough, *Mental Health Today*, April: 24–7.

23

Problems, goals and care planning

Lina Gega

Chapter overview

Care planning in mental health, irrespective of the nature of the problem or the therapeutic approaches used, becomes user-focused when the client and the practitioner develop a shared understanding of what the *problems* are and agree on *goals* to guide their working relationship. Problems and goals are the stepping-stone for an *action plan*, which describes what to be done (*action*) and why or how it may help (*rationale*). Finally, care plan *review* involves the reassessment and evaluation of problems, goals and actions within a specified period of time and with certain methods.

This chapter covers:

- care planning;
- defining problems;
- setting goals and objectives;
- outlining an action plan;
- reviewing progress.

Care planning

Care planning is the process by which the nurse arrives at:

1. a shared understanding between nurse and patient of what the problems and needs are and what priority they should take;
2. the desired or expected outcome, which is reflected on the goals and objectives;
3. the interactions/interventions which are the pathway to a certain goal

with the ultimate aim to reduce the symptoms, distress and/or disability associated with the problem (action and rationale);

4   the evaluation methods for progress and outcome (care plan review).

Three concepts are pertinent to care planning: problem solving, the nursing process and the Care Programme Approach (DH 2000). Table 23.1 shows how each part of care planning corresponds to a step in problem solving and a stage of the nursing process.

The Care Programme Approach (CPA), is the statutory framework within which bio-psychosocial needs assessment is carried out. CPA forms are set out as care plans for people with mental health problems and complex needs.

Care plans can be either standardized or individualized and uni- or multi-disciplinary. These written records usually have a format which reflects the four components of the care-planning process described above, i.e. problems and needs, goals and objectives, action and rationale, progress review (Figures 23.1 and 23.2). However, the structure and guidelines for care plans vary from one service to another to reflect the needs of specific client groups, or the working methods of a professional team. The patient should be involved in writing their care plan and ideally a copy should be kept by the patient, by the nurse, and be filed in the medical/nursing notes.

The purpose of a care plan can be summarized in six distinct but interlinked areas:

1   As a *legal document*, it demonstrates that patient care complies with national and local policies.

2   As a *means of communication*, it forms part of the patient's medical, nursing or multi-disciplinary notes and facilitates information flow and continuity of care among those involved in a patient's care.

Table 23.1 Relationship between care planning, problem solving and the nursing process

Care planning	Problem solving	Nursing process
Part 1: Problems and needs	Step 1: Defining and prioritizing problems	Stage 1: Assessment
Part 2: Goals and objectives	Step 2: Setting goals	Stage 2: Planning
Part 3: Action and rationale	Step 3: Identifying all solutions; choose best possible solution; determine tasks to arrive at the solution	Stage 3: Implementation
Part 4: Review	Step 4: Evaluating the effectiveness of the solution	Stage 4: Evaluation

```
CARE PLAN for: _____

Problem / area of need / issues to work with: _____
_____
_____

Goals / objectives:
1 _____
_____
_____

2 _____
_____
_____

Action:                              Rationale:
1 _____             1 _____
  _____               _____
  _____               _____

2 _____             2 _____
  _____               _____
  _____               _____

3 _____             3 _____
  _____               _____
  _____               _____

    Review: _____
    _____
    _____

    Completed by: _____    _____    _____

    Date:         _____    _____    _____
```

Figure 23.1 A care plan format: Example 1

3 As a *practice guide*, it provides a focus for patient needs and planning, implementation and evaluation of care.

4 As a *progress record*, it demonstrates the patient's journey within a service or across different services.

5 As a *teaching tool*, it can be used in practice-based learning to develop an understanding of the types of problems and needs that patients may have, and the way nurses may justify and deliver their interventions.

6 As a means of *user involvement*, it can guide the patient–nurse working relationship and ensure that patients participate and their views are represented in their care.

Patient/client:	CARE PLAN			

Primary nurse/keyworker:

Date:

Problem/ area of need	Goals/objectives	Action	Rationale	Review

Figure 23.2 A care plan format: Example 2

Care plans are, therefore, multi-purpose documents. However, in reality, many of these purposes may not be fulfilled at all times. Care plans can become a 'paper exercise' and their completion can be seen as just an administrative task or a legal requirement (Tunmore 1992). Also, the relationship between care plans and quality of care could be challenged on the basis that time spent writing the care plan can take away time spent with the patient. This line of argument assumes, however, that care plans are done *for* the patient rather than *with* the patient, which is too often the case in busy clinical settings.

Defining problems

Defining and prioritizing a patient's problems and needs is the first step in care planning. Information gathered during the assessment process via interviewing, observation and measurement is drawn together into succinct problem statements, which are agreed between patient and nurse. Problem statements should reflect a shared understanding of what the problems/ needs are, what maintains them and what priority they should take in the care-planning process. Prioritizing problems is not straightforward; we may choose to address the most severe problem first or, alternatively, a problem which could be resolved easily and have an associated effect on other areas of need.

An agreed definition and prioritization of a problem might not be feasible if the patient and the nurse cannot engage in a collaborative working relationship for various reasons. Such difficulties are not a reason to exclude the patient from the care-planning process, however; it is better to draw up preliminary unilateral problem statements and address the lack of a collaborative relationship as a problem in itself. Thereafter the nurse might identify the reasons for lack of collaborative relationship (for example, if the patient is severely distressed or unconscious, the nurse has not spent much time with the patient, etc.), ways to facilitate collaboration (reframing the problem in different terms or with a different focus, involving the family and other members of the team, etc.), and a date by which the problem statements should be reviewed, ideally with involvement of the patient.

If after discussing their understanding of the problem the nurse and patient have still not reached an agreed problem statement, they may have to 'agree to disagree' or 'agree to differ' (Kingdon and Turkington 1994) so to avoid prolonged repetitive discussions. In this case, the patient's understanding should still feature in the care plan; it will just be different to the nurse's. Clinicians tend to describe lack of agreement on problem statements as 'the patient lacking insight' but an alternative way of describing it from our patient's point of view could be, 'Mrs A. does not agree with what the doctors/nurses/family say about what her problem is, and she feels that the only reason for being in hospital is because she has not been behaving as she was expected to.'

Language

A way to reach agreed problem statements is to use language which is user-friendly, non-judgemental and personalized. The nurse may wish to test whether their understanding and phrasing of the patient's problem meets these criteria by asking himself or herself:

- Would this make sense to my patient?
- If this were me, would I mind someone else saying this about me?
- Would I be happy for my patient to read this?
- Does this describe my patient's personal experiences of the problem?

User-friendly language uses direct quotes or paraphrases what a person said, rather than jargon or diagnoses. Some examples of what to avoid and what to say instead are:

- 'The client is depressed' → 'Mrs Smith describes feeling low/unhappy/sad/miserable/gloomy/down.'
- 'The client exhibits bluntness of affect' → 'Mary describes feeling numb and empty, and not being able to cry even if when she wanted to get some relief.'

- 'Self-neglect' → 'John has not looked after himself for several days.'
- 'Lack of motivation' → 'Mrs Smith finds is very hard to pay the bills and do the shopping. She would like to get back to work but finds it overwhelming and does not know where to start from, so she ends up postponing and "not bothering" to fill in applications.'

Non-judgemental language describes a behaviour and the potential reasons behind it, rather than attributing a characteristic to the person based on the behaviour. The problem statement should also take into account the patient's rather than the practitioner's point of view. Here are some examples:

- 'The patient is acting out and is difficult to manage' → 'John swears and throws things around because he says "he is fed up with being in hospital and being treated like an idiot".'
- 'The patient is non-compliant' → 'Mr Smith is unhappy about taking his medication because he is worried about not having any control over it.'

Personalized statements reflect how a person experiences their illness and are specific about what symptoms mean for them. Specificity can also allow for objective evaluation of any change in the problem over time. Examples of general versus personalized statements are:

- 'The patient is lethargic and has low energy levels' → 'Mary feels sluggish and slowed down in the morning, and has a two-hour sleep in the afternoon which she never used to do. She feels exhausted when she does things such as preparing dinner or going out socializing.'
- 'The patient has poor sleep and appetite' → 'Mary sleeps 5 hours as opposed to her 8-hour normal sleep and wakes up 3–4 times during the night. She has stopped enjoying her food for the past couple of months and she has lost about 10 pounds during this time. Her everyday eating and drinking includes 5–6 cups of coffee and a sandwich.'

Apart from the appropriate language to be used, the format of problem statements depends on the model used to explain how the problem may have developed and is maintained. If the practitioner does not want to tie problem definition to a particular model, the following components can comprise a generic format for a problem statement:

1   An *experience or state (physical, emotional, mental, behavioural, cognitive, social)*, which the patient considers as the primary problem because it causes distress and disability.

   Useful questions to ask during assessment include:

   - Is anything happening at the moment that upsets you or interferes with your life?
   - Is there anything that you are particularly worried about at the moment?
   - What does your family think the problem is?

- If there was something that you could change to make your life better or more enjoyable, what would it be?
- What do you fear is the worst thing that might happen?

2 The *occurrence* of the primary problem: relevant information on what triggers or precipitates it, how often it occurs, when and where it is more likely to occur, how long it has been going on, etc.

Useful questions to ask during assessment:

- When is the problem more likely to happen?
- Is there anything that makes it better/worse?
- When did you start noticing that things were getting out of hand?
- How many times does it happen in a day/week/month?
- Is there anyone who helps or makes things worse?

3 The patient's *responses* to it and whether they are *helpful or unhelpful*.

Useful questions to ask during assessment:

- How do you make yourself feel better? Does it help? For how long?
- Is there anything that you do more of/less of because of the problem? Is what you do effective? How long does the effect last?
- Is there anything you avoid because of the problem? Is it helpful? Are there any disadvantages in avoiding things?
- Do you ever blow up because of what is happening to you/around you? What exactly do you do? Do you do anything to control it?

4 The primary problem's *impact on self, others and/or life*.

Useful questions to ask during assessment:

- How does it make you feel in yourself?
- How has it been affecting your life?
- Has it affected your relationships with others? In what way?

Problem statement: example 1

John feels unhappy and miserable (*emotional experience as the primary problem*) for most days of the week and for the past month (*occurrence*). Ever since he stopped working, he does not go out much and sits at home (*response*). This makes him feel worthless and even more miserable (*response is unhelpful*), and he worries about being able to go back to work (*impact on life*).

Problem statement: example 2

Mary sleeps less than she would like to and wakes up many times during the night (*physical experience of poor sleep is the primary problem for the patient*). This happens mainly at night when she feels other people's presence in the house (*occurrence and activating event*). She tries to cope with it by telling herself that everything is OK which makes her feel better (*helpful response*) and she occasionally shouts at them (*response*) but she is not sure whether this makes them go away (*unhelpful response*). She feels scared and helpless during the night and tired in the morning (*impact on self*); she is also unable to concentrate on doing everyday things (*impact on life*).

Note that although 'other people's presence in the house' could have been phrased as a problem (e.g. being a symptom of a psychotic illness), Mary chose 'sleep' as the experience that distresses her and interferes with her life more, therefore even if interventions address Mary's psychotic symptoms, this will be done within the context of improving her sleep.

Problem statement: example 3

Mr Smith feels severely anxious (*emotional state*) every time he is about to go out or when he is out (*occurrence*) from fear of doing something stupid and people laughing at him (*cognitive experience*). In *response*, he always goes out very early in the morning and very late at night, and avoids public transport and crowded places (*responses*). Although this prevents anxiety in the short-term (*short-term helpful response*), he never gets the chance to prove to himself that his fear is unlikely to happen (*response is unhelpful long-term*). As a result, he has very little confidence in himself (*impact on self*) and his life has been restricted significantly because he cannot work or socialize (*impact on life*).

Setting goals and objectives

Goals can be long or short term depending on the time and resources available, and the strengths and limitations that the patient is considered to have. Most importantly the nurse needs to identify the objectives to be achieved prior to the patient reaching their goal (i.e. what the person would be able to do and under what circumstances, in order to know that the problem has improved and his/her needs have been met up to a realistic point). It is helpful to include potential or actual obstacles and difficulties in meeting objectives, and to identify, also, what support or resources could assist or smooth the patient's progress. Finally, both problems and goals can be documented and rated in a standard form (Marks 1986) an example of which is given in Figure 23.3.

Questions, which may help elicit goals and objectives are:

1 What would you like to be able to do in the near future that you cannot do now because of the problem?

2 What sort of things can people without your problems do?

3 If you woke up tomorrow and the problem was gone, how would you know?

4 How could your family and friends tell if your problem improved?

PROBLEMS AND GOALS

Name: Date:

Problem: _____

_____

_____

_____

_____

_____

_____

_____

How distressing and/or disturbing is the problem?

0---------1---------2---------3---------4---------5---------6---------7---------8
not at all   slightly   moderately   very much   extremely

Goal: _____

_____

_____

_____

_____

_____

_____

_____

If I had to achieve this goal now, how difficult would it be?

0---------1---------2---------3---------4---------5---------6---------7---------8
not at all   slightly   moderately   very much   extremely

Review: _____

_____

Figure 23.3 Problems and goals form

5   How could people who know you well tell when things start getting difficult for you?

6   If there was one thing that you would like to change in your life/yourself/ the world around you, what would it be?

7   What has to change in order for you to be able to . . .?

Some examples of goals and objectives relating to the problem statements of the previous section are:

Example 1

Long-term goal: To be able to go back to work part-time within 3 months.

- This could be arranged because my boss is understanding and will not have a problem with an initial trial period of part-time work for me.

Objectives:

- To be able to get up in the morning at 8.00 a.m., have breakfast and then go out to buy my paper. (To do this every day for 2 weeks and then sleep longer during the weekends.)
- To be able to go out 2 or 3 days a week in the evening to see my friends.
- Potential difficulty could be that my friends may expect too much too soon from me because they do not understand 'what is wrong with me'.

Example 2

Long-term goal: To be able to sleep 7 hours without waking up and, if I wake up, not be scared.
Objectives:

- To be able to get back to sleep without having to shout at the people in my house and be able to do this every night for a week.
- To be able to spend 1 hour, without interruption, doing the housework every day for a week.

Example 3

Long-term goal: To be able to attend an interest group or do voluntary work in a shop within the next 6 months.
Objectives:

- To be able to walk around my local shopping area every day at lunchtime for about 30 minutes or until my anxiety goes down by 50 per cent.
- To be able to go to the local shop at lunchtime everyday to buy something and make small talk with the shop assistant while making eye contact with him/her.

Outlining an action plan

The action plan includes two elements: (a) the types of interventions or methods of support which will enable the patient to achieve their goals; and

(b) the rationale behind these interventions (i.e. why the nurse (and patient) think the intervention may help and how). The focus of interventions/support depends on the ways the nurse understands the problem (i.e. our problem statements) and what the nurse wants the patient to achieve from the interventions (i.e. our goal). Specifically:

- Using diagnostic terms to describe specific signs and symptoms (for example, ICD-10, WHO 1992) forms the basis of pharmacological or other medical interventions whose goal is to reduce these signs and symptoms and restore heath or minimize illness.

- Identifying the patient's needs and setting goals based on national policies and guidelines (for example, CPA, DH 2000) could determine areas of problem-solving priority, such as risk minimization, social inclusion, crisis management, contingency planning and relapse prevention. Apart from the therapeutic purpose of interventions, the objective is to also meet the nurse's ethical, legal and professional obligations, such as ensuring fairness and autonomy for patients, protecting the public, etc.

- Drawing on psychological models to understand the mechanisms by which a problem has developed and is maintained (for example, stress-vulnerability model, Zubin and Spring 1977) could point to effective psychological, social and family interventions. Here, the goal is to remove the distress and disability associated with a problem and to help the person function as closely as possible to how they would wish.

Reviewing progress

Reviewing progress involves evaluating other parts of the care plan, within a specified period of time and with certain methods. Thus, there are three aspects to consider in any care plan review.

What is being evaluated?

Evaluation is usually associated with 'outcome in relation to certain criteria' (that is, whether the problem has improved and goals are met against certain criteria). However, if the scope of the evaluation is broadened to include 'comparisons at different points in time' (a starting point and a review point), then any part of the care plan can be revisited as long as there are changes to be considered. For example, the nurse may choose to review the list of the patient's needs in order to update it, or rephrase the problem statements in order to include the patient's point of view, or perhaps re-examine the patient's priorities in the light of new information. The nurse might want to reconsider their interventions or whether they were successful in problem solving anticipated difficulties. Thus, the care plan review should specify the objective of the evaluation.

How is the evaluation done?

Depending on the objective of the evaluation, the nurse may use idiosyncratic descriptive methods or objective measurement tools to assess actual or required changes in the problems, goals or action plan. *Idiosyncratic descriptive methods* include diaries or verbal accounts of how someone feels or the nurse's own observations regarding the patient's progress. For example, if the objective of the evaluation is the effect of a new medication, the nurse could ask the patient to describe any side effects they experience, or the nurse could note their own observations of any side effects over time. *Objective measurement tools* include rating scales or questionnaires, which can indicate changes from baseline (*relative change*) or changes against certain criteria (*absolute change*). For example, the nurse might choose to take the patient through a standardized questionnaire, which specifies all potential side effects of medication, and rate the severity of each side effect based on the patient's response to each item of the questionnaire. Comparing this rating against a specified cut-off point could tell the nurse whether the medication is well tolerated or not by the patient (*absolute measurement*), and comparing the patient's ratings over time can indicate whether their tolerance of the medication has improved or not (*relative measurement*).

When should the evaluation be done?

Evaluation can be carried out at pre-specified time intervals (for example, weekly), or an arbitrary date can be set. Or evaluation could be triggered by critical events (such as discharge from hospital, change of medication, etc.). Most importantly, the nurse needs to specify whether the evaluation is ongoing or whether there is a cut-off point at which decisions have to be made based on the outcome of the evaluation. For example, the nurse may choose to assess the side effects of medication weekly up to a month at which point a change in medication would be considered. Or the patient's response to cognitive-behavioural therapy might be assessed weekly but an end-point might be specified (for example, the sixth session) at which to evaluate whether continuing treatment is justified.

Conclusion

There is no one definitive way of developing and writing a care plan, but whatever approach is adopted there are core components that must be included: problems and needs, goals and objectives, action and rationale, and progress review. This chapter has addressed these four components of care planning, focusing mainly on defining problems and setting goals.

In summary, the main points of this chapter are:

- The first step in care planning is to draw the information gathered during assessment into agreed problem statements that reflect a shared understanding of what the patient's problems/needs are, what maintains them and what priority they should take in the care-planning process. A way to reach agreed problem statements is to use language which is user-friendly, non-judgemental and personalized.

- The goals and objectives in care planning are the desired or expected outcomes that would indicate that the problem has improved and the patient's needs have been met up to a certain level. It is helpful to include potential or actual obstacles and difficulties in meeting objectives, as well as to identify what supports or resources could assist or smooth the patient's progress.

- An action plan includes the interventions, which will enable the patient to achieve their goals and the rationale behind these interventions (i.e. why the nurse thinks they may help and how). The action plan is shaped by the way the nurse defines the patient's problems and set targets with them (i.e. whether the nurse uses diagnostic criteria, statutory guidelines and/or psychosocial models).

- Evaluation is an integral part of care planning and need not relate only to outcomes; evaluation can involve a planned reconsideration of problems, goals and actions within a specified period of time. Care-plan review can involve idiosyncratic descriptive methods or objective measurement tools to assess any actual or required changes in the patient's progress and delivery of care.

Questions for reflection and discussion

1   Think about the language you use in your verbal and written communication with or regarding your patients:

    (a) Have you ever used terms which reflected only the diagnosis rather than the individual person's experiences?

    (b) Have you ever used statements which were vague and general, and which could not allow you to measure change?

    (c) Have you ever used value judgements in describing your patient's behaviour?

    (d) Have you ever written a care plan without your patient being involved?

    If the answer in any of the above is 'yes', what could you do differently in similar occasions, next time?

2   What framework is prevalent in your everyday practice as a guide for your care planning and delivery? Is it a diagnostic, statutory or psychosocial framework? How do these frameworks complement each other in everyday practice?

I Annotated bibliography

- Johnson, S.L. (2004) *Therapist's Guide to Clinical Intervention: The 1–2–3's of Treatment Planning* (2nd edn.) California, USA: Academic Press. A multi-disciplinary resource book which describes the assessment criteria for different types of mental health problems (using DSM-IV rather than ICD-10), and provides useful pointers for appropriate psychosocial interventions for each problem. It is an American book targeted mainly for practitioners working autonomously as therapists but it gives problem-specific goals, objectives and action plans, which makes it pertinent to care planning in mental health care.

I References

Department of Health (2000) *Effective care co-ordination in mental health services: Modernising the care programme approach – a policy booklet.* http://www.doh.gov.uk/pub/docs/doh/polbook.pdf [last updated 25 January 2000]

Kingdon, D.G. and Turkington, D. (1994) *Cognitive-Behavioural Therapy for Schizophrenia.* New York: Guilford Press.

Marks, I.M. (1986) Behavioural Psychotherapy: Maudsley Pocket Book of Clinical Management. Bristol: Wright.

Tunmore, R.G.D. (1992) Nursing care planning, in J.I. Brooking, S.A.H. Ritter and B.L. Thomas (eds) *A Textbook of Psychiatric and Mental Health Nursing.* London: Churchill Livingstone.

World Health Organization (1992) *The Tenth Revision of the International Classification of Diseases and Related Health Problems (ICD-10).* Geneva: World Health Organization.

Zubin, J. and Spring, B. (1977) Vulnerability – a new view on schizophrenia, *Journal of Abnormal Psychology* **86**: 260–6.

24

Behavioural techniques

Lina Gega

Chapter overview

Behavioural techniques are focused activities that aim to change behavioural patterns associated with the symptoms, distress and disability of mental health problems. The techniques stem from behaviour therapy, a treatment approach based on learning theories (classical and operant conditioning), that is, that people's behaviours could be sustained or extinct in the presence or absence of strong associations and positive or negative reinforcements.

The clinical application of appropriate behavioural techniques is determined by the problem they aim to treat, and choosing the right technique for the right problem is the cornerstone of evidence-based practice in behaviour therapy. Behavioural techniques have been proven effective for anxiety and stress-related problems (phobias, obsessive-compulsive disorder, post-traumatic stress disorder, panic disorder, generalized anxiety disorder), depressive disorders, some medically unexplained symptoms, impulse control problems and habits disorders. Promising results have also been reported for psychotic disorders and bipolar affective disorder.

The delivery of behavioural techniques should be considered as part of the therapeutic process underpinning most types of interventions. This therapeutic process comprises building and maintaining a working relationship, assessing the client and formulating the problem, facilitating and monitoring care, working with families and carers, measuring progress and outcome, and setting up a relapse prevention programme. The structured nature of behavioural techniques allow for flexibility in their delivery according to the client's needs and preferences. For example, professional support could be minimized if the client chooses to carry out the techniques guided by self-help materials.

The first part of this chapter outlines:

- learning theories that explain the maintenance of mental health problems and;
- the mechanisms that make behavioural techniques work.

Subsequent sections describe the practical tasks or procedures involved in five fundamental behavioural techniques:

- graded exposure and response prevention;
- controlled worry time;
- symptom management techniques;
- awareness training; and
- behavioural activation.

Behavioural explanations of problem maintenance and treatment mechanisms

Mental health problems, or physical problems influenced by mental health factors, are associated with certain experiences both *external* (for example, environmental circumstances, certain objects and situations, etc.) and *internal* (for example, automatic thoughts, bodily sensations, symptoms of an illness, etc.). These experiences trigger various responses which are either a person's way of coping with the experience or simply a reaction to urges and habits. Some of these responses could be helpful for one's problems, such as leaving the room when feeling the urge to 'lash out' and talking to people when feeling low instead of isolating oneself. Others could be unhelpful or even harmful, for example, avoiding going out because of fears and anxieties or using self-injury or substance misuse as a way of relieving tension. Problems are maintained and exacerbated when unhelpful/harmful responses to a trigger are reinforced and helpful/harmless responses are weakened or extinct.

There are three mechanisms which maintain and reinforce unhelpful/harmful responses:

- The trigger-response association becomes automatic and involuntary *(conditioned responses)*, therefore, the person has no control over the occurrence and frequency of the response. Examples include habits, tics, certain types of insomnia and some impulsive behaviours.
- The behaviours bring about a temporary relief from unpleasant feelings therefore they become more likely to occur (*negative reinforcement*, Figure 24.1). Negatively reinforced behaviours usually refer to escape, avoidance, reassurance and rituals which a person may use to prevent, reduce or manage distress (for example, in anxiety disorders or psychosis).
- The behaviours result in pleasure and reward therefore they become more likely to occur (*positive reinforcement*, Figure 24.2). Positively

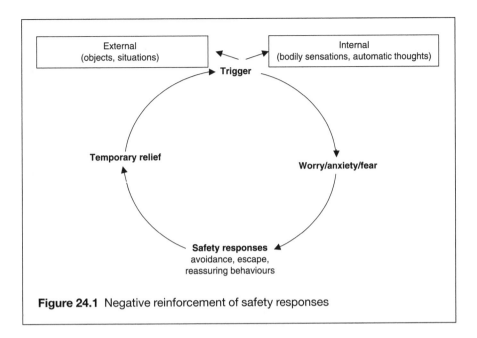

Figure 24.1 Negative reinforcement of safety responses

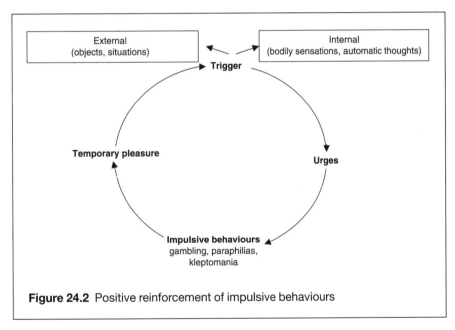

Figure 24.2 Positive reinforcement of impulsive behaviours

reinforced behaviours are usually associated with urges in impulse control problems (such as pathological gambling, kleptomania, paraphilias, etc.).

In addition, a problem may be maintained if helpful/harmless behaviours are weakened or extinct because of:

1 *Lack of practice*: For example, social skills deficits may be the result of social avoidance during which the person has not practised social interactions.

2 *Temporary unpleasant feelings*: For example, people may avoid facing up to their anxieties and problems because this can be stressful and unpleasant.

3 *Lack of response-contingent reinforcement* (reward or pleasure as expected): For example, if a person works hard and there is no reward or problem resolution, then the person may become frustrated or feel hopeless leading to feelings of despair, anger, etc.

Behavioural techniques teach people how to unlearn unhelpful/harmful behaviours and relearn more helpful/harmless responses to external and internal triggers. This is achieved by:

- breaking the association between trigger and unhelpful/harmful responses and establishing an association between trigger and helpful/harmless responses;

- interrupting the cycle of negative or positive reinforcement of unhelpful/harmful responses;

- reducing the physical symptoms and emotional distress associated with a trigger; and

- introducing a response-contingent reinforcement for helpful responses.

A diagrammatic illustration of how behavioural models explain the maintenance of a problem and the way behavioural techniques work, is given in Figure 24.3.

Graded exposure and response prevention

This technique has been extensively studied and proven effective for a range of anxiety and stress-related problems, from phobias and panic to post-traumatic stress and obsessive-compulsive disorders. Graded exposure is the process of confronting anxiety and fear-provoking triggers, starting from the least unpleasant and building up to the most dreaded one. The pre-planned grading of relevant triggers for exposure is known as 'hierarchy'. Response prevention means that the person refrains from carrying out any behaviours which 'mask' or avoid fear and anxiety (safety behaviours) during and after exposure, for example, seeking reassurance or performing rituals (Marks 1986).

The mechanism which explains how graded exposure and response prevention work is called 'habituation', this is the reduction of anxiety over time when a person encounters an anxiety/fear-provoking trigger without the use of safety behaviours. Consequently, the negative reinforcement of safety behaviours is interrupted, and with repeated exposure and response

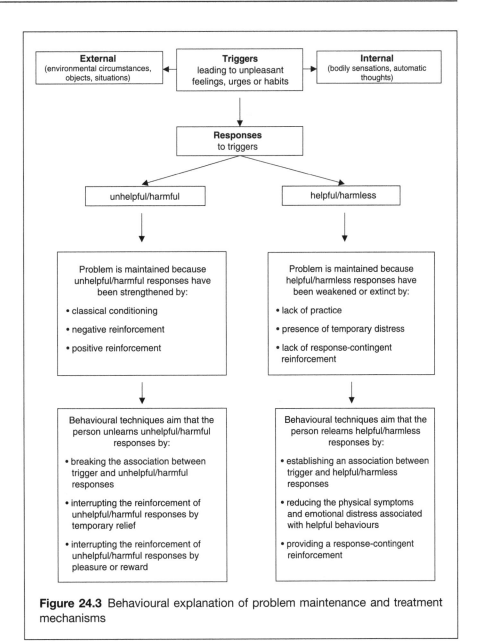

Figure 24.3 Behavioural explanation of problem maintenance and treatment mechanisms

prevention these behaviours are extinct because they no longer serve the purpose of providing relief from anxiety and fear. An explanation of the mechanism with which graded exposure and response prevention work is given in Figure 24.4.

1 Anxiety is the body's natural response to excessive adrenaline production when a person is faced with a situation which is threatening or is perceived as threatening.

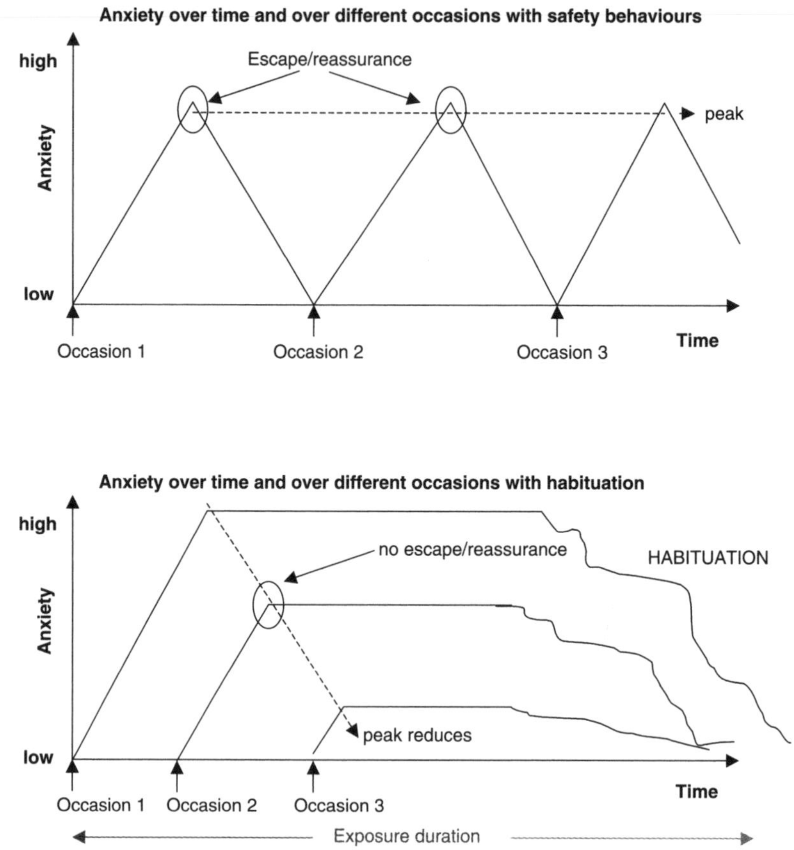

Figure 24.4 Graded exposure and response prevention

2   Adrenaline prepares the body for a flight-or-fight response to an actual or perceived threat. This means that the person experiences physiological changes resulting from increased oxygen flow and blood supply to the muscles, leading to increased heart and breathing rate, increased blood pressure, sweating, blurred vision, etc.

3   Anxiety increases until it reaches a peak when the individual tries to deal with it either by escaping from the situation or by doing certain reassuring or ritualistic things to 'mask' or avoid the anxiety.

4   With escape and avoidance, the anxiety goes down rapidly but will reappear as soon as the individual comes across the same trigger.

5   If the individual remains exposed to the trigger for a certain period of time without running away or masking the symptoms of anxiety, then the excess adrenaline in the body is gradually depleted and anxiety symptoms eventually subside.

6   Over repeated and prolonged exposure to the same or similar triggers, anxiety peaks at an increasingly lower lever and eventually fades away.

Graded exposure and response prevention involves the following steps:

1   Create a hierarchy of triggers (Figure 24.5). This is a list of all anxiety or fear-provoking experiences with ratings of distress in a 0–8 scale (0 = not at all distressing and 8 = extremely distressing). Triggers could

---

Hierarchy

List and rate all the situations which would trigger anxiety, fear or distress if you had to face them, using this scale:

0---------1----------2-----------3---------4---------5----------6-----------7----------8
  not at all   slightly   moderately   very much   extremely

Triggers	*Ratings*
Most dreaded	
1 _____	
2 _____	
3 _____	
4 _____	
5 _____	
6 _____	
7 _____	
8 _____	
9 _____	
10 _____	
11 _____	
Least dreaded	

Figure 24.5 Hierarchy of triggers associated with distressing feelings

be anything that a person avoids altogether, or situations which the person can cope with only by using safety behaviours. Questions to ask in order to elicit triggers are: 'Is there anything that you avoid because of the problem?' 'What brings your fear/anxiety/worry on?' 'What places, things or people make you feel uncomfortable?'

2   Set exposure tasks which relate to each trigger (Figure 24.6). These are exercises comprising the following components:

Exposure tasks

List all the exposure tasks according to your hierarchy of triggers. Practise each task using your daily exposure diary and when you can do your chosen task with relative ease, note the date and move to the next task up the list.

Exposure tasks	*Date achieved*
Most difficult	
1 _____	
2 _____	
3 _____	
4 _____	
5 _____	
6 _____	
7 _____	
8 _____	
9 _____	
10 _____	
11 _____	
Least difficult	

Figure 24.6 List of exposure tasks

- behaviours (what to do and in what order);
- conditions (where, with whom, when, with what response prevention);
- frequency (how often and how many times);
- duration (a specified time period or until the anxiety subsides by 50 per cent).

For example, an exposure task for someone who is anxious about going far from home and into public places could be: 'To travel a mile away from home to the nearest shopping centre, everyday for a week, alone without carrying with me my mobile phone or my anxiety pills, and stay there for 1 hour or until my anxiety reduces by 50 per cent.'

In summary, an exposure task should be:

- *Graded*: i.e. to start from the easiest to achieve and build up towards the most difficult task which could also be the final goal of the exposure programme.
- *Focused*: i.e. the person should experience the whole range of anxiety without trying to mask it or avoid it with subtle behaviours.
- *Repeated*: i.e. to carry out the same exposure task as many times as needed until it can be done with relative ease and minimal anxiety.
- *Prolonged*: i.e. to stay with the anxiety long enough without any safety behaviours to allow habituation to take place.

3 Practise each exposure task in the list for as many times as needed until the task is performed with relative ease. Keep a record of when the task is carried out, and the anxiety experienced before, during and after exposure (Figure 24.7). Distress and discomfort are part of exposure and although they are unpleasant, they are not harmful. However, if someone finds an exposure task too difficult to achieve then:

- Grade down the task by choosing a less distressing trigger to confront.
- Vary the task by either choosing a trigger with similar fear/anxiety rating or change some of the behaviours, conditions and frequency of the exposure (but not the duration as this would effect habituation).
- Use coping methods, such as controlled breathing, tension release and coping cards (described later on this chapter) which could make the task more tolerable. Such techniques should be dropped at a later stage in exposure because they could become safety behaviours which interfere with habituation.
- Use clinician-guided exposure, such as modelling, accompany the patient, etc., to demonstrate how to best carry out the task and as a way of initially managing the discomfort or embarrassment that the person carrying the exposure may feel.

It is important to note that moving too quickly up the hierarchy of triggers and its corresponding exposure tasks may be traumatic, and more harmful

Daily exposure diary

Choose one or more tasks from your list of exposure tasks, note the date and rate the anxiety/distress you felt before, during and after the task using this scale:

0---------1----------2----------3---------4--------5---------6----------7----------8
not at all   slightly   moderately   very much   extremely

If you used or did anything to make yourself feel better or to be able to carry out the task, make a note under the column 'coping methods'.

Date	Task no.	Anxiety / Distress rating			Coping methods
		Before	During	After	

Figure 24.7 Daily exposure diary

than helpful because of the excessive distress it may cause. It can also be disheartening if the person cannot achieve the task and consider themselves to have failed. However, moving too slowly could be ineffective because the person does not experience the degree of anxiety that would allow habituation to take place. Also, having to practise two or three exposure tasks of slight anxiety could be more unpleasant than having to practise one task of moderate anxiety. In conclusion, the pace of exposure should be negotiated with the person that carries it out and the fine tuning of the tasks is ongoing according to the person's strengths and preferences.

Controlled worry time

The underlying principle of this technique is that worry begins as a coping response to external or internal triggers but becomes uncontrollable and distressing, hence a problem in itself. Controlled worry time (versions of which are described by Borkovec *et al.* 1983 and Wells 1997) aims to reduce worrying thoughts and the distress associated with them by:

- giving a sense of controllability over the frequency (how often), occurrence (under what circumstances) and duration (for how long) of worrying thoughts;

- breaking the association between certain external or internal triggers and worry as a coping response to them;

- change worry from a distressing experience into a problem-solving activity.

This technique has been mainly described and applied for generalized anxiety disorder, however, the relevance of worry control strategies extends to other mental health problems in which worry is a concomitant feature; for example, a schizophrenia sufferer could interpret mental symptoms of worry (muddled thinking, lack of concentration) as a sign of relapse or a depression sufferer could have ruminatory worry about coping with everyday life. The components of controlled worry time are:

1   Identify worrying thoughts. The frequency, occurrence, duration and content of the worrying thoughts depend on the individual's experiences. The person may use a personal or standardized diary to record and monitor their worrying thoughts (Figure 24.8).

2   Establish a 'worry-time' of 30 minutes to take place at the same location every day. There is no ideal place and time; a person may choose a time in the day which allows privacy and solitude or may prefer to have a 'worry-time' when there are other people around who could offer support.

3   If catching yourself worrying on other times, postpone worrying until the designated 'worry-time' and attend to other everyday things. This could be quite difficult at the beginning, but would get easier with practice. Try to transfer your worrying thoughts from your 'head' to a piece of paper (i.e. worry record above) and put this aside until the designated worry-time.

4   Use the worry time to address your concerns; you may need to carry out a problem-solving plan to deal with factual difficulties or challenge any

---

Worry diary

Under 'situation' note what you were doing, when, where and with whom, every time you feel worried, scared or anxious. Under 'worry' write down what you were worried about, how you felt, what you were thinking, etc.

Day and time	Situation	Worry

Figure 24.8 Example of diary to be used in controlled worry time

unrealistic or overestimated fears. Alternatively, you don't have to worry at (and for) the designated time. If you choose not to worry at the designated time, be sure that you do so *not* because you want to avoid it but because you do not feel it is necessary.

Symptom management techniques

Although symptom management techniques may not produce fundamental changes, they facilitate progress by reducing distressing feelings, such as anger, anxiety, fear and worry, and making them manageable to enable other behavioural techniques to take place. Three symptom-management techniques are mentioned here: controlled breathing, tension-release exercises and coping cards.

Controlled breathing

The aim of controlled breathing is to restore the oxygen–carbon dioxide balance and acid–alkali balance which can be disrupted because of changes in the breathing rate under conditions of fear or acute stress. The key in controlled breathing is to *breathe in from the abdomen*, keep the chest still, *breathe out slowly and fully* and keep a regular pace between breathing in and out with pauses in-between. A way to know that this is done properly is when the abdomen moves out when you breathe in and moves in when you breathe out. This could be difficult to get used to, because most people breathe in from their chest and their stomach tends to move in as they breathe in. It is better to practise abdominal breathing when calm and comfortable in order to master the technique so that it can be used with the first warning signals of psychological arousal.

Tension-release exercises

Tension-release exercises (Gournay 1995) have been established as part of a comprehensive applied relaxation training programme for anxiety conditions (Ost 1987). Tension-release exercises aim to control physiological arousal symptoms, such as muscle tension, sweating, pounding heart, light-headedness, 'butterflies in the stomach', etc. The person learns to recognize these symptoms early and control them before they reach their peak. This can be achieved by systematically tensing muscle groups in the body for 5 seconds and then releasing them for about 10 seconds. The exercises are first practised for 20–30 minutes in comfortable conditions and then could be done in distress-provoking situations. It is important that:

- the muscles are only tensed until the person feels a sense of 'pulling'; too much pressure may cause injuries or the muscles may not be able to relax after releasing the tension;
- the release of the muscles should be immediate and NOT gradual.

Figure 24.9 describes in detail how to carry out tension-release exercises.

Muscle groups	Tension-release exercise	Time
Hands and forearms	First with right, then with left hand and forearm. • Clench your fist until knuckles are white and the muscles in your forearm feel tense. • Release by letting the hand fall loose.	x2 5 sec. 10 sec.
Arm	First with right, then with left arm. • Clench your fist and bend the arm to 90° trying to make your biceps muscle bulge. • Release by letting the hand and arm fall loose.	x2 5 sec. 10 sec.
Head *Forehead and eyebrows*	• Wrinkle the forehead by raising the eyebrows. • Release by letting the eyebrows relax. • Bring the eyebrows close together as in frowning. • Release by letting the eyebrows relax.	5 sec. 10 sec. 5 sec. 10 sec.
Eyes	• Screw up your eyes and hold them tightly shut. • Release by opening your eyes and letting your eyelids relax.	5 sec. 10 sec.
Jaw	• Tense the jaw by biting the teeth together. • Release by letting the jaws relax (they are *NOT* clenched).	5 sec. 10 sec.
Tongue	• Press the tongue flat against the roof of your mouth until you notice tension in your throat. • Release by letting the tongue rest (make sure your jaws are *NOT* clenched together).	5 sec. 10 sec.
Lips	• Press the lips tightly together as in a pout. • Release by letting the lips relax (make sure your jaws are *NOT* clenched together).	5 sec. 10 sec.
Neck	• Let the head fall back (towards the chair) without pushing it back and then let the head fall forward (your chin towards your chest without touching it). • Release by bringing the head in the upright position.	5 sec. 10 sec.
Shoulders	• Hunch the shoulders up towards the ears and then circle the shoulders. • Release by letting the shoulders drop.	5 sec. 10 sec.
Back	• Push your elbows into your side, push your shoulders down, push your head towards your chest and feel your big muscles across your back tense. • Release by letting your elbows relax, your shoulders drop, and your head in the upright position.	5 sec. 10 sec.
Chest	• Push your shoulders back, push your elbows down, tilt your head back and feel the muscles in your chest tighten. • Release by relaxing the shoulders and elbows and bringing the head in the upright position.	5 sec. 10 sec.
Stomach	• Tense the muscles of the stomach and push the stomach inwards. • Release by letting the muscles relax.	5 sec. 10 sec.
Buttocks and thighs	• Squeeze your thighs and buttocks together. • Release by relaxing the muscles.	5 sec. 10 sec.
Calves and shins	• Keeping the leg straight, tense the calves by pushing the feet and toes downwards. • Release by letting the feet fall loose. • Keeping the leg straight, tense the shins by pulling the feet and toes upwards. • Release by letting the feet fall loose.	5 sec. 10 sec. 5 sec. 10 sec.
Feet	• Curl over your toes, trying to make a fist with your toes. • Release by letting the feet fall loose.	5 sec. 10 sec.

Figure 24.9 Tension-release exercises

Coping cards

The person uses small index cards or pieces of paper or a certain part of their diary to write a few sentences which are:

- Encouraging: 'I have dealt with worse before, this is just fear and I won't let it get the best of me', 'I'm getting better at this all the time'.

- Challenging: 'Don't jump into conclusions or take it personally', 'There is no need to prove myself, I am good enough as I am.'

- Self-instructions or reminders: 'I must walk away now', 'Time to step back and take a breath', 'I'll make a note of this so I can take it out of my mind now and talk about it with my friend later.'

Awareness training

Awareness training can be used for actions/behaviours which are associated with impulses, urges or habits, such as eating disorders, self-injuries, habits, trichotillomania, kleptomania, anger problems, etc. The purpose of awareness training is to:

1   become aware of the stages before the behaviour occurs, so that the person can break the association between trigger–harmful response and be able to practise an alternative response on time;

2   become familiar with the behaviour itself, so that the person can develop an effective alternative response;

3   become familiar with any unpleasant (potential or actual) consequences of the harmful behaviour, so that any elements of pleasure or relief associated with it are weakened and gradually extinct.

Awareness training mainly involves self-monitoring using a diary (Figure 24.10) so as to recognize:

1   triggers, cues, warning signals and actions/behaviours associated with the urge;

2   the components of the impulsive action/behaviour itself as a response to the urge;

3   the (potential or actual) consequences of the action/behaviour.

Awareness training is the first step for the treatment of many problems that involve a certain urge of habit. The technique itself is enough to reduce the occurrence of a certain problem behaviour, but it is also combined with avoiding cues which trigger the urge–response cycle and with rehearsing alternative responses following cue exposure.

Incident awareness record

Trigger What were you doing? Who were you with, when and where?	*Urge* How strong was the urge? 0---2---4---6---8---10 **not at all extremely**	*Response* What did you do as a response to your urge? Describe in as much detail as possible.	*Consequences* What happened afterwards and how did you feel?

Figure 24.10 Self-monitoring diary for awareness training

Behavioural activation

Behavioural activation has been used to tackle problems associated with low levels of activity and lack of pleasure or satisfaction, as it may happen in depression or negative symptoms of schizophrenia. The aim of behavioural activation is to (a) increase the levels of daily activity which could have a positive effect on energy levels and motivation, (b) introduce pleasant, rewarding and interesting events as a positive reinforcement to daily routine. Behavioural activation comprises the following components: activity monitoring, activity rating, activity scheduling and graded task assignment (Fennel 1989; Greenberger and Padesky 1995).

Activity monitoring

The person needs to use a daily or weekly diary to record the time and type of activities (Figures 24.11 and 24.12). If the sleep pattern of the person is interrupted, then it may be helpful to have a 24-hour diary to monitor their pattern of sleep and what activities take place just before the person goes to bed or just after the person wakes up in the night.

Sometimes a person may write 'doing nothing' if they consider that what they do is not productive or is not what they wanted to do in the first place; things such as sleeping, lying in bed, or watching out of the window are still activities and is important that they are recorded to demonstrate their link with depressive feelings or negative symptoms.

Activity rating

In the activity monitoring diary, rate each activity using a scale 0–10; 0 meaning 'not at all' and 10 meaning 'extremely'. Intermediate ratings points could be 2 for 'slightly', 4 for 'somewhat', 6 for 'quite a lot' and 8 for 'very much'.

Put a P for PLEASURE with a 0–10 rating next to the activities that may be enjoyable (e.g. watching TV, eating). For example P0 would mean that the person did not enjoy the activity at all, P5 that they moderately enjoy it and P10 that they very much enjoyed it. The purpose of pleasure ratings is to establish (a) activities that the person used to enjoy but not any more, either because they do not have the motivation or energy to do them or because they do them but do not enjoy them; and (b) activities that the person still enjoys to some extent, and that, therefore, there is scope to build on these activities.

Put an M for MASTERY with the 0–10 rating according to the difficulty of achievement *given how the person felt at the time* (doing the housework, taking children to school). For example M0 would be that the person found the activity quite effortless and did not give them a sense of achievement, M5 that the activity was moderately difficult to achieve but the person managed it, whereas M10 would represent a difficult activity that was an achievement to complete. The purpose of mastery ratings is to demonstrate that (a) a person may achieve more things than they give themselves credit for, because achievement is not what a person *wished they achieved* but what a person *did achieve* considering their circumstances (for example, low energy because of depression, no support, etc.), and (b) if the person does things which only

Week beginning: _____

	Monday	Tuesday	Wednesday	Thursday	Friday	Saturday	Sunday
	a.m.	a.m.	a.m.	a.m.	a.m.	a.m.	a.m.
Time:							
	P=	P=	P=	P=	P=	P=	P=
M=							
Time:							
	P=	P=	P=	P=	P=	P=	P=
M=							
Time:							
	P=	P=	P=	P=	P=	P=	P=
M=							
	p.m.	p.m.	p.m.	p.m.	p.m.	p.m.	p.m.
Time:							
	P=	P=	P=	P=	P=	P=	P=
M=							
Time:							
	P=	P=	P=	P=	P=	P=	P=
M=							
Time:							
	P=	P=	P=	P=	P=	P=	P=
M=							

Figure 24.11 Weekly activity monitoring

Date: _____

Time	Activity What did I do? Where was it? Was anyone there?	Pleasure How interesting and enjoyable was it? 0----2-----4-----6----8----10 not at all very much	Mastery How difficult was it to achieve given my circumstances? 0----2-----4-----6----8----10 not at all very much

Figure 24.12 Daily activity monitoring

require little or no effort, then there is scope to schedule activities with gradually increased effort and consequently increasingly greater sense of achievement.

Activity scheduling

Using a diary similar to the one used for daily activity monitoring, the person plans in advance their hour-by-hour activities (Figure 24.13). There are two types of tasks which need to be scheduled:

- Tasks which the person *has* to do in balance with tasks that the person *wants* to do. The aim of activity scheduling is not to do as many things as possible in the time we have, but to plan the time we are going to spend on a particular activity in order to complete specific tasks.

- Sometimes people find it easier to come up with the tasks that *have* to be done rather than activities that could be just pleasurable and interesting. Pleasant/interesting activities rather than chores could crop up from the activity monitoring diary (the ones with high pleasure ratings) or from a detailed history about things that the person used to enjoy in their everyday life but stopped doing because of their depression, or from questions about things that the person always wanted to do but never did.

The person records the planned activity in detail (including what is to be done, with whom and where) and then the actual activity which took place, including whether it was similar, greater or smaller than the planned one. Then, the person records mastery and pleasure ratings as they did in the activity monitoring diary. If the planned activity was too difficult, then the person may have felt disheartened and did not do anything at all, in which case it would be useful to downgrade the task (see Graded task assignment) in order to make the activity manageable.

Graded task assignment

Graded task assignment is helpful for things that the person wants to achieve but are too difficult under their current circumstances and need to be broken down before they are introduced in the activity scheduling diary. Using the Activities list (Figure 24.14) the person could identify all the things they want to achieve during a certain period, always taking into consideration the balance between pleasures (things they *have to* do) and responsibilities (things they *need to* do). For each activity identified, there could be five potential actions:

1   omit, if the activities/tasks exceed the available time;
2   delegate, wherever possible;
3   postpone activities which are of lower priority;
4   seek help and support whenever possible;

Date: _____

Time	Planned activity What am I going to do? Where? Will anyone help/be involved?	Actual activity What did I actually do? How did it compare with the planned activity? Was it *similar*, *greater* or *smaller* than planned?	Pleasure How interesting and enjoyable was it? 0---2---4---6---8---10 not at all very much	Mastery How difficult was it to achieve given my circumstances? 0---2---4---6---8---10 not at all very much

Figure 24.13 Daily activity scheduling

Date: _____

Things to do	Action*					Time-frame
	* 1 Omit	2 Delegate	3 Postpone	4 Help/support	5 Grade task	

Figure 24.14 Activities list

5   grade the task: if, for example, the task is 'to get the children ready for school and take them there' but the person cannot do it because he or she feels exhausted or overwhelmed, then a grading could be 'prepare their packed lunch the night before – get up just before they go and just say goodbye – get up in the morning and make them drinks – get up in the morning and prepare drinks and breakfast – get up in the morning, prepare drinks, breakfast and take them to school.'

Conclusion

This chapter described 'what to do' in order to carry out some key behavioural techniques and how these techniques may work based on learning theories. Their application should be based on research evidence about what technique is proven effective for which problems and should be done with guidance by experienced clinicians. Apart from the main activities comprising each behavioural technique, their delivery in practice is more complicated and may yield difficulties because people that nurses care for could have the same problem but vastly different needs, strengths and limitations. Therefore, this chapter aimed to give the main action points and 'conceptual pegs' that practitioners could build upon with further reading, training and supervision.

In summary, the main points of this chapter are:

- Behavioural models understand mental health problems as a vicious circle of triggers (external, internal), responses (coping behaviours, habits, urges) and consequences (either strong associations, or relief from unpleasant feelings, or ensuing pleasure maintaining a problem-related response).

- Behavioural techniques are focused activities which aim to manage the symptoms, distress and disability associated with a problem by (a) reducing or removing unhelpful or harmful responses to triggers, and (b) reinforcing more helpful/harmless behaviours.

- The five fundamental behavioural techniques described were: graded exposure and response prevention, controlled worry, symptom-management techniques (controlled breathing, tension-release exercises and coping cards), awareness training and behavioural activation.

Questions for reflection and discussion

1   Considering that mental health and illness occur in a continuum, what relevance do you think the behavioural techniques described in this chapter may have for your responses to everyday life experiences? Specifically:

(a) Do you have any fears or anxieties that graded exposure and response prevention may relate to?
(b) Do you ever worry, so that controlled worry-time may be helpful?
(c) Do you ever feel miserable, sluggish or overwhelmed by daily tasks, in which case behavioural activation could apply?
(d) Do you ever act on impulse, which you would like to be more in control of by using awareness training?
(e) Do you ever get panicky and nervous, in which case symptom management techniques may be useful?

2   Focusing on one of the questions 1(a)–1(e) above, follow the relevant behavioural technique for one week. What difficulties have you experienced in trying to implement this technique and what have you learnt from it which could be useful in its application to your everyday practice?

3   Select one of the behavioural techniques which you find particularly interesting or relevant to your line of work.

(a) Explain to a colleague how the technique works, taking into account learning theories and drawing a trigger–response–consequence diagram.
(b) Find three research papers which study the implementation of this behavioural technique for mental health problems.
(c) How relevant are the papers for the clients/patients you usually care for? The type of service you work in? The expertise you have? The supervision available to you in order to implement the techniques safely and efficiently?

Annotated bibliography

- Marks, I.M. (2001) *Living with Fear: Understanding and Coping with Anxiety* (2nd edn). London: McGraw-Hill. A best-seller in many countries worldwide, this user-friendly and informative read explains the nature of fear and anxiety in relation to a range of disorders such as phobias, panic, obsessive-compulsive disorder and sexual anxieties. The book is enriched throughout with self-help instructions and case examples of people who got help by using various behavioural techniques for their problems.
- Gamble, C. and Brennan, G. (eds) (2000) *Working with Serious Mental Illness: A Manual for Clinical Practice*. London: Bailliere Tindall in association with the Royal College of Nursing. Chapter 9 has very useful applications of the triggers–responses–consequences behavioural paradigm for severe mental illness using the stress-vulnerability model and coping strategy enhancement. Chapter 13 describes behavioural strategies, such as self-monitoring and alternative-response training, in

working with people with severe mental illness and anger management problems.

* Haddock, G. and Slade, P.D. (eds) (1996) *Cognitive-behavioural Interventions with Psychotic Disorders*. London: Routledge. Chapters 2, 3 and 5 provide a theoretical background, evidence base and case examples of behavioural techniques in the management and treatment of psychotic symptoms (mostly in conjunction with cognitive theories and techniques). A comprehensive and stimulating read comprising chapters from nearly all leading specialists in the field of CBT for psychosis in the UK.

References

Borkovec, T.D., Wilkinson, L., Folensbee, R. and Lerman, C. (1983) Stimulus control applications to the treatment of worry. *Behaviour Research and Therapy* **21**: 247–51.

Fennell, M.J.V. (1989) Depression, in K. Hawton, P. Salkovskis, J. Kirk and D. Clark (eds) *Cognitive Behaviour Therapy for Psychiatric Problems: A Practical Guide*. Oxford: Oxford University Press, pp. 169–234.

Gournay, K. (1995) *Stress Management: A Guide to Coping with Stress*. Surrey: Asset Books.

Greenberger, D. and Padesky, C.A. (1995) *Mind Over Mood: Change How you Feel by Changing the Way you Think*. London: Guilford Press.

Marks, I.M. (1986) *Behavioural Psychotherapy: Maudsley Pocket Book of Clinical Management*. Bristol: Wright.

Ost, L.G. (1987) Applied relaxation: description of a coping technique and review of controlled studies. *Behaviour Research and Therapy* **25**: 397–410.

Wells, A. (1997) *Cognitive Therapy of Anxiety Disorders: A Practice Manual and Conceptual Guide*. Chichester: Wiley and Sons.

25

Cognitive techniques

Lina Gega

Chapter overview

Cognitive techniques are guided dialogues and focused activities that aim to change inaccurate, distorted or unhelpful beliefs about situations and signs or symptoms that a person may experience. The techniques stem from cognitive therapy, a treatment approach based on information-processing theories, that is, people's emotional, physical and behavioural responses to certain experiences are shaped by how people perceive these experiences and what meaning they attach to them.

This chapter describes the role of perception and thinking in the maintenance of mental health problems and outlines three groups of techniques as part of a process called cognitive restructuring; i.e. identifying misinterpretations and unhelpful ideas, generating alternative interpretations and constructive ideas, and testing and reinforcing the alternatives. This process has been applied successfully for anxiety and stress-related problems, depressive disorders, somatic problems, psychotic disorders and bipolar affective disorder. The chapter concludes by comparing cognitive and behavioural techniques in light of the integrated therapeutic approach known as cognitive-behaviour therapy (CBT).

This chapter covers:

- the role of thoughts in mental health;
- techniques to identify misinterpretations and unhelpful ideas;
- techniques to generate alternative interpretations and constructive ideas;
- techniques to test and reinforce alternatives;
- cognitive and behavioural techniques: segregation or integration?

The role of thoughts in mental health

The term 'cognitive' relates to thinking and perception, two processes by which individuals interpret their experiences and form ideas about themselves and the world around them (Beck 1976). Thoughts are formed by words and images, and their content varies according to a person's past and present experiences. Thoughts which contribute to the maintenance of mental health problems share two common characteristics:

1 they contain some form of inaccuracy or distortion;
2 they form a significant part of a person's reality and they feed into the symptoms, distress and disability associated with the problem.

The difference between 'normal' thoughts and those associated with mental health problems is not so much in their content as it is in the degree of conviction and significance that a person may attach to them. Such thoughts are considered under four groups below:

- *Negative automatic thoughts and intrusive thoughts*: They trigger distressing feelings (fear, worry, anxiety or low mood) and the person feels that he or she has no control over their occurrence.
- *Overvalued ideas and delusions*: They appear to digress from ideas that are acceptable or common within a person's environment and the person has a strong conviction in them.
- *Catastrophic beliefs and feared consequences*: They are ideas that something awful may happen if a person does not carry out certain behaviours, or does not avoid certain situations.
- *Assumptions, core beliefs, personal rules and schemas*: These are beliefs which have been developed through life experiences and shape or influence a person's views and actions in response to a critical incident.

Given that thoughts are the result of information processing in relation to past and present experiences, misinterpretations or unhelpful ideas are the result of information processing errors, as outlined below:

- *Catastrophizing*: expecting the worst to happen and overestimating the probability of it happening.
- *Emotional reasoning*: using feelings to guide our judgement and confusing how things feel with how things really are.
- *Dichotomous thinking*: thinking in absolute terms, all-or-nothing, black-or-white, not considering the middle ground.
- *Arbitrary inference*: jumping to conclusions, making judgements without evidence, believing that we know what others are thinking, predicting the future.
- *Generalizing*: making sweeping statements based on single incidents, overestimating the importance of isolated events.

- *Personalizing*: assuming that one has responsibility over everything, blaming ourselves over things that we have little control or influence on.

- *Selective focus and filtering*: Focusing on the negative and discounting the positive, looking for evidence to back up our ideas and disregarding evidence which challenges them, selecting fragments of evidence without considering the whole picture.

- *Fixed rules*: using commands rather than wishes and options as the driving force for our behaviours, such as 'I should' and 'I must', rather than 'I would like to' or 'I would prefer it'.

The key aspects of the cognitive model for mental health problems is that our thoughts shape the way we behave and feel (both emotionally and physically) and that in turn our behaviours and feelings may confirm or disconfirm these thoughts, thereby creating a cycle of interlinked thoughts, behaviours and feelings (Figure 25.1). In this chapter, thoughts relevant to mental health problems are referred to as misinterpretations (because of

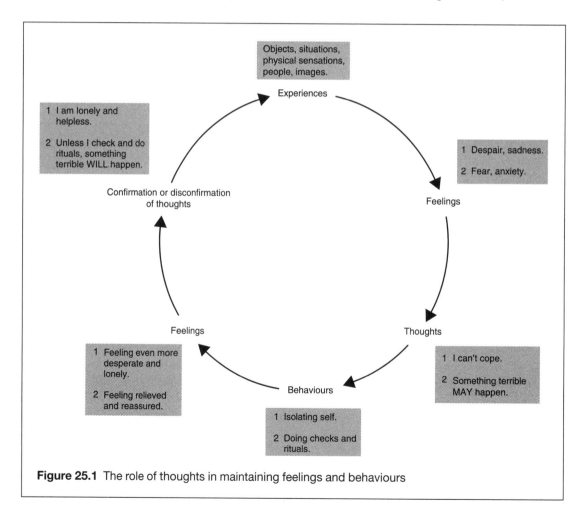

Figure 25.1 The role of thoughts in maintaining feelings and behaviours

inaccuracies or distortions in them) and unhelpful ideas (because they exacerbate and maintain the problem irrespective of their accuracy, as it may happen with some cultural or religious beliefs).

Cognitive therapy aims to produce change in a problem through a process called cognitive restructuring or reattribution (that is, reducing a person's belief in their misinterpretations and unhelpful ideas by reinforcing a person's belief in alternative interpretations and more constructive ideas). The description of cognitive techniques in three groups for the purpose of this chapter is to aid clarity, however, in clinical practice cognitive restructuring involves all three groups in a continuous process.

Cognitive restructuring is not simply about positive thinking but about expanding our thinking repertoire so that it includes other options in the way we view ourselves and others, the world around us, our life and future. Furthermore, cognitive restructuring is not so much about challenging inaccurate, distorted or unhelpful beliefs as it is about reinforcing alternatives ones. The reason for this is twofold. Firstly, someone may feel stupid or dejected if a long-held belief which had shaped a person's feelings and behaviours is crashed without an alternative being offered. Secondly, trying to challenge and undermine a person's beliefs may appear threatening and patronizing compared to suggesting and testing alternatives which may be more acceptable and unassuming.

Techniques to identify misinterpretations and unhelpful ideas

The first stage in cognitive restructuring is to identify the content and occurrence of thoughts associated with a problem and rate (a) the person's conviction in them, and (b) the person's feelings and responses to them. This could be achieved in several ways:

- Keeping thought-monitoring records (Figure 25.2) for a specific period of time, detailing the situation that a thought occurred, what the thought or range of thoughts were, how the person felt and responded at the time, and how much the person believes in that thought. The purpose of thought records is to identify a person's idiosyncratic misinterpretations or unhelpful ideas, establish a pattern of occurrence, demonstrate the link between thoughts and a person's feelings and responses, and finally rate the person's belief in them. An important point to remember while keeping a thought record is to identify which thoughts are the most potent and relevant ones by asking, 'If we could make one or two thoughts go away, which ones would you choose in order to make a real difference in the way you feel?'

- Going through a recent incident (Figure 25.3) when the person experienced emotions or symptoms associated with the problem. Starting questions could be, 'When was the last time that you felt miserable/angry/anxious/scared?' or 'Looking back during the last week, which

Thought-monitoring record

Situation	Feelings	Thoughts	Responses
What was I doing? Who was I with? When? Where?	How did I feel? How bad was it? 0---2----4-----6---8----10 not at all extremely	What was going through my mind? How much did I believe it? 0%----25%-----50%-----75%----100% not at all completely	What did I do? How did it make me feel?

Figure 25.2 A record to monitor thoughts

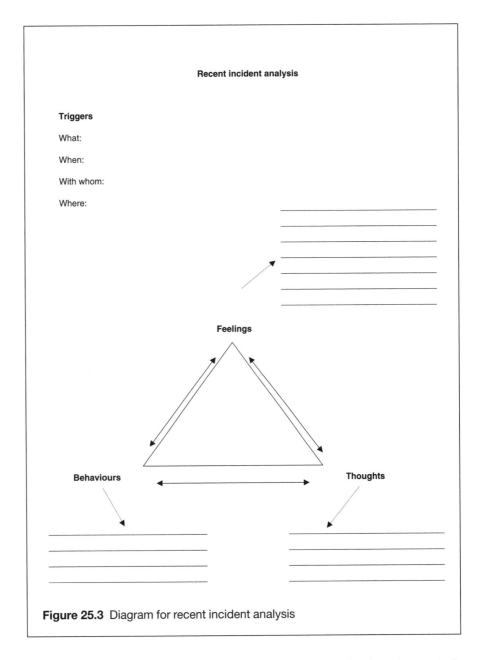

Recent incident analysis

Triggers

What:

When:

With whom:

Where:

Feelings

Behaviours

Thoughts

Figure 25.3 Diagram for recent incident analysis

was the worst day for you. What was happening at the time that made it so bad?' Then, questions such as, 'What was going through your mind at the time?' and 'Were you saying anything to yourself at the time?' could help elicit thoughts associated with the specific incident.

• Using the 'downward arrow technique' which aims to elicit the meaning of one's thoughts. The clinician starts by asking the question, 'If this were true . . .'

– What would be so bad about it?
– What would this tell you about yourself/other people/your future/ your life? and carries on by asking the same question to the patient's answer until we arrive at a statement which reflects a core belief or personal assumption. An example is given below:

I am worried I am becoming mentally ill.
↓
If this were true (you became mentally ill) what would be so bad about it?
↓
I would end up in a hospital.
↓
If this were true, what would be so terrible about ending up in a psychiatric hospital?
↓
Everyone would know and also I would never work again.
↓
If this were true, what would be so bad about it?
↓
Everyone would look down on me, feel pity on me and eventually abandon me.
↓
If this were true, what would this tell you about your life?
↓
Life will not worth living if I end up without a job and friends.

The downward arrow technique, otherwise referred to as *inference chaining*, could yield potent thoughts and powerful emotions which represent the person's ultimate fears. Therefore, this technique should be used only if the practitioner is sure about 'what to do' with the statement that lies at the end of the arrows. Some useful examples of applications of the downward arrow technique are described by Greenberger and Padesky (1995) for anxiety and depression, and Turkington and Siddle (1998) for delusions.

Techniques to generate alternative interpretations and constructive ideas

This is perhaps the most difficult part of cognitive restructuring because the practitioner may be able to see the alternatives, but needs to facilitate the individual client to arrive at these alternatives using one or more of the techniques outlined below (for some examples, see Blackburn and Davidson 1995, chapter 4). The alternative interpretation or constructive idea is phrased as a *hypothesis*, i.e. a theory or assumption for which we need to come to a conclusion about how accurate it is compared to the initial interpretations and ideas, and/or how helpful it may be in changing the way we feel and behave. At this stage, we may choose not to judge or add value to the alternatives until the next step of cognitive restructuring when we test them for accuracy and helpfulness. Remember, the objective is not to show that we are right and the other person is wrong but to show that there are other options that could be considered.

Prompt sheet

Using a prompt sheet (Figure 25.4), the client could write down their key thoughts (my interpretations and ideas are . . .), what made them think this way (these are based on the following observations and experiences . . .), and then identify whether there are any information processing errors inherent in these thoughts (In my interpretations and ideas, am I . . . e.g. overlooking some facts?). Several alternative interpretations or ideas could derive from rephrasing the initial thoughts so that they do not contain any information-processing errors.

Generating alternative ideas

My thoughts are:

My observations / experiences which influence my thoughts are:

In my thoughts, am I:

- confusing an idea with a fact?
- fortune telling or mind reading?
- confusing possibility with probability?
- overestimating the importance and significance of isolated incidents?
- confusing a 'behaviour' with the 'person'?
- taking responsibility for something that you only have a partial influence on?
- not fully appreciating some of the facts?
- letting the way I feel cloud my judgement?
- overlooking the impact that my ideas have on my mental state? my life?
- having fixed rules such as 'must, should and ought to'?

Alternative interpretations and more helpful ideas are:

Figure 25.4 Prompt sheet to generate alternative ideas

Distancing

It is difficult to see different perspectives when we are 'tangled' in a web of our own emotions and thoughts, therefore, creating some distance from our emotional state could be useful in arriving at alternative thoughts and ideas. To this end, we could ask questions such as, 'How would someone else think in your place?' or 'What advice would you give to a friend who experiences the same difficulties as you do?' Alternatively, we could advise our client to write a script of two friends talking, where one is expressing their thoughts and the other is suggesting alternatives ideas.

Role reversal

The therapist will argue in favour of a thought and the patient against it in the place of the therapist. In this way, the therapist could demonstrate an understanding of the patient's point of view and the patient would have the opportunity to identify other perspectives. The patient and therapist could swap chairs, the patient could take notes, or use a flipchart like the therapist may do, and in the end, patient and therapist assume their original positions and discuss the learning outcome of the exercise.

Metaphors

We could use metaphors or everyday examples to demonstrate that our perception of a situation is affected by our emotional state, i.e. anxiety or low mood might cloud our judgement or our ability to appraise a situation objectively. Then we could ask the person to draw parallel links to their specific situations and thoughts.

Advantages and disadvantages

Considering the advantages and disadvantages of holding a certain idea could elicit useful information not about its factual accuracy but about how helpful or unhelpful it is in light of the person's difficulties and needs. This could be very important for engaging a client to consider alternatives when their beliefs are associated with cultural or religious norms. In this case, alternatives are considered not because the beliefs are 'flawed' but because they are unhelpful for the specific problem we are addressing. Alternative ideas, which could be more helpful in overcoming the problem, are then considered within the same cultural and religious framework.

Techniques to test and reinforce alternative interpretations and constructive ideas

The aim is to *test* the alternatives interpretations or constructive ideas by either carrying out certain activities or having guided dialogues which highlight the evidence in favour of the alternatives (for some examples, see Wells 1997: 67–85). It is important that before and after testing, the client rates their belief on the alternative thoughts and their feelings in response to these alternatives using the template given (Figure 25.5).

Monitoring and testing ideas

Feelings	Initial thoughts	Alternative ideas	Test	Outcome
How bad is it? 0----2----4----6----8----10 not at all extremely	How much do I believe it? 0%----25%----50%----75%----100% not at all completely	How much do I believe it? 0%----25%----50%----75%----100% not at all completely	If the alternative idea were true, how would I behave? How could I find out more about the alternative idea?	What have I learnt? • Re-rate belief in alternative idea. • Re-rate belief in initial thought. • Re-rate feelings.

Figure 25.5 Diary to monitor unhelpful thoughts, test alternative ideas and record emotional changes

Behavioural experiments

The nature of the experiment depends on the belief it is designed to test and it should aim at reinforcing the alternative belief rather than undermining the old one. The experiments should be negotiated and the therapist should empower the patient to design and implement appropriate behavioural experiments between sessions. A good question to guide us to the appropriate behavioural experiment is, 'If the alternative were true, how would I behave?'

Corrective information

This is an exercise which could help gather factual information from various sources, such as asking trusted friends and family, looking at reliable books and journals, talking to professionals. It is important to bear in mind that people would have the tendency to filter information and focus on confirmatory evidence for their initial 'unhelpful ideas'. Therefore, we should highlight that the objective of the exercise is to gather information about the alternative thought because this was likely to be disregarded in the first place.

Rehearsing alternative responses

An observation that people often make after testing alternative thoughts is that although they may believe in them, they do not feel any better. The aim of rehearsing alternative responses is 'not just to think but feel differently', and this is achieved by repeating the same test many times and continuously monitoring one's unhelpful thoughts/ideas and gathering evidence to reinforce alternative ones.

Cognitive and behavioural techniques: segregation or integration?

Although behavioural and cognitive techniques stem from different theoretical backgrounds (behaviour therapy from learning theories and cognitive therapy from information processing theories), in practice they are inextricably bound because any changes in behaviour may influence one's thinking and any changes in thinking are usually reflected in one's behaviour. Let us take, for example, the task of asking someone to confront an anxiety-provoking situation with the aim of controlling and reducing their symptoms of anxiety. This therapeutic activity (i.e. confrontation of an anxiety-provoking situation) which leads to the same outcome (i.e. reduction in anxiety) has a different name and a different working mechanism depending on whether we consider it within a behavioural or a cognitive perspective. A behavioural explanation would use *habituation* as the anxiety-reduction mechanism, would call the anxiety-related thoughts *feared consequences* and would term the treatment activity an *exposure task*. A cognitive explanation would describe anxiety-related thoughts as *catastrophic beliefs*, would consider the *disconfirmation* of catastrophic beliefs as the anxiety-reduction mechanism and would term the treatment task a *behavioural experiment*. In practice, it is virtually impossible to differentiate what brings about the reduction in anxiety; whether it is that people get used to it over time (as in behaviour therapy's habituation) or whether it is that they no longer believe that something terrible may happen (as in cognitive disconfirmation). Therefore, the same activity used as part of a cognitive-behavioural treatment may be explained with both a behavioural and a cognitive rationale without substantial differences in its practical delivery and outcome.

Having established the crossover between behavioural and cognitive techniques, it is also important to highlight some of their dissimilarities in the way they are delivered and the emphasis they lay on different aspects of treatment. Behavioural techniques are mainly focused activities which aim to change people's pattern of responses to external and internal stimuli. These responses are the result of acquired strong associations and positive or negative reinforcement. The application of behavioural techniques is symptom-driven and depends on delivering the right technique for the right problem. In contrast, cognitive techniques use both guided dialogues and focused activities in order to change thinking processes and beliefs which are considered the mediating factors between people's experiences and their emotional state or reactions. Cognitive techniques place great emphasis on the process of therapy and their application is guided by an individualized case formulation irrespective of diagnostic classifications relating to the problem.

In summary, behavioural techniques are symptom-driven activities which explain treatment outcome in terms of learned responses, whereas cognitive techniques are process-focused dialogues and activities which explain treatment progress in terms of belief change. In practice, it is usually difficult to distinguish whether it is the behavioural or the cognitive mechanism which produces the reduction in the symptoms, distress and disability associated with a mental health problem. Investigating the differential effect of behavioural and cognitive components of CBT could lead to more efficient treatment models and specific guidelines about which techniques may suit what patients. Whether segregated or integrated, behavioural and cognitive techniques should always be considered within the wider framework of patient care which involved the interpersonal effect of clinician input, the need for risk assessment and management, and the benefits of medical, social, family and psychological interventions other than CBT.

Conclusion

The safe and effective application of cognitive techniques is determined by careful assessment and formulation of an individual's problems and needs. It is difficult to develop an understanding of cognitive techniques without putting them into the context of specific thoughts in case examples, so further reading, training and observation of experienced practitioners is recommended.

In summary, the main points of this chapter are:

- Thoughts shape the way we behave and feel, and in turn our behaviours and feelings confirm or disconfirm these thoughts, thereby creating a cycle of interlinked thoughts, behaviours and feelings.

- Thoughts which contribute to the maintenance of mental health contain some form of inaccuracy or distortion and they are significant but unhelpful for the person.

- Cognitive techniques are guided dialogues and focused activities which aim to manage the symptoms, distress and disability associated with a problem through a process called cognitive restructuring; i.e. reducing a person's belief in their misinterpretations and unhelpful ideas by reinforcing a person's belief in *alternative interpretations* and more *constructive ideas*.

- The main techniques used in cognitive restructuring are described here in three groups: techniques to identify misinterpretations and unhelpful thoughts, techniques to generate alternative interpretations and constructive thoughts, and techniques to test and reinforce the alternatives.

- Cognitive and behavioural techniques co-exist in clinical practice because any changes in behaviour influence one's thinking and any changes in thinking are reflected in one's behaviour. However, they differ in that behavioural techniques are symptom-driven activities which explain treatment outcome in terms of learned responses, whereas cognitive techniques are process-focused dialogues and activities which explain treatment progress in terms of belief change.

Questions for reflection and discussion

1 Keep a thought record for a week, noting some of your experiences at work, college or home when you felt miserable or angry or anxious. What were the thoughts and beliefs associated with these experiences? Can you identify any information-processing errors within these thoughts? Can you come up with any alternatives? How could you test these alternatives?

2 Consider some of the differences in the care of clients with common mental health problems and with severe/enduring mental illness. What do you think are the implications for the delivery of cognitive techniques for these two client groups, in terms of:

(a) pace, intensity and duration of treatment?
(b) the professional support required and type of services in which this is usually provided?
(c) the comparative benefits of cognitive techniques in relation to other interventions (e.g. medication, family work, counselling)?

3 What is your understanding of the differences between behavioural and cognitive techniques, and how do you think these are integrated for the suitable and effective delivery of CBT in everyday practice?

Annotated bibliography

- Kingdon, D.G. and Turkington, D. (1994) *Cognitive-Behavioural Therapy for Schizophrenia*. Sussex: Guilford Press. A clear and concise book which outlines the key theoretical frameworks of understanding experiences associated with schizophrenia. It also illustrates the application of specific CBT techniques with case examples, including explanations for psychotic symptoms using a normalizing rationale and stress-vulnerability model, techniques to understand and tackle delusions, and reality testing for hallucinations. Ideal as an introductory book in the field of CBT for psychosis.
- Hawton, K., Salkovskis, P.M., Kirk, J. and Clark, D.M. (1989) *Cognitive Behaviour Therapy for Psychiatric Problems*. Oxford: Oxford University Press. A classic textbook and comprehensive practical guide for students and practitioners on CBT models and methods for mental health problems. The book covers a historical overview of behavioural and cognitive treatments, and provides detailed guidelines and case examples on CBT assessment strategies, formulation and treatment methods for anxiety disorders (generalized anxiety, panic, phobias, obsessive compulsive disorder), depression, marital problems and physical problems associated with mental heath factors (e.g. sleep disorders, medically unexplained symptoms, sexual problems, etc.). In addition, one chapter refers to CBT within the context of caring for patients with high levels of dependence on psychiatric services, and another outlines the delivery and applicability of problem solving.

References

Beck, A.T. (1976) *Cognitive Therapy and the Emotional Disorders*. New York: International Universities Press.

Blackburn I. and Davidson, K. (1995) *Cognitive Therapy for Depression and Anxiety*. London: Blackwell.

Greenberger, D. and Padesky, C.A. (1995) *Mind Over Mood: Change How you Feel by Changing the Way you Think*. London: Guilford Press.

Turkington, D. and Siddle, R. (1998) Cognitive therapy for the treatment of delusions, *Advances in Psychiatric Treatment* **4**: 235–42.

Wells, A. (1997) *Cognitive Therapy of Anxiety Disorders: A Practice Manual and Conceptual Guide*. Chichester: John Wiley.

26

Medication management to concordance

Sue Gurney

Chapter overview

Medication management involves everyone who takes medication and those who care for them (NPA 1998). Since the mid-twentieth century, compelling evidence has evolved on the efficacy of a range of psychotropic medications in reducing and managing the symptoms of an array of mental health problems. As discussed in Chapter 11 the three main classes of psychotropic preparations in use for symptom relief are: anti-depressants for treating depression, anxiolytics for anxiety and anti-psychotics for treating symptoms of psychosis (WHO 2001). The development of a new generation of psychotropic preparations although not necessarily possessing improved symptom reduction-relief efficacy, generally do cause fewer side effects. Many of these preparations are also associated with increased cost (NICE 2002).

Psychotropic medications often need to be taken continuously over a sustained period of time in order to reduce symptoms and prevent relapse. Conformity to prescribed medications is often referred to as compliance or adherence. Ceasing or partial conformity to the prescription is referred to as non- or partial compliance/adherence. These are value-laden terms (Marland and Sharkey 1999) and the literature and best practice refers to a newer concept, that of concordance: promoting an equal partnership between the professional and the user (RPS 1997). The literature also consistently indicates that non-compliance/adherence with medication is common (NPA 1998). There are reports of poor professional responsibility in prescribing psychotropic medication (Taylor *et al.* 2000) and that mental health nurses are often ill prepared/equipped for aspects of medication management (Bennett *et al.* 1995; Sin and Gamble 2003).

The terms compliance, concordance and adherence are used interchangeably throughout this chapter. The term client is used to encompass service user, patient and individual. The chapter refers primarily to the literature on compliance to anti-psychotic medication. However, most issues and concepts discussed here are transferable to other forms of psychotropic and generic medication management.

This chapter covers:

- exploring the language of medication management;
- factors affecting compliance;
- the rationale for interventions;
- reviewing the evidence;
- implications for practice;
- conclusion;
- reflection.

Exploring the language of medication management

The use and understanding of the language in this area has significant meaning and impact for professional practice (Repper and Perkins 1998). The literature reveals a development in terminology reflected in a shift in the balance of power of the relationship/alliance of the prescriber and health - care workers with the client. Overall, this describes a change in value, from the client as a passive recipient of health care to an informed partner in health care decision making.

The following descriptions from the literature illustrate this development. Dodds *et al.* (2000) define compliance as the extent to which a client's behaviour regarding taking medication coincides with medical or health advice. Marland and Sharkey (1999) discuss the value-laden term 'compliance' and that interpretation varies with each individual professional. They also propose two further dimensions to the concept. The first as being process defined, influenced by the degree of conformity to the prescription. The second as being outcome defined, being determined by the maintenance of wellness. Interestingly, this latter dimension implies that wellness may not correspond with compliance.

The language of compliance then undertakes a further shift, to the concept of effective, collaborative working with clients (Kemp *et al.* 1997). These authors identify successful collaboration between professionals and the client as the most valuable approach in improving compliance, assuming that compliance is appropriate. The concept of collaboration has since shifted to one of concordance, suggesting that an equal partnership, in working harmoniously, needs to exist between health care workers and the client before clients will 'buy' in to the need to comply, if appropriate, with treatment (RPS 1997).

There is a clear relationship between compliance with prescribed medication and best practice in medication management. However, it is imperative that compliance is not the main target. In fact non-compliance for someone suffering from severe adverse reactions might be life-saving in cases of inappropriate prescription. Hence, a crucial element of best practice in medication management-concordance is about health professionals, clients and carers recognizing that a problem may be medication related.

Permeating into the literature and into current health policy is a further shift along the language continuum with the concept of choice. The power, the opportunity of clients to make informed choices about their health '. . . positive outcomes are increased if people are informed about their choices, allowed to choose and given their choice. That is the clearest finding based on the views of thousands of people with direct experience of mental illness' (Hogman and Sandamas 2000).

Compliance rates

Interpreting the literature is difficult, as there are no agreed definitions of non-compliance. These can vary from complete cessation or verbal refusal, to any significant deviation from prescription, including dosage errors or failure to attend appointments. Neither are there any valid ways of measuring compliance which may include methods of observation, self-reporting, pill counts, urine and blood assays, and these will only determine current compliance (Gray *et al.* 2002). In clinical practice, client and carer reports, clinical assessment and observation are mainly subjective measures of compliance.

Studies report rates of compliance with anti-psychotic medication ranging from 10 to 80 per cent (Kemp *et al.* 1997) with an overall average of 50 per cent (Bebbington 1995). Kisling (1994) reports that 50 per cent of people with schizophrenia relapse within the first year of illness and that this increases to 85 per cent within the first five years. The study suggests that with sound relapse-prevention programmes, which include medication compliance, rates could be reduced to around 15 per cent. More recent work by Cramer and Rosenheck (1998) suggest an average compliance rate of 42 per cent. This is similar to compliance rates for people with 'physical' disorders (Carter *et al.* 2003).

Factors which influence compliance with medication

Little work has been undertaken on the relationship of medication compliance with theoretical models of health behaviour change which might provide explanation, understanding and potential for therapeutic development (Gray *et al.* 2002). However, the literature does identify a wide variety of factors that appear to influence compliance to prescribed medications. These can be categorized into the following three themes which are illustrated below with some examples (Kemp *et al.* 1997).

1   **The person:** Culture, values, beliefs, prejudices, experience, support networks, family and carer involvement, personality, awareness and understanding of the problem, use of non-prescribed substances, e.g. cannabis or alcohol.

2   **The illness:** Cognitive impairment, thought disorder, depression, features of hallucinations.

3   **The treatment:** Value of alliance with clinicians, complexity of the treatment, the form of treatment, the treatment setting, the experience of side effects, stigma, effectiveness of the medication, polypharmacy, ease of accessing medications.

Compliance with medication is a multi-faceted issue. Decisions on whether to comply with a prescribed medication regime can be influenced by a wide range of factors, the reduction/relief of symptoms being just one.

The rationale for interventions

Although the literature exploring the benefits of improved medication compliance is limited (NPA 1998), there is a strong rationale for addressing this area for the following reasons. The first is a moral-ethical one, related to symptom reduction/relief and improving and maintaining the perceived quality/quality of life of the client; taking into account the holistic needs of the individual, a cost-benefit analysis of the prescribed medication and an awareness that improvement of health may not always be a motivating factor. The second is related to the impact of adverse reactions to medication. General studies have identified that a high proportion of all hospital admissions, general practitioner and outpatient consultations are a result of the impact of non-compliance and, or, adverse drug reactions (RPC 1996; NPA 1998). The third is related to costs of health and social care. The direct cost of schizophrenia in England and Wales is estimated to be in excess of £1 billion, with drug costs accounting for 5 per cent of this sum (NICE 2002). In 1992 £76 million was spent on 1.2 million annual prescriptions for schizophrenia, with a week on a psychiatric ward costed at £960, community support £230 and a 30-day prescription for the atypical drug olanzapine costed at £209 (Petit-Zeman 2000). In 2002 overall prescription costs rose to £6.1 billion, one-tenth of all NHS spending, with £230 million of medicines returned to pharmacies and an uncalculated cost/amount being privately disposed of (Crouch 2003).

There are also indirect costs: the costs of caring, loss of employment and the loss of active citizenship. In 1990/1 the indirect costs of schizophrenia in the UK were estimated to be at least £1.7 billion (NICE 2002). From the evidence there is obviously a clear rationale for careful, individual tailored prescribing and support in improving the quality of life for people receiving prescribed medication treatments. There is also the added potential of a positive effect in reducing direct and indirect costs.

Reviewing the evidence

A detailed systematic review of the literature on interventions to improve the taking of prescribed medication can be found in the Cochrane Library (Haynes *et al.* 2002). The review analysed 39 randomized control trials for short- and long-term interventions. Of the short-term interventions only one showed a positive effect on compliance and clinical outcome. Of the long-term interventions 18 had an improved effect on compliance, and 16 of these had improved treatment outcomes. The reviewers concluded that methods for improving compliance are generally complex, not very effective and require development.

A systematic review of randomized control trials of interventions to improve compliance with anti-psychotic medication (Dodds *et al.* 2000) yielded eight trials. The main findings were that six of the studies showed improvement in compliance rates. However, only three of these reached statistical significance; trials of individualized behavioural tailoring regimes and compliance therapy. The dominant themes of the effective interventions were counselling and psycho-education (supplying written information, offering one-to-one and groupwork) family educational programmes, cognitive-behavioural therapy (CBT), behavioural tailoring approaches (tailoring regimes to personal lifestyles), teaching problem-solving skills and working in collaboration and individualized ways with clients. The reviewers concluded, in much the same way as Haynes *et al.* (2002), that compliance could be improved through complex interventions.

A literature review on interventions to enhance compliance with anti-psychotic medication states that interventions can broadly be divided into three categories: educational, behavioural and cognitive behavioural (Gray *et al.* 2002). Educational interventions aim to provide information to clients about both their illness and medication with the goal of increasing understanding and promoting compliance. Group and individual client education has been evaluated using a variety of methodologies including a number of randomized controlled trials (Macpherson *et al.* 1996; Gray 2000). Results of these studies have consistently shown that just giving information will improve the client's understanding of their illness and medication but will not reduce the numbers who cease taking medication. Behavioural interventions aim to simplify treatment regimes and minimize side effects to help clients practically tailor their treatment to suit their daily routine. For example, clients can be encouraged to take medication last thing at night before they go to bed to minimize the sedative effects of medication, or taking medication can be linked with a routine behaviour, such as making a cup of tea first thing in the morning. There is some evidence that this approach can be useful (Boczkowski *et al.* 1985).

In recent years the focus of research into improving the taking of medication has focused on CBT approaches. These interventions focus on working collaboratively with the client to explore their beliefs about illness and treatment. Lecompte and Pelc (1996) tested a CBT programme based around five therapeutic strategies: engagement, psycho-education, identifying prodromal symptoms and developing coping strategies, behavioural strategies for reinforcing compliant behaviour and correcting false beliefs about medication. In a randomized controlled trial, clients who received the CBT intervention spent significantly less time in hospital than those in the control group, suggesting that this approach has promise.

Along similar lines Kemp *et al.* (1997) devised compliance therapy. Key principles include working collaboratively, emphasizing personal choice and responsibility and focusing on client's concerns about treatment. The therapy draws on a background of interpersonal skills, flexible approaches, education, motivational interviewing (Miller and Rollnick 1991) and CBT approaches. Paced intervention is divided into three phases that acknowledge that readiness to change is on a continuum. Phase 1 explores the client's experiences of treatment by helping them to review their illness history. In phase 2 the common concerns about treatment are discussed and explored. Phase 3 explores long-term prevention and strategies for avoiding relapse.

Compliance therapy was evaluated in a randomized controlled trial (Kemp *et al.* 1998). Seventy-four inpatients experiencing psychosis were randomly assigned to receive either compliance therapy or non-specific counselling. Patients received four to six sessions with a research psychiatrist lasting, on average, 40 minutes. Treatment adherence was significantly better in the compliance-therapy group resulting in enhanced community tenure, with patients in the compliance-therapy group taking longer to relapse than those who received non-specific counselling.

There is a growing body of work from the user movement that identifies a range of strategies that users of mental health services and those suffering with mental distress find useful. Medication may not always be a first choice. However, there is recognition of a place and value among other strategies (Faulkner and Layzell 2000; Hogman and Sandamas 2000). Non-medical interventions may include talking approaches, diet and nutrition, exercise, training, education, art, music, homeopathy, herbal medicine and supportive relationships.

In sum, medication compliance is an area of significant clinical importance and is rightly attracting increasing interest and attention. Based on the available evidence, medication concordance should aim to help maximize the clinical potential of tailored medication prescribing.

Implications for practice

There is a clear rationale related to individual needs, beliefs, quality of life, sensitive practice and tailored prescribing for implementing the evidence from the literature into practice. This is based on a fundamental premise of the approach of concordance being client-centred, client-led, and borrowing heavily from the principles, skills and techniques of the literature and particularly that of compliance therapy (Kemp *et al.* 1997).

From the literature the key areas for practice development are:

1 *Foundation skills*: reliant on interpersonal skills, partnership working, client centred-client led.

2 *Assessment*: baseline and systematic assessments of general health, lifestyle, quality of life, syndrome, symptom and side effects of medication.

3 *Pharmacology*: tailoring medication to individual needs with reference to best practice prescribing (Taylor *et al.* 2000; NICE 2002), systematic assessment of side effects utilizing valid and reliable measures (Day *et al.* 1995), and an in-depth knowledge of the prescribed medication in the following areas:

   - pharmacokinetics: how the medication biologically functions in the body through the process of absorption, distribution, metabolism and elimination;
   - pharmacodynamics: where, how and why the medication acts;
   - pharmacogenetics: awareness of the variation of ethnic and racial responses to medication;

4 *Exploring the client's illness story*: experience, attitudes, beliefs, awareness and understanding; utilizing interpersonal skills, information exchange, in normalizing and health-promotion opportunities. It is also essential to maintain awareness that there can be negative connotations to improved compliance and that it is imperative to understand the reasons for non-compliance.

5 *Exploring ambivalence towards treatment*: utilizing interpersonal, problem solving, CBT and motivational interviewing approaches, skills and techniques.

6 *Maintaining wellness*: exploring strategies, skills and techniques for managing health.

Medication concordance is a complex activity that is fundamentally about health behaviour change. Another factor, which makes this particularly pertinent to nurses, is the development of the extended role in nurse prescribing; nurses are in a key position. In the future clients are more likely to see a nurse prescriber and to see specialist nurses who recommend and influence prescribing.

Conclusion

The overall compliance rates to psychotropic medication appear similar to those of generic medication prescribing. Findings from the literature indicate that interventions to improve compliance and outcomes are generally complex and require innovation. The concept of medication concordance is that of an equal partnership with the client, a move along the continuum from a paternalistic model towards a client-centred approach. There is increasing emphasis on the role of the health worker in exploring issues and exchanging information, so that clients can make informed choices. This is a shift from an illness to a health focus model.

The mental health worker has to balance knowledge, skills, techniques and interventions based on evidence and practice development. Medication concordance requires an investment in time and money, but has major potential implications for cost and resource savings. For the future all professionals will need to accept a blurring of responsibility, to share information, joint training and identification of medication-related problems (NPA 1998). Finally, a statement, on medication concordance, from the Chief Nursing Officer states '. . . there is no doubt that there are some tricky issues, but if you enable the patient to take part in decision-making the outcome is better. Nurses have to work through the risks with patients. It's about sitting down and learning with them about the treatment' (Crouch 2003: 6).

Questions for reflection and discussion

1 Consider the rationale for the use of psychotropic medication and what negative effects there might be from improving compliance?

2 Put yourself in the position of a person taking medication, that gives you a feeling of inner restlessness, less energy and considerable weight gain. What changes would you like to make? How would you do this? What help might you need? How could you tell if things had improved?

3 Medications have side effects; there is a cost-benefit to usage. Think of a person you have known or nursed who has received a medication treatment. Make a list, one of the costs and the other of the benefits of the treatment. What is your conclusion? Now give each element in the list a weighting, say from 1 (not important) to 8 (very important) then total the figures. Are your findings the same? Has this highlighted any other issues?

Annotated bibliography

- Watson, D. (2003) The psychopharmacological treatment of schizophrenia: a critique, *Journal of Mental Health Practice*, March, (**6**)6: 10–14. Gournay, K. (2003) Drug treatments for schizophrenia: why they offer the only hope to patients, *Journal of Mental Health Practice*, March, (**6**)6: 16–17. These two articles discuss the concept of psychopharmacology in relation to differing models of mental disorder in contemporary practice.

- Rollnick, S., Mason, P. and Butler, C. (2000) *Health Behaviour Change – A Guide for Practitioners*. China: Churchill Livingstone. This book offers a patient-centred framework for any behaviour change. The authors promote the idea of a generic change method and have looked for common ground across theories and models: motivational interviewing, problem solving and brief solution-focused therapy. The result is a collection of strategies, rather than a discrete method. Some strategies have been evaluated others have not.
- Faulkner, A. and Layzell, S. (2000) *Strategies for Living: A Report of User-led Research into People's Strategies for Living with Mental Distress*. London: Mental Health Foundation. This report builds on the work of a large user-led survey and gives an understanding of how people live, cope and manage mental distress. Further reports and links can be found on the Mental Health Foundations website: www.mentalhealth.org.uk/

References

Bebbington, P.E. (1995) The content and context of compliance, *International Clinical Psychopharmacology* **9** (suppl. 5): 41–50.

Bennett, J., Done, J., Harrison-Read, P. and Hunt, B. (1995) Assessing the side-effects of antipsychotic drugs: a survey of CPN practice, *Journal of Psychiatric and Mental Health Nursing* **2**: 177–82.

Boczkowski, J.A., Zeichner, A. and De Santo, N. (1985) Neuroleptic compliance among chronic schizophrenic outpatients: an intervention outcome report, *Journal of Consulting and Clinical Psychology* **53**: 666–71.

Carter, S., Taylor, D. and Levenson, R. (2003) A question of choice-compliance in medicine taking. A preliminary review. London: The Medicines Partnership www.medicines-partnership.org/research-evidence/major-reviews/a-question-of-choice (15 December 2003).

Cramer, J.A. and Rosenheck, R. (1998) Compliance with medication regimens for mental and physical disorders, *Psychiatric Services* **49**: 196–201.

Crouch, D. (2003) Sharing medication agreements with patients, *Nursing Times* **(99)**38: 34–6.

Day, J.C., Wood, G., Dewey, M. and Bentall, R.P. (1995) A self rating scale for measuring neuroleptic side effects, *British Journal of Psychiatry* **166**: 650–3.

Dodds, F., Rebair-Brown, A. and Parsons, S. (2000) A systematic review of randomized controlled trials that attempt to identify interventions that improve patient compliance with prescribed antipsychotic medication, *Clinical Effectiveness in Nursing* **4**: 47–53.

Faulkner, A. and Layzell, S. (2000) *Strategies for Living: A Report of User-led Research into People's Strategies for Living with Mental Distress*. London: Mental Health Foundation.

Gray, R. (2000) Does patient education enhance compliance with Clozapine? A preliminary investigation, *Journal of Psychiatric and Mental Health Nursing* **7**: 285–6.

Gray, R., Wykes, T. and Gournay, K. (2002) From compliance to concordance: a review of the literature on interventions to enhance compliance with antipsychotic medication, *Journal of Psychiatric and Mental Health Nursing* **9**: 277–84.

Haynes, R.B., McDonald, H., Garg, A.X. and Montague, P. (2002) *Interventions for Helping Patients Follow Prescription for Medications (Cochrane Review)*, in *The Cochrane Library*, Issue 4, 2003. Chichester: John Wiley & Sons Ltd.

Hogman, G. and Sandamas, G. (2000) *A Question of Choice*. London: Rethink.

Kemp, R., Hayward, P. and David, A. (1997) *Compliance Therapy Manual*. London: The Maudsley Hospital.

Kemp, R., Kirov, G., Everitt, B., Hayward, P. and David, A. (1998) Randomized controlled trial of compliance therapy. 18-month follow-up, *British Journal of Psychiatry* **172** (May): 413–19.

Kisling, W. (1994) Compliance, quality assurance and standards for relapse prevention in schizophrenia, *Acta Psychiatrica Scandinavia* **89** (suppl. 382): 16–24.

Lecompte, D. and Pelc, I. (1996) A cognitive-behavioural programme to improve compliance with medication in patients with schizophrenia, *International Journal of Mental Health* **25**: 51–6.

Macpherson, R., Jerrom, B. and Hughes, A. (1996) A controlled study of education about drug treatment in schizophrenia, *British Journal of Psychiatry* **168**: 709–17.

Marland, G. and Sharkey, V. (1999) Depot neuroleptics, schizophrenia and the role of the nurse: is practice evidence based? A review of the literature, *Journal of Advanced Nursing* **30**: 1255–62.

Miller, W. and Rollnick, S. (eds) (1991) *Motivational Interviewing: Preparing People to Change Addictive Behaviour*. New York. Guilford Press.

National Institute for Clinical Excellence (NICE) (2002) Technology Appraisal No. 43: Guidance on the use of newer (atypical) antipsychotic drugs for the treatment of schizophrenia. www.nice.org.uk

National Pharmaceutical Association (NPA) (1998) Medication Management: Everybody's Problem. St Albans. www.npa.co.uk/pdf/nhsdev/mmgmnt.pdf (15 December 2003).

Petit-Zeman, S. (2000) Choice of a new life? *Guardian. Society* (6 December): 12.

Repper, J. and Perkins, R. (1998) Different but normal, language, labels and professional mental health practice, *Mental Health Care* **2**: 90–3.

Royal College of Psychiatrists (RCP) (1996) *Report of the Confidential Inquiry into Homicides and Suicides by Mentally Ill People*. London: Royal College of Psychiatrists.

Royal Pharmaceutical Society of Great Britain and Merck Sharp Dohme (1997) From compliance to concordance: achieving goals in medicine taking. London: Royal Pharmaceutical Society of Great Britain.

Sin, J. and Gamble, C. (2003) Managing side effects to the optimum: valuing a client's experience, *Journal of Psychiatric and Mental Health Nursing* **10**: 147–53.

Taylor, D., McConnell, D., McConnell, H. and Kerwin, R. (2000) The Maudsley Prescribing Guidelines, 6th edn. London: Martin Dunitz.

World Health Organization (WHO) (2001) *The World Health Report: 2001: Mental Health: New Understanding, New Hope*. World Health Organization: Geneva. www.who.int/whr2001/2001/main/en/pdf/whr2001.en.pdf (15 December 2003).

27

Therapeutic management of aggression and violence

Susan Sookoo

Chapter overview

The therapeutic management of violence and aggression is not separate to, but rather an integral part of routine care. Aggressive incidents are not isolated events, but take place within a clinical, psychological, environmental and social context. Consequently, a broad range of interventions is required in order to deal with violence and aggression and prevention is always more desirable than cure. This chapter is largely concerned with methods used to safely manage anger, aggression and violence when they occur or are imminent. As such, the techniques described can be seen as 'as required' interventions aimed at short-term management. The focus is on methods used in ward environments. Although non-physical interventions may also be applicable to community settings, safe management of aggression in the community is built on effective risk-assessment processes, multi-disciplinary team working and attention to local policies on safety when visiting clients.

However, methods for dealing with imminent aggression alone do not constitute complete management of violence and aggression: an understanding of the underlying factors that influence such behaviour and reduce the need for short-term intervention is also necessary. In addition, this chapter should be read in conjunction with Chapter 22 on engaging with clients, Chapter 9 on the creation of a therapeutic milieu and Chapter 8 on assessing and managing risk. In summary, this chapter covers:

- the factors which influence the incidence of violence and aggression in inpatient mental health services;
- mechanisms underlying anger and aggression;
- de-escalation techniques;
- physical interventions.

Some commonly used terms are defined in Box 27.1.

Box 27.1 Definition of commonly used terms

- Anger – a subjective emotional state involving physiological arousal and associated cognitions. This can be adaptive, but frequency, intensity and duration of anger can make it dysfunctional (Novaco 1983).
- Aggression – a disposition to inflict harm. This may be verbally expressed in threats to harm people or objects, or result in actual harm (Wright *et al.* 2002).
- Hostility – a personality trait, which reflects a style of appraisal in which the actions of others are seen as harmful. This can result in anger or detachment (Novaco 1983).
- Violence – acts in which there is use of force to attempt to inflict physical harm.

(Wright *et al.* 2002)

Background

There is a public perception of the psychiatric patient as dangerous to the community at large (Vinestock 1996), as well as increasing concern about the level of violence and aggression occurring within health care settings. Violence against staff in the NHS as a whole has risen at least 13 per cent in the period 2002–2003 (National Audit Office 2003) with 95,000 reported incidents during this period. The level of incidence within mental health and learning disability trusts has been reported to be three times higher than the average in all other trusts (NHS Executive 1998/1999, in Gournay 2001). A survey of care in acute psychiatric wards (Sainsbury Centre for Mental Health 1998) found that nearly a third of patients were involved in incidents of non-physical aggression, 9 per cent carried out assaults on staff or other patients without causing injury, and 5 per cent carried out assault causing minor injury. Reported rates are likely to be far less than real incidence (Gournay 2001).

This chapter does not attempt to explore the nature of the relationship between mental disorder and violence. The nature of this relationship is complex (see, for example, Monaghan 1993), and the above figures should not suggest that a relationship between mental illness and violence is inevitable. It is worth noting, though, that mentally ill people living in the community are twice as likely to be the *victim* of violent abuse as the general population (NMC press release 2003). The reasons for an apparent increase in the level of violent incidents within health services are not clear but may include a higher level of violence within society in general (Wright *et al.* 2002), the reduced number of hospital beds resulting in only the most disturbed patients being admitted to inpatient units, or the effect of non-therapeutic hospital environments (Sainsbury Centre for Mental Health 1998).

The evidence base

Violence is a complex phenomenon and it is not possible to state a theory in terms of 'violent behaviour is caused by *x, y* and *z*'. As Mason and Chandley (1999) state, there are probably as many theories of violence as there are aggressive incidents. Wright *et al.* (2002) in a report prepared for the UKCC on management of violence in psychiatric inpatient settings, summarize the literature on possible contributory factors, discussed below.

Demographic factors

Studies reporting relationships between age, gender, ethnicity and socio-economic status on violence report conflicting findings, probably because intervening variables other than demographic ones account for differences between groups. The Royal College of Psychiatrists Research Unit (1998) cautiously list several demographic or personal variables which may be risk factors for violence, as follows:

- a history of violence;
- youth;
- male gender;
- association with sub-cultures prone to violence.

Clinical factors

Wright *et al.* (2002) report an increased relative risk of violence in patients with psychotic illnesses, although once again there is no clear relationship between specific symptoms and violence, and the relationship does not seem to persist across settings. For example, one study (Lowenstein *et al.* 1990) found manic patients to have higher levels of inpatient violence than any other diagnostic group. Non-compliance with treatment and use of drugs or alcohol also complicate the picture. The Royal College of Psychiatrists Research Unit (1998), in their clinical practice guidelines for the management of imminent violence, suggest clinical factors that range across diagnosis, listed in Box 27.2.

Box 27.2 Clinical factors associated with increased risk of aggression

- substance abuse;
- agitation or excitement;
- hostility or suspiciousness;
- a preoccupation with violence;
- poor collaboration with treatment;
- delusions or hallucinations focused on a particular person;
- delusions of control with a violent theme;
- impulsive personality traits.

Wright *et al.* (2002) conclude that although symptoms may have some role in influencing violence and aggression, it is more likely that it is the effect of symptoms in reducing ability to deal with external demands and interpersonal conflict that is implicated in violent and aggressive behaviour.

Environmental factors

The Royal College of Psychiatrists Research Unit (1998) acknowledge that hospital wards are unnatural environments, which nevertheless should aim to create a safe, homely atmosphere which allows for safety and for privacy. The supporting social environment is equally important. Patients in a US maximum security facility reported that they often did not understand the reasons for ward rules and expectations (Caplan 1993), while patients in the Sainsbury Centre survey of acute wards (1998) reported disliking the refrain 'the policy is . . .'. Boredom and lack of structured activity may also contribute to violence and aggression. Katz and Kirkland examined levels of violence on psychiatric wards in the USA and concluded that, 'violence was more frequent and extreme in wards in which staff functions were unclear, and in which events such as activities, meetings or staff–patient encounters were unpredictable' (1990: 262). Shah (1993) summarized research suggesting that levels of violence increase at times when patients congregate with little structured activity, e.g. medication and meal times (see Box 27.3).

Staffing factors

Patients surveyed by the Royal College of Psychiatrists Research Unit (1998) emphasized that talking and listening are key interventions not to be undervalued. They focused on boredom, staff attitudes and staffing levels as factors affecting levels of violence. Patients in the Sainsbury Centre survey (1998) indicated that they wanted more access to staff. However, organizational and resource factors may militate against this. Shah (1993) summarized possible staff factors associated with higher levels of violence including: use of temporary staff, under-involvement of medical staff, poor communication, demoralization and incompetence among staff members and high staff turnover. It may be that these factors create a 'high expressed emotion' environment. Determining the optimum number of nursing staff in a clinical setting is complex. Owen *et al.* (1998) found an association between higher numbers of nursing staff and higher levels of violence, which may reflect increased numbers of staff as a response to violence. On the other hand, Morrison and Lehane (1995) found that over a two-year period in one psychiatric hospital, as staffing levels increased, use of seclusion fell. This study also reported that fewer seclusions took place when experienced nurses were on duty, while Owen *et al.* (1998) reported that increased violence is associated with lower levels of experience and lack of staff training in control of aggression techniques.

The Royal College of Psychiatrists Research Unit (1998), in reviewing the evidence on the influence of the physical and social environment, concluded that the quantitative evidence is too weak to draw firm conclusions about relationships between these and incidence of aggression. However, they also argue that addressing these issues makes intuitive sense. Possible influencing factors are summarized in Box 27.3.

Box 27.3 Aspects of the physical and social environment which may minimize levels of aggression

Physical environment
- clean
- allow for daylight and fresh air
- avoid overcrowding
- have controlled noise levels (for example, a separate TV room)
- allow for control of temperature and ventilation
- provide designated smoking and non-smoking areas
- allow for privacy in bedrooms, bathrooms and toilets
- provide sightlines allowing people to see what is happening in different parts of the ward

Social environment
- rationale offered for ward expectations
- open communication processes between patients, ward staff and management
- patient involvement in decision making
- planned, predictable activity
- opportunity for social and recreational activity
- clear staff functions
- adequate and consistent staffing
- effective multi-disciplinary working
- commitment to staff training and support

Royal College of Psychiatrists Research Unit's guidelines (1998) form the basis of an audit tool used to establish a baseline from which to improve standards. Findings of the national audit for the period 1999–2000 indicated that many aspects of the physical and social environment and staff training and communication fell short of the audit standards (Royal College of Psychiatrists Research Unit 2000).

Practice model

Improving services and practice in light of the factors above is likely to have a long-term and lasting impact in levels of violence. However, in the best planned environments, anger, aggression and violence will still occur, and in this case an understanding of the appropriate level of intervention matched to the phase of aggression is needed.

One model which lends itself to a range of interventions is that proposed by Novaco (1983) in his development of an anger-management treatment programme. In this model, anger is seen as a state of physiological arousal leading to tension and irritability which lead to cognitions producing antagonistic thought patterns such as attention focus, suspicious ruminations and a hostile attitude. The model is contextual in that stressors create physical arousal, which leads to irritability. As exposure continues, thought patterns become antagonistic, leading to faulty appraisal of behaviour or situations. Inappropriate coping mechanisms in response to this can cause aggression. Goleman's book, *Emotional Intelligence* (1995), describes a similar cascade of events in which a sense of threat or danger evokes the fight or flight mechanism, invoking a train of angry thoughts which in turn contribute to increased physiological arousal, rendering the person more susceptible to external triggers, each wave becoming more intense and increasing the level of physiological arousal. This suggests that one form of intervention is to engage the angry person in order to lower arousal and allow reappraisal of angry cognitions, termed 'de-escalation'.

De-escalation

The Sainsbury Centre (2001) includes understanding of de-escalation skills as a core capability for mental health nurses working in acute settings. The term 'de-escalation' refers to the 'processes by which a patient's expressed anger or aggression is defused, so that a calmer state ensues' (Royal College of Nursing, Midwifery and Health Visiting (RCN) 1997). In this position statement, the RCN (1997) describe these short-term interventions as utilizing a combination of immediate risk assessment together with verbal and non-verbal communication skills. Application is divided into several phases.

Understanding reasons for anger or aggression

As well as the clinical and social factors underlying aggression, the individual's specific situation has to be considered. The person may have experienced (or perceive that they have experienced) personal criticism, restriction or control, unfair treatment, frustration of intentions or the irritating behaviour of others. Nurses, therefore, need to be aware of what is happening both on the ward in general and for the patient in particular, and may be contributing to their anger. Stressors might also include staff behaviours. Wright *et al.* (2002) report that research shows violent incidents to be more likely when there is aversive stimulation from staff in terms of imposing limits or frustrating requests.

Assessing immediate risk

Patients in the RCP (1998) consultation felt that staff could predict incidents of aggression if they listened to what patients were saying and allowed them to discuss feelings of anger and/or symptoms without fear of restraint, restriction or medication. A study by Whittington and Patterson (1996) matched aggressive and non-aggressive patients and found that the groups were distinguished by levels of verbal abuse, threatening gestures and either very high or very low activity. Verbal abuse was the most common behaviour and preceded two-thirds of physical attacks. As ever, the caveat is that in many cases key behaviours were exhibited for long periods without being followed by violence. The RCP concluded that there was no consensus on clinically useful predictors of violence. Despite this, possible antecedents derived from the Royal College of Nursing (RCN) (1997) and RCP (1998) are indicated as shown in Box 27.4.

Box 27.4 Possible indicators of anger and aggression

Possible antecedents are indicated when the person:

- focuses attention on what is causing anger and continues to dwell on this;
- perceives threat from others or is suspicious;
- reacts in an exaggerated manner to problems;
- shows increased physical arousal – restlessness, pacing, erratic movements;
- shows increased volume of speech;
- has a tense facial expression – fixed stare, clenched jaw, makes constant eye contact;
- refuses to communicate or withdraws;
- makes verbal threats or gestures;
- reports angry or violent feelings.

Prior knowledge of the patient is also used in this risk assessment – have they been verbally abusive in the past, do they see staff as unhelpful, are they facing high levels of stress, have they used alcohol or drugs recently, have carers reported imminent violence, have these signs been present before any previous episodes of aggression?

Monitoring safety

Having identified an increased risk of violence, maintaining safety is also necessary. Practice points drawn from the RCN (1997) and RCP (1998) guidelines are listed in Box 27.5.

Once a risk assessment and safety check indicate that it is possible to approach the person safely, both non-verbal and verbal skills should be used:

Non-verbal communication

- Maintain an adequate distance – this is more than usual social distance, as when dealing with an angry person as closeness may be interpreted as threat, or may increase tension.

> **Box 27.5** Practice points for monitoring safety
>
> - Don't isolate yourself – check that colleagues know your whereabouts.
> - Check that you are familiar with mechanisms for calling for help and that you have access to these.
> - Check escape routes – avoid corners.
> - If isolated when a violent incident occurs, the priority is to get away from the situation and summon help. Do not tackle a violent person alone, whatever your or the patient's gender or size.
> - Make a visual check of the immediate area for potential weapons. (For example there may be chairs, cups or glasses in the day area or dining room; if in a kitchen there may be knives or boiling water; in a bathroom razors or aerosols may be present.) If identified, the priority is to maintain distance and offer the option to the person to leave the area and continue discussion elsewhere.

- Stand at an angle to the patient to avoid appearing confrontational and to allow for defence (put weight on back foot). Don't point and don't touch the person.
- Maintain normal eye contact – staring can be threatening, avoiding can seem dismissive.
- Appear calm and speak slowly using clear and short sentences. However, avoid being patronizing (avoid telling patient to calm down!). Be courteous, and use the person's name.
- Be aware of your own reactions, which may be fear or anger, and try to consider the patient's point of view – they might be anxious as well as angry. Don't feel that you have to win any argument or that you have to deal with this situation alone and effectively in order to be a 'good nurse'.

Verbal communication

The aim here is to continue communication and move on to problem solving. The RCN (1997) suggest the following:

- Engage in conversation and most importantly acknowledge concerns, allowing the person time to express their worries or complaints. Ask the person to sit down with you or go to a more private area (as long as other staff know where you are). Ask the person for the facts of the problem as they see them.
- Use reflective listening to acknowledge concerns. This is more skilled than it appears and is not simply stating the obvious or parroting what the person says. Imagine your own response if after a particularly

difficult day, a friend said, 'It sounds like you're angry.' Be specific –
'I can see you're disappointed and upset that you won't be able to go
home this weekend.'

- Convey that you want to help the person find a solution, e.g. 'Give
  me half-an-hour to try to find out what has happened.' Be realistic and
  do not make promises that cannot be kept. Allow the person to start
  generating options for dealing with the problem. Do not lecture or
  challenge.

Physical intervention

Verbal interventions work up to a certain point of moderate anger. Goleman
(1995) argues that after a certain stage, they have no effect as people are
unable to process information. Further, the relationship between anger and
aggression is not straightforward. Absence of overt anger does not mean
that aggression will not occur. Where aggression leads to gain – material,
social or psychological – anger is not necessary to precipitate it. If, at this
stage, aggression or violence occurs, physical intervention may be needed
to maintain safety.

Restraint

The aim here is not to describe techniques for physical restraint. These
should be taught on an approved course and involve an assessment of competence to use physical techniques. However, they should be used judiciously
with an understanding of the legal, professional and ethical context. The
Mental Health Act (1983) Code of Practice (Department of Health 1999)
makes clear that providers of inpatient psychiatric care should have policies
on the use of restraint. The RCP (1998) additionally state that there should
be local guidance as to circumstances under which it is acceptable to
use restraint (and seclusion). Their guidelines (Box 27.6) give the following
possible reasons for use of restraint.

Box 27.6 Situations in which restraint might be necessary

- serious degree of urgency and danger;
- significant physical attacks;
- significant threats or attempts at self-injury;
- seriously destructive of property;
- prolonged and serious verbal abuse, threats or disruption;
- prolonged over-activity and consequent risk of exhaustion;
- risk of serious accident to self or others;
- attempts to abscond if under Section and in an open ward.

However, restraint is a 'last resort' intervention. The RCP place it at the end of a hierarchy of interventions including verbal and communication techniques. The UKCC *Guidelines for Mental Health and Learning Disabilities* (1998) state that risk assessment and management 'must be directed to the overall best interests of your client, be based on the principle of the minimum necessary force or action to achieve the desired outcome and be carried out in a professional, competent and safe manner' (UKCC 1998: 23). However, the RCN (1997) acknowledge that use of restraint should not necessarily be seen as a failure, as people in an extreme state of anger or provocation might not be able to respond to verbal interventions. The priority in this case is to clear the area of other patients and call for help. 'Breakaway techniques' may also be used to get away from the situation when it is not possible to get help. Again, these techniques should be taught as part of an approved course.

Restraint techniques developed from Control and Restraint (C & R) training developed by the Prison Service (Wright *et al.* 2002). The term C & R should not however be used within psychiatric services as techniques have been adapted for this setting. Specific techniques have also evolved and changed in the face of deaths and injuries sustained using C & R techniques in mental health settings. Staff should attend regular updates to ensure that they are familiar with changes. In a survey of acute wards in London (Gournay *et al.* 1998) only one Trust out of 11 did not routinely train ward staff in use of physical restraint. However, it has been acknowledged that guidance is needed on the regularity of updates (Wright *et al.* 2000). Underlying principles of physical restraint are given below, incorporating guidance from the RCP (1998), RCN (1998), Wright *et al.* (2000, 2002):

- It should only be carried out by trained, competent staff as part of an agreed multi-disciplinary strategy.
- It should not involve the infliction of pain.
- The privacy and dignity of the patient should be maintained.
- A visual check for weapons should be made before restraining.
- The response should be coordinated and responsibility should be allocated to an identified team member for clear communication to the team and the patient throughout.
- There should be a hierarchical system of physical response, including the integration of physical and verbal de-escalation techniques which allow the patient a return to autonomy as quickly as possible while maintaining safety.
- Restraint should not automatically be followed by seclusion and/or medication, rather an ongoing assessment of the need for intervention should be made.
- A report should always be made of any incidence of restraint.
- Post-incident support should be offered to staff involved and the patient. The patient should be offered an explanation of why restraint was necessary.

- There should be a procedure by which patients can make a complaint about restraint.
- Mechanical restraint should not be used.

Both the RCP (1998) and the Nursing and Midwifery Council (Wright *et al.* 2002) reviews found that studies of the effectiveness of restraint in reducing levels of violence and aggression tend to be poorly designed and descriptive in nature. Many studies are from countries other than the UK and 'restraint' may have different meanings across countries. Wright *et al.* (2002) also argue that there are significant ethical and methodological issues in conducting research in this area. There are likely to be many other intervening factors apart from restraint training which influence the incidence of violence and it is arguably unethical to withhold training from some staff in order to maintain a control group. The RCP (1998) conclude that evidence suggests that injury during restraint can be reduced as a result of training although the frequency of violence may not reduce. Wright *et al.* (2002) conclude that 'it is reasonable to believe that the evidence base is sufficient to indicate what is likely to constitute good practice that is clinically, logically, ethically and medico-legally defensible' (2002: 41). What does seem clear is that the use of restraint is emotive for both patients and staff. However, patients and carers consulted by the RCP acknowledged that restraint was sometimes necessary to prevent harm to others, what was important was the judicious and rational use of physical intervention.

Seclusion

Many wards manage violence without the use of seclusion, however, its use is still widespread and remains controversial with both staff and patients expressing negative attitudes. Soliday (1985) found that patients expressed more negative feelings about seclusion than did nurses, who saw seclusion as necessary at times. As with restraint, research into the therapeutic use of seclusion lacks controlled studies. Wright *et al.* (2002) state that outcome studies are problematic because 'improvements' may be perceived as a result of a change in the patient's behaviour rather than mental state.

The *Mental Health Act (1983) Code of Practice* (Department of Health 1999) defines seclusion as: 'the supervised confinement of a patient in a room which may be locked to protect others from significant harm. Its sole aim is to contain severely disturbed behaviour which is likely to cause harm to others' (para. 18.16). In addition, it should be used as a last resort and for the shortest possible time. It should not be used as a punishment or threat, as part of a treatment programme (it should not be confused with the use of 'time out' which is a specific behavioural intervention) because of shortage of staff or where there is any risk of suicide or self-harm. The RCP (1998) additionally state that seclusion should be used 'with great care' if the patient has been heavily medicated, has physically deteriorated or has recently used drugs or alcohol. The decision to seclude should not be an automatic one following restraint. The *Mental Health Act (1983) Code of*

Practice states that the decision to seclude can be made by a doctor or the nurse in charge (para. 18.18). If seclusion is initiated, the RCP (1998) give the following guidelines (which should be read in conjunction with the Code of Practice):

- A doctor should be present within the first few minutes of seclusion.
- An observation schedule should be established to review the behaviour of the patient and identify the time at which seclusion can be terminated.
- A nurse must be in sight and sound throughout the period of seclusion.
- A nursing review should take place every 15 minutes and a medical review every 4 hours.
- If seclusion continues for 8 hours an independent doctor must review the decision to seclude.
- The patient should not be deprived of clothing and should be able to call for assistance.
- A record should be made in case notes and in specified documentation.

In addition, the seclusion room should be kept clean and free of anything that could be used as a weapon. The patient should also be checked for weapons before seclusion is initiated.

Use of seclusion is controversial and emotive. The RCP (1998) argue that service users should be involved in the development of local protocols and that patients who are secluded should always be given an explanation at the time, which is repeated later. Wright *et al.* (2002) also suggest that debriefing is offered afterwards to patients and that use of seclusion in principle should be discussed at ward or patient meetings.

Rapid tranquillization

Again the decision to use medication should not be an automatic one. As the RCP (1998) clearly state, violence is not always or only the result of symptoms of mental illness. The patients in the RCP (1998) consultation exercise expressed a need for a distinction between long- and short-acting medication, the former being used to prevent violence by treating underlying illness. They expressed concern about the use of medication in people they felt were not mentally ill, but felt that informed use of medication was preferable to physical restraint. However, it is worth noting that the *Mental Health Act (1983) Code of Practice* (1999) warns that prolonged use of medication can become a form of restraint if used solely to control aggressive behaviour. The RCP (1998) developed general guidance for the use of rapid tranquillization, the aim being to achieve sedation sufficient to minimize risk to the patient or others. The RCP (1998) concluded that research indicated that either a benzodiazepine or an anti-psychotic alone can be used in managing violent incidents. There is no evidence that combining several medications or using doses above British National Formulary

(BNF) limits has any better effect. The decision to use rapid tranquillization needs to take place within a policy context, guidelines for which are given by the RCP:

- Be aware of procedures before incidents.

- Take a history wherever possible.

- Complete a mental state examination and if possible a physical examination. Establish a provisional diagnosis.

- Be aware of the legal context before incidents (this is covered by Part IV of the Mental Health Act (1983). Sections 57 and 58 cover treatment requiring consent or a second opinion; Section 60 relates to withdrawal of consent; and Section 62 covers urgent treatment). The Mental Health Act Commission also provides guidance to nurses on the administration of medication (*Guidance note*, 2001). Decisions should be multi-disciplinary and a rationale always recorded.

- Pressure to make a decision based on inadequate information should be resisted.

More recent guidance on rapid tranquillization in schizophrenia comes from the National Institute for Clinical Excellence (NICE) (2002). Their treatment algorithm emphasizes the need for staff training in tranquillization protocols, in the properties of benzodiazepines, anti-psychotics, flumenazil (a benzodiazepine antagonist), and in cardiopulmonary resuscitation. Use should be balanced against the risks of over-sedation causing loss of alertness or consciousness and damage to the nurse–patient relationship. If the patient is secluded and rapid tranquillization used, extra vigilance is needed. Oral medication should be offered first – lorazepam, olanzepine and haloperidol are suggested (use of the latter may also require the administration of an anticholinergic). If intra-muscular (IM) administration is necessary, single use of one of the above drugs is advocated, again with the proviso that where typical anti-psychotics are used, an anitcholinergic should also be given. In contrast to RCP guidelines, NICE guidelines state that in urgent cases IM haloperidol and lorazepam can be given together. Again, the decision should be a multi-disciplinary one and a rationale clearly documented. Vital signs also need to be monitored following medication. As soon as possible, the patient should be given an opportunity to discuss the use of medication and receive an explanation for its use.

Dealing with serious incidents

Advice on dealing with situations which involve weapons is, unfortunately, unclear and contradictory. RCP (1998) guidance calls for staff to ask for a weapon to be put down rather than handed over, while the RCN (1997) advises that the area should be cleared and the police called. Wright *et al.* (2000) state that all trusts should have policies on when to involve the police. The Mental Health Act Commission (2003) argue that clear guidance is needed as police may resent being involved in minor incidents, but that nursing staff need reassurance that the necessity to prevent crime (and harm) also applies to mental health settings.

Use of physical intervention entails monitoring the safety of the patient involved. In the light of the findings of the Bennett Inquiry (2003), NICE has proposed clinical guidelines for the short-term management of violence, which incorporate staff training in life support techniques (NICE 2004).

Post incident management

Many nurses will be uncomfortable about using physical interventions as it is difficult to see them as 'therapeutic'. The Mental Health Act Commission, in their *Tenth Biennial Report* (2003) argue that restraint and seclusion are justifiable to maintain safety, but that the power to use these interventions should not be abused and they should not become punitive measures. Gunn and Rodgers (2002) argue that use of restraint and seclusion cannot be justified on treatment grounds, but that the most appropriate ethical basis is in 'common law justification', i.e. the requirement to use the least force necessary to prevent harm. The difficulty for nurses is that they may have to use these interventions while building and maintaining therapeutic relationships. It would be naive to assume that physical intervention does not affect staff–patient relationships. However, the legal, professional and ethical context which frames their use can serve to provide safety and reassurance for both patients and staff, and good post-incident management may help to reduce the longer-term effects.

The emotional impact of coping with aggression, even if managed effectively, should not be overlooked. Wykes and Whittington (1994) found that staff reactions to assault included fear, anxiety, guilt, self-blame, anger and hatred. Crichton *et al.* (1998) suggested that staff response to aggression involves an element of moral censure of the patient related to level of perceived threat and assessment of moral responsibility. Coping with these strong feelings affects relationships with patients, possibly leading to hostility, avoidance and controlling behaviour, which feeds back to levels of violence among patients (Whittington and Wykes 1994). Post-incident review is therefore vital to allow the expression of difficult emotions and enable learning from the incident (critical incident analysis is one such mechanism). Patients who have been involved in or observed aggressive incidents also need support. Neither should the impact of verbal abuse be underestimated. Community staff may be particularly affected by this, given that they often see clients alone and are often called on to make day-to-day practice decisions in isolation (ENB 1998).

Conclusion

There is no 'cookbook' approach to managing anger, violence and aggression. Interventions need to be adapted to the needs of the patient. On a positive note, research suggests that nurses do actually use a creative mixture of techniques when dealing with violence and aggression (Haber *et al.* 1997, in Wright *et al.* 2000) adopting an approach which tailors interventions to seriousness of situation. However, there is overwhelming consensus that the interventions discussed above are no substitute for competent and confident staff working as a team in a safe and therapeutic environment.

To summarize:

- The quality of the physical and social environment on mental health wards is likely to have an impact on the level of violence and aggression.
- Talking and listening to patients are basic interventions in preventing violence and aggression.
- Intervention should be matched to the level of anger or aggression; there is a hierarchy of methods from verbal to physical techniques. Restraint and seclusion are 'last resort' interventions.
- Physical intervention occurs within a legal, professional and ethical framework. Staff should make sure they understand these considerations before any incident.
- Patients and staff need to be offered support after an incident of aggression.

Questions for reflection and discussion

1 Think about wards you have worked on. Did the physical and social environment impact on levels of aggression? Were there any improvements which could have been made? (Consider the points in Box 27.3.)

2 You arrive at work for an early shift and receive a handover about Richard. He was brought to the ward during the night by the police after throwing a brick through a neighbour's window. He felt they were secretly filming him and was trying to break the recording equipment in their house. He smelt of alcohol when admitted and looked disoriented and scared. He has only slept for a few hours. After the night staff leave, Richard comes into the day area. He looks agitated; pacing the day area and talking to himself. What do you consider before approaching him? (See Box 27.4.)

3 What beliefs do you have about angry and aggressive people? What nursing skills do you think are most important when dealing with potentially aggressive situations? (See de-escalation techniques.)

4 Richard agrees to sit down and talk to you. He doesn't understand why he's in hospital and he thinks the police may have fitted him up. He'd like to go home and at least get some money and clothes. He still sounds angry when talking about his situation. What verbal interventions could you use?

5   Imagine you were told to participate in restraining a person in each of the situations in Box 27.6. Would you feel differently in each of these situations? What factors would you take into account if making a decision on whether to restrain or not? How would you feel if the person involved was elderly or an adolescent?

Annotated bibliography

- Wright, S., Gray, R., Parkes, J. and Gournay, K. (2002) *The Recognition, Prevention and Therapeutic Management of Violence in Acute In-patient Psychiatry: A Literature Review and Evidence Based Recommendations for Good Practice*. London: UKCC. This report, prepared for the NMC, provides a comprehensive review of the research on violence and aggression in mental health settings and discusses the evidence base for factors which influence violence as well as the effectiveness of management interventions.
- Royal College of Psychiatrists College Research Unit (1998) *Management of Imminent Violence: Clinical Practice Guidelines to Support Mental Health Services*, Occasional Paper OP41. London: RCP. This report provides practical guidance based on a review of research evidence and consultation with users and carers.
- Mason, T. and Chandley, M. (1999) *Managing Violence and Aggression: A Manual for Nurses and Health care Workers*, Edinburgh: Churchill Livingstone. This provides a practice-based discussion of interventions used during different phases of aggression. The sections on longer-term, structured intervention such as behavioural programmes give another perspective on management of aggression.
- Vaughan, P.J. and Badger, D. (1995) *Working with the Mentally Disordered Offender in the Community*. London: Chapman Hall, chapter 4. For guidance on managing aggression in the community, this chapter contains practical advice on maintaining safety in community mental health centres and when visiting clients.

References

Caplan, C.A. (1993) Nursing staff and patient perceptions of ward atmosphere in a maximum security forensic hospital, *Archives of Psychiatric Nursing* 3(1): 23–9.

Crichton, J., Callanan, T.S., Beauchamp, L., Glasson, M. and Tardiff, H. (1998) Staff response to psychiatric inpatient violence: an international comparison, *Psychiatric Care* 5(2): 50–6.

Department of Health (1999) *Mental Health Act (1983) Code of Practice*. London: HMSO.

ENB (1998) *Research Highlight 34: Risk Assessment and Management in Multi-agency, Multi-professional Health Care: Education and Practice*. London: ENB.

Goleman, D. (1995) *Emotional Intelligence*. London: Bloomsbury.

Gournay, K. (2001) *The Recognition Prevention and Therapeutic Management of Violence in Mental Health Care: A Consultation Document*. London: UKCC.

Gournay, K., Ward, M., Thornicroft, G. and Wright, S. (1998) Crisis in the capital: in-patient care in inner London, *Mental Health Practice* **1**(5): 10–18.

Gunn, M. and Rodgers, M. (2002) Mental health nursing. in J. Tingle and A. Cribb (eds) *Nursing Law and Ethics, 2nd edition*. Oxford: Blackwell Science.

Haber, L.C., Fagan-Pryor, E.C. and Allen, M. (1997) Comparison of registered nurses' and nursing assistants' choices of interventions for aggressive behaviours, *Issues in Mental Health Nursing* **18**: 325–8, in Wright *et al.* (2002).

Independent Inquiry into the death of Daniel Bennett (2003). Set up under MSG (94) 27.

Katz, P. and Kirkland, F.R. (1990) Violence and social structure on mental hospital wards, *Psychiatry* **53**: 262–77.

Lowenstein, M., Binder, R.L. and McNiel, D.E. (1990) The relationship between admission symptoms and hospital assaults. *Hospital and Community Psychiatry* **41**(3): 311–13.

Mason, T. and Chandley, M. (1999) *Managing Violence and Aggression: A Manual for Nurses and Healthcare Workers*. Edinburgh: Churchill Livingstone.

Mental Health Act Commission (2001) Guidance Note: Nurses, The Administration of Medicine for Mental Disorder and the Mental Health Act 1983, Commission ref: GN 2/2001.

Mental Health Act Commission (2003) *Tenth Biennial Report 2001–2003: Placed Amongst Strangers*. Trent: MHAC.

Monaghan, J. (1993) Mental disorder and violence: another look, in S. Hodgins (ed.) *Mental Disorder and Crime*. London: Sage.

Morrison, P. and Lehane, M. (1995) Staffing levels and seclusion use, *Journal of Advanced Nursing* **22**: 1192–202.

National Audit Office (2003) *A Safer Place to Work: Improving the Management of Health and Safety Risks to Staff in NHS Trusts*. London: HMSO.

National Institute for Clinical Excellence (2002) *Schizophrenia: Core Interventions in the Treatment and Management of Schizophrenia in Primary and Secondary Care*. London: NICE.

National Institute for Clinical Excellence (2004) *Clinical practice guidelines for the short-term management of disturbed (violent) behaviour in adult psychiatric in-patient settings: draft for 1st Stage Consultation Period, London: NICE*.

Nursing and Midwifery Council (2003) Press release, 3 February.

Novaco, R.W. (1983) *Stress Inoculation Therapy for Anger Control: A Manual for Therapists*. Irvine, CA: University of California.

Owen, C., Tarantello, C., Jones, M. and Tennant, C. (1998) Violence and aggression in psychiatric units, *Psychiatric Services* **49**(11): 1452–7.

Royal College of Nursing, Midwifery and Health Visiting (1997) *The Management of Aggression and Violence in Places of Care: An RCN Position Statement*. London: RCN.

Royal College of Psychiatrists Research Unit (1998) *Management of Imminent Violence: Clinical Practice Guidelines to Support Mental Health Services*, Occasional Paper OP41. London: RCP.

Royal College of Psychiatrists Research Unit (2000) *National Audit of the Management of Violence in Mental Health Settings 1999–2000*. London: RCP.

Sainsbury Centre for Mental Health (1998) *Acute Problems: A Survey of the Quality of Care in Acute Psychiatric Wards*. London: Sainsbury Centre for Mental Health.

Sainsbury Centre for Mental Health (2001) *The Capable Practitioner: a framework and list of the practitioner capabilities required to implement The National Service Framework for Mental Health*, London: Sainsbury Centre for Mental Health.

Shah, A.K. (1993) An increase in violence among psychiatric in-patients: real or imagined?, *Medical Science Law* **33**(3): 227–9.

Soliday, S.M. (1985) A comparison of patients and staff attitudes toward seclusion, *Journal of Nervous and Mental Disease* **173**(5): 282–6.

UKCC (1998) *Guidelines for Mental Health and Learning Disabilities*, London: UKCC.

Vinestock, M. (1996) Risk assessment: 'a word to the wise', *Advances in Psychiatric Treatment* **2**: 3–10.

Whittington, R. and Patterson, P. (1996) Verbal and non-verbal behaviour immediately prior to aggression by mentally disordered people: enhancing the assessment of risk. *Journal of Psychiatric and Mental Health Nursing* **3**: 47–54.

Whittington, R. and Wykes, T. (1994) An observational study of associations between nurse behaviour and violence in psychiatric hospitals, *Journal of Psychiatric and Mental Health Nursing* **1**: 85–92.

Wright, S., Lee, S., Sayer, J., Parr, A. and Gournay, K. (2000) A review of the content of management of violence policies in in-patient mental health units, *Mental Health Care* **3**(11): 373–6.

Wright, S., Gray, R., Parkes, J. and Gournay, K. (2002) *The Recognition, Prevention and Therapeutic Management of Violence in Acute In-patient Psychiatry: A Literature Review and Evidence Based Recommendations for Good Practice.* London: UKCC.

Wykes, T. and Whittington, R. (1994) Reactions to assault, in T. Wykes (ed.) *Violence and Healthcare Professionals.* London: Chapman and Hall.

28

Therapeutic management of attempted suicide and self-harm

Ian Noonan

█ Chapter overview

Working with people who harm themselves or feel and act upon suicidal thoughts can pose a dilemma: how do you help someone who is trying to hurt himself/herself or attempt to end his/her life? In health care we often assume that the person we are working with will negotiate, want, and be a partner in the care that is being provided for them, or that, at some level, we are able to find a goal that is shared in the work that we undertake.

When someone is self-harming, the behaviour itself can seem like the opposite of what we are trying to achieve, but for the client the need to cut, for example, might be so great that they fear what would happen without it. Equally, for a client who feels suicidal, they may not be able to see a future and find it very difficult to imagine a way of resolving how they feel.

For the nurse, there is a risk that we might end up resenting or feeling angry with the person who has self-harmed, as it can be perceived as deliberately undoing the work you have done.

This chapter aims to explore the range of self-harm behaviour and suicidal thoughts, feelings and actions, and show that, although the two phenomena are different, there is an overlap between self-harm and suicide. Ways of thinking about people who self-harm or are suicidal will be suggested, to help nurses understand this client group. Different treatment options will be explored using case study examples. Further details on assessment of risk in people who self-harm or are suicidal, can be found in Chapter 8.

This chapter covers:

- definition and types of self-harm behaviour;
- the relationship between self-harm and suicide;
- nursing someone who self-harms:
  - understanding – mechanism and meaning,
  - therapeutic assessment,

  – motivation,
  – harm reduction,
  – solution-focused interventions for deliberate self-harm;
* what people who self-harm want;
* nursing someone who is suicidal;
* special groups:
  – young people,
  – older adults,
  – people with psychosis;
* being safe.

Defining deliberate self-harm

The language used to describe how and why people harm themselves can reflect the judgements that are often made about this client group: 'self-abuse' and 'self-mutilation' assume emotive aspects such as guilt or self-loathing, whereas purely descriptive terms such as 'cutting' or 'blood letting' convey neither the choice that the client has made nor the fact that the act is harmful.

Weber (2002) cites several terms that have been used to describe such behaviour: self-injury, self-abuse, indirect self-destructive behaviour, para-suicide, self-inflicted injury, self-injurious behaviour, self-mutilation, as well as deliberate self-harm. The terms used often reflect the theoretical standpoint of the clinician using them rather than the client who harms himself or herself. Self-abuse, self-destructive behaviour or self-mutilation suggest a psychodynamic understanding of the motivation for the behaviour, whereas self-injury or deliberate self-harm convey some sense that the person has chosen to act in this way and that it is a behaviour rather than an illness per se.

This distinction is further emphasized if definitions of deliberate self-harm are considered. House *et al.* define deliberate self-harm as 'intentional self poisoning or self injury (such as cutting), irrespective of the apparent purpose of the act' (1999: 137) Weber, however, goes on to exclude suicidal intent as a possible purpose or meaning of the act: 'I used the term self-destruction as the broad encompassing category of behaviours that are self-inflicted, of which self-abuse, or the deliberate harm to one's own body without suicidal intent, is one type' (2002: 118). Gallop and Tully expand further on the meaning of the behaviour in their definition, 'Self-injury is often an attempt to communicate distress, relieve pain and maintain connection to oneself and others. Suicide attempts, on the other hand are directed at discontinuing all connections and ending consciousness' (2004: 236).

The Self-Harm Alliance, an advocacy, support and self-help group for people who self-harm, has identified many different ways in which people might self-harm. Table 28.1 lists these different mechanisms of injury.

Table 28.1 Deliberate self-harm: mechanisms of injury

1 *Self-harm which breaks the skin or causes bleeding*

Cutting, with knives, razor blades, broken glass	Excessive scratching by removing the top layer of skin to cause a sore	Excessive nail biting to the point of bleeding and ripping cuticles	Burning skin by chemical means using caustic liquids
Burning by physical means using heat	Friction burns to skin using abrasive materials	Gnawing at flesh	Blood letting

2 *Self-harm by more violent methods*

Pinching hard enough to cause bruises	Head banging against the floor or walls	Hitting the head with fist or hard objects	Punching windows or walls
Bone breaking	Jumping from heights without suicidal ideation	Tying ligatures around the neck, arms or legs to restrict the flow of blood	Hair pulling from head, eyelashes, eyebrows or armpits (trichotillomania)

3 *Self-harm with internal/medical effects*

Medication abuse (overdoses) without the intention to die	Poisoning by ingesting small amounts of toxic substances to cause discomfort or damage	Deliberately ingesting food to cause a known allergic reaction	Wound interference to prevent wounds from healing or to deliberately infect them
Insertion of foreign objects	Binge-eating or starvation	Alcohol misuse	Illicit drug use

(Adapted from Self Harm Alliance 2003)

Deliberate self-harm can include a wide range of behaviours that damage an individual's body, either externally or internally, with a meaning or purpose that can vary for any one client on each occasion that they self-harm, and from person to person. The act might be impulsive or planned, with immediate or long-term effect. The term only describes the behaviour and is not an illness. This does not mean that the person who self-harms will not benefit from treatment, rather that there are likely to be coexisting mental health needs which will also need to be addressed in order to help that person change their self-harming behaviour.

The relationship between self-harm and suicide

In England, around 5000 people per year kill themselves, and suicide is the most common cause of death in men under 35 (Department of Health 2003). It is important to remember that the death of an individual impacts on his community, family and society in general. One of the target groups that the government has identified for reducing suicide rates is the high-risk group of clients who commit suicide in the year following an incident of deliberate self-harm. If this group is combined with people who are currently, or have recently been, in contact with mental health services, it represents almost half of the number of people who kill themselves each year.

Bongar (2002) suggests that the 'murky' discriminations between self-harm, attempted suicide by a non-lethal method, survived and completed suicide attempts, are of more use to the researcher than the clinician. He argues that any act where someone self-harms or states their intention to do so should be treated as a communication of psychological pain, which should be thoroughly assessed. Bongar (2002) views suicide as a complex bio-psychosocial phenomenon which includes the death of those who intended to kill themselves and individuals with patterns of deliberate self-harm who accidentally die as a result of their injuries. The relationship between suicide and self-harm also depends on the client's understanding of the risk to his or her own life. Stengel defined attempted suicide as follows:

> A suicidal attempt is any act inflicted with self destructive intention, however vague and ambiguous. For the clinician, it is safer still to regard all cases of potentially dangerous self-poisoning or self-inflicted injury as suicidal attempts, whatever the victim's explanation, unless there is clear evidence to the contrary. Potentially dangerous means in this context: believed by the attempter possibly to endanger life.
>
> (Stengel 1965: 64)

Although there is some value in Stengel's definition in terms of immediate assessment, it has the potential to devalue the client's own knowledge, experience and reasons for self-harming. Without question, it is important to find out from the client what their intentions were and are, and in fact this could provide the 'clear evidence to the contrary' which Stengel seeks.

There are grounds for distinguishing between deliberate self-harm and suicidal thoughts, feelings and actions, as many people who self-harm are not suicidal. Someone who feels suicidal may not act in any way to self-harm. However, the meaning or purpose of self-harm will vary from person to person, and it may be more useful to view deliberate self-harm on a continuum with suicide.

Table 28.2 shows that self-inflicted damage to the body may be deliberate but without the intent to harm oneself – for example with tattoos, body piercing, plastic surgery or tribal marking/cutting the face. The self-harm can be deliberate and immediate, such as cutting or taking overdoses, or prolonged, such as starvation or poisoning. In turn, the intent of the person who self-harms may or may not be to end their life. Someone may feel suicidal, have suicidal thoughts but not actually make any attempt to kill himself or herself. Often referred to as attempted or parasuicide, the final group that we can nurse are clients who feel suicidal and make an attempt to end their life, but do survive.

Table 28.2 Deliberate self-harm – suicide continuum

	Any client might have suicidal thoughts, feelings or plans, whether or not they actually self-harm								
	Behaviours that may be socially acceptable, but cause harm and could result in accidental or premature death				Deliberate self-harm as a coping mechanism for psychological distress		Behaviours with varying risk of completed suicide. Remember to consider the client's view of whether an act might be lethal		COMPLETED SUICIDE
DELIBERATE SELF-HARM →	*Tattoos, body piercing, tribal cuts or scaring*	*Risk taking: driving too fast, unsafe sex*	*Smoking or drinking to excess*	*Illicit drug use or excessive use of prescribed drugs*	*Binge-eating or starvation*	*Cutting or overdosing without suicidal ideation*	*Non-lethal cutting or overdosing with the intent to kill oneself*	*Overdoses, hanging, cutting or immersion with suicidal intent*	*Attempted suicide with lethal method resulting in death* →
	Boredom, thrill seeking, frustration, experimentation, socialization, self-expression					Feeling 'out of control', angry, guilty, low self-esteem, need to punish or purge oneself	Depressed, hopeless, unable to see a future, guilty, angry, resolved to die or apathetic about living		

When considering clients who self-harm or attempt suicide it is clear that each group has different but overlapping qualities. In defining self-harm and suicide, a relationship between the two phenomena becomes evident. Displayed on a continuum, in Table 28.2, it shows that although the two acts can be separated in terms of the client's intent, there are many similarities in feelings and actions. Population studies provide the demographic data for identifying whether or not an individual falls into a high-risk group. This does not however inform the clinician of that individual's risk. Only by assessing the mechanism and the meaning of an act when somebody self-harms or attempts to commit suicide, can a plan of nursing care be made to address the behaviour.

Nursing someone who self-harms

Understanding – mechanism and meaning

The first stage in nursing someone who has self-harmed is to understand what meaning the act has for them. In order to do this we have to ask about and explore with the client what happened and how they felt, before, during and after they self-harmed. This requires us to have an attitude, and use language, that is non-judgemental. Showing that we are interested in the client as an individual and that we do not blame them for self-harming will help to establish a therapeutic relationship through which we can help the client to identify what they would like to change and how they can change their behaviour.

Therapeutic assessment

Case study: Jenny

Jenny is a 21-year-old music student training as a classical violinist. She attended the emergency department in the early hours of the morning having made ten 4 cm cuts in a row along the length of her forearm. She had played in an end-of-term concert that evening and been for a drink with her fellow students, consuming approximately 12 units of alcohol. Upon her return home she had felt an overwhelming desire to release a feeling of tension, which she described as being located in her arm. Having cut herself she felt an immediate release of tension, but very quickly felt her anxiety levels rise again as she began to fear lest she had damaged her arm, worry about what her friends, teachers and family would think, and was angry that the tension seemed to be returning. She told one of her flatmates what she had done, and was persuaded to attend the emergency department.

Although this was the first time that Jenny had cut herself, she had taken an overdose one year ago and from the age of 13 had starved herself when feeling stressed. When she was 7 years old her father, who was also a professional musician and her first teacher, left her mother. Jenny excelled at school and gained a place at the university of her choice, but always felt that she was somehow 'scraping by'. Since arriving at university she had struggled, and although passing her course, felt she was near the bottom of the class. She described in her own words a 'love–hate' relationship with her peers. Performing at university motivated her, but she resented doing it. As the end of her course approached she feared what would happen and was angry that she had failed to get onto a postgraduate course. Jenny seemed able only to see things as poles apart: she would either become a professional musician or she would be a failure; her teachers loved or hated her.

During her assessment with a psychiatric liaison nurse, Jenny was able to identify that when things went wrong she 'blamed' and 'hated' herself. She had a belief that she wasn't good enough for her father, her school or her university, and only felt better if she 'punished' herself by starving, taking an overdose or cutting herself. Jenny agreed that she wanted to do something to change this pattern of behaviour. She identified that drinking alcohol when she was feeling distressed made it more likely that she would do something to harm herself, or starve herself the following day because she felt guilty at having had too many calories in the alcohol. She also felt that she was 'testing' her body, and to some extent that she wanted 'it' (her body) to fail her so that she would be able to justify not becoming a professional violinist.

The nursing intervention as a result of this assessment was essentially pragmatic. Jenny was educated about the risks of binge drinking, and given some written information to back this up. Jenny identified that it would be helpful to speak to the careers office at her university to see if she could identify a realistic option that fell between her ideal career and her view of failure. A 'crisis plan' was devised including what Jenny would do if she felt like harming herself again. This included trying to think of a middle-ground between her extreme beliefs and feelings, asking a friend to come round rather than going to the pub, calling a student helpline, and how to access emergency mental health services.

Jenny was offered a referral for psychotherapy. However, she felt it would be 'too much to deal with' at that time, but would consider it as an option for the future.

Jenny gave permission for her case to be used as an example. Her name and other details have been changed to protect her anonymity.

The case study of Jenny illustrates the importance of this first stage. During the assessment of her self-harm, Jenny was able to formulate her own ideas about how she had come to a point where she used cutting as a coping mechanism. Even if this is your only contact with someone who has self-harmed there are treatment options available: psycho-education, solution-orientated interventions, distraction or harm-reduction techniques can all be employed in the context of a therapeutic assessment.

Anyone who self-harms and has capacity has the right to refuse treatment. In Jenny's case she did not feel able to cope with psychotherapy at that time, and so chose not to take up the offer of referral. The nurse's role includes ensuring that treatments remain accessible to their clients and acknowledging that people change their minds over time. If Jenny repeatedly attended the emergency department, the nurse could suggest to her that she needed more support to change her behaviour and re-offer the referral to psychotherapy.

Motivation

To nurse someone who self-harms we need to make an assessment of their motivation to change their self-harming behaviour. An interesting analogy can be made between models of change used in addictions nursing and nursing someone who self harms. Prochaska *et al.* (1993) demonstrate how a transtheoretical model of a cycle of change can be used to promote behavioural change in people with addictive behaviours. The six stages of change: precontemplation, contemplation, preparation, action, maintenance and termination, can equally well be applied when assessing and nursing someone who self-harms. At any stage during the cycle, an individual may relapse. Prochaska and Velicer (1997) demonstrate that when interventions are matched to the client's assessed stage of change, there is a dramatic improvement in recruitment, retention and progress in treatment programmes. Table 28.3 maps the characteristics and suggests techniques for someone who self-harms, at each stage of change.

Table 28.3 Techniques for different stages of change

Stage of change	Client characteristics	Nursing techniques
Precontemplation	Not considering change. Does not consider that self-harm is a problem. Denying that the behaviour exists and not seeking help.	Acknowledge and accept the client's lack of readiness. Respect the client's choice and that it is their decision. Encourage thinking about the meaning of self-harm rather than action. Explain and personalize the risk of self-harm.
Contemplation	Ambivalent about changing self-harm behaviour. Thinking about the role of self-harm in their life. No plans for change in the immediate future. Sitting on the fence, but interested in treatment options.	Acknowledge and accept the client is not ready to change. Respect the client's choice and that it remains their decision. Encourage evaluation of the benefits and risks of self-harming. What would it be like if you didn't self-harm? Identify possible positive outcomes of reducing or stopping self-harm behaviours.

Table 28.3 (*continued*)

Stage of change	Client characteristics	Nursing techniques
Preparation	Some experience with trying to stop self-harming – testing the waters. Feels ready to change and wants to stop self-harming. May have been finding out about self-help groups or been in touch with other people who self-harm. Enquiring about different treatment options.	Help to identify any barriers to change. Use solution-orientated techniques to diminish or remove barriers. Help to identify sources of support – self-help groups, friends and social support. Identify the client's strengths, skills and abilities to change. Set small, SMART goals.
Action	Living without self-harm. Using other coping mechanisms. Engaging with treatment. Risk of replacing self-harm with other destructive or addictive behaviours.	Acknowledge this achievement and highlight the positive outcomes of not self-harming. Identify feelings of loss and anxiety. Ask about other behaviours, drug/alcohol use, gambling, etc.
Maintenance	No self-harm for over 6 months. Continued commitment to living without self-harm. Conscious awareness of healthy management of stress and anxiety.	Plan long-term follow up. Reinforce success and internal benefits of not self-harming. Discuss techniques for coping with relapse, and that relapse does not equal failure.
Relapse (can occur at any stage of change)	Self-harming or unable to cope with the thoughts of self-harm. Feeling guilty, angry or hopeless.	Identify triggers for relapse. Explain that relapse is a part of change. Reassess motivation. Review coping strategies. Screen for depression or suicidal thoughts.
Termination	No self-harm. Reduced anxiety about not self-harming. Strong social support and interpersonal relationships.	The end of a therapeutic relationship needs to be planned. Treatment no longer required.

(After Prochaska *et al.* 1993)

In Jenny's case, she could be described as moving between the contemplation and preparation stages of changing her self-harm behaviour. She wants to change, and has been trying albeit unsuccessfully, to change her behaviour. Although she does not feel ready for psychotherapy – she has not ruled it out for the future. She is willing to try to drink less and see a careers adviser. Achieving small steps towards her goal will support her changing behaviour whereas viewing any further self-harm as a failure would reinforce Jenny's beliefs about herself. Preparing a crisis plan acknowledges that relapse is possible, moreover likely, during the process of change.

Harm minimization

In the fields of health promotion and addictions nursing the concept of harm minimization is well established. For example, in addictions, by acknowledging that someone is going to continue to use if they are in the precontemplative, contemplative or preparation stages of change, the risk of infection, accidental overdose, not knowing what they are ingesting, can be reduced by needle-exchange programmes, health education and methadone maintenance programmes. The client engages with services while still using so that the therapeutic relationships and hopefully the client's confidence in a service is established at the time they do want to change their behaviour.

It may be particularly challenging to engage with someone who is self-harming. It is possible that your client may have had previous negative experiences of health care. If you make nursing care conditional on not self-harming, you will communicate to your client that you blame them. Service users report that signing 'no self-harm' contracts is unhelpful, and that short-term tolerance of risk leads to increased honesty about deliberate self-harm (South London and Maudsley 2001). While ensuring that the responsibility for self-harm remains with the client, nurses should accept that the behaviour will continue into treatment.

Specific harm-minimization techniques such as distraction are widely used. Some people have suppressed the need to cut by snapping elastic bands against their wrist, holding ice in their hands, or punching pillows. In the short term these may reduce the risk involved in deliberate self-harm. However, they perpetuate the client's need to experience an immediate physical response to psychological distress. Positive distraction techniques that engage the client in creative rather than destructive behaviours, such as exercise, listening to music, watching television, drawing/painting, etc. are more likely to change their behavioural response to self-harm.

In Jenny's case, examining the role alcohol may have to play as an antecedent to her self-harm could be considered a harm-reduction strategy. Educating Jenny about the risks of binge drinking and finding an alternative to going to the pub may help to reduce the potential frequency and severity of her self-harm.

Solution-focused interventions

Systematic reviews of research evidence for treating deliberate self-harm have found that problem-solving therapies result in decreased repeat self-harm rates (Centre for Review and Dissemination 1998; Hawton *et al.* 2003). The lack of longitudinal studies and small numbers involved in the studies mean that these results are not statistically significant. However, they identify a clinically significant trend of reduced repetition rates, which would support the use of solution-focused techniques when working with people who self-harm. In Chapter 23 Gega explores the art of problem solving with clients.

If we apply these principles to Jenny's case, the nurse's perspective of Jenny's problem might focus on her self-harm. Jenny, however, viewed the risk to her career as her current, most important problem. Jenny's thinking about her violin playing was catastrophic; she thought that she was a failure and that she should give up, if she 'couldn't make it' as a professional violinist. The nurse's role is to help Jenny to find a solution to this dilemma. If the solution is one that Jenny can come up with, she is more likely to believe that it is achievable and, therefore, possible. However, when someone is distressed, her thinking can become very fixed and she might believe that there is no possible solution. Rather than just suggesting a solution that you think fits, questioning Jenny regarding her beliefs and feelings about her career can help her to see her situation from another perspective and to develop a solution. Once Jenny has a solution in mind, you can help her to set goals towards achieving it. Table 28.4 gives some examples of questions you might ask in order to help Jenny find her own solution.

Although in this case, Jenny's anxieties about her career may seem secondary to her self-harm behaviour, this is the problem she identifies as most significant. Jenny plans to go and see the careers adviser at her university. Although her friends had already suggested this solution, she had not before thought that she would actually go. It is not implied that this one

Table 28.4 Purpose and examples of questions for Jenny

Purpose	Examples
Defining the problem	What do you think is the main problem? What would you like help with? What do you fear will happen if you fail your course? How do you feel you are doing? How do others think you are doing? What options are there available to you?
Challenging negative thinking errors	Are you actually failing? How do your tutors think you are doing? What careers are your peers thinking of? What else would you view as being successful? What is the worst thing that could happen if you did fail?
Identifying possible solutions	What would your colleagues do in your shoes? Is there a middle ground? What would be 'good enough' for you? Can you think of alternatives? What do you think of these alternatives?
Refining solution choice	What do you think is most likely to work? Which would you like to try? What steps do you need to take to achieve this? What help would you like to achieve this? How would you feel when you achieve this?

small shift would fundamentally change Jenny's beliefs about herself, but it is achievable and very strongly linked to her own understanding of why she self-harms. It moves Jenny's focus from what she considers to be her past failures, towards what she can achieve in the future. Stevenson *et al.* (2003) suggest that nurses are required to undergo a change in their philosophy in order to work with the priorities that the client brings, and to have a solution-orientated, prospective approach rather that a retrospective 'fixing' of the underlying causes of any crisis.

What people who self-harm want

The main principles in this section should apply to all the clients whom we nurse. In the past people who self-harm have experienced judgemental, sometimes painful, treatment at the hands of health care professionals. This has been the case not only in emergency departments, but also in mental health services. Reasons for this may be that carers do not understand deliberate self-harm and therefore feel angry or frustrated with a client who may repeatedly self-harm. Two websites for people who self-harm (Self Harm Alliance 2003 and National Self-Harm Network 2003) give examples of service-users' experiences along with advice for carers, family, friends and health professionals. In general, people who self-harm want to be treated with respect and non-judgementally. This means treating injuries and assessing people in private, respecting confidentiality within the clinical team, thinking about the timing of psychosocial assessments and allowing appropriate time to recover from any injury. It is a myth that people who self-harm either enjoy, or do not feel, pain.

Conflict may arise as some people who self-harm do not wish to discuss this with a mental health professional. The Royal College of Psychiatrists (1994) advise that everyone who self-harms should have a psychosocial assessment by a trained professional before they leave the emergency department. Furthermore, the *National Suicide Prevention Strategy for England* (Department of Health 2003) states that anyone who has self-harmed within the previous three-month period should receive follow-up within seven days of discharge from hospital. As nurses we have to balance these policy requirements with the right that any capable adult has to refuse treatment. Where conflict arises, discuss with the client why they wish to refuse treatment, ensure they understand what is being offered, and whenever possible discuss the case with other members of the multi-disciplinary team.

Nursing someone who is suicidal

Many of the principles outlined above in nursing someone who self-harms, apply to nursing someone who is suicidal. Someone who is suicidal has basic needs: to be listened to, in relationship with others, cared for, under-stood and valued. Anything less risks reinforcing the hopelessness they may already feel.

The UK government's focus on the reduction in suicide as the key target in mental health (Department of Health 1990, 2001 and 2003) has contributed to a culture of risk assessment and management in mental health care. There is a growing body of evidence regarding how to assess risk of suicide, but little that supports nurses in working with clients who are suicidal.

There has been an emphasis on nursing suicidal clients on acute psychiatric wards and maintaining continuous, close observations until the risk is felt is felt to have passed. Reid and Long (1993), Cleary *et al.* (1999) and Bowers *et al.* (2000) all agree that if a client is placed under continuous observation, it provides an opportunity for the nurse working with the suicidal client, to form a therapeutic relationship. However, clients' experiences of being continuously observed are often reported as being restrictive, punishing, humiliating, and clearly far from therapeutic (Fletcher 1999; Jones *et al.* 2000). Numerous problems exist with continuous close observations:

- There is a lack of, and inconsistent application of policy, with observa-tions often being carried out by junior or agency staff (Bowers *et al.* 2000).

- People still kill themselves while on inpatient acute admissions wards (Department of Health 2001).

- It is stressful for the nurses doing the observation (Cutcliffe and Barker 2002).

- It may put the nurse at risk if the client's impulsive behaviour becomes directed towards them (Cleary *et al.* 1999).

So the question remains, how can we nurse someone safely who is suicidal?

Continuous, close observation should only be used as an emergency provision. An example of when this type of intervention might be used is given in the case study of Serena.

Case study: Serena

Serena is a 35-year-old woman who was diagnosed with bipolar affective disorder in her early twenties. She has tried to kill herself on four occasions, each shortly after a depressive episode. Her suicidal behaviour has been impulsive and high risk: trying to hang herself, running out in front of oncoming traffic, and jumping from a high building. Over the past fortnight, her community nurse has been increasingly concerned about Serena. She had been depressed, and although her mood was still low, she was becoming increasingly irritable and angry. In the days before her admission, she started telephoning staff at the hospital stating she was going to 'be with God' as 'He wanted her back at his right side' and that she was 'ready to die'. The community nurse arranged a mental health act assessment at Serena's home, and they found that Serena had tied a noose with her dressing gown cord, which was hanging from the banisters on her landing. She did not want to come into hospital, was assessed as being at risk of harm to herself and was admitted to an acute psychiatric admissions ward under Section 3 of the Mental Health Act (1983).

Serena gave permission for her case to be used as an example. Her name and some other details have been changed to protect her anonymity.

In such an emergency situation as Serena's, the assessment of risk should be multi-disciplinary, and the purpose, level and duration of the observation made explicit. Where possible, the client should be involved in the decision about whether observation will be helpful and reduce the identified risk, and should always be informed about why and how they will be observed. The nursing staff doing the observation must be appropriately trained, know the local observation policy and should not be expected to continuously observe a client for more than two hours at a time. When it is decided that someone should be continuously observed, the team should also agree when this will be reviewed, and what changes in the client's thoughts, feelings and behaviours will result in the observation level being reduced.

The aim of continuous, close observation should be to engage with the client, to try to form a relationship with them, so that they can express their suicidal thoughts and feelings and be prompted to identify what else would be helpful. This can be achieved by listening to, and talking with, the person you are observing. However, constant focus on being 'nursed' can be exhausting – so negotiating activities, and doing them with the client, will help to form the therapeutic relationship as well as provide a break for both the client and the nurse.

For observation to be of any value, the nurse's observations of their client must be documented and discussed with the multi-disciplinary team responsible for his or her treatment. An example of how this might be done in Serena's case is given in Box 28.1.

Observation is limited. An example from the author's experience may serve to introduce an alternative way to safeguard someone who is suicidal. When assessing a client in the emergency department, even if they are actively suicidal, they are very rarely placed on continuous close observation. The process of being listened to, accepted, consulted regarding treatment options, actively involved in their care seems to be sufficient to engage the client in their treatment and successfully manage their risk in the department. It seems ironic that if admitted to an acute psychiatric ward, that this personal, relationship-based treatment is often replaced with observation. Observation may protect an individual's physical safety but may risk damaging their psychological safety.

Cutcliffe and Barker (2002) suggest that there are two approaches to the care of suicidal clients: 'observation' and 'engagement and inspiring hope'. They argue that the observation approach limits the role of the nurse to that of a custodian, and has little therapeutic value. Using the

Box 28.1 An example of an observation care plan and monitoring for Serena

Care need

Serena has a history of violent suicide attempts and today was found at home with a noose tied to her banister. Serena is also known to act impulsively. She is expressing a desire to die in order to 'be with God' and appears irritable in mood.

Plan

Serena will be closely observed at all times by registered nursing staff. The purpose of this observation is to maintain her safety by preventing her from impulsively harming herself and de-escalating any conflict that arises with other clients. The nurse in charge and duty psychiatrist will review this level of observation in 6 hours' time, once an initial risk assessment has been undertaken. During this period of observation, the nurse observing her will explain the purpose of her observation, show her around the ward, introduce her to the other staff and clients, explain emergency procedures, and document Serena's mood, suicidal thoughts, behaviour and any other concerns she may raise.

Observations

Time	Observations
14:00–16:00	Serena appears frustrated at being back on the ward. She feels angry that we won't leave her alone, and has been slamming her room door and asking me to sit outside. I have explained that we will try to keep this period of observation as short as possible and that our aim is to make sure she is safe on the ward. Serena says that there are times when she wishes she were dead. She says she tied the noose to her stairs to 'wind up' her CPN and denies any suicidal plans at present. In the coffee room she was laughing when telling other clients she was 'on special'.
16:00–18:00	Spent half an hour in the quiet room telling me that she feels angry with herself for coming back into hospital. On reflection, Serena thinks she knew she was becoming unwell again and that she did think about killing herself because she feels stuck in a cycle of 'hospital, depression, hospital, depression'. She finds it hard to look forward to anything, because although she is beginning to feel 'happy' and 'powerful', she knows it won't last. From 16:30 until 18:00 Serena was with the duty psychiatrist and her named nurse, doing her admission assessment.
18:00–20:00	Serena felt tired after her assessment and wanted to eat her supper in her room. She spent time in the day room, watching TV and talking to other clients in the smoking room. Her mood seemed irritable when another client asked her for a cigarette, and she knocked the ashtray over before running out of the room. Serena did not want to talk about this. In the garden, she mentioned that she enjoyed gardening and asked if the OT still worked with people in the garden.

Evaluation

The duty psychiatrist, named nurse and charge nurse met to discuss Serena's observation. Assessment reveals she is thinking about suicide and displaying impulsive behaviour such as slamming her door and knocking over the ashtray – however, these have been in response to the frustration of being observed and being asked for a cigarette. She has made no attempt to harm herself or leave. She has no specific plan at present, and her own belief is that she will not harm herself on the ward. She has been prescribed 7.5 mg zopiclone at night.

The process of observation may be exacerbating Serena's irritable mood. However, a moderate risk of an impulsive suicide attempt still exists. If the zopiclone is effective, and Serena sleeps well tonight, the observation level can be reduced to general observation, and then reviewed when she awakens in the morning.

If she has slept well, and her impulsive behaviours have not increased, it is agreed that the team will consider reducing the observation level.

interpersonal processes of engagement and inspiring hope may help to address the problem of how to nurse someone who is feeling suicidal.

They describe the engagement process as forming a relationship, conveying acceptance and tolerance, and hearing and understanding. If the client is valued by their nurse, this sense of worth can be conveyed to the client who may be experiencing feelings of hopelessness and worthlessness. In the absence of a relationship with a client, the mental health nurse is inhibited from doing anything else, and in itself the relationship is valuable. As with deliberate self-harm, acknowledging, accepting and tolerating the client, without conditions supports the process of engagement. Thurgood discusses engaging clients in detail in Chapter 22.

Engaging with someone who is suicidal can itself inspire hope. There is a sense of expectation created in the relationship – you expect your client to live, to recover. Imagine the contrast with continuous close observation, where you are expecting your client to do something harmful. In their study of what relatives of suicidal people found hope-inspiring, Talseth *et al.* (2001) identified six themes:

- being seen as a human being;
- participating in an 'I–You' relationship;
- trusting staff, treatment and care;
- feeling trusted by staff;
- being consoled;
- entering into hope.

These themes were fundamental for the relatives to feel that they had 'been met' during the crisis of their relatives being suicidal. Being met, Talseth *et al.* (2001) propose, is a passageway to hope. This could equally be applied to the client as the relative or carer. Table 28.5 shows what Collins and Cutcliffe (2003) describe as the key elements of hope and hopelessness.

Cutcliffe and Barker (2002) suggest that the same processes involved in engaging with a client, demonstrating unconditional acceptance, tolerance

Table 28.5 Key elements of hope and hopelessness

Hope	Hopelessness
Multi-dimensional	Multi-dimensional
Dynamic	Dynamic
Empowering	Disempowering
Central to life	A threat to the quality and longevity of life
Related to external help	Related to the absences of caring, or
Related to caring	uncaring practitioners
Orientated towards the future	Orientated towards the past
Highly personalized towards each individual	Highly personalized towards each individual

(Source: Collins and Cutcliffe 2003)

and understanding, inspire hope because of the relationship between caring and hope.

For Serena, her main emotions appear to be anger and frustration at being readmitted to hospital and a fear of being depressed again when she is eventually discharged. It will be important for staff to listen to, accept and tolerate her anger, frustration and help her to explore these feelings. Although Serena fears her future, she does envisage it. She has also demonstrated a positive interest in her sharing a joke with another client, and enquiring about the occupational therapy gardening group. Promoting or facilitating these interpersonal relationships and experiences will help to create purpose, and therefore diminish hopelessness in Serena's life.

Although there is a gradual shift in focus in the care of people who are suicidal, the majority of NHS trusts have policies and an expectation that people at high risk of attempting suicide are closely observed. As Bowers *et al.* (2000) have shown, where these policies exist they differ greatly across the country. As you will be expected to closely observe clients, it is important that you consult the local policy in your clinical area. Ideally, continuous, close observation should only be used as an emergency provision, but where it is required, you must be clear of what is expected of you, and wherever possible use it as an opportunity to engage with, form a relationship, accept, tolerate, listen to and understand the person with whom you are working.

Special groups

When working with people who self-harm or are suicidal, there are groups of the population who need special consideration: young people, older adults, and people with psychosis who are self-harming in response to psychotic experiences.

Young people

The Royal College of Psychiatrists (1998) have made specific recommendations for the management of deliberate self-harm in young people. In summary, they recommend that all young people under the age of 16 who self-harm should be admitted to an appropriate paediatric or medical ward so that a comprehensive assessment of risk and the young person's mental health can be undertaken. This assessment will involve the young person, their family, mental health, social and education services, and, therefore, will take some time. Ideally an agreed local protocol should exist in order to manage these cases.

Older adults

Older adults are less likely to self-harm, but those that do are at an increased risk of suicide (Marriott *et al.* 2003) and are identified as one of the target groups for the promotion of mental health in the National Suicide Prevention Strategy (Department of Health 2003). Marriott *et al.* (2003) found that people over the age of 55 who had self-harmed were more likely than those under 55, to be admitted to a mental health unit for further assessment and treatment. When working with an older adult who is either suicidal or who has self-harmed, it is important to consider this increased risk.

People with psychosis

There is a markedly increased risk of suicide for clients with psychotic illnesses (Harris and Barraclough 1997) and this risk is further elevated in those who have a co-morbid psychosis and personality disorder (Moran *et al.* 2003). There is the potential for a further exacerbation of risk if an individual's experience of psychosis includes command auditory hallucinations (instructing them to self-harm or commit suicide) or beliefs that they should harm or kill themselves. While the risk is high, nurses can help clients to identify the strengths and strategies the client has used to resist these instructions or beliefs. If the client is in such distress that they are compelled to act on the instructions they hear or believe, emergency measures such as continuous close observation in an inpatient setting may be necessary to try to protect the individual's physical safety.

Being safe

Rather than addressing risk-assessment issues, this section is concerned with maintaining the physical and psychological safety of nurses who work with people who self-harm or are suicidal. Any mental health work can be stressful, but the added pressure of working with someone with potentially life-threatening behaviour, means that extra support is required. Furthermore, this chapter has emphasized the importance of the relationship between client and nurse as the key to any therapeutic intervention. Relationships are not risk free. People who self-harm have often had traumatic relationships in their past, and the ways in which they form and break relationships may mirror the impulsivity displayed in their self-harming behaviour. Not only do suicide attempts often follow the loss of an interpersonal relationship (Hall *et al.* 1999), but people who self-harm may have had previous negative experiences of their relationships with health care workers (Smith 2002).

There is also a risk when trying to de-escalate someone who is in the process of self-harming. If someone is using a knife, razor blade or glass to cut themselves, there is a risk that this could be used against a nurse trying to intervene. It is not suggested that someone who self-harms is likely to be violent to others, rather that at the point of self-harming, they might be emotionally charged and acting impulsively. This combination can put health care professionals at risk of being injured.

The following key points may help nurses to maintain their physical and psychological safety:

- The responsibility for self-harming behaviour always remains with the client.
- Supervision is essential, both as an individual nurse working with clients who self-harm, and as a team.
- Risk assessments should be made by the multi-disciplinary team, and risk-management plans agreed.
- Continuous close observation should only be used as an emergency provision.
- Ask clients to hand in any sharp objects they may have and do not attempt to remove any sharps by force.

If someone self-harms, it is neither a failure on the nurse's part, and nor should the client be blamed. Incident reporting may help to highlight other contributory factors that have influenced the client's distress as well as monitoring the rates and type of self-harm in any clinical area. Also, if there is an incident where someone self-harms or attempts suicide, part of the purpose of incident reporting is to ensure that the health care professionals involved receive appropriate support from their manager or supervisor.

Summary

This chapter has given an overview of the different types of self-harm behaviour and explored the relationship between self-harm and suicide. In summary, the main points are:

- Self-harm is a behaviour not an illness. However, there is a strong association between self-harm and suicide, and nurses have a health-promoting role to try and help reduce the psychological distress that underlies the behaviour.
- Viewing self-harm and suicide on a continuum may help nurses to understand the emotional context of such behaviour.
- In all cases, the therapeutic relationship is the key to working with these client groups.
- Models of care from addictions nursing have scope for application to working with people who self-harm: assessing motivation, considering where someone is in a cycle of change (Prochaska and Velicer 1997), and harm-minimization techniques have been suggested as ways of engaging clients who self-harm.
- The science, or research evidence, suggests that techniques such as problem solving are likely to reduce the frequency of further self-harm,

though there are insufficient, large-scale, longitudinal studies to advocate one particular treatment (Hawton *et al.* 2003).

- The art is to use interpersonal skills of engagement (forming a relationship, conveying acceptance and tolerance, and hearing and understanding), and inspiring hope to help clients who may be suicidal shift their position from one of hopelessness to possibility (Cutcliffe and Barker 2002).

- People who self-harm want to be treated with respect, and conveying acceptance and tolerance is a key to understanding how and why they are using self-harm as a coping mechanism.

- Risk assessment is a dynamic process, and it is the author's opinion that there is still a role for continuous close observation, as an emergency provision while risk is assessed.

- Anyone who works with people who self-harm or are suicidal must have clinical supervision in order to manage the anxiety, frustration and anger that may arise from being in a therapeutic relationship with clients for whom relationships are difficult.

Questions for reflection and discussion

1   What are your beliefs about and attitudes towards people who self-harm?
2   In relation to Table 28.2, what behaviours do you do that might damage your health in the short or long term?
3   Consider Jenny's case, outlined in the case study. If you were nursing Jenny, how might you encourage her to engage with treatment?
4   Serena still feels suicidal. Reflecting on the brief details given in the case study and Table 28.5, think about how you could 'inspire hope' with Serena.
5   What do you think about continuous close observation? Try to imagine having someone with you 24 hours a day and list the different feelings you might have.

Annotated bibliography

- Barker, P. and Cutcliffe, J.R. (2000) Creating a hopeline for suicidal people: a new model for acute sector mental health nursing. *Mental Health Care* 3(6): 190–3. Barker and Cutcliffe outline a new model of care for suicidal people. They propose a combination of restoring hope through individual, in-depth assessment and developing a personalized 'security plan'. The model can be applied to other aspects of acute psychiatric care.

- Hawton, K., Townsend, E., Arensman, E. *et al.* (2003) Psychological and pharmacological treatments for deliberate self-harm. *The Cochrane Library*, Issue 2. Oxford: Update Software. A systematic review of randomized control trials relating to the treatment of deliberate self-harm. Raises issues of the lack of longitudinal follow-up and large-scale studies in deliberate self-harm research. This text provides summaries of the effectiveness of problem-solving interventions, short- and long-term therapy, intense intervention plus outreach, emergency card provision, dialectical behaviour therapy, general hospital admission and treatment with anti-depressants.
- National Institute for Clinical Excellence (2004) Self Harm: short-term physical and psychological management and secondary prevention of self-harm in primary and secondary care. Draft for second consultation. National Collaborating Centre for Mental Health, Commissioned by the National Institute for Clinical Excellence. http://www.nice.org.uk/pdf/ SelfHarm_full_guideline_secondcons.pdf

  This draft guideline has been developed by a multidisciplinary team of health care professionals, clients, their carers and other representatives. It outlines national guidelines recommending short-term physical and psychological management of self-harm as well as recommending strategies for preventing self-harm. It includes evaluations of the assessment and treatment of people within the first 48 hours following an episode of self-harm, as well as considering ongoing pharmacological and psychological treatments in primary care and in mental health services.
- National Self-Harm Network (2003) National Self-Harm Network website: http://www.nshn.co.uk and Self Harm Alliance (2003) Self Harm Alliance website: http://www.selfharmalliance.org. Both of these websites provide an invaluable resource in terms of service user experience and opinion, links to self-help groups and other support agencies, information for health care professionals, people who self-harm and their carers. They are regularly updated and have links to other online resources and organizations.

References

Abba, K., Church, E. and Webster, J. (1999) What happens to patients who attend A & E with deliberate self-harm? – tracking the follow-up they receive, *Journal of Clinical Governance* **7**: 68–73.

Barker, P. and Cutcliffe, J.R. (2000) Creating a hopeline for suicidal people: a new model for acute sector mental health nursing. *Mental Health Care* **3**(6): 190–3.

Bongar, B. (2002) *The Suicidal Patient. Clinical and Legal Standards of Care* (2nd edn). Washington, DC: American Psychological Association.

Bowers, L., Gournay, K. and Duffy, D. (2000) Suicide and self-harm in inpatient psychiatric units: a national survey of observation policies, *Journal of Advanced Nursing* **32**: 437–44.

Centre for Review and Dissemination (1998) Deliberate self-harm, *Effective Health Care*. **4**(6) NHS Centre for Review and Dissemination: University of York http://www.york.ac.uk/inst/crd/ehc46.htm

Cleary, M., Jordan, R., Horsfall, J., Mazondier, P. and Delaney, J. (1999) Suicidal patients and special observation, *Journal of Psychiatric and Mental Health Nursing* **6**: 461–7.

Collins, S. and Cutcliffe, J.R. (2003) Addressing hopelessness in people with suicidal ideation: building upon the therapeutic relationship utilizing a cognitive behavioural approach, *Journal of Psychiatric and Mental Health Nursing* **10**: 175–85.

Cutcliffe, J.R. and Barker, P. (2002) Considering the care of the suicidal client and the case for 'engagement and inspiring hope' or 'observation', *Journal of Psychiatric and Mental Health Nursing* **9**: 611–21.

Department of Health (1990) *Health of the Nation*. London: HMSO.

Department of Health (2001) *Safety First – Five Year Report of the National Confidential Inquiry into Suicides and Homicides by People with Mental Health Problems*. London: HMSO.

Department of Health (2003) *National Suicide Prevention Strategy for England* http://www.doh.gov.uk/mentalhealth/suicideprevention.htm

Fletcher, R.F. (1999) The process of constant observation: perspectives of staff and suicidal patients. *Journal of Psychiatric and Mental Health Nursing* **6**: 9–14.

Gallop, R. and Tully, T. (2004) The person who self-harms, in P. Barker (ed.) *Psychiatric and Mental Health Nursing: The Craft of Caring*. London: Arnold.

Hall, R.C.W., Platt, D.E. and Hall, R.C.W. (1999) Suicide risk assessment: a review of risk factors for suicide in 100 patients who made severe suicide attempts: evaluation of suicide risk in a time of managed care, *Psychosomatics* **40**(1): 18–24.

Harris, E.C. and Barraclough, B. (1997) Suicide as an outcome for mental disorders. A meta analysis, *British Journal of Psychiatry* **170**: 205–28.

Hawton, K., Townsend, E., Arensman, E. *et al.* (2003) Psychological and pharmacological treatments for deliberate self-harm. *The Cochrane Library*, Issue 2. Oxford: Update Software.

House, A., Owens, D. and Patchett, L. (1999) Deliberate self-harm, *Quality in Health Care* **8**: 137–43.

Jones, J., Ward, M., Wellman, N., Hall, J. and Lowe, T. (2000) Psychiatric inpatients' experiences of nursing observation. A United Kingdom perspective, *Journal of Psychosocial Nursing* **38**(12): 10–19.

Marriott, R., Horrocks, J., House, A. and Owens, D. (2003) Assessment and management of self-harm in older adults attending accident and emergency: a comparative cross-sectional study, *International Journal of Geriatric Psychiatry* **18**: 645–52.

Melville, A. and House, A. (1999) Understanding deliberate self-harm. *Nursing Times* **95**(7): 46–7.

Moran, P., Walsh, E., Tyrer, P. *et al.* (2003) Does co-morbid personality disorder increase the risk of suicidal behaviour in psychosis? *Acta Psychiatrica Scandinavica* **107**: 441–8.

National Self-Harm Network (2003) http://www.nshn.co.uk

Prochaska, J.O. and Velicer, W.F. (1997) The transtheoretical model of health behaviour change. *American Journal of Health Promotion* **12**(1): 38–48.

Prochaska, J.O., DiClemente, C.C. and Norcross, J.C. (1993) In search of how people change: applications to addictive behaviours. *Addiction Nursing Network* **5**(1): 2–16.

Reid, W. and Long, A. (1993) The role of the nurse providing therapeutic care for the suicidal patient. *Journal of Advanced Nursing* **18**: 1369–76.

Royal College of Psychiatrists (1994) *The General Hospital Management of Adult Deliberate Self-harm: A Consensus Statement on Standards for Service Provision (Council Report CR 32)*. London: Royal College of Psychiatrists.

Royal College of Psychiatrists (1998) *Managing Deliberate Self-harm in Young People (Council Report CR 64)*. London: Royal College of Psychiatrists.

Self Harm Alliance (2003) http://www.selfharmalliance.org

Smith, S.E. (2002) Perceptions of service provision for clients who self-injure in the absence of expressed suicidal intent, *Journal of Psychiatric and Mental Health Nursing* **9**: 595–601.

South London and Maudsley (2001) *Crisis Recovery Service: A Service for Individuals who Self-Harm. Philosophy and Protocols for the Management of Self-Harm*. London: South London and Maudsley NHS Trust.

Stengel, E. (1965) *Suicide and Attempted Suicide*. Bristol: MacGibbon & Kee.

Stevenson, C., Jackson, S. and Barker, P. (2003) Finding solutions through empowerment: a preliminary study of solution-orientated approach to nursing in acute psychiatric settings, *Journal of Psychiatric and Mental Health Nursing* **10**: 688–96.

Talseth, A., Gilje, F. and Norberg, A. (2001) Being met – a passageway to hope for relatives of patients at risk of committing suicide: a phenomenological hermeneutic study. *Archives of Psychiatric Nursing* **15**(6): 249–56.

van der Sande, R., Buskens, E., Allart, E., van der Graaf, Y. and van Engeland, H. (1997) Psychosocial intervention following suicide attempt: a systematic review of the literature, *Acta Psychiatrica Scandinavica* **96**: 43–50.

Weber, M.T. (2002) Triggers for self-abuse: a qualitative study, *Archives of Psychiatric Nursing* **16**(3): 118–24.

PART 5

Future directions

29

Functional teams and whole systems

Steve Onyett

This chapter adopts the time-honoured approach of defining terms ('functional teams' and 'whole systems') before then describing the teams in question and looking briefly at the research on what they can achieve for users. It then considers team working itself before looking at the whole service system and how teams within it need to interrelate. The penultimate section considers how to achieve effective whole systems working before looking at some of the specific implications for nurses.

I describe what the *Mental Health Policy Implementation Guide* (MHPIG) (DH 2001a, 2002a,b) says about various forms of teams but from a critical perspective, since the guide itself is an excellent reference with which readers should be familiar. It is the definitive government guidance on how teams should be developed in line with the *National Service Framework (NSF) for Mental Health* (DH 1999) and the *NHS Plan* (DH 2000), and is being revised and added to. The chapter covers:

- the meaning of functional team;
- types of mental health teams;
- key issues about the operation of all teams;
- effects of team provision on outcomes for service users;
- engaging service users and their social networks;
- assertive Community Treatment and the 'team approach';
- whole systems thinking, care coordinators, and inter-team relationships;
- teams for various groups of service users;
- the case for service integration;
- whole systems service improvement;
- implications for mental health nursing.

What do we mean by 'functional teams'?

The phrase 'functional teams' does not appear in the MHPIG or the *NSF for Mental Health* (although the rather alarming word 'functionalized' appears once). Nonetheless, the phrase has emerged to distinguish teams that are established to fulfil a specific function. The implication is that 'functional teams' are different from existing community mental health teams (CMHTs). This itself could be seen as fairly damning, implying that CMHTs either have no function or are 'dysfunctional'. This was perhaps true of many CMHTs of the 1980s and 1990s (Onyett 2002), although many CMHTs had learned the lessons of the international case management and assertive community treatment literature prior to the *NSF for Mental Health* and had accordingly become more targeted and clear about their operations.

The MHPIG was keen to dispel the notion that the newer teams are to usurp existing CMHTs, stressing that:

> The new services outlined in this guide are designed to enhance the local mental health systems. It is not intended that where good services are in place, like well functioning CMHTs, that these services should be abandoned ... [CMHTs] should provide the core around which newer service elements are developed. The responsibilities of CMHTs may change over time with the advent of new services, however they will retain an important role. They, alongside primary care will provide the key source of referrals to the newer teams. They will also continue to care for the majority of people with mental illness in the community.
>
> DH (2002a: 6–7)

Given the unambiguous targets and rigorous performance management that accompanied the development of the newer teams, it is interesting to note that the *NSF for Mental Health* had a permissive tone regarding service configuration, stating that:

> CMHTs may provide the whole range of community-based services themselves, or be complemented by one or more teams providing specific functions. This latter model is most common in inner city and urban areas. Whichever model is used, the mental health system will need to provide the range of interventions and integration across all specialist services.
>
> (DH 1999: 47)

The full range of interventions referred to in the MHPIG covers 'early intervention; assertive outreach; home treatment; the needs of those with comorbidity; black and minority ethnic communities; homeless people; or mentally disordered offenders'. The guidance refers also to rehabilitation teams focusing on the housing, income, occupational and social needs of people with 'serious disabilities resulting from their mental illness'.

This functional approach is helpful in thinking about team design in a locality. The overriding imperative to bear in mind is that whatever the fashion for new teams may be, our task is to ensure that the right functions are fulfilled for the right people. In parts of the Avon area the *Developing Individual Services in the Community* framework (DISC) (Smith, H. 1998) was used to provide an even more comprehensive approach to local needs assessment and service development. The use of such a framework with a broad range of stakeholders serves to establish some key values and a shared language about what mental health services should be achieving for people. Team functions explored using the DISC framework are listed in Box 29.1.

It is important to consider how teamworking *across the patch* provides the right range of functions for service users. This teamworking within the locality will include a range of service configurations, the design of which needs to be informed by local needs assessment, existing strengths in local provision, and the unique history, geography and demography of the patch.

The newer teams may be the key to achieving this range of functions. However, we should not be dazzled by novelty. Rather we should build on existing strengths, particularly on those parts of the existing system where mental health service users have built strong and effective relationships with staff. To ensure a comprehensive, effective and well-targeted local service system we should be informed about service models, the specific components of their implementation that appear to be effective, and evidence for their effectiveness.

It is unhelpful to restrict the term 'functional teams' to the newer service models only. All local teams need to be functional, including inpatient teams. The existing research evidence reviewed below suggests that even the most intensive community service will not completely eliminate the need for inpatient care. The principles of effective team design and teamworking are applicable equally to inpatient teams, and indeed it may be at admission and discharge that effective whole systems working is *most* essential to promote continuity of care and effective communication. Continuity of practice between the hospital and the community is critical, and it is encouraging

---

Box 29.1 The functions explored using the DISC framework

With respect to the following key functions, how are the needs of local people currently being met, and how might they be better met:

- Needs for equitable and fair access and good information.
- Needs for individual planning.
- Meeting needs in crisis.
- Needs for treatment and support with mental distress.
- Needs for ordinary living and long-term support, for example regarding employment, housing and money.
- Needs for personal growth and development.

to see the emergence of teams (often crisis-resolution teams) that span inpatient and community care by having members that provide both.

Whole systems working demands 'whole systems thinking', a term that highlights the need to design, plan and manage organizations as living, independent systems while working to achieve 'seamless' care for those they aim to serve. In turn this begs an awareness of the multitude of factors involved in health and social care and the lives of users and their social networks. Complex health and social problems lie beyond the ability of any one practitioner, team or agency to resolve. Whole systems thinking emphasizes also the need to develop shared values, purposes and practices within and between organizations, and uses large group interventions to bring together the perspectives of a wide range of stakeholders across a wider system (Iles and Sutherland 2001).

Types of mental health team

This section outlines policy guidance and research findings with respect to the different types of mental health team featured in the *NSF for Mental Health* and *NHS Plan* and described in detail in the MHPIG.

'Assertive outreach' teams

These are teams aiming to serve people with 'A severe and persistent mental disorder (for example, schizophrenia, major affective disorders) associated with a high level of disability' (DH 2001a), who are heavy users of inpatient or intensive home-based care, and who have difficulty also in maintaining lasting and consenting contact with services. These people are likely to have multiple complex needs including risk of harm to others or themselves, persistent offending, concurrent substance misuse and unstable accommodation or homelessness. The MHPIG identifies key aspects of service design and implementation as the critical ingredients of assertive outreach teams. These teams should:

- be self-contained and responsible for providing a wide range of interventions (these are specified in detail in the MHPIG);
- have a single responsible medical officer who is an active member of the team;
- provide treatment on a long-term basis with an emphasis on continuity of care;
- deliver most services in community settings;
- emphasize maintaining contact and building relationships with service users;
- provide care coordination by the team; and
- maintain small caseloads of no more than 12 service users per staff member.

Some teams have sought to avoid the term 'assertive' because it over-emphasizes the potentially coercive nature of intensive community treatment. Words such as 'intensive' or 'active' community treatment have been proffered as alternatives. It is also unhelpful that these teams are described as 'assertive outreach' teams in the Guidance. Assertive outreach has been used to describe the practice of taking services to where people need them in their own environment, regardless of the type of team. It is also a key feature of the crisis resolution and early intervention teams described below. The more commonly used term in the international literature on these kinds of teams is 'assertive community treatment' (ACT). The defining characteristic of ACT is not the location of care but the *intensity* of service provision provided in community settings in order to achieve effective working relationships with people with whom this can be a challenge. The acronym 'ACT' will therefore be used here because of its widespread currency.

The efficacy of ACT in a UK context remains contested and large UK studies of service structure are underway. The prevailing view appears to be that the successes of ACT as practised in the USA have not been replicated in Europe, although there are examples of successful services, as described below. This failure is attributed on the one hand to a failure to implement ACT with sufficient fidelity to the model (Marshall *et al.* 1999), and on the other to the fact that standard mental health care in Europe is far superior, therefore, making the contrast with ACT less measurable (Tyrer 2000).

Marshall and Lockwood's (1998) review of randomized controlled trials concluded that significant and robust differences between ACT and standard community care could be found on accommodation status, employment and patient satisfaction but not for mental state or social functioning. Other key reviews, that take less account of UK studies (Mechanic 1996; Mueser *et al.* 1998), make modest claims for improvements in symptomatology, functioning and quality of life although more recent studies have shown greater gains (Johnston *et al.* 1998). Assertive, targeted teams can reduce inpatient bed use (Merson *et al.* 1992; Burns *et al.* 1993; Dean *et al.* 1993; Marks *et al.* 1994; Marshall and Lockwood 1998) and as a result it has been judged to be cost-effective (Burns *et al.* 1993; Knapp *et al.* 1994; Mechanic 1996).

The UK experience, as elsewhere, has shown that when ACT is discontinued improvements are lost, for example in social functioning and reduced time in hospital (Audini *et al.* 1994). This has important implications for when and how a step down to less intensive provision takes place. Burns and Firn (2002) suggest that ACT teams need to reduce support gradually to that which users will receive in step-down care. They ensure that service users are stable on one contact per month for at least three months, and their experience is that the whole discharge process usually takes around six months.

The possibility of step-down care to other services, such as the CMHT, continuing care teams or the primary care team, is a feature of ACT that may be lacking in other countries. Burns and Firn's (2002) account is unusual in that it is based upon the experience of running the Wandsworth

ACT team, one of our few mature teams. Their expectation is that the team will have a client turnover of about 10 per cent a year, which, with a caseload of around 100, equates to one user being admitted and one discharged per month. Potentially, users could be served by the team for around 10 years though the team aspires to an ideal turnover of 15–20 per cent and an average time for users to work with the team of around five years. The team also allows a minimum of one year to achieve effective engagement. Usually it would take one or two years of concerted effort for the team to decide that the team is not appropriate for the user's needs.

Crisis resolution (or 'home treatment') teams

These teams provide a 24-hour service to users in their own homes to avoid hospital admissions where possible and provide the maximum opportunity to resolve crises in the contexts in which they occur. Their role in the mental health system is to ensure that individuals experiencing severe mental distress are served in the least restrictive environment, and as close to home as possible.

Although the MHPIG advocates local flexibility regarding client groups, crisis teams are most commonly targeted on people with severe mental distress who might require hospital admission. These teams therefore need to sit in the pathway between community-based referrers and inpatient care and be able to act as a point of assessment and as a gatekeeper to other parts of the mental health system for people in severe distress. They will therefore usually need the capacity to provide immediate home treatment 24 hours a day, 7 days a week.

Clients will often be people with an existing diagnosis of severe mental disorder such as schizophrenia, manic depressive disorder, or severe depressive disorder. The guidance recommends excluding people with mild anxiety disorders, a primary diagnosis of alcohol or other substance misuse, an exclusive diagnosis of personality disorder, and a recent history of self-harm in the absence of a diagnosis of psychosis. It also advocates not responding to crisis related solely to relationship issues. How realistic it is to apply these exclusion criteria out of hours and in crisis remains to be seen. Other key features of crisis resolution team operation includes:

- remaining involved with the service user until the crisis has resolved and they are linked into ongoing care;
- where hospitalization is necessary, being actively involved in discharge planning and providing intensive care at home to enable early discharge; and
- working to reduce future vulnerability to crisis.

From prior experience, the MHPIG highlights the following key principles of care:

- a 24-hour, 7-day a week service;
- rapid response following referral;

- intensive intervention and support in the early stages of the crisis;
- active involvement of the service user, family and carers;
- an assertive approach to engagement (i.e. assertive outreach as described above);
- time-limited intervention with sufficient flexibility to respond to differing service user needs;
- an emphasis on learning from the crisis with the involvement of the whole social support network.

Joy *et al.*'s (2001) review of crisis intervention reported only a limited effect on admissions but found home care to be as cost effective as hospital care with respect to loss of people to local services, deaths and mental distress. Crisis services reduced the burden on families, and were preferred by both users and families. Routing all referrals for inpatient care through the crisis service appears to be critical to their success in offering a realistic alternative to admission. They are, therefore, likely to be highly dependent on support from those practitioners who can circumvent the system by making direct admissions to inpatient care.

Early intervention teams

These teams work proactively to serve people in the early stages of developing psychotic symptoms in order to reduce their longer-term dependency on services and promote better outcomes. They are targeted on people aged between 14 and 35 with a first presentation of psychotic symptoms, and people aged 14 to 35 during the first three years of psychotic illness.

Increased delay between the first onset of psychotic phenomena and receiving treatment produces negative longer-term consequences (Drake *et al.* 2000). It may also be that the early stages of psychotic experience are a critical phase during which key psychological and biological changes occur (Birchwood *et al.* 1998). The first few years of psychosis carry the highest risk of social disruption and suicide. It therefore follows that providing help as soon as possible should have a positive longer-term impact. The guidance highlights that it can take up to two years after the first signs of psychosis for an individual to begin receiving help. Lack of awareness, ambiguous early symptoms and stigma all contribute to the delay in appropriate help being offered. Service systems need to be able to identify people early in the course of their distress by working closely with primary care, ACT teams, and other people who are likely to encounter young people with psychotic experiences (for example, college counsellors, police, agencies for homeless people).

Garety and Jolley (2000) highlight encouraging early evidence for the efficacy of psychological interventions in the early phases of psychotic experience, but suggest that they need to be highly attuned to the recovery style of the individual and embedded within a service response that combines pharmacological interventions, family work and vocational and social programmes. A wide variety of interventions are described in the MHPIG. In summary, the guidance suggests that an early intervention service should:

- reduce the stigma associated with psychosis and improve professional and lay awareness of the symptoms of psychosis and the need for early assessment;

- reduce the length of time young people remain undiagnosed and untreated;

- focus on managing symptoms rather than the diagnosis;

- develop meaningful engagement, provide evidence-based interventions, and promote recovery during the early phase of psychotic experience;

- increase stability in the lives of service users, facilitate personal development and provide opportunities for personal fulfilment (for example, through education and meaningful employment);

- provide a seamless service for those aged 14–35, that integrates child, adolescent and adult mental health services and works in partnership with primary care, education, social services, youth and other services;

- provide culture, age and gender sensitive family-orientated services in the least restrictive and stigmatizing setting. This will include separate, age-appropriate facilities for young people (see, for example, Box 29.5 on page 809: the Plymouth Early Intervention Service).

- at the end of the treatment period, ensure that the care is thoughtfully and effectively transferred. The maintenance and re-establishment of the integration of young people with age-appropriate, mainstream services is an ongoing aim of early intervention services. Therefore, there is a need to establish a wide range of links, for example, with primary care, education, youth agencies, leisure providers and other relevant services across the voluntary and statutory sectors.

Community mental health teams

CMHTs appear to be that crucial part of the whole service system that is left when the other newer service models have become operational. The MHPIG update on CMHTs (DH 2002a) is, therefore, not prescriptive about team structure but rather focuses on the functions that the team should achieve. However, it also stresses that even these functions may be fulfilled in other ways. It highlights three major functions:

1 giving advice on the management of mental health problems by other professionals – in particular advice to primary care and a triage function enabling appropriate referral;

2 providing treatment and care for those with time-limited disorders who can benefit from specialist interventions;

3 providing treatment and care for those with more complex and enduring needs.

The guidance acknowledges that the first two may be fulfilled by CMHTs in the form of primary care liaison teams. There are also a rich variety of other primary care or community-based services that may fulfil this function, not least the UK government's own plans for 1000 new graduate workers in primary care to help GPs manage common mental health problems, and the 500 new 'Gateway' workers to respond to people requiring immediate help. The NHS Plan requires that both types of worker are to be trained and deployed by 2004.

The MHPIG also highlights that 'rehabilitation and recovery teams' may fulfil the third function. Where there are complex issues such as difficulty establishing effective working relationships with users, and multiple diagnoses this function is also likely to be fulfilled by the local ACT team.

We are, therefore, left in a problematic situation regarding social policy on teams. We have recommendations for CMHTs that acknowledge that many of their functions will be carried out in other ways, and recommendations for newer team models that key commentators continue to suggest are already carried out by existing CMHTs (Tyrer *et al.* 2001). Some have felt it nonsensical to reconfigure already effective services to accord with newer service models where existing teams have already evolved to fulfil the required functions (for example, Tyrer 1998; Thornicroft *et al.* 1999; Simmonds *et al.* 2001).

In this context it has to be questioned whether it is helpful to restrict the term CMHT to a specific *type* of team since in practice it may be impossible to reliably define and recognize from one locality to the next. It is notable that mature UK ACT teams tend to stress their continuity of practice with existing CMHTs rather than differences (Burns and Firn 2002) and this has been substantiated by Simmonds *et al.*'s (2001) review of CMHTs which found them to be achieving many of the functions claimed for the newer service models, such as reducing inpatient treatment, reducing costs, less dissatisfaction with care, better engagement and fewer suicides. Any team providing coordinated multi-disciplinary input in community settings through a team process is by definition a 'community mental health team'.

The MHPIG describes the CMHT 'function' as being to: increase capacity within primary care through collaboration, reduce stigma, ensure that care is delivered in the least restrictive and disruptive manner possible, and stabilize social functioning and protect community tenure. However, there is nothing in the description of how CMHTs work that gives them a privileged role in achieving these functions. People with 'time limited disorders (who can) be referred back to their GPs after a period of weeks or months' are described as the major client group of CMHTs. It is very questionable whether involvement in a dedicated team process is the best way to serve such individuals. Instead, people could be effectively served through individual practice-based counselling or therapy (Gask *et al.* 2000; Mellor-Clark 2000). More radically, Box 29.2 describes a service to primary care that works to keep individuals involvement in specialist services to a minimum by building capacity to respond to mental health problems within

Box 29.2 The Mental Health in Primary Care team. Gloucestershire

The team has developed free open access Stress Management Workshops in cooperation with Cirencester College. The workshops are delivered continuously to meet demand, last six weeks and are provided in non-health settings. Information about the workshops is obtained from members of the primary care team, CMHTs, the college brochure and leaflets on stress. People who are identified as being significantly anxious or depressed are advised to see their GP. The workshops are facilitated by an occupational therapist with co-facilitators from primary care who thus acquire the skills to run groups themselves.

The team has also developed a Certificate in *Professional Studies: Mental Health in Primary Care* for primary care clinicians who have not undertaken specific mental health training. It is a six-day module at level two. Each participant produces a resource, such as a self-help leaflet, assessment tool or awareness poster. Some of these are selected for countywide distribution. This focus on products is felt to promote 'ownership' of mental health issues in primary care.

These workshops and training are integrated with assessment and signposting from an experienced mental health worker; a full range of psychological therapies available in primary care, including computerized CBT; primary care team facilitation and training; and full evaluation.

Whole systems working has been seen as an important part of the project. The team has had to develop information about resources and assist neighbourhood projects in enabling their own staff to be more responsive to the mental health needs of their community. As well has the local primary care teams, the Mental Health in Primary Care team works with specialist mental health services, colleges of higher education, a mental health project for black and minority ethnic groups, Health Promotion, voluntary agencies, the District Council, the local Health Authority and other community resources.

The team obtained funding to employ a mental health service user to develop a resource directory and ensure that self-help information is available at every Primary Health Care team across the county. Links with the non-statutory sector and education providers have dramatically enhanced service delivery, for example, by being able to provide crèche facilities. Assistant psychologists were found to be an extremely useful workforce in the delivery and evaluation of initiatives.

The project has improved access to cognitive behavioural therapy and other evidence-based treatments and doubled the number of adults seen over a year with stress related difficulties. From the outset the Project had steering group representation from service users, primary care, the Health Authority and secondary care staff. This has been crucial to ensuring ownership and change in practice.

Contact: Jackie Prosser, Primary Mental Health Coordinator, Hadwen Medical Practice, St Michael's Surgery, St Michael's Square, Gloucester, Gloucestershire GL1 9HX. Tel: 01452 505 362. email: Jackie.Prosser@egnhst.org.uk the primary care team and providing psychological help through less stigmatizing routes such as further education.[1]

The MHPIG also describes a 'substantial minority' of CMHT caseloads as requiring 'ongoing treatment, care and monitoring for periods of several years'. This includes people with:

- severe and persistent mental disorders associated with significant disability (such as schizophrenia and bipolar disorder);
- longer-term disorders of lesser severity but which are characterized by poor treatment adherence requiring proactive follow-up;
- a significant risk of self-harm or harm to others;
- needs for a level of support that exceeds that which a primary care team could offer (for example, chronic anorexia nervosa); and
- disorders requiring skilled or intensive treatments (for example, CBT, vocational rehabilitation, medication maintenance requiring blood tests) not available in primary care.

Except where they have been taken on by local ACT teams or specialized personality disorder teams the guidance also suggests that CMHTs may serve people with severe disorders of personality where these can be shown to benefit by continued contact and support, and people with problems of 'management and engagement' of such complexity and severity that the powers of the Mental Health Act (1983) are invoked.

The guidance makes efforts to describe a valued role for CMHTs as separate services from the new 'functional' teams. However, it is easy to see how CMHT staff may come to feel devalued and demoralized. They are being described as the place where primary care addresses its capacity problems regarding people with more minor mental health problems, while simultaneously being the repository for all the community-based clinical provision that the newer teams decline; and in many cases offering step-down care where these teams feel they have fulfilled their role. CMHTs may also have least control over their caseloads while continuing to serve very challenging clients.

Issues of definition and lack of fidelity in implementation make outcome research on CMHTs as with any teams problematic. CMHTs are also so ubiquitous it is difficult to envisage a site where a standard care would not include CMHT provision of some kind. We have described above how the systematic review of CMHTs by Simmonds *et al.* (2001) found that CMHTs achieved some of the benefits of ACT but to a lesser extent. For example, the impact on reducing inpatient bed use was interpreted by the authors as less than ACT but greater than case management. As with much of the ACT literature (for example, Marshall and Lockwood 1998) they found no evidence of gains in social functioning and clinical symptomatology. Again as with the ACT reviews definition problems abound in that some of the teams covered may, in practice, be as close to ACT teams as many of the teams covered in ACT reviews. For example, the team described by Merson *et al.* (1992) (which used to be managed by the author) included many of the features of an ACT team, including home visiting and clinical co-working with colleagues within and outside the team.

Borrill *et al.* (2000) examined 113 CMHTs as part of a large-scale study of health care teams in the NHS. They found that effective CMHTs were more likely to have few part-time workers, a positive team climate (described below), a single, clear leader, and relatively low stress levels. The biggest contributor to poor functioning of teams was unclear team objectives. It will be important that local team members, in whatever part of the local health and social care system, can see their team's contribution to the whole and understand and agree how the local population is to be served. This requires approaches to local service development in mental health that have hitherto been unusual, and which are described later. Clarifying the role of the team is also a key task of team leaders and managers. It is notable that in the Borrill study a lack of clear objectives was associated with the absence of a clear team leader or coordinator or where there was conflict about leadership.

Teams with the labels disregarded

Whatever type of team we are thinking about there are some key issues about the operation of any team that need to be considered. In the past team working was seen merely as what people do in teams. Ovretveit (1986) noted how 'Just calling a group of practitioners a team has become a way in which managers and planners avoid the real problems and work needed to coordinate an increasingly complex range of services in the community'.

Whenever thinking about team design we need to keep in mind why and if teamworking is needed. Shea and Guzzo describe a work group as 'three or more people employed by an organisation who see themselves as a group, are seen by others in the organisation as a group and *who depend on each other for resources to accomplish a task or set of tasks*' (1987: 327, emphasis added). Teams need to look hard at this issue of interdependence between team members to get the job done. It bears on what types of decisions can be best made within the user–staff member relationship alone by pooling their shared expertise and experience, which require the involvement of others in the team or beyond, and which require the involvement of the whole team. These detailed issues are beyond the scope of this chapter but are explored in detail in Onyett (2002) and through the national *Action learning for improved team working and leadership in mental health* programme.[2]

We need to look to the broader social psychology literature to get a view of what constitutes effective teamworking. For example, West *et al.* (1998) have produced a large body of research culminating in the study of NHS health care teams (Borrill *et al.* 2000) which found effective teamworking to be associated with clearer objectives, higher levels of team member participation in decision making, a stronger commitment to quality and better support for innovation. Working in effective teams was also associated with improved mental health among staff, perhaps because they serve to buffer team members from the worst impacts of wider organizational change.

West *et al.*'s (1998) formulation of what constitutes a 'complex decision-making team' such as a mental health team captures some of the dynamic nature of the environment in which teams have to operate:

- *They operate in uncertain, unpredictable environments.* Perhaps the only predictable quality of the policy context in which teams operate is that it will be constantly changing.

- *They work with uncertain and unpredictable technology.* For CMHTs the uncertain nature of risk assessment and management is a key example (see Chapter 8 in this volume).

- *It is unclear how tasks should be performed on a day-to-day basis.* Not only is there often a contested evidence base for much that is provided to users, but also there are often ideological schisms within the team concerning the very nature of mental distress and its care and treatment.

- *Team member interdependence is high.* Where teams are targeted on people with the complex health and social care needs there is an obvious need for team members with different backgrounds to combine their efforts to achieve successful outcomes.

- *Autonomy and control for the teams are relatively high.* This is true despite the highly prescriptive nature of the *NSF for Mental Health* and the MHPIG. This issue is explored below.

- *The tasks that the team are required to perform are complex.* Work in mental health teams may require high levels of technical knowledge, for example, in terms of the application of complex psychological theory, the effects and side effects of prescribed drugs, and unravelling the vagaries of the benefits system. In addition practitioners may experience ethical and intellectual tensions, for example, regarding their roles as caring professionals responding to need alongside their increasingly explicit role as an agent of social control.

- *There are multiple components of effectiveness, and the team is responsible to multiple constituents.* For example, in order to develop a tool to evaluate CMHT effectiveness, Richards and Rees (1998) had to systematically map what a range of stakeholders expected CMHTs to achieve. The stakeholders involved in developing these effectiveness criteria included users, carers, advocates, practitioners, policy makers, managers and researchers.

We cannot assume such teams will be effective because of a magical 'synergy' that arises when people are organized into groups. Team effectiveness can be achieved only through premeditated design and good team process that both take thorough account of the context of the team's work. This in turn requires a clear understanding of the tasks that the team has to perform for the people it is established to serve, and some consideration of the knowledge, skills and experience that individuals need to bring to the team. We cannot assume teams will be effective unless we very specifically design them to be effective, and recruit and train their members accordingly.

Does teamwork work?

We have seen above how the outcome of different team models remains contested because of uncertainty about the fidelity of implementation to specific models, the different contexts in which teams are implemented and the extent to which they constitute an improvement on the existing local service system. Spindel and Nugent (1999) also expressed concern about:

- the problem of researchers evaluating their own services, including the problem of data being collected by team members themselves;
- over-reliance on staff accounts rather than independent assessment of user perspectives and direct observation;
- poor definition of the service that was actually being delivered;
- neglect of the effects of social inequalities arising from race, gender, poverty and previous involvement in the criminal justice system;
- failure to take adequate account of the effects of high drop-out rates, and views on the adequacy of the service among those who dropped out;
- the short time-span (often two to three years) of many studies. Given that this is such a short time in the life of someone with severe mental health problems, results gained from such evaluations may have limited validity.

Determining the effect of team provision on outcomes for users is also problematic because of the user's involvement with other services and other 'uncontrolled' aspects of their lives. To judge services properly we need to take account of the net benefit of running the service in a way that encompasses outcomes for users, the effects on their social supports, service use, hospitalization, involvement in the criminal-justice system and other indicators of community mental health. Very few studies have achieved such comprehensive evaluation although the Madison experiment (Stein and Test 1980) and the study of the Crisis Intervention Service in New South Wales (Hoult 1986) provide notable exemplars. Both supported the development of intensive community interventions. Provan and Milward (1995) also looked at the whole system of community support. They examined the 'network effectiveness' of four community mental health services. Networks were evaluated rather than specific organizations, recognizing that outcomes for users will depend on the actions of a range of agencies. This study found that integration of providers was unlikely to improve outcomes unless the network was stable, resourced adequately and centrally and directly controlled.

In the USA evaluations of several national service demonstrations have shown that although reforms in the system occurred the impact on individual service users was very limited (Goldman *et al.* 1994; Ridgely *et al.* 1996). These changes have been seen as necessary but insufficient for improving the lives of people with severe mental distress and attention has shifted to content and quality of services (Goldman *et al.* 2001).

Sashidharan *et al.* (1999) argued, from the perspective of an experienced clinician informed by the existing research, that it is common sense to expect more intensive and targeted community services to make a difference but that different team types should, therefore, be evaluated in terms of the extent to which they provide an effective platform for the delivery of care (Gournay 1999). The achievement of positive outcomes for users will be determined by the quality of that care. In order to get the care at all, users will need to remain effectively involved with teams. It, therefore, makes sense to evaluate teams principally in terms of the extent to which they successfully involve users and their social networks in change.

Engaging users and their networks

The working alliance between users and staff has a significant impact on outcomes for people with severe mental health problems (see Onyett 2000 for review and Chinman *et al.* 2000). This is more likely to be achieved if they are getting a service they want (see Chapter 5 of this volume).

People receiving ACT, case management and crisis resolution services are more likely to remain in contact with services than people receiving standard community care (Marshall and Lockwood 1998; Marshall *et al.* 1998; Joy *et al.* 2001). Intensive community teams are also better able to ensure that difficult-to-serve people maintain contact following discharge from hospital (Ford *et al.* 1995; Holloway and Carson 1998; Johnston *et al.* 1998). This may be explained by the balance of evidence which suggests that these services are preferred by users and their social networks (Hoult *et al.* 1983; Merson *et al.* 1992; Marks *et al.* 1994; Holloway and Carson 1998; Joy *et al.* 2001). This tends to be because of the high quality of their relationships with staff (McGrew *et al.* 1996). McGrew *et al.* (2002) found that even when asked specifically about aspects of ACT that users disliked least 44 per cent were unable to identify a negative aspect. However, such research needs to be interpreted in light of the obvious power relationships that exist between staff and users. Another 21 per cent expressed concern about home visits and intrusiveness, although others complained about the lack of intensity of contact.

Regarding users' social networks, Mueser *et al.* (1998) concluded that there was an emerging trend towards increased satisfaction among relatives and speculated that this was associated with the community-orientated locus of care.

Overall, it can be concluded that where teams are intensive, proactive and focus on developing good working relationships by providing support to achieving outcomes valued by users themselves, they can effectively engage them, keep them out of hospital and in many cases improve important aspects of their lives. However, there is a risk that these good working relationships will become soured if intensive approaches are implemented insensitively or are too strongly identified with a coercion and control.

Smith *et al.* (1999) warn against the more coercive aspects of ACT as practised in parts of the USA and Canada becoming manifest in the UK. The withholding of welfare payments unless users accept treatment in particular. Deci *et al.* (1995) found that 82 per cent of the 303 US ACT teams they surveyed provided 'financial management' of users' income.

Spindel and Nugent (1999) also criticized ACT teams role in collaborating with other agencies to enforce treatment, particularly medication, and expressed concern about ACT staff collaborating with probation and parole officers to reincarcerate users when they were found to be non-compliant. Diamond also expressed concern about the nature of some inter-agency working and communication:

> This communication, even when done with the client's permission, allows enormous pressure to be applied for the client to take medication, stay in treatment, live in a particular place, or 'follow the plan' in any number of ways. This pressure can be almost as coercive as the hospital in controlling behaviour, but with fewer safeguards.
>
> (1996: 58)

The *NSF for Mental Health* tended to frame ACT as part of a risk reduction and crisis prevention strategy rather than as a way of providing users with better quality care on their own terms. Indeed, the most explicit *NSF for Mental Health* standard for ACT concerns suicide prevention. It is too early to draw firm conclusions about the advantages or disadvantages of ACT with respect to risk of harm to users themselves or to others (Marshall and Lockwood 1998). Burns and Firn caution against ACT's role in reducing risk being 'overplayed' stating that 'teams work best when they engage patients collaboratively rather than attempting to control them' (2002: 295). While not neglecting the important role that ACT can have in helping to assess and manage risk they also make the point that untoward incidents happen in the contained environment of a hospital ward and so it would be an unrealistic 'hostage to fortune' to suggest that ACT represents a panacea for risk management.

It remains to be seen how ACT will be regarded by both users and staff if it becomes associated with the more coercive measures that may be introduced with a new mental health act. There is a risk for all of us that the advantages of working actively and intensively with individuals and agencies can become oppressive because they are embedded in ideologies and practices that fail to pay enough respect to users' views, aspirations and rights. In this context the emphasis being paid by the National Institute of Mental Health for England on the recovery approach and an explicit set of values to underpin mental health work is very welcome (see Chapter 5, this volume).

ACT and the 'team approach'

Its adherents advocate the 'team approach' as the key feature that separates ACT from other intensive community approaches such as case management. It advocates that all service users should have a relationship with all members of the team, rather than a single worker in a care coordinator role. Advantages claimed include:

- improved continuity of care because strong relationships with staff have not come and gone;
- reliable weekly contact because workloads are shared;
- opportunities for more intensive and flexible responses as staff can be called upon to respond to changing clinical need;
- a better response to crises that is not reliant on one worker's availability;
- peer support and consultation;
- reduced stress for staff, partly because of the greater containment of the emotional responses of staff to clinical work (Navarro 1998);
- better access for users to staff who may share or be sensitive to their unique cultural and ethnic background; and
- the avoidance of 'pathological dependency' whereby the therapist's competence at improving the mental health of the user paradoxically reinforces their low self esteem, and sense of inadequacy and personal failure.

This approach is now widespread among ACT teams after having been pioneered by the Tulip project in Haringey and the Impact team in Hammersmith, London. Evaluating the former team, Gauntlett *et al.* (1996) found effective engagement with users and good morale among staff.

However, users have also identified negative implications of this approach. Spindel and Nugent identified difficulties 'for any human being to establish warm, supportive, and trusting relationships with a "team"' (1999: 7). The same experience was reported by Burns and Firn (2002) who found that it simply did not accord with their experience of working with people with severe and long-term mental health problems who were often shy or mistrustful. They advocated building up one relationship through time, commitment and consistency and only then working to expand the network of people involved. In their experience some people may never accept contact with more than one or two staff members. Indeed, some users of the Tulip service expressed a preference for individual relationships with fewer staff (Gauntlett *et al.* 1996). Burns and Finn (2002) reported that far from always being 'pathological', their experience suggested that periods of dependence are part of a normal pathway to independence.

Spindel and Nugent also expressed concern that the 'team' approach could creates barriers to social inclusion because it gives the impression that

> a client is so abnormal, bad, or different that a whole team of people is needed to work with him or her . . . Far from seeing a person as having strengths, and creating a context for their empowerment, this kind of overprofessionalized, stigmatising approach may destroy what little self-worth, sense of belonging, and hope a client has.
>
> (1999: 8)

They argue also that teams are not easy for family and friends to work with, and that high-profile professional responses may lead others to drop their involvement. They complained of having to tell the same story to different team members and experienced a lack of continuity among staff in the way they managed tasks over time. Some teams have overcome these practical difficulties using ongoing task sheets (for example, Greenwich) or a shared team diary to ensure that tasks do not get lost. However, even on this point the Wandsworth ACT team has rejected this task-centred approach in favour of a more person-centred approach akin to care coordination where individuals have primary responsibility for ensuring that tasks get done. They argue that the task-centred approach takes too much time to administer and supervise and produces information overload for staff. They also report that users 'want the security of knowing that some recognisable individual has an overview of their needs and bring continuity to ensuring their welfare' (Burns and Firn 2002: 48–9). Even staff at Tulip sought this role with some missing the opportunities to develop individual responsibility for a holistic approach to their work with users. Some reported practical difficulties, for example, in establishing effective liaison with other agencies where the task was shared within the team (Gauntlett *et al.* 1996).

The exact opposite of the team approach is the 'generic' keyworker approach where individual workers supply all one-to-one contact themselves. This is clearly nonsensical and negates the point of having a multidisciplinary team staffed with people with a variety of knowledge, skills and experience. In other words, if the keyworker can do it all themselves why work in a team at all? This approach was characteristic of some community mental health centres of the late 1980s where valued notions of democratic team structures and flat hierarchies served to fudge the need to examine individual practice, skill mix within the team and individual team members different levels of authority to make decisions (Patmore and Weaver 1991).

In practice, if the user in question really does need contact with only one worker in the team then they probably do not need to be seen by a multidisciplinary team at all. At the other extreme the dogmatic application of the 'team approach' may be just as inappropriate and insensitive. Burns and Firn (2002) note that many teams claiming adherence to the team approach in reality operate more flexibly in response to the needs of users. The most pragmatic and sensitive response is usually to consider the user and their social networks as the centre of a virtual team and build the required supports and relationships around them on the basis of their preferences, needs and experience of what works. This normally means at least three members of the team being fully familiar with them.

Many of the claims for the whole team approach described above could also be regarded merely as features of effective multi-disciplinary team working (Onyett 2002). We have for too long assumed that effective team working will be an emergent property of bringing people together in teams. Experience has shown that this is far from the case and pre- and post-qualifying education and training needs to regard it as necessary, problematic and an area that requires expert attention.

‘Whole systems thinking’

‘Whole systems thinking’ has a high profile within the policy rhetoric within the *NSF for Mental Health* and the subsequent MHPIG. It is worth taking these documents as our starting point while acknowledging that systems thinking has much deeper roots and important implications that reflect ways of thinking about mental health service design and implementation that may be both new and fruitful.

At its most prosaic, whole systems thinking is about ensuring that all the component parts of a mental health system are in place and ‘in balance’ (*NSF for Mental Health*, DH 1999: 7). The MHPIG emphasizes ‘the need for whole systems development which will address the most conspicuous gaps in service provision. We cannot afford to focus on any single aspect of the mental health system and hope that this will provide a solution’ (3). Achieving the stated ‘balance’ referred to in the *NSF for Mental Health* requires new priorities, new investment and reinvestment of existing resources. Unacceptable variations in service use, for example, in the use of hospital beds, are interpreted as ‘a sign that not all mental health services are operating a whole systems approach’ (ibid. 49).

One implication of this is that change needs to involve a broad spectrum of people in a variety of roles. The MHPIG stated that:

> Such a comprehensive programme of change cannot be achieved by a single agency or a single profession working in isolation. One of the defining characteristics of mental health services is the range of disciplines who frequently need to be involved in the care plan of a single individual; suitable accommodation, adequate income, meaningful occupation, and family support all play a part alongside competent diagnosis, treatment and care.
>
> (DH 1999: 7)

This demands high levels of joint working and communication both between individuals in teams, and across teams working in different settings.

The MHPIG also makes clear the requirement for new information systems to improve both direct care and our overall understanding of the quality of care being delivered. This will also be needed to inform and monitor the de facto rationing that goes on through team referral and allocation processes (Griffiths 2001).

Care coordination as the glue that binds

As soon as we begin to think about what is required to achieve a high level of joint working between elements of the whole service system, we need to acknowledge the complexity of the system involved. Systems are embedded within each other. The nature of complex systems is such that a change in one element has implications for many other elements. Taking the obvious need for service elements to work effectively together means looking at the system of care at the individual level – the level described by the integrated care programme approach (or 'care coordination'). Care coordinators should be the glue that binds the system together in a coherent way for service users and their supports: 'It is critical that the care co-ordinator should have the authority to co-ordinate the delivery of the care plan and that this is respected by all those involved in delivering it, regardless of agency of origin' (NHSE/SSI 1999: 22). This objective is supported by strong inter-agency agreements between health and social care on the use of pooled budgets to support the implementation of the care plan. Care coordinators need to work with families and other natural supports, as well as liaising with other agencies such as employers, housing providers, primary care, inpatient facilities, education providers, leisure services, the Benefits Agency and criminal justice agencies. The role should also include 'inreach' into inpatient settings and prisons. Indeed, the multi-agency nature of the work is such that the MHPIG states, 'No one service or agency is central [to the system of relevant agencies involved]. Service users themselves provide the focal point for care planning and delivery' (DH 2000a: 3). It therefore follows that teams need to be built around their needs to support the exercise of care coordination and that these teams need to be commissioned as part of a coherent whole system.

MHPIG guidance on inter-team relationships

For care coordinators and other team members to be able to work effectively across teams there needs to be clarity about who is being served and how and when they can achieve access. Figure 29.1 describes *only* those direct referral relationships described in the MHPIG. In reality the referral network will be even more complex. The figure captures just some of the complexity at service level and the need for clarity about how parts of the system will interrelate. It highlights also the importance of an inter-team care coordinator role that will smooth transitions and ensure continuity.

Box 29.3 describes the respective service responses that the MHPIG advocates from the different teams. Extended hours, rather than a 24-hour

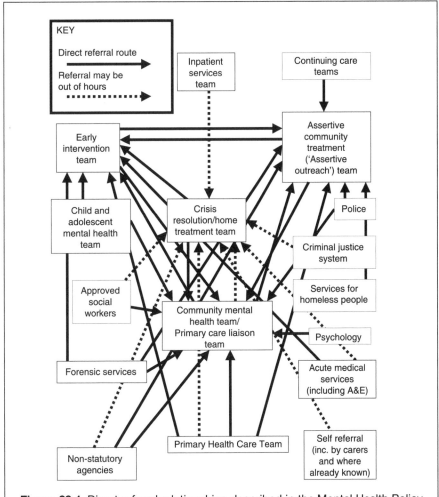

Figure 29.1 Direct referral relationships described in the Mental Health Policy Implementation Guide: Community Mental Health Teams (DH 2002a)

response is advocated for ACTs. Burns and Firn (2002) found the introduction of a seven-day working week particularly valuable in that it covered weekend periods when users were particularly vulnerable to relapse arising from lack of activity, contact and increased substance misuse. Contrary to expectations, these periods are not used for dealing with crises and mainly comprise planned visits and phone calls.

The MHPIG envisages that crisis resolution teams will usually be providing the crisis response for clients of the ACTs and early intervention teams out of hours. However, it is important to stress that the MHPIG does not propose that crisis response work would be restricted to the crisis resolution service. Where the ACT team is involved with the individual concerned they should offer the community-based response within working hours. Where continuing input is needed following a crisis the ACT team,

---

Box 29.3 Mental Health Policy Implementation Guidance (DH 2002a) on service responses around the clock

Team type	Core working hours	Out of hours response
Assertive community treatment	8 a.m. to 8 p.m., 7 days a week.	One member of staff on call for phone advice. No provision for home visits. If visit are required, referral should be made to the crisis resolution team.
Early intervention	8 a.m. to 8 p.m., 7 days per week.	A member of staff on call for phone advice, or alternatively from staff at a linked community respite facility (either by telephone or by visiting the unit). No provision for home visits. If visit are required, referral should be made to the crisis resolution team or the CAMHS out-of-hour service.
Crisis resolution/ home treatment	A shift system is required to ensure a minimum of two trained caseworkers available 24 hours a day, 7 days a week. Home visits to known service users require two caseworkers. The 24-hour assessment team for assessment of new referrals should also include a senior psychiatrist.	The evening/through the night service is usually accessed through an on-call system. The medical on call rota should allow a senior psychiatrist to undertake home visits 24 hours a day.
CMHT/Primary care liaison team	9 a.m. to 5 p.m. weekdays with flexible out-of-hours working for specific tasks (for example, evening work for a relative support group). Some teams may chose to work with moderately extended hours, for example, 8 a.m. to 7 p.m. to accord with GP surgery times. This is strongly recommended for improved primary care liaison.	No crisis provision is made out of hours by the CMHT and patients and carers would access the local emergency services (crisis resolution teams, help lines, A&E, etc.).

---

crisis resolution team and the other parts of the local service system should work together to ensure that the least restrictive and stigmatizing setting for care is arranged. The whole system should work together to avoid hospitalization and restrictive care wherever possible, and opportunities to provide care in the community or service user's own home should be grasped.

The MHPIG stresses that effective joint working requires links to be established between the teams within a locality so that:

- Handover and referrals are made easily.
- Crises are anticipated and contingency plans are known to all involved in care.
- Early intervention and assertive outreach service users are aware of whom to contact out of hours.
- Staff from the assertive outreach team and/or early intervention team can participate in the crisis resolution/home treatment team out of hours rota. It may also be advantageous to involve inpatient staff in these rotas so that they do not feel like an excluded part of the wider system and are able to contribute their skills, expertise and knowledge of the user to promote continuous and effective care.
- If inpatient care is needed for ACT clients, the team can maintain contact during the user's stay, contribute to decision making concerning discharge planning and ensure that the home environment is ready for discharge. Regular joint, formal reviews should aim to promote transfer to the least stigmatizing and restrictive environment as soon as clinically possible.
- Local arrangements are made between the crisis resolution team, the early intervention team and child and adolescent mental health services to ensure rapid access to an out of hours crisis service for users under 16 years old.

Once again, however, no matter how clear the inter-team relationships and protocols are, the key tool for helping individual users navigate the system is an up-to-date care plan developed through the care coordination process. This care plan should include individually tailored contingency plans that specify what works well for this individual in a given circumstance and what actions should be specifically avoided.

Teams for who?

What team design or development is needed in a given context needs to be informed by how the current service is meeting the needs of a range of service users with varying needs. This requires some shared language for who is being served. This can be uncomfortable as it groups people together into broad, crudely defined groups for the purposes of service development. However, Rubin and Panzano (2002) argue that this lack of more holistic descriptions, beyond diagnosis or diagnosis-related groups, has been a barrier to the development of recovery-orientated community support systems. They identified five meaningful subgroups among over 3600 service users in Ohio using multivariate statistical analysis and have reorganized services accordingly.

In the absence of a comparable UK study the following framework was developed from Shepherd (1999) (see Onyett 2002) and further developed by

Schneider (2002)[3] as a tool for caseload auditing and weighting. Although unsupported by statistics it appears to have face validity for clinicians and begins to describe how people presenting with different needs and histories might best be served within a whole system of care. This does not mean, of course, that people fitting these descriptions will always have the same needs and will remain dependent on the services described.

Groups of local service users and possible service responses

Group A: Long-term users who place a high level of demand on services

Effective and well-coordinated multi-agency programmes are needed to help Group A users out of the 'revolving door' of hospital admissions, and other chaotic service contacts. Shepherd stressed the need for the 'right kinds of interagency links (for example with housing, day provisions, etc), and the right kind of attitudes and "philosophy" to provide consistent long term support' (1999). Group A service users are likely to have other specific treatment needs (for example, regarding substance misuse, reduction of self-harm, anger management). They are a highly visible group who will be known to staff on acute wards, social workers, GPs, police, probation, and other agencies. As well as diagnoses of severe mental illness, people in this group may also have been assessed as having a personality disorder. Although heavy users of services, people in this group may often have lower levels of enduring disability than people in Group B below. Group A users most closely fit the client group definitions for ACT set out in *Keys to Engagement* (Sainsbury Centre for Mental Health 1998). This estimated the number of people requiring intensive service provision, for example, through ACT at around 45 per 100,000 of the population but with considerable variation (14–200) depending on the locality.

Group A users need to be served by a team that has many of the features of ACT teams as described above. Thornicroft *et al.* (1999) argued that a well-functioning CMHT offers most of the advantages of such intensive community treatment while also offering more long-term support, increased flexibility and a simpler service structure. However, other commentators have found that incorporating assertive outreach as a function of existing CMHTs can give rise to problems in maintaining the level of coordination, skill development, and cross-support needed. Burns and Firn also expressed concern about ACT workers who are 'dislocated from like-minded colleagues and a consistent model' (2002: 299) as a result of this approach. However, in some rural catchments the geographical dispersal of clients may mean that attempting to preserve a single ACT-style team with an adequate caseload may be at the expense of other key aspects of team working.

There is consensus that to meet the needs of Group A users the team and its caseload should be restricted. If it becomes too large, staff have difficulty getting to know all the users being seen by the team and the intensity of the service drops. Practitioners should have no more than 12 on their caseload and the whole team of around seven to eight members should have no more than 60–100 cases in total. If the number of Group A users within a locality is low, then incorporating users fitting the profile of Group B below into the work of the team can have advantages. The style of work is similar in that team members, often in their roles as care coordinators, will need to work very closely with other agencies to ensure that users' needs are regularly assessed, addressed, monitored and reviewed.

Group B: Long-term users with high levels of disability but low levels of demand

People in this category usually have low motivation to continue with programmes of care and treatment. Considerable input is needed to maintain community living for this group; without this they fall out of follow-up care and can live a very marginalized existence with poor quality of life. They are likely to live in a variety of sheltered and supported housing. Some may live in their own homes cared for by families or support staff.

Service users in Group B are easy to overlook in a busy 'acute' or primary care orientated service. Without input from a specialist team they are likely to deteriorate, particularly socially, and lose contact with services. Some lose contact with specialist services completely and are seen in primary care, if at all. Local needs assessment should include working with the primary care team and their practice registers (reviewing by diagnosis and therapeutics) to ensure that people in this category who are registered with GPs are having their care reviewed regularly.

Group C: Long-term users with lower levels of disability, but intermittent high demand

People in Group C are more likely than those in Groups B and C to have a stable level of adjustment, for example, they are more likely to be able to hold down a job and maintain key relationships. However, they are likely to have complex care plans and require regular support and monitoring of the plan in order to remain stable. They may be vulnerable to occasional relapses that require effective crisis intervention and in some cases inpatient admission.

Group D: Long-stay service users who have been resettled into the community as part of a programme of hospital closure

The basic needs of people within this group are likely to be met within the residential setting in which they have been placed. These settings will normally be operated by non-statutory, private or 'not for profit' organizations. There is nonetheless a need for regular contact with statutory services, not least because of the highly variable quality of care in such settings (Shepherd *et al.* 1996).

The stable functioning and secure accommodation of people in this group means that they can be incorporated within larger caseloads, albeit with mechanisms to ensure regular and routine review. They are unlikely to require the same service response as people who are less easy to involve effectively in services. Achieving effective working relationships may, nonetheless, be a challenge and practitioners need to be able to work flexibly with them over long periods. This may be an area where the greater deployment of community support workers, such as the new Social Time and Recovery workers (WAT 2001) may be able to make a substantial contribution (Murray *et al.* 1997), either as part of CMHTs or more specialized community rehabilitation teams.

Group E: New users with severe mental health problems (for example, psychosis) who do not have major problems with effective engagement

This category was advocated by psychiatrists who felt that a proportion of people that they saw as outpatients had severe mental health problems (for example, a diagnosis of psychosis) yet could be assessed, treated and discharged without an expectation that they would need long-term involvement with specialist mental health services. Group E users are similar to those in Group F below, but are distinguished from them by their psychotic illness diagnosis and the increased likelihood that they will be seen mainly by a psychiatrist. This group could be amalgamated with Group F described below if uni-disciplinary psychiatric outpatient services are perceived as outdated, and so not provided.

Group F: People with severe health care or social care needs whose difficulties can be resolved through contact with one discipline or agency within specialist mental health services

Users in Group F require input from practitioners with considerable training and expertise in health or social care provision, who will need to communicate effectively with each other in order to work most efficiently. However, this need *not* require a dedicated team approach, where expensive professional staff meet frequently to allocate and review cases. Such care could be provided through a more open multi-disciplinary, multi-agency network of practitioners. The network may have a regular weekly or fortnightly forum for peer consultation on particularly difficult cases, but routine review of all cases is unlikely to be necessary. Peer consultation meetings would be in addition to the practitioner's own consultation or supervision from a nominated person.

Such a service could operate as a psychological therapies and counselling service in primary care or other community settings. Examples of referrals might include people diagnosed with agoraphobia, panic disorder, moderate depression, people with sexual dysfunctions, and *some* people diagnosed with borderline personality disorders or eating disorders.

Group G: People with less severe health or social care needs whose needs do not require specialist mental health services to resolve

Increasingly, people presenting with minor to moderate mental health problems have their needs met within primary care settings or the independent sector, for example, by GPs, counsellors, practice nurses, health visitors or community workers. Examples of the kinds of mental health problems experienced by this group include minor degrees of anxiety, depression or emotional disturbance related to life stressors, personality problems in the absence of other mental health or social care needs, substance misuse problems in the absence of mental health service needs, or referrals for counselling, anger management, assertiveness, social skills or anxiety management training.

Practitioners working with Groups E, F or G above will generally be used to a linear style of work with users whereby people's needs are formulated, addressed and then resolved. In contrast, work with people in Groups A to D demands a more iterative approach with constant assessment, reassessment (or review) and concurrent adjustment of provision to ensure the best configuration of treatment, care and support.

Crisis-resolution staff are most likely to be involved with users in Groups A, B, C or E, and will need to be able to link effectively to the parts of the service that are more routinely involved in their care.

Service integration

There is a need for clarity about how people with the most long-term mental health problems should be served. Both ACT and rehabilitation services focus on this client group and ACT teams have evolved both within mainstream adult services and within rehabilitation services.

Rehabilitation services have their own coherent ideology, based upon a 'disability' model that emphasizes managing one's entire life, rather than just being treated for an illness. This is closer to the recovery approach than the ideologies that have prevailed traditionally in mainstream adult mental health services. The classic definition of psychiatric rehabilitation from Douglas Bennett as a 'process of helping a physically or psychiatrically disabled person make the best use of his or her residual abilities in order to function at an optimum level in as normal a social context as possible' (1978), is as relevant today as ever it was and captures the positive emphasis on social inclusion that is so much a part of the current policy Zeitgeist.

There may now be strong arguments for abandoning the traditional boundaried style of rehabilitation services in order to make better use of the invaluable resource of knowledge, skills and experience contained therein and apply the more socially informed ideology of care that has characterized rehabilitation services to all users of mental health services. The same spirit of realistic optimism and hope that characterizes the recovery approach (see Chapter 5), should shape the support that people receive, regardless of their age and service history. There is a danger that separate rehabilitation services:

- create enclaves that promote dependence and exclusion (for example, reliance on sheltered work and clubhouses, rather than promoting supported employment in real jobs);
- perpetuate long-standing problems of trying to generalize skills learnt in a therapeutic setting to real-life situations (for example, regarding social skills training, vocational training programmes);
- exacerbate poor and inequitable access to the most relevant provision creating delays for people in getting the right help at the right time because of meaningless service eligibility criteria. For example, Burns and Firn (2002) describe how whether a user is served by the main ACT team or the rehabilitation outreach team depends upon whether the user is in independent accommodation or staffed residential accommodation. This may be the best division of labour in the interests of preserving and promoting existing relationships. But in some contexts it may create inflexibility in the deployment of valuable skills, knowledge and experience. Similarly, some rehabilitation services operate eligibility criteria to the effect that individuals have to be in the local mental health system for a year without improvement before they are considered to be eligible for rehabilitation. By the time they access the right service, their ability to benefit from it may be substantially impaired.

The MHPIG advocates that so long as there is evidence of benefit, ACT should continue indefinitely. Nonetheless there will be a continuous need for 'step-down' care for those people who require less intensive interventions to maintain their stability. The capacity for step-down might again be better coordinated and deployed if rehabilitation teams and CMHT combine their resources to provide it.

Dual diagnosis

The imperative to integrate care within mainstream mental health services also extends to people with a dual diagnosis of mental distress and substance misuse. Models of assertive community treatment that integrate mental health and substance misuse services appear to hold much promise (Gournay *et al.* 1997; DH 2002b) and some ACT teams include dual diagnosis workers (for example, Greenwich, Cheltenham).

The MHPIG update on good practice in dual diagnosis (DH 2002b) advocates:

- providing care for dually diagnosed individuals within mainstream mental health services through close working with drug and alcohol services;

- deploying specialist teams of dual diagnosis workers to provide support to mainstream mental health services;
- training all staff in ACT teams in work with dual diagnosis, as well as staff in crisis resolution teams, early intervention teams, inpatient services and CMHTs; and
- ensuring that care coordination extends to people with dual diagnosis and all the services that work with them.

Whole systems service improvement

One feature of complex systems is that you can define them as narrowly or as widely as you wish. It is a question of utility in terms of the issues you need to address and just how much you and your colleagues can hold in your heads and work with effectively.

Capturing the whole complexity of 'whole systems'

Figure 29.2 illustrates a local whole system. At the centre are users themselves and their social networks. The latter phrase is used advisedly. Bainbridge (2002) provides a powerful critique of how the term 'carers' makes a range of assumptions about the role of relatives, friends and others

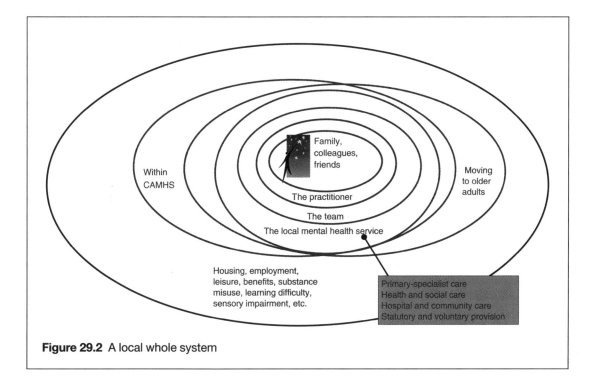

Figure 29.2 A local whole system

in users' lives while also making unhelpful assumptions about how they define their role with respect to the user concerned. In the main it is this social system that teams should be working with rather than taking an overly individualistic view (see Smith, M. 1998).

Working outwards, there is then the question of how practitioners relate to that complex social system and how in turn they are supported in their work by the team (or teams) of which they are a member. There is then the question of how the team fits into the local service system which in turn is influenced by how other interconnected systems concerned with the relationship between health and social care, primary and specialist care, the statutory and voluntary sector and hospital and community care interact. For many service users there are then issues concerning how they transfer to or from related systems of care for children and adolescents or older adults. All this is similarly embedded within other systems concerned with the provision of housing, employment, benefits, and, in many cases, a range of other specialist services. These systems themselves operate in ways that are influenced by wider societal perceptions of people with mental health problems.

It is perhaps unsurprising in this context that today there is greater recognition of the need to disseminate knowledge and understanding about how complex systems work. This must go beyond abstract theorizing, to understanding and managing change, which is crucial if care environments for service users are to improve. Many care environments are very resistant to change. Hutchison (1999) makes the point that, from a user perspective, the most remarkable thing about mental health services and their repeated policy reforms is how little the lot of service users within these systems improves.

Plsek and Greenhalgh defined a complex system as 'a collection of individual agents with freedom to act in ways that are not always totally predictable, and whose actions are interconnected so that one agent's actions changes the context for other agents' (2001). We have explored this with respect to the way teams in a locality interrelate. Other systems with which we should be concerned include those that influence how different professionals relate to the experience of team working, the training and education system that supplies team members, systems that create family-friendly work policies, so that staff are supported in managing the interface between their work and home lives (for example, with respect to picking children up from school), and systems that influence how society views people with mental health problems and in some cases acts to exclude them from the rightful roles as citizens (for example, by threatening their status as employees or tenants). Each system has its own rules that shape the behaviour of its members, and which may not be understood or comprehensible to other actors within it. However, because actors and their behaviour can change, a complex system can evolve over time, and different systems that may be connected, or embedded one in the other, can evolve and co-evolve.

The evolution of one system influences and is influenced by other systems. For example, tabloid scandal-mongering and misrepresentation has fed social concerns about risk of violence from service users, which have almost certainly influenced politicians, and, in turn, social policy and new legislation. At a team level this has influenced the profile of risk assessment and management for clinicians and increased personal anxieties about responsibility and accountability. More positively, the disability rights movement and the political rhetoric of social inclusion has influenced the mental health user movement, academic debate and those working in mental health services and has helped shaped the new recovery-orientated ideology of care promulgated vigorously by the National Institute of Mental Health for England. These developments in turn influence practice in ways that lead to tensions and paradoxes that can never be fully resolved. For example, team members are likely to find themselves working in contexts that are concerned with risk reduction while advocating an ideology of care that gives primacy to issues of self-determination, independence, autonomy and choice. Working with mental health systems requires that practitioners seek to understand them. This is not easy since changes in complex systems cannot be attributed simply to the actions of individuals and the rules they follow. Whole systems thinking informs us that systems are best understood by observing them over time, to see what works and what doesn't.

Working with complexity

Change gurus such as Senge *et al.* (1999) use observations of biological growth as a metaphor for organizational change. For example, a growing tree develops through a reinforcing process of water and nutrients allowing root systems to expand to draw in more water and nutrients while simultaneously being constrained by limiting factors such as the availability of space and the effect of population and insects. New limitations may emerge as the growth gets to different levels. Observing and understanding the world as it is, rather than imposing reductionist, linear, mechanistic models is a key feature of working effectively with complexity. As Leonardo da Vinci said, 'Those who take for their standard anyone but nature – the mistress of all masters – weary themselves in vain.' You cannot make a tree grow through encouragement or threats, and you need to attend to removing the limiting factors as much if not more than promoting those factors that reinforce change and growth. Moreover, growth and change take time; achieving one stage of development is a requirement to achieving the next stage of development.

The certainty-agreement diagram in Figure 29.3, derived from Stacey (2000), provides a useful guide. It describes continua of certainty about how things are and agreement about how things should change. Most of the time we are somewhere in the middle of these continua which defines a 'zone of complexity' (Plsek and Greenhalgh 2001). Here it is not obvious what to do, as in the simple zone, but there is not so much disagreement and uncertainty as to throw the whole system into chaos.

If the aim is to move the system more towards the simple zone where groups of stakeholders can jointly partake in planned action, then measures

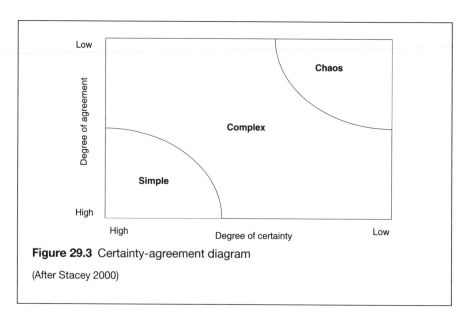

Figure 29.3 Certainty-agreement diagram
(After Stacey 2000)

to increase certainty about the current situation and agreement about what should be done are desirable. The first stage in planned developments involving a range of partners, whether they are agencies working to implement strategy, or team members working together, is to develop a shared vision of how things should be and achieve a shared understanding of how things are at the moment. There is, therefore, a need to focus explicitly on articulating basic values about what services should be achieving for people and developing an effective local needs assessment at the individual, service and locality level.

The development of standards and guidelines (for example, through user-led clinical governance or quality assurance processes), approaches to the spread of best practice, and team-based training and educational interventions, can all be thought of as ways of promoting agreement about how things can be changed. It is, however, important not to rush to this before a shared understanding of the current situation is achieved. Fraser and Greenhalgh (2001) noted that 'checklist driven' approaches to clinical care such as critical appraisal, clinical guidelines and the implementation of care pathways are important tools, but are only useful once the issues have been understood.

Working in the zone of complexity places a high value on intuition and imagination. It requires multiple approaches that make effective use of experience, experimentation, freedom to innovate and working at the edge of knowledge and experience. Tools for this include the use of action learning (Smith 2001) and the plan-do-study-act cycle of quality improvement (Berwick 1998). Increasingly, these take place in the context of improvement work that involves large groups of participants with a strong emphasis on working bottom-up so that the involvement and influence of users, their networks and front-line staff is maximized.

One key perspective on systems is how service users experience them. As the MHPIG states, 'All elements have to interact as a system, so that the service user experiences continuity during their pathway through care, with each element offering added value' (DH 2001a: 86–7). Process redesign (Locock 2001) is a method for exploring this experience with users and front-line staff in a systematic manner (see http://www.modernnhs.nhs.uk for guidance). Mental health services have also begun to experiment with 'collaboratives' where a large number of working teams come together supported by an expert reference group and explicit standards to work on incremental change with an emphasis on cross-team comparison, measurement of outcomes and the use of plan-do-study-act cycles aimed at incremental change. All such approaches need to start with the experience of users as the foundation from which to develop services.

Another feature of working with complexity is the need to use only minimum specifications for change that allow maximum freedom for creativity. This contrasts somewhat with the highly specified approach embodied within the MHPIG and the performance management that accompanies it. This bears on the issue of local commissioning, described below, which requires performance managers to support local innovation by allowing local solutions to emerge that both achieve the functions sought by centrally prescribed models while not over-specifying the means such that local ownership, interest and commitment is sacrificed.

Where does the power lie in complex systems?

If we again apply the principle of only being able to understand systems by looking at how they work, some key insights emerge about where power lies in complex systems to make things different. Changes proposed in *Shifting the Balance of Power* (DH 2001b) were premised on the need to devolve power to front-line staff and users. However, our experience of how policy is translated into practice, suggests that power has always resided with front-line staff.

Wells (1997) provides a comprehensive analysis of the ways in which CMHT staff translate policy and priorities drawing upon Lipsky's (1980) notion of the 'street level bureaucrat'. This work seeks to explain why service organizations behave in ways that are counter to policy frameworks and imperatives. The experience of previous highly prescribed policy imperatives, such the care programme approach, would suggest that change will occur only where practitioners support the change (Bindman *et al.* 1999). Lipsky (1980) argued that we need to understand the routines, perceptions and behaviours of these 'street level' agents to understand how policy will be operationalized. Their ways of coping with the tensions and role ambiguities created by policy imperatives largely define the experience of policy for users and their networks. Wells's (1997) analysis describes the tensions arising from perceived personal implications of change, managing imperatives from local managers, and living in professional and peer cultures. He suggests that managers and policy makers may have a vested interest in not scrutinizing practitioners implementation of policy too rigorously as this deflects responsibility for its consequences. He states:

> If a discipline or clinical team set their face against implementing the new legislation there maybe little the manager can do, particularly as any such interference could be portrayed as an attack on clinical discretion, with all the attendant politic fallout and bad publicity this would generate. It can be argued that local managers deal with this issue by setting in place the necessary systems to meet the agenda of central government but only purse the question of practitioner compliance in general ways.
>
> (Wells 1997: 5)

This may reflect why the high aspirations of clinical governance to achieve a radically user-led and accountable framework for quality assurance have still to be fully realized (DH 1998).

Carrots are more powerful than sticks in influencing practitioners' behaviour. The achievement of meaning in one's work through feeling clinically effective appears to be a central source of personal reward and job satisfaction for staff (Onyett 2002). A wide range of people in leadership and management roles have a key role to play in developing work contexts where staff can stay effective and feel that their work has social value. Team effectiveness research (for example, Borrill *et al.* 2000) provides practical guidance on how this can be achieved which is why in Mental Health South West we have sought in our training to bring leadership and teamworking together in an action learning programme and why we teach people how to apply the principles of motivational interviewing, which has a strong evidence base in work with users, to their efforts to involve their colleagues in change (see Rollnick *et al.* 1999).

Commissioning within a whole system

Achieving effective care coordination and provision requires that individuals and the organizations of which they are members have a complementary vision of what they should be achieving for users and their supports, alongside agreed access criteria, referral systems and protocols. This in turn requires them to have a shared view on the needs of local residents and how to allocate resources to meet these needs. This takes us into the realm of joint working to achieve effective commissioning, a term which has been defined as 'the assessment of health needs, the development of strategies to meet those needs, the purchasing of services for users and the monitoring of the quality of the services provided' (Lester and Sorohan 2002: 6).

Peck and Wigg's (2002) summary of findings from five annual surveys of senior mental health service managers in London reveals that developing joint CMHTs was the top priority for implementation over this whole period. Partnership working is embodied at strategic level through joint commissioning arrangements and Health Improvement Plans at managerial level (for example, through the joint management of CMHTs), and at practice level through integrated care coordination roles. Partnership working is therefore multi-layered with systems operating within systems. It is also not an end in itself but a means to strong inter-agency care planning, assessment and provision at the point where providers meet to assist service users. Box 29.4 sets out the objective partnership working (from Poxton 1999). Perhaps unsurprisingly it provides a good manifesto for what teams within local whole systems might aspire to.

Changes introduced by *Shifting the Balance of Power* (DH 2001b) radically reduced higher-level commissioning structures in order to locate the bulk of commissioning responsibility with primary care trusts (PCTs). In 2002, eight regional offices of the NHS Executive were reduced to four directorates, and strategic health authorities within these directorates have assumed responsibility for managing the performance of providers against national policy objectives.

As the title suggests, the stated rationale for the *Shifting the Balance of Power* changes was to decentralize power such that users and front-line staff exercised greater influence. PCTs certainly have the potential to help develop primary mental health care and integrate it with secondary care and, in some cases, the provision of specialist care. However, there are concerns about the capacity of PCTs to commission mental health care and this is where considerable development support will need to be focused (Lester and Sorohan 2002; Sainsbury Centre for Mental Health 2002).

Often social services and PCT commissioning come together in joint commissioning boards. Increasingly, these will become synonymous with or advised by the local implementation teams (LITs) established in 1999 to implement the *NSF for Mental Health*. LITs are variously configured to cover the old health authority catchments, counties, local authorities or PCTs. They include representation from health and social care managers, clinicians, statutory and voluntary sectors, professionals, service users and their networks.

Box 29.4 The purposes of partnership working

- One point of entry to health and social care systems.
- Assessment process that focuses on needs in the round and involves as few assessors as is practicable.
- Single care management/planning approach that is sensitive to changing needs of the user and includes all necessary sharing of information between agencies.
- Shared approach that positively promotes the maintenance and recovery of independence wherever possible.
- No unnecessary admissions to hospital.
- Discharge from hospital as soon as is medically and socially appropriate to a setting of the user's choice.
- End to arguments about distinction between health and social care needs and hence respective funding responsibilities.

LIT capacity has been largely dedicated to responding to performance management imperatives whereby they have to plan and report back on specific targets embodied within annual phases of their local implementation plans. These plans include clear targets that LITs must assess themselves, using a simple traffic-light rating system. The MHPIG highlights that 'Whilst current policy, and the specifications in this guide, aim to give a clear sense of direction, it is important that this is balanced by the flexibility to respond to differences in local needs' (DH 2001a: 8). This has not been felt easy to achieve to date.

As they mature as organizations and draw support from the NIMHE development centres there is an expectation that LITs will place increasing emphasis on the other key elements of whole systems working such as local needs assessment, and other key underpinning functions such as workforce planning and development, and financial planning. Joint commissioning through LITs should also help to ensure that commissioning is not skewed too far towards primary care, neglecting people with the most complex health and social care needs. It will be important that LITs, perhaps through their support from the new strategic health authorities, have the skills, capacity and credibility to ensure equitable and participative joint working between PCTs and other providers.

LITs are also well placed to support future developments in local partnership working. *The NHS Plan* (DH 2000) introduced the possibility of care trusts aimed at achieving even closer integration of health and social services. They will be able to commission and deliver primary and community health care as well as social care for older people and other care groups.

LITs will need to work creatively with new partners to involve the wider community, which may include groups and individuals whose needs are not being met by current services (for example, as a result of highly specialized needs or, more usually, because of the effects of age, sex, geography, disability or ethnic background). Local partnership working for mental health also needs to take increasing account of the other broad 'Local Strategic Partnerships' through which the local authority can work with other bodies. These cross-sectoral, umbrella partnerships bring together public, private, voluntary and community agencies within a single overarching local coordination framework. This provides a context within which more specific partnerships can work. The aims of these partnerships are broadly stated but particular reference is made to deprivation, social exclusion, poor quality environment and health inequalities, as well as the national strategy for neighbourhood renewal. Box 29.5 describes the development of a functional team aimed at early intervention that has emerged through strong inter-sectoral working in the form of a health action zone. Phase four of the local implementation planning requirements for LITs includes, for the first time, the expectation that local strategic partnerships will focus on the needs and circumstances of people in mental distress. Whole systems research methodologies have to be developed to accommodate these new ways of working (for example, Proctor *et al.* 2000).

Box 29.5 The Plymouth Early Intervention Service

The mental health programme board of the health action zone took a bottom-up approach to the development of the mental health stream of work. Early in the process a stakeholder day was held to consider how to take forward projects and to agree the formation of the programme board. Users and carers were in the majority on the day, which also included front-line professionals. It was agreed that the number of carers/users should at least equal the number of professionals on the board. The user/carer members would be drawn from a think tank of users and carers and the stakeholder day participants would become a reference group for the programme board to maintain contact with as large a group as possible.

The Early Intervention Service (EIS) focuses on young people aged 16–25 who are making contact with mental health services for the first time with a severe mental illness. The service has developed through an innovative partnership of Plymouth Social Services, Plymouth Primary Care Trust and the Youth Enquiry Service (YES). This partnership has been supported through funding from the health action zone. The EIS is led by YES which is a street-level organization looking after the needs of young people within the Plymouth area, not a mental health organization.

The staff of the EIS includes a number of generic workers as well as social services and trust staff and input from a psychiatrist. Staff emphasize engagement, developing early signs plans, working with educational, employment and leisure agencies and specific medical and psychological interventions. The service is provided in a non-stigmatized environment and is accessible seven days a week 24 hours a day.

Where people who access the service are thought not to have a severe mental illness they are referred on and engaged with more appropriate mental health services and/or other YES services.

The Plymouth Early Intervention Service was one of three key programmes being fully and independently evaluated. The others were:

- A one-stop employment shop to support people with mental health problems back into work or further training. This was established in partnership between Plymouth Community Services NHS Trust and Routeways, a voluntary sector provider of support to people seeking employment.
- A short-term, 48- to 72-hour, assessment area for people who present as homeless. This was established by seconding mental health nursing staff to a special needs project run by Devon and Cornwall Housing Association. Its aim was to overcome the problem of people being admitted to in-patient facilities for assessment rather than because of distress or social need.

Contact: Phil Confue, Director, Mental Health and Learning Disabilities, Plymouth Primary Care NHS Trust. Tel: 01752 268011, email: Phil.Confue@pcs-tr.swest.nhs.uk

The potential role of LITs remains to be realized. There is much local variation and potential confusion between the roles of LITs, strategic health authorities, commissioning consortia/networks and PCTs regarding the scope of their commissioning role and their role in 'signing off' service and expenditure plans. The National Institute for Mental Health for England appears committed to supporting LITs as the main focus for local partnership working through its local development services.

What does it all mean for nursing, and their training and education?

Community mental health nurses (CMHNs) were at the forefront of more intensive approaches to community teamworking before the advent of the *NSF for Mental Health* and the MHPIG. Home visiting ('assertive outreach' by another name) has been central to this. Thus, CMHNs have been working more holistically and autonomously than some other staff in the past. In some cases autonomous working has been associated with increased morale (Collins *et al.* 2000), and clinical experience suggests that it has resulted in greater self-confidence within the discipline leading to a more egalitarian and productive dialogue with other disciplines (Burns and Firn 2002). In common with other mental health disciplines, a greater focus on the operational management of more tightly designed teams has also been experienced by nurses as a threat to their professional autonomy and identity. However, greater emphasis on operational management may prevent the frequency of poor practice that has been associated with freedom and lack of accountability (Morrall 1997). The role of inpatient nurses, hitherto neglected, is now also being given the attention that such a central and skilled role demands (DH 2002c).

However, counter to the move towards strengthening professional identification and practice, the *NSF for Mental Health* and the work of its Workforce Action Team (DH 2001c) has stressed the need to recruit and retain staff with the right range of competencies, regardless of their background. Features such as their attitudes and life experiences, and whether they reflect the diversity of the communities being served are coming to be seen as equally important as the individual's professional training. Indeed, Holmes (2001) argued that we are in 'postdisciplinary' world where people have hitherto unimaginable access to knowledge and technical skills leading to increased specialization and an erosion of the link between one's profession or discipline and the actual work activity undertaken. Complexity requires 'solutions accommodating the unpredictability, irrationality and serendipity of everyday life' (Holmes 2001: 232) which have to be achieved collaboratively by a range of parties each bringing particular and specific insights and skills. Holmes criticizes as reactionary nurses' desire to protect and strengthen professional identify while embracing inter-professional collaboration and extended roles. He argues for purposefully designed generic mental health worker roles.

This proposal was rejected by the *Pulling Together* review conducted by the Sainsbury Centre for Mental Health (Sainsbury Centre for Mental Health 1997) and perhaps for good reason. Blanket genericism may erode the diversity that is needed to ensure effective multi-disciplinary team-working. While it is important that some core aspects are shared across disciplines (such as basic human values, an ability to form effective working relationships and skills in assessment), the elements that separate us as disciplines should be celebrated in the interests of promoting a wide and flexible skills mix. In CMHTs the best outcomes in terms of staff morale are achieved when staff can simultaneously feel a valued sense of belonging (or 'identification') with both their team and their discipline (Onyett 1997). This is not to argue against new roles that address gaps in provision that have been identified, or changes in the way that the professions are training to provide more interprofessional work experience and exposure to different cultures and mental models.

With increased professional self-determination and diversity of role comes an imperative for nurses to place greater emphasis on lifelong learning. The increasingly inter-dependent nature of education and training requires a focus in increasing whole systems' capability to improve. Fraser and Greenhalgh (2001) describe a range of education and training interventions aimed at developing systems. They tend to be self-directed, team focused, and based upon story telling and other narratives, particularly from users of the service.

Conclusion

In summary, the key points that emerge from this chapter are as follows:

- We need to be mindful of, but not dazzled by, the guidance on functional teams and the research to support it. This information needs to be integrated with what we know to be local needs and circumstances and existing strengths and deficits in team.

- All teams needs to be functional. Not just the new models.

- If we can achieve effective team working and the full implementation of care coordination many of the complex issues of how local teams interrelate would be solved. Effective team working requires clear objectives, effective leadership and management, support for change, an expectation of excellence and good team member participation in decision making.

- Whole systems working is more than a way of thinking about how services work together. It requires bottom-up approaches that take full account of the complexity of systems, the nature of change, recognition of where power lies to make things different, and incorporates the experience of a wide range of stakeholders.

- Education and training for mental health staff needs to reflect this postmodern environment in which disciplines become less defined, increased collaboration is required, there is an increased emphasis on learning by experience, and recognition that change is best achieved from the bottom up by focusing on the experience of users, their social networks and staff.

Questions for reflection and discussion

1   What types of mental health teams operate in your work context and what are their defining characteristics?

2   How 'functional' is the current organization of teams in your area of work? How far do they ensure that the right functions are fulfilled for the right people?

3   How 'functional' is the multi-disciplinary team within which you currently work? Where does the power lie within the team? What might be done to improve the ability of the team to meet service users' needs?

4   With reference to service users that you know in receipt of community mental health services, consider the benefits or otherwise of adopting the 'team approach'.

Notes

1   The example in Box 29.2 and the Plymouth Early Intervention Team in Box 29.5 are edited from the Best Practice Resource compiled and edited by Vida Field for Mental Health South West.

2   The programme was developed for the Leadership Centre (which forms part of the NHS Modernization Agency) by the author and Carol Borrill of the Organizational Studies Group at Aston Business School. For details contact paul.adams@doh.gov.uk.

3   We are grateful for the input of Andrew Quarry, clinical psychologist at the Somerset Partnership, and others for their input into developing this tool.

Annotated bibliography

- Department of Health (2001–2) *Mental Health Policy Implementation Guide*. London: DH. As the definitive government guidance on teams this is required reading. The astute reader will embed it within an informed view of what is important for local service development and implementation.

- Onyett, S.R. (2002) *Teamworking in Mental Health*. London: Palgrave. This text takes a deeper look at teamworking itself, regardless of the service model in which it takes place. It has a strong emphasis on practice within teams as well as giving a historical perspective and further guidance on the leadership, management and improvement of teams.
- Burns, T. and Firn, M. (2002) *Assertive Outreach in Mental Health: A Manual for Practitioners*. Oxford: Oxford University Press. Although about ACT this book can be read as a grounded, accessible and common-sense guide about working in any mental health team context. Its big strength is that it draws directly from the experience of running a mature ACT team. Highly recommended even if you do not agree with their position on compulsion.
- Pilgrim, D. and Rogers, A. (1999) *A Sociology of Mental Health and Illness*, 2nd edn. Buckingham: Open University Press. The effects of social inequalities on access to services and the ways in which services respond are a neglected part of this commentary. Understanding teams also requires an appreciation of the wider sociology of mental distress and the ways in which professions exercise power in their own interests.
- NHS Executive and Social Services Inspectorate (NHSE/SSI) (1999) *Effective Care Coordination in Mental Health Services: Modernising the Care Programme Approach*. London: DH 16736. This really is useful guidance, which takes account of the consistent failure of services to implement the care programme approach and care management as separate enterprises. It is both practical and aspirational. If we can fulfil this guidance adequately at local level we will have achieved a transformation in how users navigate complex systems and teams work together to support them.

References

Audini, B., Marks, I.M., Lawrence, R.E., Connolly, J. and Watts, V. (1994) Home-based versus out-patient/in-patient care for people with serious mental illness. Phase II of a controlled study, *British Journal of Psychiatry*, 165: 204–10.

Bainbridge, M. (2002) Carers are people too, *Mental Health Today*, June, 24–7.

Bennett, D. (1978) Social forms of psychiatric treatment, in J.K. Wing (ed.) *Schizophrenia: Towards a New Synthesis*. London: Academic Press.

Berwick, D.M. (1998) Developing and testing changes in delivery of care, *Annals of International Medicine* 128: 651–6.

Bindman, J., Beck, A., Glover, G. *et al.* (1999) Evaluating mental health policy in England: Care programme approach and supervision registers, *British Journal of Psychiatry* 175: 327–30.

Birchwood, M., Smith, J., Macmillan, F. and McGovern, D. (1998) Early intervention in psychotic relapse, in C. Brooker and J. Repper (eds) *Serious Mental Health Problems in the Community: Policy, Practice and Research*. London. Bailliere Tindall.

Borrill, C.S., Carletta, J., Carter, A.J. *et al.* (2000) *The Effectiveness of Healthcare Teams in the National Health Service.* Birmingham: Aston University.

Burns, T. and Firn, M. (2002) *Assertive Outreach in Mental Health: A Manual for Practitioners.* Oxford: Oxford University Press.

Burns, T., Beadsmoore, A., Bhat, A.V., Oliver, A. and Mathers, C. (1993) A Controlled Trial of Home-based Acute Psychiatric Services I: Clinical and social outcome, *British Journal of Psychiatry* **163**: 49–54.

Chinman, M.J., Rosenheck, R. and Lam, J.A. (2000) The case management relationship and outcomes of homeless persons with serious mental illness, *Psychiatric Services* **51**: 1142–7.

Collins, K., Jones, M.L., McDonnell, A., Read, S., Jones, R. and Cameron, A. (2000) Do new roles contribute to job satisfaction and retention of staff in nursing and professions allied to medicine?, *Journal of Nursing Management* **8**: 3–12.

Dean, C., Phillips, E.M., Gadd, E.M., Joseph, M. and England, S. (1993) Comparison of community based service with hospital based service for people with acute, severe psychiatric illness, *British Medical Journal* **307**: 473–6.

Deci, P.A., Santos, A.B., Hiott, D.W., Schoenwald, S. and Dias, J.K. (1995) Dissemination of assertive community treatment programs, *Psychiatric Services* **46**(7): 676–8.

Department of Health (1998) *A First Class Service.* London: HMSO.

Department of Health (1999) *National Service Framework for Mental Health: Modern Standards and Service Models.* London: DH.

Department of Health (2000) *The NHS Plan.* London: DH.

Department of Health (2001a) *Mental Health Policy Implementation Guide.* London: DH.

Department of Health (2001b) *Shifting the Balance of Power within the NHS.* London: DH.

Department of Health (2001c) *Mental Health National Service Framework (and the NHS Plan). Workforce Planning, Education and Training Underpinning Programme: Adult Mental Health Services. Final Report by the Workforce Action Team.* London: DH.

Department of Health (2002a) *Mental Health Policy Implementation Guide: Community Mental Health Teams.* London: DH.

Department of Health (2002b) *Mental Health Policy Implementation Guide: Dual Diagnosis Good Practice Guide.* London: DH.

Department of Health (2002c) *Mental Health Policy Implementation Guide: Adult acute in-patient care provision.* London: DH.

Diamond, R.J. (1996) Coercion and tenacious treatment in the community: Applications to the real world, in D.L. Dennis and J. Monahan (eds) *Coercion and Aggressive Community Treatment. A New Frontier in Mental Health Law.* Plenum Press: New York.

Drake, R.J., Haley, C.J., Akhtar, S. and Lewis, S. (2000) Causes and consequences of duration of untreated psychosis in schizophrenia, *British Journal of Psychiatry* **177**: 511–15.

Ford, R., Beadsmore, A., Ryan, P. *et al.* (1995) Providing the safety net: case management for people with a serious mental illness, *Journal of Mental Health* **1**: 91–7.

Fraser, S.W. and Greenhalgh, T. (2001) Coping with complexity: educating for capability. *British Medical Journal* **323**: 799–803.

Garety, P. and Jolley, S. (2000) Early intervention in psychosis. *Psychiatric Bulletin* **24**: 321–3.

Gask, L., Rogers, A., Roland, M. and Morris, D. (2000) *Improving Quality in Primary Care: A Practical Guide to the National Service Framework for Mental Health.* Manchester: University of Manchester, National Primary Care Research and Development Centre.

Gauntlett, N., Ford, R. and Muijen, M. (1996) *Teamwork: Models of Outreach in an Urban Multi-cultural Setting.* London: SCMH.

Goldman, H.H., Morrissey, J.P. and Ridgely, M.S. (1994) Evaluating the program on chronic mental illness. *Millbank Quarterly* **72**: 37–48.

Goldman, H.H., Ganju, V., Drake, R.E. *et al.* (2001) Policy implications for implementing evidence-based practices, *Psychiatric Services* 52(12): 1591–7.

Gournay, K. (1999) Assertive community treatment – why isn't it working?, *Journal of Mental Health* **8**: 427–9.

Gournay, K., Sandford, T., Johnson, S. and Thornicroft, G. (1997) Dual diagnosis of severe mental health problems and substance abuse/dependence: a major priority for mental health nursing, *Journal of Psychiatric and Mental Health Nursing* **4**(2): 89–95.

Griffiths, L. (2001) Categorisation to exclude: the discursive construction of cases in CMHTs, *Sociology of Health and Illness* **23**(5): 678–700.

Holloway, F. and Carson, J. (1998) Intensive case management for the severely mentally ill: controlled trial, *British Journal of Psychiatry* **172**: 19–22.

Holmes, C.A. (2001) Postdisciplinarity in mental health-care: an Australian viewpoint, *Nursing Inquiry* **8**(4): 230–9.

Hoult, J. (1986) Community care of the acutely mentally ill, *British Journal of Psychiatry* **149**: 137–44.

Hoult, J., Reynolds, I., Charbonneau-Powis, M, Weekes, P. and Briggs, J. (1983) Psychiatric hospital versus community treatment: The results of a randomized controlled trial, *Australian and New Zealand Journal of Psychiatry* **17**: 160–7.

Hutchison, M. (1999) Still singing the same old blues, *Health Matters* **34**: 16–17.

Iles, V. and Sutherland, K. (2001) *Organisational Change.* NCCSDO.

Johnston, S., Salkeld, G., Sanderson, K. *et al.* (1998) Intensive case management in Australia: a randomized controlled trial, *Australian and New Zealand Journal of Psychiatry* **32**: 551–9.

Joy, C.B, Adams, C.E. and Rice, K. (2001) Crisis intervention for those with severe mental illness, in *The Cochrane Library*, Issue 4, Oxford: Update Software.

Knapp, M., Beecham, J., Koutsogeorgopoulou, V. *et al.* (1994) Service use and costs of home-based versus hospital-based care for people with serious mental illness, *British Journal of Psychiatry* **165**: 195–203.

Lester, H. and Sorohan, H. (2002) *The Organisational Development Needs of PCTs in Mental Health Commissioning and Service Provision.* Birmingham: Inter-disciplinary Centre for Mental Health, University of Birmingham.

Lipsky, M. (1980) *Street-level Bureaucracy.* New York: Russell Sage.

Locock, L. (2001) *Maps and Journeys; Redesign in the NHS.* Birmingham: Health Services Management Unit, University of Birmingham.

Marks, I.M., Connolly, J., Muijen, M. *et al.* (1994) Home-based versus hospital-based care for people with serious mental illnesses, *British Journal of Psychiatry* **165**: 179–94.

Marshall, M. and Lockwood, A. (1998) Assertive community treatment for people with severe mental disorders (Cochrane review), in *The Cochrane Library*, Issue 4, Oxford: Update Software.

Marshall, M., Lockwood, A. and Green, R. (1998) Case management for people with severe mental disorders (Cochrane review), in *The Cochrane Library*, Issue 4, Oxford: Update Software.

Marshall, M., Bond, G., Stein, L.I. *et al.* (1999) PRiSM Psychosis Study: Design limitations, questionable conclusions. *British Journal of Psychiatry* **175**: 501–3.

McGrew, J.H., Wilson, R.G. and Bond, G.R. (1996) Client perspectives on helpful ingredients of assertive community treatment, *Psychiatric Rehabilitation Journal* **19**(3): 13–21.

McGrew, J.H., Wilson, R.G. and Bond, G.R. (2002) An exploratory study of what clients like least about assertive community treatment, *Psychiatric Services* **53**: 761–3.

Mechanic, D. (1996) Emerging issues in international mental health services research, *Psychiatric Services* **47**(4): 371–5.

Mellor-Clark, J. (2000) *Counselling in Primary Care in the Context of the NHS Quality Agenda: The Facts*. Rugby: British Association for Counselling and Psychotherapy.

Merson, S., Tyrer, P., Onyett, S. *et al.* (1992) Early intervention in psychiatric emergencies: a controlled clinical trial, *The Lancet* **339**: 1311–14.

Morrall, P.A. (1997) Professionalism and community psychiatric nursing: a case study of four mental health teams, *Journal of Advanced Nursing* **25**: 1133–7.

Mueser, K.T., Bond, G.R., Drake, R.E. and Resnick, G. (1998) Models of community care for severe mental illness: A review of research on case management, *Schizophrenia Bulletin* **24**(1): 38–73.

Murray, A., Shepherd, G., Onyett, S.R. and Muijen, M. (1997) *More than a Friend: The Role of Support Workers in Community Mental Health Services*. London: SCMH.

Navarro, T. (1998) Beyond keyworking, in A. Foster and V.Z. Roberts *Managing Mental Health in the Community: Chaos and Containment*. London: Routledge.

NHSE/SSI (1999) *Effective Care Coordination in Mental Health Services: Modernising the Care Programme Approach*. DH 16736.

Onyett, S. (2002) *Teamworking in Mental Health*. London: Palgrave.

Onyett, S.R. (1997) Collaboration and the community mental health team, *Journal of Interprofessional Care* **11**(3): 257–67.

Onyett, S.R. (2000) Understanding relationships in context as a core competence for psychiatric rehabilitation, *Psychiatric Rehabilitation Skills* **4**: 282–99.

Ovretveit, J. (1986) *Organisation of multidisciplinary community teams*, BIOSS Working paper. Uxbridge: Brunel University.

Patmore, C. and Weaver, T. (1991) Unnatural selection, *Health Service Journal* **10** October, 20–2.

Peck, E. and Wigg, S. (2002) Policies, priorities, opportunities and barriers in mental health services: five years of the London managers' survey, *Health Services Management Research* **15**: 55–66.

Plsek, P.E. and Greenhalgh, T. (2001) The challenge of complexity in healthcare. *British Medical Journal* **323**: 625–8.

Plsek, P.E. and Wilson, T. (2001) Complexity, leadership and management in healthcare organisations, *British Medical Journal* **323**: 746–9.

Poxton, R. (1999) *Partnerships in Primary and Social Care*. London: Kings Fund.

Proctor, S., Watson, B., Byrne, C. *et al.* (2000) The development of an applied whole-systems research methodology in health and social service research: a Canadian and United Kingdom Collaboration, *Critical Public Health* **10**(3): 331–42.

Provan, K.G. and Milward, H.B. (1995) A preliminary theory of interorganisational network effectiveness: a comparative study of four community mental health systems, *Administrative Science Quarterly* **40**: 1–33.

Richards, A. and Rees, A. (1998) Developing criteria to measure the effectiveness of community mental health teams, *Mental Health Care* **21**(1): 14–17.

Ridgely, M.S., Morrissey, J.P., Paulson, R.I., Goldman, H. and Calloway, M.O. (1996) Characteristics and activities of case managers in the RWJ Foundation Program on Chronic Mental Illness, *Psychiatric Services* **47**(7): 737–43.

Rollnick, S., Mason, P. and Butler, C. (1999) *Health Behaviour Change: A Guide for Practitioners*. Edinburgh: Churchill Livingstone.

Rubin, W.V. and Panzano, P.C. (2002) Identifying meaningful subgroups of adults with severe mental illness, *Psychiatric Services* **53**(4): 452–7.

Sainsbury Centre for Mental Health (1997) *Pulling Together. The Future Role and Training of Mental Health Staff*. London: SCMH.

Sainsbury Centre for Mental Health (1998) *Keys to Engagement*. London: SCMH.

Sainsbury Centre for Mental Health (2002) Response to the consultation document *Shifting the Balance of Power within the NHS*. London: SCMH.

Sashidharan, S.P., Smyth, M. and Owen, A. (1999) PRiSM Psychosis Study: Thro' a glass darkly: A distorted appraisal of community care, *British Journal of Psychiatry* **175**: 504–7.

Schneider, J. (2002) *Caseload Profiling Audit Key. Somerset Partnership Health and Social Care NHS Trust*. Available from the author.

Senge, P., Roberts, C., Ross, R. *et al.* (1999) *The Dance of Change*. London: Nicholas Brealey.

Shea, G.P. and Guzzo, R.A. (1987) Groups as human resources, *Research in Personnel and Human Resources Management* **5**: 323–56.

Shepherd, G. (1999) *Review of Specialist Mental Health Rehabilitation Services. Avon and Western Mental Health Trust*. London: Health Advisory Service 2000.

Shepherd, G., Muijen, M., Dean, C. and Cooney, M. (1996) Residential care in hospital and in the community – quality of care and quality of life, *British Journal of Psychiatry* **168**: 448–56.

Simmonds, S., Coid, J., Joseph, P., Marriott, S. and Tyrer, P. (2001) Community mental health team management in severe mental illness: a systematic review, *British Journal of Psychiatry* **178**: 497–502.

Smith, H. (1998) Needs assessment in mental health services: the DISC framework. *Journal of Public Health Medicine* **20**(2): 154–60.

Smith, M. (1998) Social systems intervention, *Nursing Standard* **13**(1): 35–6.

Smith, M., Coleman, R., Allott, P. and Koberstein, J. (1999) Assertive outreach: a step backward. *Nursing Times*, 28 July–3 August, **95**(30): 46–7.

Smith, P.A.C. (2001) Action Learning and Reflective Practice in Project Environments that are related to Leadership Development, *Management Learning* **32**(1): 31–48.

Spindel, P. and Nugent, J.A. (1999) The Trouble with PACT: Questioning the increasing use of assertive community treatment teams in community mental health. http://www.madnation.org/pacttrouble.htm.

Stacey, R.D. (2000) *Strategic Management and Organisational Dynamics*, 3rd edn. Harlow: Pearson Education.

Stein, L.I. and Test, M.A. (1980) Alternative to mental hospital treatment I, *Archives of General Psychiatry* **37**: 392–7.

Thornicroft, G., Becker, T., Holloway, F. *et al.* (1999) Community mental health teams: evidence or belief? *British Journal of Psychiatry* **175**: 508–13.

Tyrer, P. (1998) Cost-effective or profligate community psychiatry? *British Journal of Psychiatry* **172**: 1–3.

Tyrer, P. (2000) Effectiveness of intensive treatment in severe mental illness, *British Journal of Psychiatry* **176**: 492–3.

Tyrer, P., Simmonds, S., Coid, J., Mariott, S. and Joseph, P. (2001) A defence of community mental heath teams (letter), *British Journal of Psychiatry* **179**: 268.

Wells, J.S.G. (1997) Priorities, 'street level bureaucracy' and the CMHT, *Health and Social Care in the Community* **5**(5): 353–41.

West, M.A., Borrill, C.S. and Unsworth, K.L. (1998) Team effectiveness in organisations, in C.L. Cooper and I.T. Robertson (eds) *International Review of Industrial and Organisational Psychology*. Chichester: John Wiley and Sons.

Workforce Action Team (WAT) (2001) *Mental Health National Service Framework (and NHS Plan); workforce planning, education and training (adult mental health services underpinning programme)*. Final Report of the Workforce Action Team. London: Department of Health.

30

Reflections

Ian Norman and Iain Ryrie

Chapter overview

In the preface to this book we suggested that any contemporary account of mental health nursing needs to establish its case within three broad parameters: national policy, service user expectations and professional diversity. In this final chapter we return to these themes, with reference to preceding chapters, and outline our vision for the future of mental health nursing. We begin by placing *the National Service Framework (NSF) for Mental Health* (DH 1999a) within the context of the 1997 incoming UK Labour government's strategy for assuring and maintaining high quality health services and highlight the opportunities it offers to mental health nurses. This leads us to argue for integration of the art and science of mental health nursing which we see as crucial if nurses are to deliver the *NSF for Mental Health* in ways that empower service users and help them regain control of their lives. In summary this chapter covers:

- perceived problems with mental health services in the UK at the end of the 1990s;
- key elements of the *NSF for Mental Health*;
- recovery-oriented mental health nursing;
- unity in professional diversity.

Perceived problems with mental health services in the UK at the end of the 1990s

In general terms the greatest problem with the NHS was perceived by the incoming 1997 Labour government to be unacceptably large variations in clinical practice and outcomes for patients. There were perceived to be four main reasons for this:

- The negative effects of the internal market introduced by the previous Conservative administration, shattered the unity of the NHS into hundreds of small competing businesses where there was no incentive to share best practice.

- Predating the internal market, there were no clear national standards for care that the NHS was expected to achieve; the National Service Frameworks, for different service user groups, provide these standards.

- In the history of the NHS there had been no clear assessment of which treatments work best for which patients.

- As a public service the NHS had not been sufficiently open or accountable for the quality of services it offers the public (DH 1998).

What about the government's more specific 'diagnosis' of what was wrong with the mental health service? For some, community care was perceived to have failed for five reasons:

- The presence of a vulnerable group of mentally-ill people who are socially isolated, difficult to engage and in need of long-term care. They were and continue to be a focus of great public concern fuelled by media reports of the link between mental illness and homicide.

- Families that are overburdened and poorly supported in their role as informal carers for mentally-ill people.

- Under-funding and poor management of existing resources, which had resulted in an inadequate range of available services.

- An outdated legal framework that failed to support effective treatment outside hospital.

- Problems of recruiting and retaining staff, including nurses.

(Peck, personal communication)

The government's general 'prescription' for remedying these problems and driving up quality is now in place. It comprises standards set by the National Institute for Clinical Excellence, Social Care Institute for Excellence and national service frameworks:

- delivered by clinical governance, underpinned by professional self-regulation and lifelong learning;

- monitored by the Commission for Healthcare Audit and Inspection and the Commission for Social Care Inspection.

The specific prescription for the problems of mental health services is presented in the *NSF for Mental Health* published in 1999 that set out national standards for mental health, what they aim to achieve and how they are to be developed, delivered and measured. This was supported by reform of the Mental Health Act (1983) (covered in Chapters 4 and 6) and proposals to improve the mental health workforce (discussed in Chapter 4), and the *NHS*

Plan (DH 2000) that set out the government's plans for investment and reform. For mental health nurses these reforms were supported too by the White Paper, *Making a Difference* (DH 1999b), which outlined the government's plans to strengthen the nursing contribution to health care. In Chapter 4 Ford discusses the providence and place of the *NSF for Mental Health* within the UK government's policy for mental health care services. We summarize the main elements of the Framework below.

Key elements of the *National Service Framework for Mental Health*

The *NSF for Mental Health* (DH 1999a) focuses on the mental health needs of adults up to age 65. It also touches on the needs of children and young people in areas where services for children and adults interact, for example, services for mentally-ill parents and services for 16- to 18-year-olds. The *NSF for Mental Health* is an important policy document, which sets the agenda for mental health services for the next decade and will exert continuing influence on the direction of mental health services in the years ahead. The *NSF for Older People*, published in 2001, covers the mental health needs of those aged 65 and over; Standard 7 of this policy document, entitled 'Mental health in older people' is the focus of Keady and Ashton's chapter (Chapter 19).

The *NSF for Mental Health*:

- sets national standards and defines service models for promoting mental health and treating mental illness;
- put in place five programmes (on finance, workforce, research and development, clinical decision-making support systems, and information) to underpin and support local delivery of services; and
- sets milestones and performance indicators against which progress within agreed time-scales will be measured.

The document sets out values and principles to help shape decisions on service delivery. According to these, people with mental health problems may expect services that will:

- involve service users and their carers in planning and delivery of care;
- deliver high quality treatment and care which is known to be effective and acceptable;
- be well suited to those who use them and non-discriminatory;
- be accessible so that help can be obtained when and where it is needed;
- promote their safety and that of carers, staff and the wider public;
- offer choices which promote independence;
- be well coordinated between all staff and agencies;

- deliver continuity of care for as long as this is needed;
- empower and support staff;
- be properly accountable to the public, service users and carers.

(DH 1999a: 4)

Value-for-money, or efficiency, is not listed – but the rest of the *NSF for Mental Health* makes it clear that cost-effectiveness and rigorous performance management are to be important drivers to the direction of services.

At the heart of the *NSF for Mental Health* are seven standards (specified later in this chapter) that provide a guide for investment and together purport to offer a vision of a comprehensive high-quality mental health service. The standards set global objectives for mental health delivery rather than precise targets, and rather than prescribe a rigid national service model advocate local development of care which is sensitive to local variations in need, culture and resource. The standards are presented as the means towards 'whole systems' working (discussed in Chapter 29) across all agencies responsible for mental health care, that is, primary and specialist services, and services located in the NHS, social services and the independent sector.

In summary, the *NSF for Mental Health* is an important policy document which, for the first time in our professional lifetimes, sets out a comprehensive agenda for mental health services which incorporates mental health promotion, primary care and secondary care, and acknowledges that the whole system of mental health care must be made to work if there are to be real benefits to service users.

Together with related mental health policy reforms, the *NSF for Mental Health* has major implications for the work of mental health nurses. Ford (Chapter 4) highlights the following implications for future mental health nursing practice:

- increased partnership working with service users, their families and communities;
- increased specialization and identification with the specialist setting rather than the profession;
- increased inter-professional working, as a normal requirement of practice;
- a decreasing role as direct providers of hands-on care and an increased role as supervisors and enablers of new staff groups;
- an expectation of lifelong learning; and
- increased reliance and use of information management and technology.

Reaction

As with most policy documents, the *NSF for Mental Health* received a mixed reaction on publication. For some commentators it did not fulfil its remit by failing to provide an overall model of mental health services, related to different areas of need. For others, including ourselves, the fact that the *NSF for Mental Health* did not set out a model was a strength; it set out a direction of travel and identified objectives along the way, but not how to get there – which staff and many service users may prefer to a more prescriptive approach. Others commented on the fact that its proposals were not fully costed, although many would now acknowledge that it has been accompanied so far by substantial additional investment by the UK government in the future of mental health services.

The NSF for Mental Health is underpinned by a set of values concerning social inclusion, user choice, and support for carers that most service users and staff would support, and it also pays attention to the evidence for particular service models within which care plans might be pursued, i.e. crisis intervention, home treatment and assertive community treatment. Thus, the document is evidence-based, although an important limitation here is that the evidence cited is almost entirely from the psychiatric literature and virtually none from the social care field. Further, the evidence is graded for quality using a standard evidence-based hierarchy (discussed in Chapter 3) which places systematic reviews, which include at least one randomized controlled trial at the top of the hierarchy and expert opinion, including the opinion of service users and carers at the bottom. Thus, in spite of the values and principles on which it is based, the *NSF for Mental Health* places insufficient emphasis, in our view, on service-user perspectives and, in particular, to the evidence which demonstrates the potential of users for 'recovery', a concept which is the focus of Chapter 5 by Perkins and Repper, and one that is gaining ground in the mental health field.

The evidence for recovery is contained primarily in first-hand accounts of service users of their illness experience and those things that aided them in their recovery, or impeded them. Service-users' accounts of their recovery, tend to emphasize their own self-determination and the important role of key supporters. There is little mention of formal carers and mental health nurses in particular and our conclusion is that hitherto (and certainly with exceptions), mental health nurses have had little impact on recovery processes. Service-users' accounts of recovery would be ranked at the bottom of most standard hierarchies of evidence, but they hold important lessons for the work of mental health nurses (see also Chapter 3).

It is encouraging that the National Institute for Mental Health (England) (NIMH-E) supports the development of recovery-oriented services for people who experience mental illness/distress. We understand Vick (personal communication) that NIMH-E has commissioned a discussion paper on the subject, although at time of writing this is not yet available.

Recovery-oriented mental health nursing in the context of the *National Service Framework*

Below we set out the implications for the practice of mental health nurses committed to delivering the *NSF for Mental Health* standards in ways that promote service users' recovery.

Standard 1: Mental health promotion

Standard 1 requires that health and social services:

- promote mental health for all, working with individuals and communities;
- combat discrimination against individuals and groups with mental health problems, and promote their social inclusion.

This standard supports the rights of service users and facilitates their access to life domains that others take for granted – work, education, social networks. It alerts nurses to the importance too of intervention at the levels of whole populations through promoting healthy neighbourhoods, at the level of individuals at risk (new parents, the unemployed, distressed families), vulnerable groups (Black and minority ethnic communities, rough sleepers), as well as action to combat discrimination and promote positive images of mental ill health.

Nursing to promote mental health involves promoting lifestyles that enhance emotional as well as physical health and spiritual and sexual well-being. It involves also ensuring access of service users and carers to information on self-management techniques (some of which are discussed in Chapters 10, 24 and 25), and self-help/recovery groups, which involve peer support.

Combating discrimination and reducing stigma require nurses to become familiar with local media and use this knowledge to promote positive stories and images. It might involve too, supporting recovered service users who want to 'come out' about their experiences and also education activities targeted at those groups who through their contact with service users influence service users' self-image and their lives; for example, those working in the criminal justice system (police, magistrates), and those involved in administering state benefits. Promoting social inclusion is likely to involve nurses facilitating service users' access to mainstream services (employment, education and housing services) and supporting and promoting their social networks.

Standards 2 and 3: Primary care and access to services

Standard 2 requires that any service user who contacts their primary health-care team should:

- have their mental health needs identified and assessed;
- be offered effective treatments, including referral to specialist services for further assessment, treatment and care if they require it.

Standard 3 requires that any individual with a common mental health problem should:

- be able to make contact round the clock with the local services necessary to meet their needs and receive adequate care;

- be able to use NHS Direct, as it develops, for first-level advice and referral on to specialist help-lines or to local services.

These standards emphasize access, identification, treatment and communication. Primary care is placed at the heart of the system, as it must manage the large majority of people with what are referred to as 'common mental health problems' – that is depression (discussed in Chapter 14), eating disorders (discussed in Chapter 16) and anxiety disorders (discussed in Chapter 15) – and many with severe mental illness (discussed in Chapter 13). This implies a greatly increased role in primary care for mental health nurses, particularly those who can prescribe correctly and provide evidence-based psychological therapies.

From a recovery perspective early detection and intervention within primary care is crucial to minimizing mental distress and keeping as many people as possible away from specialist care services. The quality of the service user's first contact with nurses may have important implications for their recovery process. It is an opportunity for nurses working in primary care services to instil hope, give positive messages about recovery, provide relevant and timely information to dispel negative myths about mental disorders and outline treatment alternatives. Information on medication is important, including its possible side effects, as is information and advice on lifestyle changes (diet, exercise, stress management), which may increase service users' capacity for self-management. If referral to specialist services is needed, this should be accompanied by referral also to self-help and other sources of peer support.

Standard 3 states that any service user should be able to make contact round the clock with local services necessary to meet their needs and receive adequate care. A major role is anticipated for NHS Direct to complement specialist mental health help-lines. Another key point of contact for people who use mental health services are local Accident and Emergency departments. Here, staff see, routinely, a range of problems linked with mental health conditions including alcohol misuse, deliberate self-harm and homelessness. The *NSF for Mental Health* is clear about the value of mental health nurses working in a liaison capacity both in assessing service users and training Accident & Emergency department staff.

Crucial to nursing practice is that front-line staff within these services have access to information on peer support and self-help networks, and are trained to provide positive messages about recovery to those in distress.

Standards 4 and 5: Effective services for people with serious mental health problems

The Care Programme Approach (CPA) provides a framework for assessment, care planning and review by a designated care coordinator. The *NSF for Mental Health* recommended that this be fully integrated with care management, the framework used previously by social services, to create: a standard CPA for those not posing a risk to themselves or others and requiring care from only one agency, and an enhanced CPA for those with complex needs, including those considered at risk. Integration of these two frameworks has been widely welcomed.

Standard 4 requires that all mental health service users on the CPA should:

- receive care, which optimizes engagement, prevents or anticipates crises, and reduces risk;
- have a copy of a written care plan which:
  - includes the action to be taken in a crisis by service users, their carers and their care coordinators;
  - advises the general practitioner (GP) how they should respond if the service user needs additional help;
  - is regularly reviewed by the care coordinator;
- be able to access services 24 hours a day, 365 days a year.

Standard 5 requires that each service user who is assessed as requiring a period of care away from their home should have:

- timely access to an appropriate hospital bed or alternative bed or place, which is:
  - in the least restrictive environment consistent with the need to protect them and the public;
  - as close to home as possible;
- a copy of the written after-care plan agreed on discharge, which sets out the care and rehabilitation to be provided, identifies the care co-ordinator, and specifies the action to be taken in a crisis.

These standards focus on effective services for people with severe mental illness, who are at the heart of specialist mental health service provision. They demand comprehensive services, including 24-hour access, engagement, crisis intervention and access to hospital. They also clarify the role and content of the care plan. These standards highlight the importance of core nursing skills required by engagement and crisis intervention. It also focuses attention on the relatively neglected speciality of inpatient care. We need to be clear about the role and function of inpatient wards, and also how we can work to create within these hard-pressed wards a therapeutic milieu for both service users and staff (discussed in Chapter 9).

Mental health nursing in the context of these standards emphasizes engagement of service users as true partners in the CPA. This would include: an assessment process, which is not problem dominated but incorporates also people's strengths and aspirations (discussed in Chapter 7); a care plan owned by the service user which is, in effect, a recovery plan, directed towards their desired lifestyle; a plan in which the role and responsibility of the service user in making the plan work is emphasized (including their responsibilities in preventing and responding to crises) and in which the nurse's role is primarily one of support and acting as a sounding board to help the service user think through their actions; planning and review meetings scheduled at a time and location which is convenient to the service user (perhaps at home) and which involves not simply the service user and professionals, but all those identified by the service user at the time as important people in their life.

Standard 6: Caring about carers

Standard 6 specifies that all individuals who provide regular and substantial care for a person on CPA should:

- have an assessment of their caring, physical and mental health needs, repeated on at least an annual basis;
- have their own written care plan, which is given to them and implemented in discussion with them.

This standard targets people looking after persons on the CPA and is based on the Carers (Recognition and Services) Act (1995) (DH 1995) which gave carers the right to request an assessment when the service user's needs are also being assessed. Conflicts of interest may arise between users and carers and it is important that their plans and interest are considered together. Nurses need to recognize that carers are not the only people who are significant in service users' lives, and that these other 'significant others' also need to be kept well-informed and treated as sources of expert advice on treatment and care. Being a significant person in the life of a mentally distressed person is likely to exert a personal cost; nurses may need to provide support and education to assist these people to recover their own lives.

Standard 7: Preventing suicide

Standard 7 specifies that local health and social care communities should prevent suicides by:

- promoting mental health for all, working with individuals and communities (Standard 1);
- delivering high quality primary mental health care (Standard 2);
- ensuring that anyone with a mental health problem can contact local services via the primary care team, a help-line or an Accident & Emergency department (Standard 3);
- ensuring that individuals with severe and enduring mental illness have a care plan which meets their specific needs, including access to services round the clock (Standard 4);
- providing safe hospital accommodation for individuals who need it (Standard 5);

- enabling individuals caring for someone with severe mental illness to receive the support which they need to continue to care (Standard 6);

and in addition:

- supporting local prison staff in preventing suicides among prisoners;
- ensuring that staff are competent to assess the risk of suicide among individuals at greatest risk;
- developing local systems for suicide audit to learn lessons and take any necessary action.

Standard 7 is a composite, combining elements of the other six. Its aim is to ensure that health and social services contribute to the target set out in the White Paper, *Saving Lives: Our Healthier Nation* (DH 1999c), which is to reduce the suicide rate by at least one fifth by 2010.

Preventing suicide is important, but is a negative objective from a nursing perspective. Important too are life-enhancing interventions, which highlight the importance of the relationship between the nurse and the service user as a medium for promoting hope and helping the service user grow beyond the confines of their illness. Thus, this standard emphasizes the importance of working in partnership with service users to help them achieve their goals and ambitions and linking them with responsive and flexible services and peer support and recovery groups which are sensitive to their changing needs.

Pathways to recovery

Although the process of recovery is unique to each individual and so can take many paths, Perkins and Repper's discussion in Chapter 5 suggests that for service users recovery has the following elements:

- grieving what has been lost;
- learning about their difficulties;
- redefining themselves and what they might become;
- finding new meaning and purpose;
- finding new sources of hope;
- taking responsibility for their problems and for their life again.

Service users are faced often with a philosophical or spiritual crisis. One day they are a person, often a young person, with friends and great possibilities. On the next they have been diagnosed with a mental illness, and face a lifelong disability that limits all life's possibilities. They are forced to question what their life is all about – what is its meaning? A common reaction at such times is to want to go back – back before the illness, to happier days. But there is no way back – only forward. The person needs to grieve what has been lost, learn about their difficulties and redefine themselves and what they might become. Mental health nurses are well placed to lend a helping hand to service users through this difficult process.

Above all, people in recovery need hope, and fundamental to this is the belief of the people around them in their capacity to recover, however serious their problems. Nurses need to have more faith in service users – not blind faith, but a faith based on a realistic but optimistic assessment of the person's situation in which they themselves are most closely involved. Therapeutic pessimism has no place in mental health nursing practice; it is self-defeating and robs service users of hope and self-confidence, which are crucial to their recovery process. A common factor in service users' accounts of recovery is of people who believe in them, who stand by them, who try to listen and understand, who encourage their recovery without forcing it or becoming frustrated when nothing seems to change. These are important lessons for nurses in their relationships with patients. People in mental distress need around them positive nurses who recognize that life is about trying and failing and trying again, and who encourage and support service users to try and try again to take active responsibility for their problems and their lives. Important here is providing opportunities for those in a process of recovery to give – to share their knowledge and skills with others. As Perkins and Repper point out (Chapter 5), service users are too often simply recipients in relationships.

Finally, accounts of recovery show that service users need contact with others who have experienced mental distress and who have not simply survived but have flourished. Famous people who have recovered from mental illness provide important positive images, but the lives of the famous are far removed from the lives of most of us. More important as positive role models are ordinary people who have suffered mental distress but who have recovered sufficiently to lead ordinary lives, have ordinary relationships and bring up ordinary children successfully. Nurses are well placed to foster these recovery networks and link service users to them.

Conclusion

In sum, a limitation of the *NSF for Mental Health* is its neglect of the recovery literature, most of which would, if included, be ranked at the bottom of most hierarchies of evidence, being relegated to the domain of 'expert opinion'. However, the experts in this case are service users themselves with first-hand experience of mental distress and suffering and how this can be alleviated. Their accounts hold important lessons for the work of mental health nurses who strive to work beyond the *NSF for Mental Health* in a way that empowers service users and helps them to regain control of their lives.

Unity in professional diversity

Recovery-oriented practice does not require mental health nurses to abandon their existing theoretical frameworks or evidence bases. Rather it requires a shift in emphasis when applying our knowledge and skills, which places the service user's experience at the very centre of care. In Chapters 1 and 7 we introduced a schema for understanding the totality of human experience, which we used to examine models of mental disorder and the scope of assessment. We reproduce it here in Figure 30.1.

Thus, the experience of being human consists of an *objective* and *subjective* sense of *self* (upper quadrants) and a *subjective* and *objective* sense of *self in community* (lower quadrants). Jacobson's (1993) account of the frameworks employed by service users to understand the nature of the difficulties they experience (discussed in Chapter 5) have been entered onto the schema. It is striking, as we suggested in Chapter 1 through the work of Rose (2001), that service users appear to hold an integrated view of their experience of mental distress incorporating all four quadrants. Thus, a shift in mental health nursing's focus towards the service user's experience needs to be accompanied by an integrated understanding of human experience that can accommodate its subjective and objective components at the individual and community level.

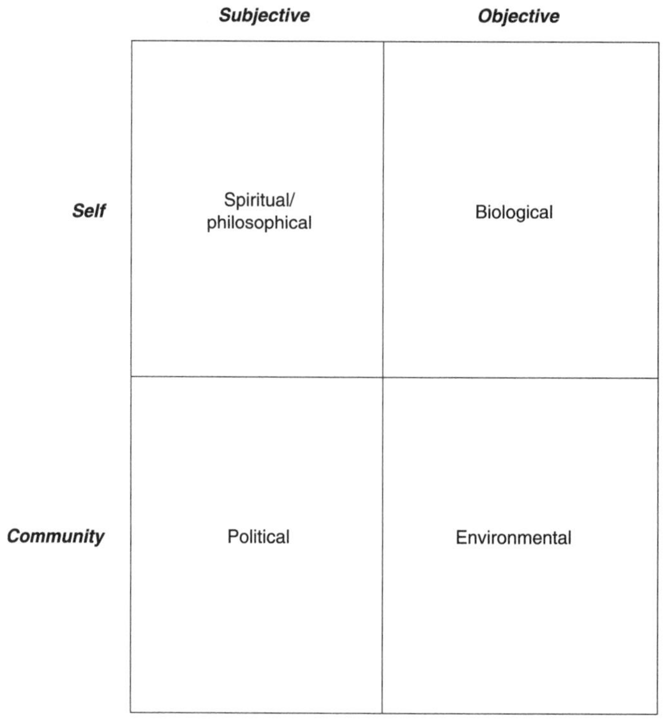

	Subjective	Objective
Self	Spiritual/ philosophical	Biological
Community	Political	Environmental

Figure 30.1 Jacobson's (1993) service users' frameworks mapped onto the schema

(After: Wilber 2000)

In practice this requires recognition of both the 'art' (left-hand quadrants) and the 'science' (right-hand quadrants) that underpin mental health nursing (and human experience). These have been evident to varying degrees in the preceding chapters. For example, Chapter 11, which deals with pharmacological interventions predominantly reflects the upper-right quadrant (objective self), while Chapter 9 (therapeutic milieu) is concerned with both lower quadrants (subjective and objective community). Chapter 13 (disorders of perception) uses medical terminology to describe symptoms that stem from the upper-right quadrant (objective self), but describes the experience of hallucinations and delusions in a way that accommodates an individual's subjective experience of self (upper-left quadrant).

Mental health nurses are, we believe, well placed to develop an integrated understanding of a person's experience of mental health and illness. Mental health nurses are not psychologists (upper quadrants only) or social workers (lower quadrants only), nor are they psychiatrists (primarily upper-right quadrant). The profession can cover all bases as the content of this book has demonstrated, though we need not all be competent practitioners in all four areas. Individuals are likely to specialize and have preferred areas and methods in which they work. The key is to maintain an integrated perspective predicated upon the service user's experience. In so doing we can recognize the need for and work alongside other professionals and lay carers with skills that are complimentary to our own, and which are necessary to provide holistic care.

Questions for reflection and discussion

1   What practical steps can you take today to make your nursing practice more recovery oriented?

2   What are the implications of a recovery-based approach to mental health nursing for the selection and education of mental health nursing students?

3   Does the schema for understanding the totality of human experience, which we present in this and in previous chapters, help you to understand your role as a mental health nurse? How might the schema be developed or improved?

Annotated bibliography

- Repper, J. and Perkins, R. (2003) *Social Inclusion and Recovery. A Model for Mental Health Practice*. Oxford: Elsevier Science. This text provides a detailed analysis of recovery and inclusion by the authors of Chapter 5 of this book. It draws on service users' experiences of living with mental health problems, and their accounts of recovery to construct a model for practitioners seeking to promote recovery and inclusion.

References

Department of Health (1995) Carers (Recognition and Services) Act (1995). www.doh.gov.uk

Department of Health (1998) *A First Class Service: Quality in the new NHS.* London: DH.

Department of Health (1999a) *National Service Framework for Mental Health: Modern Standards and Service Models.* London: DH.

Department of Health (1999b) *Making a Difference: Strengthening The Nursing, Midwifery and Health Visiting Contribution to Health and Healthcare.* London: DH.

Department of Health (1999c) *Saving Lives: Our Healthier Nation.* London: The Stationery Office (CM 4386).

Department of Health (2000) *NHS Plan.* London: DH.

Department of Health (2001) *National Service Framework for Older People.* London: DH.

Jacobson, N. (1993) Experiencing recovery: A dimensional analysis of recovery narratives, *Psychiatric Rehabilitation Journal* **24**(3): 248–55.

Rose, D. (2001) *Users' Voices: The Perspectives of Mental Health Service Users on Community and Hospital Care.* London: SCMH.

Wilber, K. (2000) *Sex, Ecology and Spirituality: The Spirit of Evolution.* Boston, MA: Shambhala.

Index

Page numbers in *italics* refer to figures, tables and boxes; *passim* indicates scattered references within page range.

rationale for 722
systematic review 723–4
see also compliance
Melia, P. and Moran, T. 603
Mental Health Act (1983) 154–5,
  166
  Code of Practice 156–66 *passim*,
    737, 739–40
  compulsory hospital admission
    159–62
  compulsory treatment, Part IV
    (Sections 57–63) 154–5,
    169–71, 176, 741
  definition of psychopathy 626–7
  mentally disordered offenders 606
  risk management 212, 214
Mental Health Act Commission
  741–2
Mental Health Care Group
  Workforce Team
  (MHCGWT) 118
mental health and mental illness 4,
  35–6, 45
  continua 45–51
  policy issues 54–6, 100–3
  see also mental illness
mental health policy 106–16
  capable practitioner 117–23
  failures/problems 54–6, 819–20
  forensic mental health services
    605–8
  implementation guide (MHPIG)
    110–12, 774, 776–83 *passim*,
    791–5, 800–1, 805, 808
  mental health/mental illness 54–6,
    100–3
  practitioner implementation
    805–6
  risk assessment/management
    212–14
  see also Department of Health
    (DH); *National Service
    Framework (NSF) for
    Mental Health*; *National
    Service Framework for Older
    People* (NSFOP); *NHS Plan*
mental health promotion 35–61
  NSF 17, *108*
  older people 556–8
  policy 57–8
  practice 58–9

prevention of eating disorders
  458–61
recovery 138–46, 824
theory 57
mental health services
  child and adolescent (CAMHS)
    113–14, 546–7
  current 105–6
  future 123–4
  historic development 104–5
  integrated teams 799–801
  principles 103, *104*
  service-related factors in non-
    engagement 653–5
  severe mental illness 18, *108–9*,
    798, 825–7
  see also forensic mental health
    services; service users
mental illness
  factors in compliance 722
  factors in non-engagement 652–3
  multi-faceted aspect 129–30
  see also mental health and mental
    illness
mentoring 145
metaphors, cognitive technique 712
methadone 489, 506–7
MIND 12, 242
mind–body interventions 330
mind–body relationship 356–7, 360
minor/moderate needs, primary care
  799
mixed states, bipolar disorder 404–5
modelling procedures, exposure
  therapy 441
models of mental disorder 4–14
  integrating 14–18
monitoring
  medication in schizophrenia 378
  moods in depression 398–9
  safety, violence management 735,
    736
  self- 286–7, *288*, 693, *694*
  thoughts 707, *708*, 712, *713*
  see also diaries
monoamine oxidase inhibitors
  (MAOIs) 310, 321–2, 393
monoamines/monoamine oxidase
  309, 343
mood disorders, *see* bipolar disorder;
  depression; mania

mood stabilizers 322–3
  bipolar disorder 406–7
  personality disorder 636
moral therapy movement 68–9
Morgan, S. 211, 221, 222, 223, 224,
  231, 233, 235
motivational interviewing 279–84
  case study 281–4
  characteristics *280*
  in substance misuse 506
Mullen, P.E. 595
multi-agency approach 133, 287,
  659, 788
  NSF 107
  see also Care Programme
    Approach (CPA)
multi-disciplinary approach, *see*
  teams/teamworking
multi-faceted aspect of mental
  illness 129–30
mutuality/reciprocity 139, 575–6
myths, challenging 140–1

naltrexone 508
National Association for the Care
  and Rehabilitation of
  Offenders (NACRO) 594
National Institute for Clinical
  Excellence (NICE) 114, 820
  anti-psychotics 320–1
  childhood/adolescence 544
  cost of schizophrenia 722
  dementia 557–8
  eating disorders 466
  ECT 324–5
  rapid tranquillization (RT) 741
National Institute of Mental Health
  (England) (NIMHE) 117,
  118
National Self-Harm Network 218
*National Service Framework (NSF)
  for Mental Health* 107–10,
  821–9
  anxiety disorder 416, 436, 440
  complementary/alternative
    therapies 348
  delivery of modernization agenda
    107
  depression 397–8
  forensic mental health services
    605–6

THINKING NURSING

Tom Mason and Elizabeth Whitehead

● Important new nursing theory textbook

This major new text seeks to provide nursing students with an accessible overview of the theory which informs the application of nursing activity. The key disciplines that contribute to the nursing curriculum – such as sociology, psychology, public health, economic science and politics – are comprehensively discussed, with each chapter offering both a theoretical discussion and a section showing how the topic in question applies to nursing practice. Particular attention has been paid to pedagogy with brief boxed case studies, chapter summaries, glossaries of key words and further reading lists enabling easy use by students.

Contents:
Introduction – Thinking Sociology – Thinking Psychology – Thinking Anthropology – Thinking Public Health – Thinking Philosophy – Thinking Economics – Thinking Politics – Thinking Science – Thinking Writing – Conclusions – References – Index.

432pp   0 335 21040 6 (Paperback)   0 335 21041 4 (Hardback)

COMMUNITY MENTAL HEALTH NURSING AND DEMENTIA CARE
PRACTICE PERSPECTIVES

John Keady, Charlotte L. Clarke and Trevor Adams (eds)

A rounded account of Community Mental Health Nurses' practice in dementia care has been long overdue. This is the first book to focus on the role of Community Mental Health Nurses in their highly valued work with both people with dementia and their families.

This book:

- Explores the complexity and diversity of Community Mental Health Nurse work
- Captures perspectives from along the trajectory of dementia
- Identifies assessment and intervention approaches
- Discusses an emerging evidence base for implications in practice.

Contributions to this collection of essays and articles are drawn from Community Mental Health Nurse practitioners and researchers at the forefront of their fields.

It is key reading for practitioners, researchers, students, managers and policy makers in the field of community mental health nursing and/or dementia care.

Contents
Contributors – Acknowledgements – Editorial note – Foreword by Professor Mike Nolan – Introduction – Part One: Setting the scene: the landscape of contemporary community mental health nursing practice in dementia care – Voices from the past: the historical alignment of dementia care to nursing – Integrating practice and knowledge in a clinical context – Multidisciplinary teamworking – 'We put our heads together' – Risk and dementia – Part Two: Dementia care nursing in the community: assessment and practice approaches – Assessment and therapeutic approaches for community mental health nursing dementia care practice – Cognitive-behavioural interventions in dementia – Turning rhetoric into reality – From screening to intervention – The community mental health nurse role in sharing a diagnosis of dementia – Group therapy – Psychosocial interventions with family carers of people with dementia – Admiral nurses – Normalization as a philosophy of dementia care – Assessing and responding to challenging behaviour in dementia – Part Three: Leading and developing community mental health nursing in dementia – Clinical supervision and dementia care – Multi-agency and inter-agency working – Higher level practice – Index.

Contributors
Trevor Adams, Peter Ashton, Gill Boardman, Angela Carradice, Chris Clark, Charlotte L. Clarke, Jan Dewing, Sue Hahn, Mark Holman, John Keady, Kath Lowery, Jill Manthorpe, Anne Mason, Cathy Mawhinney, Paul McCloskey, Anne McKinley, Linda Miller, Gordon Mitchell, Elinor Moore, Michelle Murray, Mike Nolan, Peter Nolan, Tracy Packer, Sean Page, Marilla Pugh, Helen Pusey, Assumpta Ryan, Alison Soliman, Vicki Traynor, Dot Weaks, Heather Wilkinson

306pp   0 335 21142 9 (Paperback)   0 335 21143 7 (Hardback)

PALLIATIVE CARE NURSING
PRINCIPLES AND EVIDENCE FOR PRACTICE

Sheila Payne, Jane Seymour and Christine Ingleton

This innovative interdisciplinary textbook reviews current research and examines the evidence base for palliative care practice. Focusing on palliative care for adults, the first three sections use a novel framework – the trajectory of life-limiting illness – to cover key issues including:

- What happens to people as they become ill
- How individuals cope as they near death and are dying
- How families and friends deal with bereavement and loss

The final section addresses contemporary issues in nursing and inter-professional working. The book contains helpful overviews and is written in an informative and reader-friendly style.

Palliative Care Nursing is essential reading for post-qualifying nursing students and all nurses and health/social care professionals who provide care to people with advanced illness and those who are near the end of life.

Contributors
Julia Addington-Hall, Hilde Ahmedzai, Sam H Ahmedzai, Sanchia Aranda, Liz Barker, Jon Birtwistle, Katie Booth, Bert Broeckaert, Margaret Camps, David Clark, Mark Cobb, Jessica Corner, Karen Cox, Sue Davies, Deborah Fitzsimmons, Katherine Froggatt, Merryn Gott, Elizabeth Hanson, Sue Hawkett, Matthew Hopkins, Christine Ingleton, Veronica James, Nikki Jarrett, Gail Johnston, Jeanne Katz, David Kissane, Jonathan Koffman, Carol Komaromy, Mari Lloyd-Williams, Sian Maslin-Prothero, Kay Mitchell, Margaret O'Connor, Sheila Payne, Silvia Paz, Marilyn Relf, Liz Rolls, Jane Seymour, Paula Smith, Margaret Sneddon, Magi Sque, Vanessa Taylor, Joanne Wells, Michael Wright.

Contents
List of Contributors – Acknowledgements – Introduction – **Part 1: Encountering illness** *– Overview – History, gender and culture in the rise of palliative care – What's in a name? – User involvement and palliative care – Referral patterns and access into specialist palliative care – Acute hospital care – Transitions in status from wellness to illness, illness to wellness – Communication, the patient and the palliative care team – Approaches to assessment in palliative care –* **Part 2: Transitions into the terminal phase** *– Overview – Good for the soul? – Working with difficult symptoms – Pain – Emotions and cognitions – Working with family caregivers in a palliative care setting – Supporting families of terminally ill persons – Social death – No way in – Ethical issues at the end of life – The impact of socialization on the dying process – Palliative care in institutions –* **Part 3: Loss and bereavement** *– Overview – Nursing care at the time of death – Organ and tissue donation – The care and support of bereaved people – Bereavement support – Risk assessment and bereavement services – Bereavement support services – Families and children facing loss and bereavement –* **Part 4: Contemporary issues** *– Overview – Professional boundaries in palliative care – The cost of caring: surviving the culture of niceness, occupational stress and coping strategies – Specialist professional education in palliative care – Information and communication technology in nursing – Research and scholarship in palliative care nursing – Developing expert palliative care nursing through research and practice development – Policy, audit, evaluation and clinical governance – Leading and managing nurses in a changing environment – Conclusion – Indexes.*

800pp   0 335 21243 3 (Paperback)   0 335 21492 4 (Hardback)